Law and Medical Ethics

Fourth Edition

J K Mason CBE MD LLD FRCPath DMJ

Regius Professor (Emeritus) of Forensic Medicine
at the University of Edinburgh

R A McCall Smith LLB PhD

Reader in Law
at the University of Edinburgh

Butterworths
London, Dublin, Edinburgh
1994

This book is dedicated to
two Elizabeths

United Kingdom	Butterworth & Co (Publishers) Ltd, Halsbury House, 35 Chancery Lane, LONDON WC2A 1EL and 4 Hill Street, EDINBURGH EH2 3JZ
Australia	Butterworths, SYDNEY, MELBOURNE, BRISBANE, ADELAIDE, PERTH, CANBERRA and HOBART
Canada	Butterworth Canada Ltd, TORONTO and VANCOUVER
Ireland	Butterworth (Ireland) Ltd, DUBLIN
Malaysia	Malayan Law Journal Sdn Bhd, KUALA LUMPUR
New Zealand	Butterworths of New Zealand Ltd, WELLINGTON and AUCKLAND
Puerto Rico	Butterworth of Puerto Rico Inc, San Juan
Singapore	Butterworths Asia, SINGAPORE
South Africa	Butterworth Publishers (Pty) Ltd, DURBAN
USA	Butterworth Legal Publishers, CARLSBAD, California and SALEM, New Hampshire

A CIP Catalogue record for this book is available from the British Library.

ISBN 0 406 02478 2

Typeset by Doyle & Co, Colchester
Printed and bound in Great Britain by Thomson Litho, East Kilbride

DS

1000231544

0

Preface

Major interests in medical jurisprudence tend to be cyclical and this has become evident as the various editions of this book have reached the market. At the time of our original publication, selective non-treatment of the newborn was dominating the medico-ethical scene; the second edition coincided with the explosion in assisted reproductive techniques; and, by the time the third edition arrived, the broad issue of consent to medical treatment overshadowed the whole medico-legal arena.

It seems to us that we have now reached the age of the euthanasia debate. Across the Atlantic, Nancy B has won and Ms Rodriguez has lost a right to die by one's own choosing; at home, Dr Cox has made medico-legal history and Anthony Bland has been allowed to end his existence. It is within the context of euthanasia that the Hippocratic ethos, the autonomy of the individual and the interests of the state – both moral and economic – are currently conjoined and we make no excuse for the fact that the chapter on euthanasia is now almost the largest in the book, for it is here that the most recent developments are to be found.

This is not to say that other issues have become dormant. Rather, we have felt, throughout, that we have been re-writing – rather than re-editing – the previous edition. And it is this which makes medical jurisprudence such an exciting and vibrant field of study – of which it might surely be said: 'Those behind cried "forward" and those in front cried "back".'

We hope that we have been able to convey this feeling in our current edition. Perhaps the most obvious monument to the importance and viability of the subject lies in the fact that, despite our efforts to the contrary, the text of this edition is more than twice the size of that of the first.

Once again, we thank our publishers and the Faculty of Law of the University of Edinburgh for making this continuing project possible. We have received much helpful advice from colleagues and we would like, in particular, to thank our post-graduate students who have been outstandingly supportive.

Edinburgh,
January 1994

JKM
RAMcS

Authors' note: In general, this book follows the Interpretation Act 1978, s 6 in that, unless the contrary intention appears, words importing the masculine gender include the feminine and words importing the feminine gender include the masculine.

Contents

Table of statutes

References in this Table to *Statutes* are to Halsbury's Statutes of England (Fourth Edition) showing the volume and page at which the annotated text of an Act may be found.

Table of foreign enactments

The enactments in this Table are listed in order of countries and their respective territorial jurisdictions.

List of cases

Introduction

1 The evolution of medical ethics

The influence exerted by the doctor is, in many ways, unique. Whether he is undertaking open heart surgery or simply saying 'there is nothing wrong with you', he is making decisions which, if not of life and death significance, at least represent the difference between fitness and ill-health. The two sides of the doctor/patient relationship are not, however, always equally balanced. Just as the lawyer knows more about the law than does his client, so the doctor knows more about medicine than does his patient. The patient's attitude, therefore, is poised between trust in the learning of another and the general distrust of one who is in a state of uncertainty. Such ambivalence leads naturally to a sense of inferiority; it is the function of medical ethics to ensure that the potential superiority of the doctor is not abused.

The progress of medicine

A limited review of the history of medicine is needed if the development of the doctor/patient relationship is to be understood properly. Very early medicine was, of course, a matter of mystery; there being no apparent natural reason why disease struck one person rather than another, the answer had to be found in the supernatural and, supernatural powers being sparingly distributed, healing became a prerogative of a few whose power depended largely on the ignorance of others. At its inception, therefore, the medical profession was elitist and it is easy to conceive of the transference of healing powers from the isolated tribal witch doctor to the priest of organised religion.

Priestly medicine extended the principle of supernatural power. Since the Gods were the arbiters of life and death, those in association with them could reasonably be expected to intervene successfully on behalf of the outsider. Disease was caused by evil spirits at war with the Gods who were, themselves, protectors of the person. Religion and medicine had the same objectives in that they were defences against evil which expressed itself in either a spiritual (disease of the mind) or a material (disease of the body) form. However, the priests comprised a relatively closed community who could learn from each other and who could appreciate the advantages of organisation and codification. They could also teach and, by virtue of their privileged position, they could attract students from the higher reaches of society. Medicine thus developed both priestly and secular practitioners and in doing so preserved the image of superiority.

Medicine in the Middle East

The first effective example of organised medicine is to be found in Egypt where Imhotep, widely regarded as the father of medicine, practised. He was the archetypal combination of physician, priest and court official.[1] The papyri discovered in the nineteenth century indicate that Egyptian medicine was comparatively advanced as early as the second millennium BC.[2] Some features of its organisation can be related to modern practice. In the first place, the concept of a national health service seems to have been well developed, with patients not being charged for visits to the healers who, themselves, were supported by the community. Second, rather rigid rules were laid down as to experimental treatment. There was no culpability in failure to cure provided that the standard textbooks were followed. Severe penalties were, however, threatened for those who ignored such instructions, the reason being that very few men would be expected to know better than the best specialists who had gone before – an interesting attitude towards negligence which was still being adopted by the courts at the turn of this century (see chapter 9, below). More importantly, the notion of specialisation was deeply instilled although medical treatment remained very much the practice of the priest caste. Indeed, the aura of mystique which surrounded the physician as compared with appreciation of the technical expertise of his surgical colleagues has persisted until recent times.

The extension of surgical practice into lay hands was steady and was demonstrated in the parallel practice of Babylonian medicine. It is from here that the first known legal code originated – the Code of Hammurabi (c 1900 BC). This contained an element of medical ethics and laid down, inter alia, a system of payment which was based on results and, to some extent, on the ability to pay and on the status of the patient. It also tabled penalties for negligent failure, some of which were draconian to an extent which must have deterred many from entering the profession.

Greek medicine

For the origin of our modern ethics, however, we must look to Greece where, by 500 BC, the originally strong influence of the priest had waned. This had been taken over by the philosophers who, through the processes of logical thought, observation and deduction, transformed the practice of medicine. Inevitably, this led to the formation of schools involving close association, paternalism and the elements of the 'closed shop'. A code of intra-professional conduct evolved – the dawn of what has become known as medical etiquette. In addition, the new concepts of practice dictated that the physician went to the patient rather than the patient to the temple. A standard of practice relevant to the new ideals was required and has survived as the Hippocratic Oath (Appendix A).

Hippocrates remains the most famous figure in Greek philosophical medicine but he was not alone and it is probable that the Oath predates his own school. It therefore indicates a prevailing ethos rather than a professorial edict and it is still regarded as

1   A W Beasley believed that Imhotep made a special study of trauma arising in the workers employed in building the Saqqara pyramid under his direction. If true, it would seem to be a very early example of an unethical research project ('The Origins of Orthopaedics' (1982) 75 J Roy Soc Med 648).

2   Our major source is A Castiglioni *A History of Medicine*, trans and ed E B Krunghaar (2nd edn, 1947).

the fundamental governance of the medical profession. We are not, here, concerned with medical etiquette. As to medical ethics, the Oath lays down certain guidelines. First, it implies the need for the co-ordinated instruction and registration of doctors. The public is to be protected, so far as is possible, from the dabbler or the charlatan. Second, it is clearly stated that a doctor is there for the benefit of his patients. To the best of his ability he must do them good and he must do nothing which he knows will cause harm. Third, euthanasia and abortion are proscribed. The reference to lithotomy probably prohibits mutilating operations (castration) but has been taken by many to imply the limitation of practice to that in which one has expertise. Fourth, the nature of the doctor/patient relationship is outlined and an undertaking is given not to take advantage of that relationship. Finally, the Oath expresses the doctrine of medical confidentiality.

In fact, the Hippocratic Oath did not become an integral part of ethical teaching until well into the Christian era; it lapsed with the decline of Greek civilisation and was restored with the evolution of university medical schools. It is doubtful if any British medical school now requires a reiteration of the Oath at graduation – although Edinburgh, for one, requires assent by students to a modified version – but, avowed or not, all doctors would admit to its persuasive influence. The language of the Oath is, however, archaic and a modernised version was introduced by the World Medical Association as the Declaration of Geneva. This was amended at Sydney in 1968 (Appendix B) and provides the basis of an International Code of Medical Ethics (Appendix C).

The Judaeo-Christian influence

Before leaving this early evolutionary phase, one must return to a brief consideration of the Jewish influence on medical ethics. There were two main sources. First, medicine was governed by the law and the law was administered by the priests. Religious and medical practices were, therefore, inseparable and religious hygiene was of general benefit to the community. Second, the principle was accepted that the rights of the individual must sometimes be sacrificed for the good of the community. There was strong emphasis, for example, on the isolation of infectious cases, including those of venereal disease, on the regulation of sewage disposal and the like and the principles of public health medicine were born. Much of this attitude passed to the Christians who were also forced into the group life-style and were fortified by the concepts of equality, charity and devotion to the less fortunate – concepts which still underlie the ethical practice of medicine in Christian countries. It is small wonder that, during the Dark Ages, medicine was virtually kept alive in the monasteries which provided the template for the voluntary hospitals of later years.

A basis for medical ethics

The academic moral philosopher would hold that the pragmatic emergence of a Hippocratic-based code of medical practice is an inadequate basis for decision making in medicine. What is needed is a solid philosophical foundation to which appeals can be made when making moral evaluations. Put another way, medical morals dictate the particular actions and beliefs which regulate the day to day judgments of doctors while medical ethics analyse the universal principles on which the decisions are made.[3]

The identification of such a starting point is not easy. Almost every school of philosophy has its contribution to make but none is wholly satisfactory. The utilitarianism of J S Mill fails as a model because it is virtually impossible in medicine to define the distribution of 'happiness' in terms of either quality or numbers – is a little happiness derived by large numbers of mentally subnormal patients any greater or less than a lot of pleasure experienced by a small number of liver transplant recipients? Campbell clearly leans towards the Kantian ethos based on respect for persons. Total benevolence may be the ideal, but it can hardly be adduced seriously as the motivating force behind all medical practice. The student black humour which suggests that a given specialisation is to be preferred because one's patients 'never get better and never call one out at night' is an indication of self-interest. More seriously, it would be foolish to deny that medical doctors enjoy a relatively high standard of living the world over.

The concept of autonomy now pervades the whole of medical practice mirroring its general importance in contemporary moral philosophy. In one view, the extent to which the autonomy of the individual is enhanced provides the touchstone against which all ethical solutions should be measured. This criterion at least provides a clear answer. In the abortion debate, for instance, the mother's right of autonomy – her entitlement to control her own body – is taken as 'trumping' any argument against the moral permissibility of abortion. In the same way, the autonomy argument can be used in an issue such as surrogacy in that the exercise of reproductive powers is a matter for the autonomous decision of the individual and this fact outweighs any moral objection to the commercialisation of human reproduction. But this vision of autonomy depends on the acceptance of an individualistic ethos which all may not share. Even if self-fulfilment does shine through the development and the exercise of autonomy, there is a social dimension to life which is potentially equally enriching.[4] Autonomy must be qualified by the legitimate interests and expectations of others, as well as by economic constraints. In the medical context, the claims of autonomy must be moderated so as to accommodate the sensitivities of others, including those of the doctor who is, after all, also an autonomous agent. It may be that respect for individual autonomy points in the direction of allowing voluntary euthanasia, but another moral agent has to administer the drug that ends life, and that person may be affected by the task. There are also the interests of others in being protected against involuntary euthanasia and it is possible that, in providing such protection, we may have to deny self-determination to those who are truly volunteers.

3   We have relied very much on A V Campbell *Moral Dilemmas in Medicine* (3rd edn, 1984) for the development of our ideas in this section. T L Beauchamp and T F Childress *Principles of Biomedical Ethics* (3rd edn, 1990) is a fundamental source. There is a growing body of works which focus on particular, sometimes narrowly defined, issues in medical ethics. See, for example, A E Buchanan and D W Brock *Deciding for Others* (1989) (surrogate decision making); K W M Fulford *Moral Theory and Medical Practice* (1989) (the concept of illness, especially mental illness); and F M Kamm *Creation and Abortion* (1992) (abortion and the permissibility of killing).

4   For discussion, see D T Meyers *Self, Society, and Personal Choice* (1989). Also of interest is T E Hill 'The Importance of Autonomy' in his *Autonomy and Self-respect* (1991).

An alternative autonomy-based approach involves appeals to rights. The concept of rights has many proponents and, like autonomy, rights theory plays an important part in contemporary moral debate. Yet the language of rights may also become unduly assertive and combative and may hinder, rather than promote, moral consensus.[5] This is not to suggest that rights are unimportant. Many of the central moral positions defended in this book, and recognised by the law, can be couched in terms of rights. Once again, however, rights-talk is peculiarly suited to an individualistic moral tradition and conflicts of rights tend to lead to moral impasse. Most discussion centres on the rights of the patient – but has the doctor no rights when choosing treatment in accordance with his Hippocratic principles and his training? Consideration of the reverse proposition indicates that this must be so, at least in part – the autonomy or rights of the patient cannot be allowed to relieve the doctor of his duty to treat to the standard of his best knowledge and belief. Certainly, they provide no excuse for a retreat into therapeutic inertia.[6]

We must go behind these contemporary shibboleths if we are to identify the values which should inform ethical medical practice. This process may be eclectic, with values and formal principles being drawn from different sources. It is likely to come up with moral propositions which will find favour with a fairly wide range of people, even if they are not universally acceptable; this is probably the best that can be achieved in a modern pluralistic society in which there will often be disagreement on moral issues which might well be regarded as being of a fundamental nature.

For many doctors, the first practical guide to morality is likely to be 'conscience' which is a somewhat vague concept but one which roughly accords with what the philosopher terms 'moral intuition'. Intuition has a limited appeal as a basis for moral philosophy but it should not be wholly discounted. This especially so in the field of health care where the practical fact is that each doctor/patient encounter is played out on a different pitch – and the goal-posts move imperceptibly with each consultation within that relationship.[7] Intuitions may point in the direction of a value which the individual may not be able to articulate formally but which can be defended properly. The moral significance of human life is one such matter. We know intuitively that it is wrong to kill but we may find difficulty in locating exactly why this should be so, particularly when we may be depriving a person of no more than a few minutes' existence. Some degree of taboo may be operating here but there is something more important besides – there is an intuitive awe that we feel for the

5   In the view of some philosophers, rights can be reduced to principles which form the real content of morality. For a sceptical view, see R Frey *Rights, Killing and Suffering* (1983); to be contrasted with L W Sumner *The Moral Foundation of Rights* (1987) and with the outstanding contribution of K Cronin *Rights and Christian Ethics* (1992).
6   A G M Campbell 'The Right to Be Allowed to Die' (1983) 9 J Med Ethics 136. The same issue contains a series of papers devoted to 'the competently made irrational decision': R Sherlock 'Consent, Competency and ECT: Some Critical Suggestions' (1983) 9 J Med Ethics 141; H Lesser '. . . A Philosopher's Comment', p 144; P J Taylor '. . . A Psychiatrist's View', p 146.
7   For expression of this view, see T B Brewin 'How Much Ethics Is Needed to Make a Good Doctor ?' (1993) 341 Lancet 161. Also G Gillett 'Euthanasia, Letting Die and the Pause' (1988) 14 J Med Ethics 61.

sheer fact of human life, an awe which loses its force when expressed in the bland language of rights.

Even so, the practice of medicine is constrained by outside influences; the conduct of doctors is circumscribed by the pubic conscience and, whether the public conscience fashions the law or whether the law moulds the public's attitudes, the latter are inevitably reflected in the law. Whether the law has a right to impose morality is a well-known and controversial issue in jurisprudence.[8] That it has not hesitated to do so in the medical context is shown by the willingness of legislatures to enact statutes limiting private choice, for example, in the field of reproductive medicine.[9]

Thus we see the general rules of medical practice as being developed within a moral framework which is constantly being restructured by contemporary society. Doctors, as might be expected, play an important part in this process. This role is emphasised in the words of Farquharson J in his charge to the jury in *R v Arthur*:[10]

> I imagine that you will think long and hard before deciding that doctors, of the eminence we have heard, representing to you what medical ethics are, . . . have evolved standards which amount to committing crime.

Often, the doctor's individual conscience may be specifically involved. A good example lies in the Abortion Act 1967 which contains a conscience clause but, simultaneously, withdraws this when the public attitude is clear – that is, when the life of the mother is in question.

In general, the urgency of the medical ethos in relation to a particular issue is proportional to the interest taken by the public in that issue. Modern reproductive techniques do not form a major part of medicine as a whole but widespread public anxiety led to an energetic and prompt medical response in the form of rules and guidelines. By contrast, public apathy breeds medical insecurity – an expression of which lies in the confusion and contradictory attitudes relating to the treatment of the aged.

Reliance on legal precept is, however, by no means a perfect answer to the foundation of medical ethics and may, indeed, be a two-edged weapon. No matter how principled may be the doctor in making a specific value judgment, he may sometimes have difficulty in dissociating himself completely from the implications of that judgment for himself. The 'cool self love' described by Joseph Butler may avoid impulsive decision making but it can hardly be regarded as a sound ethical model when it is invoked. Thus, in defending himself against potential litigation, the practitioner may over-treat or over-investigate in ways which are unnecessary or, even, frankly unethical. As a further example, it is asking a great deal of the doctor, when faced with a life or death decision, to be completely certain that he entertains no notion of balancing the relative demerits of litigation for personal injuries against the possibility of criticism by the coroner or the sheriff. Lord Denning's rather unusual implication that it would have been better if an accidentally brain-damaged woman had

---

8   For a discussion of this, including many medico-legal examples, see S Lee *Law and Morals* (1986).
9   See, for example, the Surrogacy Arrangements Act 1985; the Infertility (Medical Procedures) Act 1985 (Victoria) and the Human Fertilisation and Embryology Act 1990.
10 (1981) The Times, 6 November, pp 1, 12; (1981) 12 BMLR 1 at 22.

died[11] prompts the question 'better for whom?'. The sad aspect is that the question need be raised. Clearly, the patient's interests – or the consequences to the patient – should be of prime importance, yet an element of self-interest is difficult to eradicate completely.

The organisation of modern medicine

The age of medical research can be said to have begun with the Renaissance and, since that time, the practice of medicine has become increasingly scientifically based. New dimensions are, thus, introduced and new dilemmas posed. It is obvious that scientific medicine cannot improve without extensive research while, on the other hand, that process tends to turn medical practice into a series of problem-solving exercises – a diversion which, even now, stimulates some of medicine's severest critics.

The practical effect of the scientific approach has been to convince doctors that they have an expertise worth preserving and, as early as the sixteenth century, we find the establishment of the Royal College of Physicians of London together with a general tightening of the rules governing the practice of surgery. The early Royal Colleges had considerable powers of examination and registration. The latter function has now gone and the major purpose of the Colleges (which now represent some eight specialities with additional Faculties) is to maintain a standard of excellence among specialised practitioners – a matter of current importance to which we return at p 11.

As organisation proceeded, fortune began increasingly to depend upon fame, and fame in its turn upon academic superiority over one's colleagues. From all accounts, British medicine in the eighteenth and early nineteenth centuries was not the happiest of professions, power being secured by practitioners not so much through the scientific merit of their writings but rather by their content of deprecatory comment. Even so, it was not so much medical ethics, as they are understood today, that were found wanting but, rather, medical etiquette. Something had to be done to ensure the status of the profession and this need was first met by the formation of the British Medical Association in 1832. The BMA has always been deeply concerned with the way medicine is practised but its present main function is the protection of the doctors' interests. Today, it is a non-affiliated registered Trade Union.[12] Clearly, an interested party could not represent the public need for control of a profession with such power and it was largely due to the lobby of the BMA itself that the General Medical Council was established by the Medical Act 1858.[13]

---

11 In *Lim Poh Choo v Camden and Islington Area Health Authority* [1979] QB 196, [1979] 1 All ER 332.
12 Trade Union and Labour Relations Act 1974.
13 The General Medical Council at present consists of 102 members. Fifty-four of these are elected (by statute, the number of elected members must exceed the combined total of all others). A further 35 are appointed by the universities which have medical schools, by the Royal Colleges and Faculties and by the Society of Apothecaries. Thirteen further members are nominated by the Queen in Council, of whom the majority must be lay people. By convention, 11 of the 13 are lay people and the other places are filled by two of the Chief Medical Officers. For a review of the status of the General Medical Council, see a series of articles by R Smith 'Profile of the GMC' (1989) 298 BMJ 1241 to (1989) 299 BMJ 40. The President answered some of the criticisms in R Kilpatrick 'Profile of the GMC: Portrait or Caricature?' (1989) 299 BMJ 109.

The control of medical practice

It is emphasised that, while the GMC is the governing body of the medical profession,[14] its essential function is to regulate the standards of the profession rather than professional standards. As things stand, negligence is of no direct concern to the Council unless it brings the profession of medicine into disrepute.[15] The primary function of the GMC is to maintain the official register of medical practitioners and, thus, to protect the public from those who have not undergone recognised training. Unlike the practise of dentistry, no specific offence lies in an unqualified person practising medicine in the United Kingdom – the offence is that of pretending to be a registered medical practitioner[16] or of usurping functions which are statutorily limited to registered practitioners – such as prescribing 'prescription only' medicines.[17] Other functions include supervision of standards of education, the laying down of standards of fitness to practise and the exercise of discipline over the medical profession. As to the last, the Council has, until recently, refused to comment on the propriety of specific intended or past actions; although guidelines have been issued, detailed advice has been a matter for the doctors' protection or defence societies. Since the passing of the Medical Act 1978, however, the Council itself has undertaken to advise when so requested by registered practitioners. The Professional Conduct Committee (PCC) is the ultimate tribunal in respect of discipline and is subject only to appeal to the Privy Council.[18] A doctor appearing before the PCC may be found guilty or not guilty of 'serious professional misconduct'. This has been defined as conduct such as 'would reasonably be regarded as disgraceful or dishonourable by his professional brethren of good repute and standing' – a definition which is so wide as to be virtually non-exclusive.

The GMC has been subject to considerable criticism which has been but little allayed by the changes in structure – both imposed and self-regulatory – that have

14 Professions allied to medicine have their own controlling bodies (see, for example, the Nurses, Midwives and Health Visitors Act 1979 as amended by s 1 of the 1992 Act of the same name) as do those offering 'alternative Medicine'. The latter are gaining increased official recognition (see the Osteopaths Act 1993, s 1).

15 In addition to actions for negligence as a tort (ch 9, below), professional standards may be regulated through the National Health Service legislation (National Health Service (Service Committees and Tribunal) Regulations 1974, SI 1974/45). Incompetence by hospital practitioners is investigated under the terms of Ministry of Health circular HM(61)112(1961) as amended by HC(90)9(1990). The actions of a disciplinary inquiry are subject to judicial review (*R v Department of Health and Social Security, ex p Darnell* (1986) 293 BMJ 322, unreported).

16 Occasionally, the GMC lapses in this respect. A recent example is that of an unqualified person from overseas who managed to obtain registration with the GMC. He received £450 000 in salary payments from the NHS before being detected through the vigilance of a pharmacist (J Ironside 'Five Year Sentence for Fake General Practitioner' (1992) 304 BMJ 1652).

17 A further case, prosecuted and convicted under the Medicines Act 1968, has come to light: C Dyer 'Bogus British Professor Sentenced to Prison' (1993) 306 BMJ 1499.

18 The conduct of the GMC is also open to judicial review both as to its 'advice' (*Colman v General Medical Council* [1989] 1 Med LR 23, QBD; sub nom *R v General Medical Council, ex p Colman* (1989) 4 BMLR 33, CA) and as to the actions of the PCC (*R v General Medical Council, ex p Gee* [1987] 1 All ER 1204, CA; on appeal [1986] 1 WLR 226, QBD). It is of passing interest that the conduct of the PCC is governed by English law irrespective of where the Committee is sitting; save in unusual circumstances, the standard of proof required is that applicable to civil proceedings: *McAllister v General Medical Council* [1993] 1 All ER 982, PC.

arisen in the last 15 years. Much of this criticism centres on the belief that such a form of 'peer control' provides inadequate protection for the public.[19] To a large extent, this stems from the widely held misconception of the Council's fairly limited responsibility for the control of the British medical profession. The pressure to extend its role is strong but seeks to impose responsibilities which are probably too much for a single organisation to discharge. It could be better to strengthen those controls on poor medical practice which already exist. Thus, the doctor is as much subject to the criminal law as is any other citizen, remedies are available at civil law for the aggrieved patient and the doctor who breaks the terms of his contract can be disciplined through the National Health Service. The Royal Colleges are responsible for certification of specialist status and there seems little reason why their remit should not include greatly increased powers to remove accreditation from specialists shown to be in need of re-training. The GMC, at present, fills a gap in constraining such conduct as is not actionable yet which would not be expected of the ethical practitioner. Thus, the law on medical confidentiality is in many ways unclear but few doctors would wish to tangle with the GMC on the issue of professional secrecy. There is nothing criminal in adultery; yet the public cannot expect family relationships to be destroyed as a result of the doctor's privilege to enter the bedroom and, accordingly, adulterous conduct with a patient is dealt with exceptionally severely by the Professional Conduct Committee.

It is, perhaps, unsatisfactory that the power of the GMC itself to institute disciplinary proceedings is very strictly limited. Effectively, the Council can act only on complaints received. Something of a lacuna develops when the only likely informants would be fellow doctors – for example, when treatment of doubtful validity is being dispensed.[20] Most professional men are inherently unwilling to denounce their colleagues and the distinction between disparaging the skill of another doctor, which the GMC would regard adversely, and informing of behaviour which raises a question of serious professional misconduct, which is approbated, may be tenuous. This restriction does not, however, apply when other health care professionals are involved and, indeed, most reports of dubious behaviour on the part of doctors stem from outraged nursing staff. Many such protests are based on grounds of conscience, these being related especially to life or death decisions. The informants in such cases seem to attract little public sympathy – a relic, perhaps, of the consultant's autocracy in the health care hierarchy – and they have been described as 'moralist groups pursuing their own ends by threatening doctors with criminal prosecution'.[1] We prefer the view that the great majority genuinely believe they are protecting the public against undisclosed violations of the moral and criminal codes.

A more recent development stems from the increasing dichotomy between the clinical and managerial arms of the health service. Public criticism – predominantly of the latter by the former – is now known popularly as 'whistle blowing'. Whether

---

19 A major review is to be found in M Stacey *Regulating British Medicine* (1992).
20 R Smith 'Doctors, Unethical Treatment, and Turning a Blind Eye' (1989) 298 BMJ 1125. See also criticism of the management of a case of doubtful practice associated with advertising: A B Kay 'Alternative Allergy and the General Medical Council' (1993) 306 BMJ 122; R Smith 'GMC in the Dock Again' (1993) 306 BMJ 82.
1 J D J Havard 'The Influence of the Law on Clinical Decisions Affecting Life and Death' (1983) 23 Med Sci Law 157.

disclosure of defects in the system, which may be real or imaginary, is regarded as a legitimate duty in the public interest or as a breach of a contract of employment entered into in mutual good faith is open to debate and the answer may depend very much on the particular community's attitude to freedom of information.[2]   The government has now issued draft guidelines which stress that, in so far as the interests of patients are of paramount importance, NHS staff have a right and a duty to raise issues concerning patient care.   The right depends, however, on following a prescribed procedure which, for example, relegates contact with the press to a last resort.[3]   Clearly, there are difficulties in distinguishing genuine concern from malcontent but, here, we are moving some way from the doctor/patient relationship. There is little more to say on the point other than that we believe, in general, that patients' rights may be better safeguarded through managerial self-audit than through legislation.

Public relations

The importance of the overall relationship between the medical profession and the public cannot, however, be gainsaid.   Support for patient autonomy and self-regulation has escalated within the past 25 years and has carried with it a parallel claim to a right to personal assessment of one's doctor's expertise and quality. This has added a new dimension to the GMC's attitudes to advertising by the medical profession.   Time was when, for example, a doctor discussing medical matters of public interest on the radio had to do so anonymously for fear of disciplinary action on the part of the GMC.   There is little doubt that such restrictions were based on a fear of competitive doctors 'touting' for patients; the advent of the National Health Service virtually eliminated any need for such behaviour and the antipathy of the GMC was steadily relaxed.

The solution of the matter was, however, catalysed by the reference of the GMC's prohibition to the Monopolies and Mergers Commission who held that the rule forbidding advertising in the press by general practitioners was against the public interest.[4]   At the same time, the Commission recommended considerable restraint – including a prohibition on disparaging other doctors and on claiming special

2   D Greene and J Cooper 'Whistle Blowers' (1992) 305 BMJ 1343; R Smith 'Whistle Blowing: A Curse on Ineffective Organisations' (1992) 305 BMJ 1308.
3   J Warden 'New Guidance for Whistleblowers' (1992) 305 BMJ 977; 'Speaking Out in the NHS' (1992) 305 BMJ 1180; S Handysides 'Health Workers who Protest Face Disciplinary Action' (1993) 306 BMJ 1710. An interesting study of the effects on the informant may be found in K J Lennane '"Whistleblowing": A Health Issue' (1993) 307 BMJ 667.
4   T Delmonthe 'GP's May Advertise (1989) 298 BMJ 774. Interestingly, the Court of Appeal subsequently held that the recommendation did not render the GMC's advice unreasonable (see *R v General Medical Council, ex p Colman* (1989) 4 BMLR 33, CA, fn 18, above). An important issue was whether or not the English courts should apply the principles of the European Commission on Human Rights in reaching decisions despite the fact that the latter had not been incorporated into United Kingdom law.   The claim, which is still sub judice, was rejected by the European Commission on Human Rights: C Dyer 'Ban on Newspaper Advertising by Doctors Upheld' (1989) 299 BMJ 1482; A Rogers 'Court Case Rejected' (1993) 341 Lancet 366.

aptitudes. The Commission, fearing exploitation, declined to extend its recommendations to advertising to the general public by specialists – although it allowed specialists to inform their medical colleagues of the services that they offered.

These recommendations, which were designed for the benefit of patients and for the improvement of specialist services, were opposed by the British Medical Association[5] but seem logical and in accord with modern custom. They have been accepted by the GMC[6] whose advice currently reads:

> The Council encourages doctors to provide factual information about their professional qualifications and services . . . , in any form, to the public or other members of the profession.
>
> . . .
>
> General practitioners publishing information about their services should not abuse the trust of patients or attempt to exploit their lack of medical knowledge . . . Advertising material should contain only factual information.[7]

Even so, the GMC remained opposed to the public recognition of medical specialists and, together with the Royal Colleges, has resisted the publication of a distinct 'specialist register'. The current United Kingdom compromise of accreditation of specialists by the Royal Colleges could be seen as breaching the directives of the European Commission and this was admitted in the case brought by Dr Goldstein.[8] The present situation is unsatisfactory from the points of view of both specialists and the public and changes are being considered urgently.[9] The case for the publication of background information on practitioners is unassailable especially in the light of increasing reciprocity of national medical registrations.

Modern medical technology and the law

The late twentieth century picture of medical practice is one of rapidly advancing technology which is effected in a strongly research oriented environment and which exists within an increasingly hedonistic and materialistic society. Society, for its part, demands more and more esoteric methodology and personal involvement in

5   J D J Havard 'Advertising by Doctors and the Public Interest' (1989) 298 BMJ 903.
6   L Beecham 'Advertising – No Longer a Dirty Word' (1990) 300 BMJ 1420. The history of the GMC's changing attitude is outlined in D H Irvine 'The Advertising of Doctors' Services' (1991) 17 J Med Ethics 35.
7   General Medical Council *Professional Conduct and Discipline: Fitness to Practise* (1993), paras 59-61, 97-115.
8   *R v Secretary of State for Health, ex p Goldstein* (1993) Times, 5 April. Even so, the applicant failed to secure publication of a specialist list: D Brahams 'EC Directives and Specialists' (1993) 341 Lancet 1017. Dr Goldstein's case is complicated by the fact that he is taking more than one set of proceedings against the Secretary of State: *R v Joint Committee on Higher Medical Training and Specialist Advisory Committee on Rheumatology, ex p Goldstein* (1992) 11 BMLR 10 and is also suing for loss of earnings: (1993) The Times, 8 June, p 2.
9   Department of Health *Hospital Doctors: Training for the Future* (1993). See S Hunter and P McLaren 'Specialist Medical Training and the Calman Report' (1993) 306 BMJ 1281.

medicine is encouraged on all sides. The law, however, moves more slowly than either medicine or the public mores. As a result, doctors frequently find themselves operating in an atmosphere of legal uncertainty which promotes confrontation. This is typified by such comments as:

> It is a crushing indictment of our legal system that men such as Aleck Bourne [who was found not guilty of illegal termination of pregnancy] and Leonard Arthur [who was acquitted of attempted murder] should be subjected to criminal prosecution for carrying out with great devotion and skill procedures which are accepted by the profession as in the best interests of patients.[10]

Whether or not one agrees with this view, it cannot be denied that it reveals an unsatisfactory state of affairs – a state which self-perpetuates as new attitudes and new techniques evolve.

Legal intervention in medicine

We have argued that the public conscience, as embodied in the law, provides a useful foundation for medical ethics. This, however, is not to say that the law should dictate to the profession and, particularly, not that it should dictate by means of restrictive statute. Effectively, we are suggesting that medicine must operate within broadly stated legal rules – such as those embodied in the common law – and, as Lord Scarman has indicated,[11] the law must be flexible in the absence of Parliamentary direction.

The crucial question, then, is that of determining the *extent* to which medical decisions should be the object of legal scrutiny and control. At one extreme there are those who hold that the medical profession should be left to regulate itself and that it alone should decide what is acceptable conduct. According to this view, intervention by the law is too blunt a way of tackling the delicate ethical dilemmas which doctors have to face; the individual, guided by personal experience and by prevailing public and professional standards, must confront and resolve the day-to-day ethical issues of medical practice.

The contrary view, frequently expressed just as firmly, denies that there is any reason why doctors alone should regulate their relationship with their patients. In this view, reserving to the medical profession the right to decide on issues of life and death is an improper derogation from an area of legitimate public concern and an encroachment by clinicians into what is, properly, social policy. According to the proponents of this opinion, the law, even if it is an imperfect and often inaccessible weapon, is at least one means of controlling the medical profession in the interest of the community as a whole.[12]

10 J D J Havard 'Legal Regulation of Medical Practice – Decisions of Life and Death: A Discussion Paper' (1982) 75 J Roy Soc Med 351.
11 In *Gillick v West Norfolk and Wisbech Area Health Authority* [1986] AC 112, [1985] 3 All ER 402, HL.
12 'I would expect medical ethics to be formed by the law rather than the reverse' *Airedale NHS Trust v Bland* [1993] 1 All ER 821, (1993) 12 BMLR 64, per Hoffman LJ at 103.

Yet it is difficult to read the numerous judgments which have emanated from the courts of the United States in, say, 'right to die' cases without feeling that these are matters which it would have been far better not to have litigated. The spectre of prolonged courtroom action over the appropriate treatment of terminally ill people is not edifying and it seems wrong to have reduced such issues to, effectively, legal checklists. The case of *Airedale NHS Trust v Bland*, which is discussed in greater detail at p 341, came perilously close to importing that process into this country. The intrusion of the law into such a private tragedy may have been inevitable for it was a case in which there was real doubt as to the legality of the course of action which the doctors and the next-of-kin wished to pursue. It is also one which raises starkly the relative positions of the courts and the legislature in face of the speed of evolution of modern technology – as Lord Browne-Wilkinson put it: 'Existing law may not provide an acceptable answer to the new legal questions [raised by the ability to sustain life artificially]'.[13] He went on to question whether judges should seek to develop new law to meet a wholly new situation and to suggest that it was a matter which required society, through the democratic expression of its views in Parliament, to reach its decisions on the underlying moral and practical problems and then reflect those decisions in legislation. In this, he was strongly supported by Lord Mustill.[14]

It is clearly unacceptable that doctors should have to work in a 'legal vacuum' in which they may be uncertain as to whether or not they face the prospect of a civil action or, again in the words of Lord Mustill, they take the risk of having to validate their conduct after the event in the context of a trial for murder. For these reasons, it may be preferable to have certain general rules set out clearly as can be done by way of statute and we have, in fact, concrete examples of the benign effect of legislative involvement in medical issues – it is through statute, for example, that the legal uncertainties which once surrounded the new reproductive technology have been largely dispelled. The way in which this has been achieved varies according to jurisdiction. In Victoria, for instance, the relevant statute[15] spells out in relative detail what the clinician may or may not do. The British approach, by contrast, has been for Parliament to state its general aims and to remit their refinement to officially appointed authorities on which the profession and the public are adequately represented.[16]

This approach serves to circumvent one of the most cogent arguments against introducing legal rules into human affairs – namely that, once rules acquire a specific meaning, they allow little room for manoeuvre and can turn out to be more restrictive than was originally intended by the framer of the rule. The effect of this, as we have intimated above, can be to distort people's behaviour through the fear of litigation or prosecution. One may then be concerned not with doing what one feels to be right but with what one feels to be the legally safest thing to do.

But when there are no alternative methods of resolving disputes between doctors and patients, other than complaints procedures which have no financial implications

---

13 [1993] 1 All ER 821 at 878, (1993) 12 BMLR 64 at 124.
14 *Airedale NHS Trust & Bland* [1993] 1 All ER 821, (1993) 12 BMLR 64 at 135.
15 Infertility (Medical Procedures) Act 1984, amended in 1987.
16 Eg, see the Human Fertilisation and Embryology Authority established under the Human Fertilisation and Embryology Act 1990.

for the patient, the courts are bound to find themselves drawn in to act as mediators in complex and frequently distressing matters. There seems, however, to be little enthusiasm for the task and judicial hostility to medical negligence claims in this country has occasionally been overt. In *Whitehouse v Jordan*,[17] for example, Lord Denning MR took the somewhat controversial step of considering an individual claim for damages in general terms. It was clear that in making his decision he had one eye on the picture of medical litigation in the United States:

> There, the damages are colossal . . . Experienced practitioners are known to have refused to treat patients for fear of being accused of negligence. Young men are even deterred from entering the profession because of the risks involved . . .

Similar remarks were made in the same case by Lawton LJ[18] who expressed the view that the system of fault-based litigation was compelling judges to make decisions 'which they prefer not to make'. The legal system, then, is faced with the classic problem of doing justice to both parties. The fears of the medical profession must be taken into account while the legitimate claims of the patient cannot be ignored.

Medical negligence apart, the various chapters in this book will indicate that, in practice, the courts are increasingly reluctant to interfere in clinical matters. What was once perceived as a legal threat to medicine has disappeared a decade later.[19] While the courts will accept the absolute right of a patient to refuse treatment,[20] they will, at the same time, refuse to dictate to doctors what treatment they should give.[1] Indeed, the fear could be that, if anything, the pendulum has swung too far in favour of therapeutic immunity.[2]

The doctor's position

There is no doubt, too, that the defining of a relationship, such as that of doctor and patient, in legalistic terms leads to a subtle but important change in the nature of the relationship. Trust and respect are more likely to flourish in one which is governed by morality rather than by legal rules and, no matter how appropriate the law may be for the regulation of many of the other ordinary transactions of life, the injection of formality and excessive caution into the relationship between doctor and patient cannot be in the patient's interest if it means that each sees the other as a potential adversary.

Where, then, does the doctor stand today in relation to society? To some extent, he is a servant of the public, a public which is widely (though not always well) informed on medical matters. Society is conditioned to distrust paternalism and the

---

17 [1980] 1 All ER 650 at 658, CA.
18 [1980] 1 All ER 650 at 661-662.
19 Compare J D J Havard 'The Legal Threat to Medicine' (1982) 284 BMJ 612 and J K Mason 'The Legal Threat to Medicine Reconsidered' (1993) 22 Ann Acad Med Singapore 95.
20 *Re T (adult: refusal of medical treatment)* [1992] 4 All ER 649, (1992) 9 BMLR 46.
 1 *Re J (a minor)(wardship: medical treatment)* [1992] 4 All ER 614, (1992) 9 BMLR 10.
 2 For a general overview, see J K Mason 'Master of the Balancers: Non-voluntary Treatment Decisions under the Mantle of Lord Donaldson' [1993] Juridical Rev 115.

modern medical practitioner has little wish to be paternalistic. The new talk is of 'producers and consumers' and the concept that 'he who pays the piper calls the tune' is established both within the profession and in its relationships with patients. The competent patient's inalienable rights to understand his treatment and to accept or refuse it are now well established.

Changes in the doctor/patient relationship are also much affected by the economic context in which it exists. Doctors and patients will undoubtedly view one another differently when medical treatment is provided free by the state as compared with when it is obtained on a commercial basis. Attempts to graft a consumerist philosophy on to the former may be made[3] but are unlikely to have any real impact on the altruistic ethic of care which, despite early opposition from the medical profession, has motivated the National Health Service over the past four decades. By contrast, the development of medical care along business lines in the United States appears to have led to dubious practices such as costly over-investigation and the unnecessary referral of patients to facilities owned by the doctors themselves. Rodin's analysis[4] of this problem concludes bleakly that money's corrupting role is difficult to avoid, even by a profession which acknowledges a high degree of responsibility for the welfare of the community. It is not surprising that, in a climate where the doctor is seen as a businessman, eager to make as much profit as possible, the patients should view themselves as being in potential conflict with him and should be ready to claw back, through litigation, what might be seen as the profession's undue gains.

A relationship of conflict – or of mutual suspicion – is in the interests of neither doctor nor patient. What is needed is one of mutual respect in which doctors acknowledge the interests of patients while patients, for their part, reciprocate this respect while appreciating the pressures, both physical and mental, under which a health carer must work. The public has also to understand the broader issues in medicine. The profession must experiment and research if it is to improve its art and many would hold that a slight loss of autonomy on the part of patients is a small price to pay for a useful advance in therapeutic skills. The profession must also teach or there will be no doctors to serve future generations; some loss of confidentiality can be looked upon as a return for the best treatment and the best investigative facilities. Clearly these opposing attitudes cannot be reconciled so long as they are polarised. A middle way, based on respect and trust, must be found and this is the function of medical jurisprudence.

The darker sides of medicine

Even so, society itself occasionally demands questionable practices of doctors. The extreme ethical problem of the late twentieth century relates to what are described as cruel, inhuman or degrading treatments or punishments. Political violence is all around us and the doctor cannot wholly dissociate himself from this. An international attempt to define his position is to be found in the Declaration of Tokyo (Appendix D) which shows well the difficulties of drafting ethical codes of an academic nature

3 National Health Service *The Patients' Charter* (1993).
4 M A Rodin *Medicine, Money and Morals* (1993).

– definitions of principle can only be interpreted in the mind of the individual. Who is to define a degrading procedure? Whether or not a caning is ethically preferable to deprivation of liberty is a matter of personal opinion. Is it self-evident that the well-being of an indiscriminate terrorist bomber is as valuable as is that of his potential victim? Granted that unethical biological measures are to be used in interrogation, could it not be that a doctor's presence, although disapproving, might be to the benefit of the victim? And one might ask by what right can the doctor command complete clinical independence when, in some circumstances, he may be ignorant of the widespread effect his decision may have on others? The motivation of the Declaration of Tokyo is impeccable in condemning the excesses of politically motivated punishment and torture but it fails in its general purpose because it was drafted with that rather narrow end in view. Clause (8) states that the doctor 'shall in all circumstances be bound to alleviate the distress of his fellow men and no motive . . . shall prevail against this higher purpose'. Carried to its logical conclusion, this would ostracise all those who assist in bringing criminals to justice and punishment yet forensic medicine must be seen as providing an ethical service to the community.

An exception to this rule should, however, be drawn in respect of the death penalty. We have some sympathy with the argument that life imprisonment in present day conditions is, itself, classifiable as inhumane and degrading treatment; yet, on balance, it must be preferable to the barbarism (and uncertainties) of the death penalty. The doctor's position in this respect is certainly less acute in areas still permitting judicial hanging than it is in the federal prisons of the United States where the preferred method of execution by lethal injection must involve medical or paramedical intervention. However, if one can legitimately recruit a hangman, it should also be possible to engage a lethal phlebotomist and, following extensive lobbying by medical organisations, the US Department of Justice has now dropped its requirement for physician participation in an execution. Although the American Medical Association accepts that doctors may attend to certify death, this absolute need has also been dropped in the United States. Here, the physician who objects for ethical reasons is, surely, on less firm ground – the horror of premature disposal of a body is as least as great as that of the execution itself.[5] We feel, however, that an obligatory autopsy examination is a further and unnecessary indignity and that pathologists should not be involved to this extent.[6] All codes of medical ethics should be carefully guarded but they are subject to interpretation and adaptation.

On a more prosaic level, there has always been something of an armed truce between the medical profession and the police as to confidentiality. The anxiety engendered here has been summed up:

'Although doctors in general wish to co-operate with the police, they must be sure that any information divulged *in confidence* will not be used in court unless they are aware at the time of interview that that information might be so used'.

The problem is discussed further in chapter 8.

5   R Rhein 'American Doctors Do Not Have to Attend Executions' (1993) 306 BMJ 813. See also G R N Jones 'Judicial Execution and the Prison Doctor' (1990) 335 Lancet 713.
6   For a very strong view, see The Lancet 'Doctors and Death Row' (1993) 341 Lancet 209 discussing, inter alia, S Trombley *The Execution Protocol* (1993).

The matter of the professional relationship between doctors and the police came to a head during the prolonged debate on what emerged as the Police and Criminal Evidence Act 1984. The major issues revolved round both confidentiality and the problems associated with intimate body searches. As to the latter, the British Medical Association considered that, in the absence of consent, they should be carried out only by medical practitioners and, then, only when there was a possibility of the secreting of a dangerous article. It could not, however, approve of compulsory searches for evidentiary reasons:

> The ethical position of a doctor invited to carry out an intimate body search for the purpose of providing evidence in support of a criminal prosecution is that it should be done only with the full, free and informed consent of the subject

wrote the Secretary of the British Medical Association, who further thought that written consent was insufficient to protect the doctor in the absence of confirmation that an 'informed' consent had been obtained[7] (see chapter 10).

The controversy exemplifies the difficulty of relying on individual conscience as a guide to ethical medical practice. The leadership of the BMA agreed with those politicians who regarded the legal permit to make searches as 'an oppressive and objectionable new statutory power [which was] a serious affront to a person's liberty.'[8] Many others, including ourselves, would consider drug peddling, with its potential catastrophic effect on many young people, as being a crime which merits draconian preventive methods. In the event, honours can be said to have been even. The British Medical Association – and other interested groups – succeeded in protecting medical records from the powers of police search; the Act retained the legal right of the authorities to ask for an intimate search but the actual operation must be performed by a medical practitioner when it is related to a Class A drug offence (PACE, s 55). The fact that s 55 has not been challenged in the European Court of Human Rights suggests that it has been operated reasonably well.[9]

The small cadre of police surgeons comes into closest contact with the police[10] but it is, perhaps, the prison medical service which most magnifies and brings into focus many of the problems associated with codified ethics. Given an abnormal population, is it possible to apply to it normal methods? One would have hoped that this would be so but there is little doubt that prison doctors are under considerable stress that results, in summary, from attempting to answer the question: are they there to serve the prisoners or the prison?[11] Smith believed that those in the service who regard their problems as exaggerated delude themselves and the frequent allusions to prisoners made in this book – particularly as to consent to examination and treatment – testify to the strength of this suggestion. The number and proportion of mentally disordered prisoners has increased steadily over the years and are likely to

---

7 J D J Havard 'Doctors and the Police' (1983) 286 BMJ 742.

8 W Russell 'Intimate Body Searches – for Stilettos, Explosive Devices, et al' (1983) 286 BMJ 733.

9 The Police and Criminal Evidence Act 1984 does not run to Scotland where the framework for police powers lies in the common law as supplemented by the Criminal Justice (Scotland) Act 1980.

10 For a critical editorial comment, see The Lancet 'Three-faced Practice: Doctors and Police Custody' (1993) 341 Lancet 1245.

11 R Smith 'Prison Doctors: Ethics, Invisibility, and Quality' (1984) 288 BMJ 781.

escalate still further with the current encouragement of community care.[12] It is hard to imagine that sedative treatments are never given without the consent of the prisoner and the procedure may be justifiable on occasion. We would suggest, however, that any fault to be found in such practices lies not so much in their doing, which is a matter of clinical judgment, but, rather, in their secrecy – and that is a criticism which can also be applied to the introduction and use of many modern medical techniques. In such circumstances, medicine may be said to be 'shooting itself in the foot'.

Every now and again, however, events overtake the medical profession and do so with such an impact as to enforce a radical alteration to its relationship with the public. The epidemic of infection by the human immunodeficiency virus (HIV) is archetypal of such an occurrence and merits special consideration.

The acquired immune deficiency syndrome (AIDS)

It is remarkable – and something of a reflection of the extraordinary mystique accorded to the condition – that the causative relationship between the human immunodeficiency virus (HIV) and AIDS should be seriously questioned more than a decade after the syndrome was first described.[13] Nonetheless, for the purposes of this review, we will keep Professor Duesberg's unorthodox views at a respectful distance and will accept the commonly held theory of HIV infection as being factual.[14] In this, sexual intercourse remains the main method of transmission of the responsible virus although this depends to a large extent on the local social ambience. Male homosexual intercourse retains its pre-eminent importance although, again, this is not universal – heterosexual spread is increasingly significant and may predominate in some areas. The second major route of transmission is through the transfer of infected blood or blood products. The result is to place at high risk those who *court* transfer – essentially, the intravenous drug abusers – and those who *need* it – for example, haemophiliacs; the catastrophic epidemic among Romanian children being a prime example of this last category.[15] Congenital infection is said to occur in some 30% of infants born to infected mothers;[16] the role of breast-feeding in transmission is currently uncertain. HIV infection is, of itself, symptomless despite the fact that the virus is transmissible. However, after a long incubation period (a mean of seven years),[17] 30-50% of those infected will develop clinical

12 R Bluglass 'Mentally Disordered Prisoners: Reports but No Improvements' (1988) 296 BMJ 1757.
13 M Y Schechter, K J P Craib, K A Gellon et al 'HIV-1 and the Aetiology of AIDS' (1993) 341 Lancet 658.
14 A further disturbing newspaper article has recently appeared: N Hodgkinson 'New Doubts over Aids Infection as HIV Test Declared Invalid' (1993) The Sunday Times, 1 August, p 1.1.
15 B S Hersh, F Popovici, R C Apetrei et al 'Acquired Immunodeficiency Syndrome in Romania' (1991) 338 Lancet 645.
16 See, for example, European Collaborative Study 'Mother-to-child Transmission of HIV Infection' (1988) 2 Lancet 1039.
17 R M Anderson and G F Medley 'Epidemiology of HIV Infection and AIDS: Incubation and Infection Periods, Survival and Vertical Transmission' (1988) 2 AIDS 57. For the American scene, see N Mueller 'The Epidemiology of the Immunodeficiency Virus Infection' (1986) 14 Law Med Hlth Care 250.

AIDS or pre-AIDS. The mortality of the full-blown disease is probably 100% and hopes for an effective treatment before the onset of symptoms have recently been set back.[18]

The almost inevitable result has been that scientific attempts to control the disease have been clouded by emotion and the process has been amplified by reason of the unusual sexual connotations of the disease. In addition, however, there is a political dimension – the homosexual lobby is powerful and suspicious of discrimination on the grounds of illness with the result that civil rights and AIDS have become inseparable issues in the United States.[19] Thus, the bid to control the disease is being made in difficult circumstances and there is less than complete agreement that all the measures taken are ideal. In essence, this dilemma stems from the need, on the one hand, to protect the public from infection and, on the other, to ensure that patients are not deterred from seeking medical help for fear of the consequences of diagnosis. The issue has crystallised into one of balancing the individual's right to privacy against the degree of coercion which the state may properly impose.

In theoretical terms, this is nothing new. All public health measures embody an involuntary element which has been accepted without protest since the middle of the last century. In practice, however, the politicisation of AIDS has led to a small number of countries taking what can only be described as draconian measures – as in Cuba where the result of testing positive for HIV may be detention for an indefinite period.[20] Such a response generally attracts little support from public health workers; indeed, it would be impossible to enforce such a simplistic and crude policy in most societies. There may, however, be more support – and possible justification – for less coercive but, still, compulsory measures such as submission to obligatory, and intrusive, blood tests in certain cases. If, for example, a person is known to be engaging in promiscuous sexual activity, the diagnosis of infection may help to impress the need for prophylactic measures and may also play a role in contact tracing. It might also be argued that detention was justified in the extreme case, despite the civil rights implications of such a measure.

The Australian response to this issue has been to endorse restriction of freedom of those HIV carriers who pose an unreasonable threat to the safety of others.[1] The Legal Working Party of the Intergovernmental Committee on AIDS has recommended that supervision and, indeed, detention may be ordered when a person has knowingly exposed others to a risk of infection, has failed to change his or her behaviour when counselled to do so and when, as a result, there is a danger to others. Powers of this sort already exist in the individual states where procedures have been developed to

18 B G Gazzard 'After Concorde' (1993) 306 BMJ 1016.
19 For a general review, see P Sieghart *AIDS and Human Rights* (1989).
20 R Bayer and C Healton 'Controlling AIDS in Cuba: The Logic of Quarantine' (1989) 320 New Engl J Med 1022. Many other countries provide for quarantine of those who pose a health risk to others but these are rarely invoked. For United States provisions, for example, see L Gostin 'Public Health Strategies for Controlling AIDS: Legislative and Regulatory Policy in the United States' (1989) 261 J Amer Med Ass 1621.
 1 For discussion, see H Watchirs 'HIV/AIDS and the Law: The Need for Reform in Australia' (1993) 1 J Law Med 9.

ensure that those affected have rights of review and of appeal against their exercise in an inappropriate way.[2]

Criticism of compulsory measures has been directed mainly from a liberal position which, at times, has given the impression of defending individual rights to sexual privacy irrespective of the social implications.[3] Such an impression may be misleading; liberal objections to compulsory measures may well be based on the premise that the behaviour in question is almost always consensual and that people should be free to take risks should they so wish. Alternatively (and more usually) they are based on a conviction that the real protection of others is more likely to be brought about by fostering voluntary restraint. Education, rather than compulsion, then becomes the key to limiting the spread of infection.

In general, Western public health authorities have opted for education and persuasion as the preferred methods of attacking the HIV epidemic. The policy of co-operation with at-risk groups has involved the use of hard-hitting and, to some, offensive advertisements and literature as well as the provision of needle exchange schemes for intravenous drug abusers and condoms for prisoners.[4] The latter ploys have been criticised as amounting to aiding and abetting drug abuse or precisely those forms of sexual behaviour which contributed to the dissemination of the disease in the first place. Yet such concerns seem dwarfed by the public interest in the containment of a public health disaster of such magnitude.

For present purposes, however, the most important concern lies in the relationship between the doctor and the HIV-positive patient and that between the HIV-positive doctor and his patient. It is the latter problem which has resurfaced only recently with the publication of the names of several doctors suffering or dying from AIDS.[5] All the health authorities involved emphasised the negligible risk to their patients and the simultaneous setting up of incident rooms and helplines testifies to the illogical thinking that is so often applied to the disease. Calls for the routine testing of health care workers have arisen and these have, to a considerable extent, been implemented in the United States.[6] The British government has set its face against such a policy and puts its faith in those health workers who are infected or who have been exposed to infection appreciating and acting upon their responsibilities. The imposition of an ethical duty to inform the employers of any invasive contact with patients is balanced by the admonition that information as to the HIV status of health care personnel should be kept confidential. However; practical experience indicates that

2   Watchirs, fn 1, above, p 20.
3   R Bayer *Private Acts, Social Consequences* (1989). The author analyses the response of public health policy in the United States to the libertarian rejection of intervention in individuals' sexual practices. For critical review, see P Illingworth 'AIDS and Liberalism' (1990) 4 Bioethics 340 and response by Bayer 'AIDS and Liberalism: A Response to Patricia Illingworth' (1992) 6 Bioethics 23.
4   R P Brettle 'HIV and Harm Reduction for Injection Drug Users' (1991) AIDS 125.
5   A further case has recently been given banner headlines in a quality newspaper: B Christie 'Hunt for AIDS Scare Patients' (1993) Scotsman, 27 May, p 1. It seems that the doctor's name was published by the paper despite the fact that the Health Board intended to preserve anonymity – a far cry from *X v Y* [1988] 2 All ER 648, (1987) 3 BMLR 1 (see p 175). The privacy of AIDS patients has also been protected by the Australian courts: *T K v Australian Red Cross Society* [1989] WAR 335.
6   M Morris 'American Legislation on AIDS' (1991) 303 BMJ 325.

this is scarcely possible. The revised guidelines also distinguish contacts by way of exposure-prone invasive procedures from those of normal 'social' type between physician and patient; it has been recommended that patients in the former category should be offered HIV testing.[7]

It is fair to say that these guidelines have not gone uncriticised, particularly as to the true extent of the risks. Simply to deny the presence of a risk is not to ensure that none exists.[8] We feel, however, that there is sufficient negative evidence to indicate that widespread testing of contacts with infected doctors would be unjustified and would be suspiciously like random testing through the back door (see p 366). Whatever the precise danger to patients may be, all authorities will agree that the risk to health care workers from infected patients is far greater; we return to this subject at p 234.

The HIV positive patient, the doctor and the law may, however, become interconnected in other fields. One such area is employment law which, because of its close association with discrimination, is particularly emotive. There is no anti-discrimination legislation in the United Kingdom directly related to either homosexuality or physical disability. In the previous edition, we suggested that an employer would be entitled to refuse to engage a known HIV carrier. There have been no recent cases in point in the United Kingdom but it now seems more likely that discrimination on the grounds of HIV status would be regarded as indirect sex discrimination – and this despite the fact that the imbalance between male and female infection is narrowing.[9] No offence would be committed, however, if the employer was able to justify his action, and such justification would be judged on the balance between the degree of discrimination and the employer's need.[10] The issue would be very much to the present point were a health authority to insist on pre-employment screening of health carers but the proposition has not been tested. Considerable public interest was aroused, however, when it was disclosed that British Airways was operating such a policy in relation to its aircrew.[11] This has not been challenged in the courts; it can be assumed that at least part of the justification lies in the possibility that the change from asymptomatic to symptomatic HIV infection may

7 UK Health Departments *AIDS-HIV Infected Health Care Workers: Practical Guidance on Notifying Patients* (1993); Department of Health *AIDS-HIV Infected Health Care Workers: Guidance on the Management of Infected Health Care Workers (interim)* (1993). Infected doctors who do not abide by the guidelines may be subject to the GMC's disciplinary procedure ((1993) 341 Lancet 1407). The risks have been analysed in Royal College of Pathologists *HIV Infection: Hazards of Transmission to Patients and Health Care Workers during Invasive Procedures* (1992).

8 See, for example, A G Bird, S M Gore, A J Leigh-Brown and D C Carter 'Escape from Collective Denial: HIV Transmission during Surgery' (1991) 303 BMJ 351 and A G Bird and S M Gore 'Revised Guidelines for HIV Infected Health Care Workers' (1993) 306 BMJ 1013. Two allied papers giving full discussion of the US attitudes are: L Gostin 'The HIV-Infected Health Care Professional: Public Policy, Discrimination, and Patient Safety' (1990) 18 Law Med Hlth Care 303 and M Barnes, N A Rango, G R Burke and L Chiarello 'The HIV-Infected Health Care Professional: Employment Policies and Public Health' (1990) 18 Law Med Hlth Care 311. Neither paper supports routine testing.

9 N Fagan and D Newell 'AIDS and Employment Law' (1987) 137 NLJ 752; J Kelly 'The AIDS Virus at the Workplace' (1991) 141 NLJ 88. This is not, however, agreed everywhere: B W Napier 'AIDS, Discrimination and Employment Law' (1989) 18 ILJ 84.

10 Cf *Hampson v Department of Education and Science* [1991] 1 AC 171, [1990] 2 All ER 513.

11 J Ashworth 'Charter Condemns Jobseekers' Aids Test' (1992) The Times, 10 July, p 1.

first manifest itself in the central nervous system.[12]   Such an argument is less applicable to cabin crew and there is no doubt that it would be unlawful to discriminate on the grounds that men are *more likely* to be HIV positive than are women.[13] Whether or not an employee could be discharged on being discovered to be HIV positive is even more difficult to prejudge. It is, however, a problem that is most likely to arise as a result of breach of confidentiality and is better discussed under that head. (See chapter 8.)

A major ethical problem associated with pre-employment testing would lie in what to tell the prospective employee in the event of a positive finding. The effects on the life-style of the subject are such that it may, in fact, be detrimental for him to be made aware of his status. This is an issue which is most vividly illustrated in the field of life insurance.

British insurers take a more interventionist stance than do their trans-Atlantic counterparts who cannot take into account any negative or unknown result when assessing their premiums and who may be statutorily barred from asking about any previous tests at all.[14] The Association of British Insurers has attempted to soften its attitude in saying: 'having had a negative HIV test will not, of itself, prevent someone from obtaining life insurance or even affect the cost, providing there are no adverse factors present'[15] – but, clearly, the qualification implies an enduring right to investigate the appellant's life-style. The doctor is in some difficulty if questioned on the point; the British Medical Association has advised doctors not to speculate on their patients' life-styles or risks of infection on behalf of insurance companies – such things are for the patient himself to disclose. Any reports of this type are, of course, subject to the provisions of the Access to Medical Reports Act 1988 (see p 186).

There have been no British cases where an insurer's decision has been challenged in court. A leading Australian ruling has, however, shown the courts' reluctance to interfere with the insurers' right to manage their own affairs.[16]   Since anti-discrimination policy in this respect is far stronger in Australia than it is in the United Kingdom, it is unlikely that an appellant would fare any better here. By and large, the problem of insurance provides a prime example of the need for adequate counselling before anyone subjects himself to testing.

Even if courts and legislatures have been at pains to protect the rights of HIV/ AIDS patients within their own jurisdictions, little restraint has been shown in limiting the rights of infected outsiders.   It was revealed in a Canadian study

12 In support, see, for example, M E Appleman, D W Marshall, R L Brey et al 'Cerebrospinal Fluid Abnormalities in Patients without AIDS who are Seropositive for the Human Immunodeficiency Virus' (1988) 158 J Infect Dis 193. There are, however, as many papers to the contrary: see, for example, A O Seines, E Miller, J MacArthur et al 'HIV-1 Infection: No Evidence of Cognitive Decline during the Asymptomatic Stages' (1990) 40 Neurology 204.

13 Eg Equal Opportunities Commission *Formal Investigation Report: Dan Air*, January 1987.

14 B Simon and P Roth 'Life Insurance and HIV Antibody Testing' (1992) 305 BMJ 902.

15 L Dillner 'Asking about HIV' 303 BMJ 327. See also N Hulme, R Smith and S E Barton 'Insurance and HIV Antibody Testing' (1992) 339 Lancet 682.

16 *Australian Mutual Provident Society v Goulden* (1986) 160 CLR 330. The case was brought under the Anti-Discrimination Act 1977 (NSW) which deals with physical and mental impairment in general. It was not associated with HIV infection.

conducted in 1989 that over 50 countries restricted the entry of HIV positive persons.[17] In some cases, the main purpose of the regulations is to prevent immigration of HIV positive persons and, in several of these, deportation follows a seropositive test. Once again, the issue is by no means novel or specific to HIV infection. For years, it has been well recognised that a state may insist on minimum health standards in its immigrants – particularly in relation to infective disease. In most countries, permission to immigrate has depended upon the likelihood that the immigrant will not tax the local resources unduly. Yet the politically charged nature of the AIDS debate has resulted in that specific issue being treated in isolation. At the Pan-Commonwealth meeting on 'AIDS and Human Movement' in 1989, the policy of denying entry to HIV positive applicants was roundly condemned even when the purpose of entry was permanent residence.[18] It was resolved that such a policy amounted to an abuse of the would-be immigrant's human rights and, in the words of the meeting's resolution: 'could have consequences for the enjoyment of the rights of other members of [the immigrant's] family and obstruct the implementation of the fundamental human rights principle of respect for family unity'. It is difficult to accept such a position unless one chooses to regard AIDS as an infective disease to which exceptional rules are applicable.

In practice, there is little doubt that much of the public's fear of AIDS stems from the belief that it is a highly infectious disease. This is not so – a fact which justifies, for example, infected children attending school; the benefits of normal schooling greatly outweigh the risks of transmission of the disease.[19] One senses a widespread, albeit vague, mistrust of many aspects of modern medicine but the greater part of that distrust, be it of AIDS or of genetic engineering, is founded upon ignorance. There is a need for publicity in these matters but, in its provision, the medical and legal professions must shed some of their essentially paternalistic seclusion and take the lead themselves – the alternatives are subjective television and radio presentations which often do little more than pile confusion on misunderstanding. The eventual resolution of these questions should be the product of open medico-legal debate – unhampered by political considerations.

17 M Duckett and O J Orkin 'AIDS-related Migration and Travel Policies and Restrictions: A Global Survey' (1989) AIDS, supp 3, s 231.
18 Commonwealth Secretariat *AIDS and Human Movement: Report of a Pan-Commonwealth Meeting* (1990).
19 For a general exposition, see A Orr 'Legal AIDS: Implications of AIDS and HIV for British and American Law' (1989) 15 J Med Ethics 61. For an American view, see W E Parmet 'AIDS and the Limits of Discrimination Law' (1987) 15 Law Med Hlth Care 61.

Reproductive Medicine

2 A reform of sex law?

Sexuality is so integral a part of human nature that its influence pervades the doctor's surgery and its importance as a factor in emotional tension is increasing. At the same time, public attitudes to sex are changing rapidly – and, indeed, are fluctuating as responses to the HIV epidemic are modified. Medical knowledge and expertise are moving to serve the altered needs of young people and it is arguable that medicine is, if anything, ahead of its time. But can the same be said of the law? It is doubtful if our present sex laws do accurately reflect current public mores and, even if the legal principles are agreed, questions are raised as to the effectiveness of traditional methods in dealing with the issues at the present time. Probably the most frequently quoted reference in jurisprudence is to Mill,[1] who said:

> The only purpose for which power can rightfully be exercised over any member of a civilised community against his will is to prevent harm to others. His own good, either physical or moral, is not a sufficient warrant. He cannot rightfully be compelled to do or forebear because it would be better for him to do so, because it would make him happy or because, in the opinion of others, to do so would be wise, or even right.

Applying these criteria to sex law, it is clear that they distinguish those sexual acts which are consensual from those in which one of the parties is non-consenting. In the latter, the aggrieved party obviously needs the protection of the criminal law. The only problem to be decided is how best can that protection be given with justice to all. In the former case, the law should only intervene if it is believed that autonomous consent cannot or, as a matter of public policy, should not be given.[2] The ability to consent depends to some extent on age but the effect of age is greatly influenced by the social environment and by education; we need to consider whether the time has come to reappraise the woman's age below which sexual intercourse is unlawful.[3] The reasons for regarding other sexual activities – such as incest or homosexuality – as being anti-social or criminal may be questioned either because there have been changes in public standards or as a result of advances in medical knowledge.

---

1 J S Mill *On Liberty and Representative Government* Blackwell's Political Texts (1st edn, 1948) p 8.
2 See the condemnation of sexual sado-masochism in *R v Brown (Anthony)* [1993] 2 All ER 75, [1993] 2 WLR 556. For a critique of this judgment, see E Edwards 'No Defence for a Sado-masochistic Libido' (1993) 143 NLJ 552.
3 Lord Brandon, in *Gillick v West Norfolk and Wisbech Area Health Authority* [1986] AC 112, [1985] 3 All ER 402, HL, pointed out that it is incorrect to speak of 'the age of consent to sexual intercourse' ([1985] 3 All ER 402 at 431). For early comment see Humphreys J in *R v Harling* [1938] 1 All ER 307 at 308, CCA.

Consent to sexual intercourse

The law makes a very evident distinction between, on the one hand, the wide spectrum of sexually motivated behaviour and, on the other, sexual intercourse which is carefully defined in the criminal law as penile penetration of the vulva. Regulation of the former is relatively unbiased as between men and women – at least in England and Wales. Thus, indecent assaults can be perpetrated by both men and women in either a homosexual or heterosexual configuration[4] and neither a boy nor a girl below the age of 16 can consent to such action. The Indecency with Children Act 1960, covering indecent practices short of indecent assault, refers to both boys and girls under the age of 14. In Scots law, the use of 'lewd, indecent or libidinous practices' against all children is an offence when they are below the age of puberty (12 for a girl and 14 for a boy). Above the age of puberty, however, the offence can only be committed against girls and then only if they are aged less than 16 years.[5] Other sexual acts involving young persons could be prosecuted under the umbrella of shameless indecency[6] or as acts of gross indecency. The principle is clear – everyone has a right to be protected against unsolicited sexual advances. And when public opinion is outraged – as it is when children are abused – the factors of consent or error as to age should be, at most, marginally mitigating.

By contrast, the control of sexual intercourse is highly discriminatory. Only the general law of assault protects the male from non-consensual sexual intercourse, whereas protection of the female is one of the most emotive aspects of the criminal law. This may be no more than a recognition of physiological reality – the circumstances in which a man can be forced to have sexual intercourse per vulvam must be very unusual. It is to be noted, however, that the consenting young male suffers no recognisable anatomical damage following such intercourse whereas the consenting girl is deflowered and may be at risk of pregnancy. At the same time, there is not much to inhibit a precocious young boy from satisfying his urges with the help of an older woman although she might be criminally liable by way of indecent assault.[7] Nevertheless, it has to be emphasised that these considerations apply to sexual intercourse as it is currently defined in the United Kingdom; the concept of sexual intercourse is being extended to include extragenital and homosexual acts in the United States and in Australia where the alternates are embodied in statute.[8]

4 *R v Hare* [1934] 1 KB 354, CCA,
5 Sexual Offences (Scotland) Act 1976, s 5.
6 *McLaughlan v Boyd* 1934 JC 19. See C Gane *Sexual Offences* (1992), pp 68, 137.
7 *Faulkner v Talbot* [1981] 3 All ER 468, [1981] 1 WLR 1528. It has been suggested that the woman commits no offence in such a case if she is merely a passive partner in sexual intercourse in which there is no genital handling by her – see J C Smith and B Hogan *Criminal Law* (7th edn, 1992) p 473. The Criminal Law Revision Committee was unwilling to add to the number of offences in this area. See B Hogan 'The Fifteenth Report of the Criminal Law Revision Committee: Sexual Offences (2) Sexual Offences other than Rape' [1985] Crim LR 425.
8 See, for example, Crimes (Sexual Assault) Amendment Act 1981 (NSW) and Acts Amendment (Sexual Assaults) Act 1985 (WA).

Intercourse with a girl between the ages of 13 and 16 years

The very specific attitude adopted both to rape and to consenting intercourse with young girls is probably associated with the importance attached throughout history to pre-marital virginity. While it is true that the Criminal Law Amendment Act 1885, in introducing the offence of having intercourse with a woman between the ages of 13 and 16 years, was largely inspired by a revulsion to child prostitution, the concept of lawful sexual intercourse was, nevertheless, still closely allied to the idea of marriageable age and, thus, to virginity. The importance of defloration was emphasised when it was established that emission was not essential to sexual intercourse[9] and, while it has long been agreed that sexual intercourse, in the context of the criminal law, can be achieved without full penetration,[10] the significance attached to the integrity of the female genitalia remains and marks the difference between potential imprisonment for life or for two years. Whether this emphasis is valid or, indeed, desirable in the late twentieth century is open to debate.

An increasing number of adolescent females below the age of 16 indulge in sexual intercourse at least occasionally. The pregnancy rate in England and Wales for girls under the age of 16 was 10.1 per thousand in 1990 and in the same year, the conception rates in England and Wales were 6.6 per thousand for girls aged 14 and a remarkable 21.6 per thousand for those aged 15.[11] There were 8,634 conceptions in girls under the age of 16 and, perhaps surprisingly, 49% of these progressed to maternity. 3,622 legal abortions were performed on girls resident in England and Wales under the age of 16 in 1990.[12] Against this tide, the number of prosecutions under section 6 of the Sexual Offences Act 1956 or section 4 of the Sexual Offences (Scotland) Act 1976 is miniscule. The experience of many doctors in examining the 'victims' of the offence is that they are usually candid, unrepentant and unaffected by the intervention of the law. To find that a statute is widely ignored is not to show that it should be repealed but a case for reform may be made out if it can be shown that such disrespect results in no public harm and, even more so, if it is not disapproved by responsible society. That such might be the case in respect of the age of lawful sexual intercourse was shown by judicial attitudes as long ago as 1976 when prosecutions under s 6 of the 1956 Act were trivialised by the judiciary on the grounds that attitudes had changed in the previous decade and girls below the age of 16 were now considered capable of organising their own sexual mores.[13]

There are, however, some cogent reasons for, at least, discouraging sexual intercourse below the age of 16 years. The facts that this age coincides with that for lawful marriage or that it is the age of consent adopted by many EC countries are, perhaps, of lesser importance than that it is the same as the current school-leaving age. The law thus alleviates one major problem for the headteacher. Yet under-age sex *is* practised and the difficulty then becomes that of distinguishing the love-play

---

9 *R v Marsden* [1891] 2 QB 149, now incorporated in the Sexual Offences Act 1956, s 44.
10 *R v Nicholls* (1847) 2 Cox CC 182.
11 Office of Population Censuses and Surveys (1991), *Birth Statistics 1991*.
12 Office of Population Censuses and Surveys (1991), *Abortion Statistics 1990* .
13 Referred to and explained with little approbation by Lawton LJ in *R v Taylor; R v Simons; R v Roberts* [1977] 3 All ER 527 at 529, [1977] 1 WLR 612, CA. See also the earlier observations by Lord Parker LCJ in *R v Howard* [1965] 3 All ER 684 at 685, CCA.

of adolescence from anti-social criminal activity and the exploitation of young people. There is, therefore, much to be said for adopting the concept of differential age which has been championed, among others, by the National Council for Civil Liberties and by the Howard League. Under the latter's scheme, which is aimed at protecting young people from sexual exploitation by their elders, the offence of unlawful indecency with a child, which already exists in the Indecency with Children Act 1960, would be extended to cover any sexual act committed with a young person between the ages of 14 and 18 years. This would be subject to the provisos that the offender was at least two years older than the child and that there had been some form of abuse of trust or of exertion of undue influence. Undue influence is, of course, a notoriously vague concept to apply in a criminal context and to avoid this problem, the League's Working Party suggests that there should be a presumption of such influence where, for example, there is material inducement or there is a relationship of trust or dependence.[14]

The record of prosecutions indicates that, in practice, the law pays major attention to such factors as similarity of age or the youth of both participants; it seems unfortunate that what is de facto cannot also be de jure as it is, with variations, in all the Australian States and in Canada. Perhaps Professor Hogan had the problem best identified when he wrote:

> ... the fact of the matter is that there is at best less than a furlong of political mileage in lowering the age and absolutely none in abolishing it altogether.[15]

Rape

Sexual intercourse without consent is, however, a different area in which it is beyond dispute that women deserve full protection. What is at issue is whether they are, in fact, receiving that protection. Society is torn between rightful anger at the thought of women being abused and horror of condemning an innocent man to jail for many years. Society's compromise is, like so many compromises, unsatisfactory. Moreover, discussion of the criminal law's response to rape has become intensely politicised, to the extent, perhaps, where a central value of the system of criminal justice – the protection of the innocent from conviction – is threatened. Certainly, male insensitivity to the seriousness of rape, and regrettable instances of unwarranted scepticism as to allegations of rape, should have no place in modern criminal law. Yet what continues to have a place – and a place that must be defended – is the principle that the only persons who should be convicted of rape are those who have knowingly, or recklessly, had non-consensual intercourse with a woman.

In England and Wales, a man commits rape if he has unlawful sexual intercourse with a woman who, at the time of the intercourse, does not consent to it and, at that time, he knows that she does not consent or he is reckless as to whether she consents to it.[16] Unlawful sexual intercourse clearly does not refer to what is unlawful by

---

14 Howard League Working Party Report 'Unlawful Sex' (1985).
15 See B Hogan 'The Fifteenth Report of the Criminal Law Revision Committee: Sexual Offences (2) Sexual Offences other than Rape' [1985] Crim LR 425.
16 Sexual Offences (Amendment) Act 1976, s 1(1).

reason of statute law; were it to do so, it would not be possible to commit rape on a mentally normal woman over the age of 16. Since this is an absurdity, the phrase 'unlawful sexual intercourse' has been taken to express the common law as it once stood and, thus, to exclude 'lawful sexual intercourse' – that is, sexual intercourse within marriage – from the definition.[17]

The anomaly in modern times of 'marital immunity' to a charge of rape has come under special attack in Scotland where Gordon has written:

> 'The idea that the husband has an 'irrevocable privilege to have sexual intercourse during the marriage' of which he can be deprived only by a decree of judicial separation . . . [is a concept that] has only to be stated to be seen to be archaic.[18]

A steady line of exceptions to the rule was developed by the courts[19] and the principle was further undermined by regarding rape as a crime of violence rather than being primarily sexual in nature.[20] The marital exemption was finally laid to rest in *Stallard v HM Advocate* in which it was said in the Inner House:

> Whether or not the reasons for the husband's immunity given by Hume[1] was a good one in the eighteenth or early nineteenth centuries, it has since disappeared altogether . . . . The fiction of implied consent has no useful purpose to serve to-day in the law of rape in Scotland.'[2]

English law has followed Scots law and a very similar line of exceptions evolved.[3] The matter came to a head, however, at the start of this decade when a number of conflicting rulings were given. In *R v R*, the trial judge ruled that an agreement to

---

17 Indeed, the Criminal Law Revision Committee Working Paper on Sexual Offences, October 1980, inserted 'extra-marital' by way of explanation of the term 'unlawful' in the 1976 Act. See also *R v J* [1991] 1 All ER 759.

18 G Gordon *The Criminal Law of Scotland* (2nd edn, 1978) p 889.

19 In *HM Advocate v Duffy* 1983 SLT 7 a libel of rape by a husband on his wife, with whom he was not living at the time, was held to be competent; the accused was acquitted. The principle was extended in *HM Advocate v Paxton* 1985 SLT 96, 1984 SCCR 311 to include amicably separated couples who were still seeing each other socially. *Stallard v HM Advocate* 1989 SCCR 248, sub nom *S v HM Advocate* 1989 SLT 469 involved a husband and wife who were still cohabiting; as in *Paxton,* the trial resulted in a not proven verdict. For an overview, see D Kelly and R S Shiels 'Marital Rape in Scots Law' (1988) 28 J Forens Sci Soc 253; T H Jones 'Marital Rape' 1989 SLT 279; and D Kelly 'The Reassessment of Rape in Marriage' (1990) 35 J Law Soc Scot 89.

20 *Stallard v HM Advocate* 1989 SCCR 248 at 250 per Lord Mayfield. The same result was arrived at by diametrically opposed reasoning in the South African case *S v H* 1985 (2) SA 750 (N) – see J R L Milton 'Rape in Marriage and Assault in Rape' (1985) 102 SALJ 367.

1 Baron Hume *Commentaries on the Law of Scotland Respecting Crimes* (4th edn, 1884) i. at 306.

2 *Stallard v H M Advocate* 1989 SCCR 248 at 254 per Lord Emslie L J-G.

3 In *R v Miller* [1954] 2 QB 282, [1954] 2 All ER 529, Lynskey J refused, with obvious reluctance, to accept that an extant petition for divorce provided an exception to the rule. Husbands have, however, been sent to trial when a decree nisi had already been granted (*R v O'Brien* [1974] 3 All ER 663); when a separation order was in force (*R v Clarke* [1949] 2 All ER 448); when an undertaking had been given not to molest the wife (*R v Steele* (1976) 65 Crim App Rep 22 – but see the conflicting opinion in *R v Sharples* [1990] Crim LR 198); and when an ouster order had, in fact, expired (*R v Roberts* [1986] Crim LR 188).

live apart – or even withdrawal of cohabitation without agreement – sufficed to revoke the immunity.[4] The following year, however, Rougier J found himself unable to extend the exceptions beyond those existing at the time of the 1976 definition of rape.[5] Yet again, in the same year, Simon Brown J concluded that the only logical approach to the problem was to follow the law in Scotland to the effect that there was no marital exemption from rape.[6] The commentator on this case concluded that the solution lay in the hands of the legislature but that the apathy of Parliament was such that the judges should take such initiative as was left open to them. The nettle was grasped both by the Court of Appeal and by the House of Lords in the appeal stages of *R v R*. In the Court of Appeal, Lord Lane LCJ regarded the word 'unlawful' in the 1976 Act as mere surplasage.[7] In the House of Lords, Lord Keith engaged in some semantic juggling, including an opinion that 'unlawful' could not ordinarily be ascribed to sexual intercourse outside marriage in modern times, so as to restrict the definition of rape to simply having sexual intercourse with *any* woman without her consent. He concluded that s 1(1) of the 1976 Act presented no obstacle to the House and declared that, in modern times, the supposed marital exemption in rape formed no part of the law of England.[8]

The courts, therefore, appear to have done what was expected of them[9] and, broadly, the decision in *R v R* must be applauded.[10] Certainly, *Stallard v H M Advocate* and *R v R* bring the United Kingdom into line with – and perhaps beyond – other common law jurisdictions which have incorporated the principle into statute[11]. Nevertheless, there *are* doubts as to whether 'stranger' rape can be fully equated with enforced intercourse within marriage. Williams, in particular,[12] has suggested, on the one hand, that a charge of rape is too powerful a weapon to put into a wife's hand and, secondly, that a summary offence of assault within marriage would be sufficient to protect a wife from unwanted advances. Williams has justified this on the grounds that : 'marital "rape" cannot be nearly so traumatic for the wife as stranger-rape' – and suggested that the difference should be reflected in differential

4 *R v R* [1991] 1 All ER 747.
5 *R v J* [1991] 1 All ER 759.
6 *R v C* [1991] 1 All ER 755.
7 *R v R* [1991] 2 All ER 257, CA per Lord Lane at 265.
8 *R v R* [1991] 4 All ER 481, HL per Lord Keith at 489. By reinterpreting the wording of the Act, the courts avoided the charge that they were interfering with statutory legislation – something which is difficult, though not impossible, to do. See A H T Smith 'Law Lords' Ruling on Marital Rape' (1991) The Times, 26 October, p 13; R Egerton 'Changing the Law on Marital Rape' (1991) The Times, 5 November, p 17. For further discussion: K Harrison 'No Means No – That's Final' (1991) 141 NLJ 1489; M Giles 'Judicial Law-making in the Criminal Courts: The Case of Marital Rape' [1992] Crim LR 407.
9 R Brooks 'Marital Consent in Rape' [1989] Crim LR 877.
10 See Law Commission Working Paper 116 'Rape within Marriage' (1990).
11 For the USA, see A F Schiff 'Rape; Wife vs. Husband' (1982) 22 J Forens Sci Soc 235 and 'Husband versus Wife: Rape' (1987) 27 J Forens Sci Soc 193. For New Zealand see Crimes Amendment (No 3) Act 1989 (New Zealand). The Criminal Law Consolidation Act Amendment Act 1976, cl 12(5) of South Australia, however, provides that a husband could be guilty of rape only when intercourse was accompanied by, inter alia, assault occasioning actual bodily harm, gross indecency or humiliation.
12 G Williams 'The Problem of Domestic Rape' (1991) 141 NLJ 205, 246; see also G Williams 'Rape is Rape' (1992) 142 NLJ 11.

sentencing. By and large, the courts have regarded cohabitation or a previous relationship as mitigating factors[13] and, judging from the Scottish experience, juries are reluctant in the extreme to convict in cases involving a close relationship. Williams has some lay feminine support[14] but the majority view, nevertheless, must be one of relief that an archaic absolute rule has been discarded in favour of one which, it is to be hoped, will be based on enlightened pragmatism.

The recognition of consent outside marriage is currently unsatisfactory from the point of view of both the man and the woman. Concern for the position of the woman was raised in *DPP v Morgan*.[15] This bizarre case involved a husband who convinced his friends that any resistance his wife might put up to sexual intercourse was simulated. It was established – and widely accepted – that, given an honest belief that the woman consented, the reasonableness of the accused's mistake was irrelevant to the law of rape unless he was reckless. The jurisprudential concept of recklessness underwent modification in the twin cases of *Caldwell* and *Lawrence*[16] and there was some doubt as to whether the principles established in the circumstances of causing criminal damage could be extrapolated to rape. Two lines of authority developed. In *Pigg*[17] and *Thomas*[18] it was held that reckless rape was committed when a man did not care as to whether or not the woman consented ; in *Satnam*,[19] which the Court of Appeal decided slightly later, reckless rape was deemed to be committed in any case in which the man did not actually believe that the woman consented. This latter approach, which is the one chosen by the Law Commission for embodiment in the Draft Criminal Code, makes it reckless rape whenever the man failed to think about the woman's state of mind. There is no reasonable man test here; the inconsiderate are put on notice of the need to address the issue of their partner's consent.[20] A man cannot be reckless if he has a genuine belief – including an objectively unreasonable belief – that the woman is consenting to sexual intercourse. He is, however, reckless if he could not care less whether the woman consents and presses on regardless. The test, therefore, is subjective – what matters is the individual accused's state of mind. Clearly, it may be difficult for the prosecution to eliminate the defence of belief but, at the same time, the limits of consent seem to be narrowing and a state of what might be regarded as resigned acquiescence now qualifies as lack of consent.[1] Casual sexual intercourse is becoming more hazardous for men and concepts such as that of 'contributory negligence' on the part of the victim have not found favour. The law is now far removed from requiring 'resistance to the utmost' from a reluctant woman.

13 *R v Berry* (1988) 10 Cr App Rep (S) 13; *A-Gs Reference (No 7 of 1989)* (1990) Times, 16 January.
14 Eg B Amiel 'Why Law Lords Got It Wrong on Marital Rape' (1991) The Sunday Times, p 2.4. Cf
   L Waller and C R Williams *Criminal Law* (1993), p 92 for the opposite view.
15 [1976] AC 182, [1975] 2 All ER 347, HL.
16 *Metropolitan Police Comr v Caldwell* [1982] AC 341, [1981] 1 All ER 961, HL; *R v Lawrence*
   [1982] AC 510, [1981] 1 All ER 974, HL.
17 *R v Pigg* [1983] 1 All ER 56, [1983] 1 WLR 6, HL.
18 *R v Thomas* (1982) 77 Cr App Rep 63.
19 *R v Satnam, R v Kewal* (1983) 78 Cr App Rep 149, CA. For criticism of the purely subjective stance,
   see commentary on *R v Bashir* [1982] Crim LR 687, CA.
20 S Gardner 'Reckless and Inconsiderate Rape' [1991] Crim LR 172.
 1 *R v Olugboja* [1982] QB 320, [1981] 3 All ER 443, CA.

Nevertheless, a prosecution for rape is less likely to succeed in the absence of evidence corroborating lack of consent. Clearly, the best of such evidence is the presence of injury resulting from force. Rape is defined in Scotland as the carnal knowledge of a female by a male person obtained by overcoming her will. This leads to some interesting paradoxes as regards English and Scottish practice. It is not rape in Scotland, for example, to have intercourse with a woman who is in a voluntary drunken stupor because she has no will to overcome,[2] whereas it would clearly be rape in England because she had not consented.

The fact of intercourse itself may be difficult to establish. Defloration as a result of rape is relatively uncommon these days and the only evidence of intercourse may be the finding of spermatozoa. Not only is emission not essential to rape but, the event having occurred, it may be difficult to demonstrate sperm after the several hours which may have elapsed since the offence. There may, thus, be no evidence of resistance and no evidence of intercourse yet the woman has been subjected to a harrowing experience. She may, indeed, have been degraded in one of many deviant ways yet there is no rape, for rape, in the United Kingdom, requires intercourse per vulvam.[3]

The result is that rape is very difficult to prove and it is arguable that women are not adequately protected against the man who acts unreasonably. There is a good case, therefore, for abandoning the out-dated concept of rape in favour of one of assault with sexual intent. The Heilbron Committee looked briefly at such a proposal[4] and rejected it for two main reasons. First, the committee objected on the grounds that all of the existing problems – for example, proof of consent – would re-emerge with any new system. This attitude, however, continues to emphasise the act of vulval penetration as the essential element of rape, whereas we prefer the notion that 'rape' is essentially an act of violence. Whether or not evidential difficulties would still arise, they could not be worse than those associated with rape as it is currently defined. Juries who, by nature, tend to an all or nothing policy in rape trials, and who are generally very reluctant to send men to prison for very long periods, would, in practice, be more likely to reach a verdict of guilty of assault, the severity of which could be reflected in sentencing. The de facto protection of women would, thereby, be improved. The committee's second main objection was that the concept of rape is well established in popular thought and that the law should reflect contemporary ideas and categorisations. We are unconvinced by this argument. A major problem appears to be that neither the public nor the media appreciate the legal limitations set upon the crime of rape and this has at least two adverse consequences. First, they find it difficult to understand why rape is so seldom charged and, second, why the conviction rate is so low in cases which come to trial. The result is frustration and anger at what seems to be undue lenience in prosecution, conviction and, occasionally,

---

2 See C Gane *Sexual Offences* (1992).
3 The interesting defence that consent withdrawn *after* penetration was, therefore, irrelevant to rape has been rejected (*Kaitamaki v R* [1985] AC 147, [1984] 2 All ER 435). There has been at least one similar plea in England: F Gibb '"No" means No at Any Point' (1993) The Times, 26 February, p 3.
4 Report of the Advisory Group on the Law of Rape (Cmnd 6352) para 80.

sentencing. The National Council for Civil Liberties has suggested that 'to take the emotion out of rape trials is to ignore the very nature of the crime'[5] – and this may well be so. None the less, we feel that the introduction of an offence of assault with sexual intent as discussed above – even if only as an interim measure – would result, overall, in increased protection of women, notwithstanding a very probable reduction in sentences imposed on the individuals convicted.

The laissez-faire attitude which persists in the United Kingdom has been found unacceptable in many parts of the Commonwealth and in the United States. Thus, the definition of rape in both South Australia and Victoria now includes non-consensual penetration of the penis into the vagina, anus or mouth of any person, male or female, or the introduction of any other part of the body or of an inanimate object into the vagina or anus.[6] Similar regulations are in force in many of the United States.[7] It still seems illogical, however, to attempt to extend the meaning of rape which, as a term, is well established in law and in history. We have suggested above that the more practical approach is to abandon the use of the term and this policy has been adopted both in Canada[8] and in New South Wales[9] where rape is assimilated into a category of aggravated criminal assault. The fears of the Heilbron Committee appear to have been partially realised in Canada where the definition of sexual assault has caused some difficulty. It now seems to have a wide interpretation including any assault which is 'gender-based' and includes, for example, assault to the female breasts.[10] The New South Wales approach has been to redefine sexual intercourse in a very broad way but so as to exclude mere touching of the breasts from sexual assault. Western Australia has abandoned the term rape in favour of sexual assault which may be both homosexual and heterosexual and which includes sexual penetration of all orifices by natural or artificial means. An offence of aggravated sexual assault is committed, inter alia, if penetration is accompanied by force or the threat of force, if the circumstances involve degradation or humiliation of the victim, if there are multiple assailants or if the victim is very old or very young.[11] It is hard to doubt that such forward-looking legislation represents an improvement on the somewhat archaic British law and the Scottish judiciary is moving in that direction. Thus, in *Duffy*, Lord Robertson specifically disdained the English cases and said:

> . . . in modern times it is quite illogical and unreasonable to treat the question of rape as if it was in some way different from assault . . . [I]t is really an aggravation of an assault.[12]

---

5 'Sexual Offences' (1976) NCCL Rept no 13.
6 Criminal Law Consolidation Act 1935-1985 (S Aust); Criminal Law Consolidation (Rape) Amendment Act 1992 (S Aust); Crimes Act 1958 (Vic) as amended by the Crimes (Rape) Act 1991 (Vic).
7 See the useful surveys by Schiff at fn 11, p 34 above.
8 Criminal Code, ss 246.1-246.3.
9 Crimes Act 1900 (NSW) as amended by the Crimes (Amendment) Act 1989 (NSW) and the Criminal Legislation (Amendment) Act 1992 (NSW).
10 *R v Ramos* (1984) 42 CR (3d) 370; see also *R v Alderton* (1985) 17 CCC (3d) 204. For discussion, see *Martin's Criminal Code* (1985).
11 Acts Amendment (Sexual Assaults) Act 1985 (W Australia).
12 *HM Advocate v Duffy* 1983 SLT 7. See also fn 19, p 33 above.

In the more influential case of *Stallard v H M Advocate,* Lord Mayfield, at first instance, held:[13]

> It would . . . be illogical and unconscionable . . . to hold [that] the libel was not relevant to what is an aggravation of assault, namely rape.

and, finally, Lord Emslie LJ-G:

> . . . rape has always been essentially a crime of violence and, indeed, no more than an aggravated assault.[14]

How far this attitude will extend, in the face of considerable opposition, remains to be seen.

Homosexuality

Attitudes to homosexuality have changed in the last quarter-century. The Sexual Offences Act 1967, permitting male homosexual practices by two consenting adults in private, was passed amid considerable public concern.[15] Twenty five years later, homosexuals constitute significant political pressure groups but the law in respect of sexuality remains, in many respects, ambivalent. It is not illegal in the United Kingdom to refuse employment on the grounds that a person has homosexual tendencies[16] but to refuse to employ only male homosexuals would almost certainly contravene the Sex Discrimination Act 1975, s 1(1)(a).[17] Once employed, however, the fairness of dismissal on the grounds of homosexuality would be a matter of proof which would be governed by the Employment Protection (Consolidation) Act 1978, ss 57(1)(b) and (3).[18] Here, much would depend upon the nature of the employment. In *Nottinghamshire County Council v Bowly,*[19] a male schoolteacher was dismissed fairly having been convicted of gross indecency although this was unrelated to his pupils. In *Boychuk v Symons Holdings Ltd,*[20] an employer was found to have acted reasonably in dismissing a lesbian who refused to remove her Gay Liberation badge. However, in *Bell v Devon and Cornwall Police Authority,*[1] a homosexual canteen

13 *Stallard v H M Advocate* 1989 SCCR 248 at 250, sub nom *S v H M Advocate* 1989 SLT 469 at 471.
14 Footnote 13, above, at 1989 SCCR 24 at 253.
15 Scotland, despite its traditional resistance to ecclesiastically unacceptable practices, came into line with England and Wales through an obscure clause (s 80) in the otherwise unrelated Criminal Justice (Scotland) Act 1980. The impact on the public was minimal.
16 B W Napier 'AIDS, Discrimination and Employment Law' (1989) 18 ILJ 84. In many common law jurisdictions (eg Australia, United States) homosexuals are specifically protected by anti-discrimination laws (for further discussion, see p 23).
17 *James v Eastleigh Borough Council* [1990] 2 All ER 607, HL.
18 As amended by Employment Act 1980, s 6.
19 [1978] IRLR 252
20 [1977] IRLR 395.
 1 [1978] IRLR 283. See also *Saunders v Scottish National Camps Association Ltd* [1980] IRLR 174, EAT; on appeal [1981] IRLR 277.

worker was found to have been unfairly dismissed because, inter alia, there was insufficient evidence to show that customers would have been upset by knowing he was homosexual.

The keys to any legislation lie, of course, firstly in privacy and, secondly, on the age of consent to homosexual practices. As to the first, the European Court of Human Rights has confirmed that it regards legislation restricting the rights of adults to act as they please in private as an infringement of the European Convention on Human Rights, art 8 – which bars interference by a public body in the right to respect for private and family life, home and corrspondence. The mere fact that prosecutions have not been taken in recent years under such legislation is considered immaterial – the threat is sufficient to affect peoples' private lives and is disproportionate to any aims that might be sought to be achieved.[2] The European Court of Human Rights acknowledges that it is for individual jurisdictions to fix for themselves any appropriate extension of the age of consent in relation to homosexual conduct.

In the UK, Parliament has recently voted to amend the current Criminal Justice and Public Order Bill to reduce the age of lawful consent to 18. A motion to reduce the age of lawful consent to 16 was narrowly defeated. Since reproduction is necessarily a heterosexual matter, homosexual intercourse is regarded by the majority as somehow unnatural; and, despite the controversy which surrounds the issue, homosexuality is commonly seen as an acquired, rather than instinctive habit.[3] Resistance to further relaxation in the protection of the young is to be anticipated.

There is, however, a variation on the current law which, we feel, must be generally acceptable. The law should have regard to teenage experimentation and there is much to be said for a differential age system such as has been discussed above in relation to heterosexual activity. This, while not necessarily approving the practice, would decriminalise that which might in certain cases be merely an aspect of growing up.

Of the other reforms which have been suggested, that concerning the definition of privacy seems least controversial; there is little logical reason why group homosexual sex should be proscribed any more than are heterosexual parties – public decency is neither less nor more outraged provided the restraints of consent and age are respected and the blinds are drawn. The problem of special relationships, particularly in respect of a duty of care, deserves closer attention than it has received – should there, in other words, be a particular homosexual offence analogous to incest? There does seem to be much merit in such a proposition and this is discussed further below. Finally, there is the suggestion, strongly argued by Honoré,[4] that the law and, particularly, its terminology should be tidied up. Archaic words such as buggery are emotive and, as has been discussed in relation to rape, may well be self-defeating. The only homosexual deserving of criminal censure is one who forces

---

2 *Modinos v Cyprus* (1993) Times, 17 May. Confirming *Dudgeon v United Kingdom* (1981) 4 EHRR 149 – a case which arose out of the fact that the Offences Against the Person Act 1861, ss 61 and 62 was not repealed in Northern Ireland. The matter was corrected in Homosexual Offences (Northern Ireland) Order 1982 (SI 1982/1536 [NI 19], art 3).

3 The age of consent issue must involve debate as to the extent to which sexual orientation is determined by adolescent experiences. For discussion of this, and related matters, see the excellent study by M Ruse *Homosexuality* (1988).

4 T Honoré *Sex Law* (1978) p 109.

himself on those who do not or cannot in law consent to his attentions. The concept of the offence of assault with sexual intent again has its attractions.

Female homosexuality within the limits of consent, and outwith the military sphere, has never been regarded as criminal save in respect of public indecency. Even here, attitudes are changing, with many films on public display including explicit lesbian activity. Quite why this is acceptable in circumstances where simple full frontal exposure of the male body would cause anxiety is difficult to understand. It is possibly a powerful example of male chauvinism, the dominant class of male heterosexuals being content to condone such voyeurism while feeling unsettled by their own sex being exposed to such objectification.

Incest

Incest, which is defined in the *Oxford English Dictionary* as 'Sexual commerce of near kindred', is, perhaps, the most illogical of sexual offences.

The primary difficulty lies in its scope. 'Near kindred' must be interpreted before any law is applied. Most jurisdictions which maintain the concept limit the offence to intercourse between three generations of relations in the direct line of descent or ascent and between siblings; the relationship persists in the illegitimate state and siblings of half blood are also included. This is the situation in England and Wales, with a curious dispensation for grandmothers and grandsons.[5] But around this norm there are variations ranging from an absence of the offence as such in France to the relatively wide relationships which are proscribed in Scotland.[6] No-one can be happy when a relationship is legal to the South of the River Tweed but attracts a potential sentence of life imprisonment to the North. In the face of such variations, it is pertinent to question the rationale of the offence for which there is, undoubtedly, an innate public distaste. Few of the common reasons adduced for the so-called 'incest-taboo' provide good grounds for legislation in modern times.

Socio-anthropological theories depend, in many ways, on the supposed advantages to the tribe or clan of 'breeding out', but such imaginings have no place in modern society with its easy access to the opposite sex outside the immediate family. More often, the case against incest is based on genetic grounds. This, we suggest, is a fundamental misunderstanding. In the first place, genetics can have no place in the historic development of an incest taboo because genetic considerations would only have been apparent to those communities who regularly practised in-breeding and, therefore, suffered from no restrictive 'horror'. Second, genetics are related to procreation while incest is a matter of sexual intercourse; hence, genetic considerations are more properly directed at the marriage laws. Third, there is no certainty that an isolated incestuous pregnancy will result in congenital abnormality. In the worst conceivable case – that of father/daughter incest with both carrying a deleterious recessive gene – the chances of a manifestly abnormal offspring are 1:4. Even so,

---

5 Sexual Offences Act 1956, ss 10, 11.
6 Sexual Offences (Scotland) Act 1976 as amended by Incest and Related Offences (Scotland) Act 1986.

this, taken with the intermediate possibility of multi-factorial disease (see chapter 6, below) would be sufficient to render an incestuous pregnancy legally terminable under s 1(1)(*d*) of the Abortion Act 1967 – in addition to the obvious indications under s 1(1)(*a*); many jurisdictions specifically include pregnancy arising from rape or incest as a justification for legal termination but the wide scope of the 1967 Act makes this unnecessary in Great Britain. Far more cogently in relation to the present era, incest must be disruptive of the family. The same can, however, be said about adultery yet we do not judge it as a criminal offence. A high proportion of the wives of men indulging in incest will say that they are quite prepared to resume normal family relationships 'if only he will stop it'. Here, the argument is edging towards what must be the family's and society's basic revulsion to incest, namely that it exemplifies the exploitation of those in the care of or under the authority of the perpetrators. Not even apparent consent can be truly autonomous in such circumstances and, therefore, incest is effectively an insidious form of rape.

Once that is accepted, the way to modernising the law becomes very much clearer. Age becomes a significant factor; it seems irrational to allow of consenting homosexual practices between adults in private yet to criminalise consenting normal intercourse between two adults who are closely related yet in a loving relationship.[7] On the other hand, increasing disparity in age increases the degree of subordination and, thus, the severity of the offence. But this is not the only feature bearing on authority. A father, in effect, has inherent authority which persists through life; a prohibition on father/daughter intercourse should, therefore, be absolute. Similar authority, albeit only until approximately school-leaving age, rests in the stepfather or the mother's common law husband and the same can be said of the foster father – the authority of an adopting father, indeed, corresponds closely to that of the genetic father. None of these are related in blood to the child yet intercourse is, in every case, within the family and the effect on the child is the same – she is being sexually abused by someone she trusts.

Scottish legislation[8] provides an example of how some of these principles may be effected. Prohibited relationships are now defined and are restricted, as regards the offence of incest, to those which are consanguineous and adoptive – sexual intercourse between a man and his adopted daughter or former adopted daughter is now characterised as incest, as are the other permutations of the adopting state; half-blood relationships are now included, as are illegitimate relationships. A separate offence of having intercourse with a step-child is created when the step-child is either under the age of 21 or has, at any time before attaining the age of 18, lived in the same household and been treated as a child of the step-parent. A further offence of having intercourse with a child under the age of 16 who is a member of the same household and over whom a position of trust or authority exists is also enacted provided that the

---

7   As suggested by the Criminal Law Revision Committee, 15th Report *Sexual Offences* (Cmnd 9213) para 8.22.

8   Sexual Offences (Scotland) Act 1976 as amended by Incest and Related Offences (Scotland) Act 1986. Prohibitions under Scots law still include uncle/aunt and great-grandparent relationships. Otherwise, the CLRC (fn 7 above) was clearly concerned to avoid major deviations between the English and Scots law of incest. The Scottish offence under 'trust and authority' was not, however, accepted.

person concerned is over 16 years old. A number of defences, including that of ignorance as to relationship or age, are specified.

These provisions are a compromise between strict logic and current public opinion. Thus, the potential right of adult brothers and sisters to act in private as they please is not yet recognised while uncles or aunts could equally well be caught in the 'trust and authority' net. More importantly, the legal obsession with defloration is perpetuated. We cannot help feeling that to force deviant sex on a young girl or homosexual acts upon a young boy is as offensive as it is to enforce natural sex; they all become of the same nature once the overall importance of trust and authority is recognised and they should, accordingly, be treated as a group.[9] The use of the word incest to cover a wide spectrum of relationships may also be considered unwise and it should, if retained, be limited to that act which is objectionable on any rationale, namely a sexual relationship between parent and child. Rape, buggery and incest are all subject to restrictive definitions which probably fail in their objectives. As a result, we would continue to argue in favour of an all-embracing concept of assault with sexual intent.

Transsexualism

Although the civil law currently takes little note of sex, the problems of transsexualism – or the gender dysphoria syndrome – are being raised with increasing frequency and carry serious issues of medical jurisprudence in their wake. The transsexual does not necessarily demonstrate any anatomical or physiological abnormality but, nevertheless, suffers from an intense wish to be of and be accepted as being of the opposite sex. Thus, while a proportion of transsexuals pass through a phase of homosexuality, the two states differ in that homosexuals are content with their own sexuality and the manner in which they express it; transsexuals are convinced that nature has made a mistake in their case and are intent on rectifying it.

The fully developed syndrome must lead to severe distress. Nevertheless, living with a problem is a personal matter and, in the absence of identification cards, National Service and the like, society is scarcely concerned to regulate the outward trappings of transsexualism such as transvestism. But rectification becomes very desirable to the subject and the public morality is then concerned at three heads – the treatment of the condition, the recognition of treatment and, perhaps most particularly, the final legal status of the transsexual. Psychiatric treatment, as opposed to simple support, of the fully fledged syndrome is generally ineffective; the patients need to change their sex organs and this goal can be achieved only by radical surgery. This includes castration in both males and females and, whereas an artificial vagina can be fashioned in the male, the biological alternative in the female is scarcely practical. In 1970, Meyers[10] questioned the legality of these operations on the grounds that consent to such physical invasion was legally impossible. Certainly, castration as

---

9 As, indeed, they are in many jurisdictions. For US experience, see D H Browning and B Boatman 'Incest: Children at Risk' (1977) 134 Amer J Psychiat 49; and D A Batten 'Incest – A Review of the Literature' (1983) 23 Med Sci Law 245, which indicates how the definition has been widened in the medical literature.

10 D W Meyers *The Human Body and the Law* (1970) p 66.

such would be a common law maim in England. Some countries have legislated for this. Swedish law on transsexualism puts the age of consent at 18 and in Germany it is 25.[11] Elsewhere, legal consent is generally based on a tacit understanding between medicine and the law. 'Sex change' operations are, today, justified nearly everywhere under the doctrine of 'necessity' or of 'genuine medical treatment' and the ethical problem then becomes one of case selection. Roth[12] has emphasised how small a number of applicants should, in fact, be recommended for operation. Nevertheless, over 2,000 cases, including 360 females, have been operated upon within the British National Health Service while some foreign national centres have a very high turnover – of anything up to 800 cases per year.

The success of treatment of a condition such as this must depend to some extent on society's reaction. Outside Scandinavia, and, particularly, Sweden, this has not been all that helpful – especially as it is exemplified by the law. Essentially, one can hope to determine a person's sex from their genital organs, from their gonads or from their chromosomal make-up. Their gender, or role, can be determined from their secondary sex characteristics and their psyche.[13] These vary from person to person. The genitalia may be congenitally malformed in the male or they may be grossly masculinised in the female (the adrenogenital syndrome); at one extreme, rudimentary female genitalia together with well-developed secondary characteristics may be present in a chromosomal male with non-functioning testes (the testicular feminisation syndrome) and, rarely, one sees a true hermaphrodite with the gonads of both sexes present in one body. Faced with a conflict of evidence, the medical solution is to 'assign' a person to the sex which they are most likely to be able to support in society, the function of the chromosomal sex being then relegated to that of an indicator of the direction in which to steer an infant's upbringing. In later life, the one characteristic of sex or gender which is apparent to no-one, including the principal, is the state of a person's chromosomes. Unfortunately, because of its immutability, that is the feature which appeals most to the lawyer.

The law has resolutely turned its face against 'sex change' and only a genuine mistake at birth can justify the alteration of a birth certificate.[14] In practice, this matters surprisingly little. Ormrod has pointed out the relative lack of concern of the law with sex[15] and that several 'corrected' transsexuals have been officially re-registered for National Insurance and employment purposes.[16] The ultimate test, however, lies in marriage which is the union between a man and a woman. The

---

11 A Cremona-Barbaro 'Medicolegal Aspects of Transsexualism in Western Europe' (1986) 5 Med Law 89. For a resumé of the current legal confusion at international level, see A Rogers 'Legal Implications of Transsexualism' (1993) 341 Lancet 1085.

12 M Roth, 'Transsexualism and the Sex Change Operation: A Contemporary Medico-legal and Social Problem' (1981) 49 Med-leg J 5. For a more recent appraisal of the difficulties, see P Snaith 'Gender Reassignment Today' (1987) 295 BMJ 454.

13 It is suggested that the brain is basically female and that its 'masculinity' depends on the development of the testes: C N Armstrong and T Walton 'Transsexual Metamorphoses' (1992) 142 NLJ 96.

14 *X Petitioner* 1957 SLT (Sh Ct) 61.

15 R Ormrod 'The Medico-legal Aspects of Sex Discrimination' (1972) 40 Med-leg J 78.

16 In *White v British Sugar Corpn* [1977] IRLR 121, a woman who was treated as a 'man' for national insurance needs was regarded as a woman for the purposes of the Sex Discrimination Act 1975.

leading British case in this context is *Corbett v Corbett*[17] in which it was held that, irrespective of reconstructive surgery, the so-called wife was not a woman for the purposes of marriage and had at all times been a biological male. This was decided on the three-pronged basis of the chromosomal make-up and the pre-operative gonadal complement and genital appearances. It was the last of these factors which it was thought would probably take precedence in the event of incongruence of the criteria. More controversially, it was held that, notwithstanding the validity of the marriage or the sex of the 'wife', she was physically incapable of consummating a marriage by the use of an artificial cavity. The case was thus distinguished from *SY v SY*[18] in which a decree of nullity had been refused on the grounds that a vestigial vagina could have been corrected by forming an artificial passage. In *SV v SY* Wilmer LJ commented:

> If a woman with an artificial vagina is incapable of true sexual intercourse she cannot be raped or commit adultery. I would regard such a result as bordering on the fantastic[19] . . .

The irony of the distinction between the two cases is that it would seem to have been made on the basis that SY was an imperfect woman. Today it is likely that she would have been diagnosed as a case of testicular feminisation and, accordingly, as a chromosomal male.

The decision in *Corbett* has since been followed both in industrial and criminal law.[20] It has, however, been criticised on the general grounds that it is unfeeling and fails to take into account the total sexual ambience of an individual. In a discussion of *Corbett* in association with *Re C and D*,[1] it has been proposed that a transsexual marriage should be valid if the transsexual is found to be capable of fulfilling the essential role of the sex that he or she has assumed and that this should include the ability of the two partners to love and understand one another. This attitude has fairly wide modern academic legal support.[2]

The attitude of the European Court of Human Rights, which is of major concern to British medical law, is, inevitably, complex but, nevertheless indicates a trend. In the original British case – *Rees v United Kingdom*,[3] the court came to a clear decision that the current English law does not transgress an individual's right to privacy and to marriage. It is to be noted that this case concerned a female to male translation – a change which might well be more difficult to support on physiological grounds.

---

17 [1971] P 83, [1970] 2 All ER 33. The 'marriage' took place in Gibraltar. An unreported case, *Franklin v Franklin (otherwise Jones)*, is said to have been the first involving a 'marriage' in England; it was annulled: (1990) Scotsman, 9 November, p 2.
18 [1963] P 37, [1962] 3 All ER 55, CA.
19 [1963] P 37 at 60.
20 *White v British Sugar Corpn* [1977] IRLR 121; *R v Tan* [1983] QB 1053, [1983] 2 All ER 12 – a prosecution under the Sexual Offences Act 1956, s 30.
  1 *Re C and D* (1979) 53 ALJ 659; H A Finlay 'Sexual Identity and the Law of Nullity' (1980) 54 ALJ 115.
  2 J M Thomson 'Transsexualism: A Legal Perspective' (1980) 6 J Med Ethics 92; A Samuels 'Once a Man, Always a Man: Once a Woman, Always a Woman – Sex Change and the Law' (1984) 24 Med Sci Law 163; J Taitz ' The Law Relating to Consummation of Marriage when One of the Spouses is a Post-operative Transsexual' (1986) 15 Anglo-Amer L Rev 141.
  3 (1986) 9 EHRR 56; [1987] 2 FLR 111.

Even so, the precedent was followed in *Cossey v United Kingdom*,[4] where the physical conditions were reversed. In both cases, the grounds for rejection of the suit were that birth certification in the United Kingdom was a matter of historical fact while there were few, if any, other impediments to a British citizen claiming to be of the sex opposite to that registered. Nevertheless, the majority decision in *Cossey* was very much narrower than that in *Rees* and the court commented forcefully on the fact that medical and social science changed with the times; as a consequence, several jurisdictions were amending their practices in this field. The European Court of Human Rights followed this line further in *B v France*,[5] a case in which the originally male applicant had failed through the French courts to obtain a declaration that she was now of female sex. Here, it was held that refusal to recognise B's true status was a breach of art 8 of the European Convention for the Protection of Human Rights. The court was, undoubtedly, strongly influenced by the changing attitudes to and understanding of transsexualism (including the full acceptance of the testicular feminisation syndrome) but would not overrule the *Rees* and *Cossey* judgments – essentially on the grounds that birth certificates in England and in France served different purposes, the latter being intended to be updated throughout the life of the person concerned. The arguments put forward in *B v France* have something of a sophistical flavour. Nevertheless, there are strong indications that common law jurisdictions, as well as European, are taking a more pragmatic, and perhaps more humane, approach than that maintained in the United Kingdom. Thus, in the American case of *MT v JT*,[6] the transsexual partner to a marriage was held to be capable of acting within marriage as a female. In rejecting *Corbett*, Handler J could perceive:

> no legal barrier, no cognisable social taboo, or reason founded in public policy, to prevent that person's identification, at least for the purposes of marriage, to the sex generally indicated.

The reasoning in this case cannot, however, be applied to the female to male transsexual and such 'marriages' have been annulled in the United States.[7] Even in the unlikely event of the law being changed so as to validate a marriage between a converted transsexual and a person of the same chromosomal complement, such a 'marriage' between a female to male transsexual and a female would, in the absence of additional legislation, be voidable in both England and Scotland on the grounds of incurable impotency.[8]

---

4   [1991] 2 FLR 492, (1991) 13 EHRR 622.
5   [1992] 2 FLR 249, (1993) 16 EHRR 1.
6   *MT v JT* 355 A 204 (NJ, 1976).
7   *B v B* 355 NYS 2d 712 (1974).
8   See K McK Norrie 'Transsexuals, the Right to Marry and Voidable Marriages in Scots Law' 1991 SLT 353.

More recently, attention has been drawn to two Australian cases, *R v Cogley* and *R v Harris, R v McGuiness*,[9] (albeit arising in the field of criminal law), in which *Corbett* was specifically disclaimed. Both are of interest individually and comparatively. In *Cogley*, circumstances very similar to those envisaged by Wilmer LJ in *SY v SY*[10] were tested and the converted transsexual complainant was considered to possess a vagina. The trial judge followed the reasoning in *MT v JT* and found the conformity of the current genitalia and the 'core' identity as constituting the essential ingredient for establishing the 'sex' of a person. The Court of Appeal, however, in an obiter opinion, thought that judges' expressions in such cases laid down no legal principles and that the determination of disputed sex was a matter for the legislature.[11] *Harris* exhibited remarkably controlled conditions. Two male to female transsexuals were accused of attempting to procure an act of indecency by a male. One had undergone reassignment surgery and was held to be a female within the meaning of the Crimes Act 1900 (NSW); the other, although psychologically a female, had not had surgery and was considered male. The importance of the existing genitalia was, thereby, emphasised, Mathews J saying:

> The criminal law is concerned with the regulation of behaviour . . . I cannot see that the state of a person's chromosomes can or should be relevant . . . in the determination of his or her criminal liability . . . How can the law sensibly ignore the state of [the external] genitalia . . . simply because they were artificially created or were not the same at birth?

Although the New South Wales' Court of Appeal conceded that there was some doubt as to whether a similar test would be applied in civil litigation, the implications are that the Australian courts will apply the same reasoning to family law when asked.[12]

There are, however, dangers in moving too fast. Kennedy,[13] in putting the case for legalising converted transsexual marriage, went on to extrapolate this to the authorisation of homosexual marriages – 'I have no doubt it will occur', he said, 'later if not sooner'. We feel that this stretches logic too far. Marriage is defined at common law as the union between a man and a woman but, problems of consummation excepted, the anatomic/physiologic *completeness* of either party is seldom of major importance. A man with infantile or undescended testes is still capable of a legal

---

9 *R v Cogley* [1989] VR 799; *R v Harris*; *R v McGuinness* (1989) 35 A Crim R 146. Discussed in H Finlay 'Transsexuals, Sex Change Operations and the Chromosome Test: *Corbett v Corbett* not Followed' (1989) 19 UWAL Rev 152 and in R Bailey-Harris 'Sex Change in the Criminal Law and Beyond' (1989) 13 Crim LJ 353 – which includes the appeal stage in *Cogley*. For an opinion published in a UK journal, see J L Taitz 'Confronting Transsexualism, Sexual Identity and the Criminal Law' (1992) 60 Med-leg J 60.
10 [1963] P 37, [1962] 3 All ER 55, CA.
11 For pioneer Commonwealth legislation in the field, see the South Australian Sexual Reassignment Act 1988. Section 7(8)(b) states that a recognition certificate may be issued to an adult who has been reassigned.
12 For a comparison of the cases with *R v Tan* [1971] QB 1053, [1983] 2 All ER 12 (fn 20, p 44, above), see Taitz 'The Law Relating to Consummation of Marriage when One of the Spouses is a Post-operative Transsexual' (1986) 15 Anglo-Amer L Rev 141.
13 I M Kennedy 'Transsexualism and Single Sex Marriage' (1973) 2 Anglo-Amer L Rev 112.

marriage with his sexual opposite. Similarly, a woman without a uterus and unable to bear a child would rightly expect to be treated as a woman for the purposes of marriage to a man. It is at least arguable that the gap between this situation and that involving the converted male to female transsexual is bridgeable. A homosexual 'marriage', by contrast, is a bond based on the union of like with like. While few would deny the potential social and emotional benefits flowing from an institutional union of such type, it would surely warrant a label separate from what we now know as marriage. The plights of the transsexual and the homosexual are different in this context; to consider them together can lead to misunderstanding and may, consequently, inhibit social progress in either case.

Deliberate transmission of sexually transmitted disease

The liability for deliberately infecting another person with sexually transmissible organisms has received considerable attention recently. Although the principles would be the same in respect of any such disease, the problem is amplified in the case of HIV infection as, here, the scenario includes the possibility of death and of unlawful killing.

Public health aspects have been discussed in chapter 1. Here, we are concerned only with issues surrounding the knowing transmission of disease from one individual to another. These can be viewed either from the perspective of the criminal law – one purpose of which is to deter by way of threatened punishment – or of the civil law – which is concerned to compensate individuals for injury done to them or to prevent acts or omissions likely to result in its occurrence.

It is difficult to accommodate such an action within any existing principles of criminal law and, for this reason, several common law jurisdictions have enacted a statutory offence of knowingly transmitting AIDS or other serious diseases.[14] Surprisingly, the only English precedent lies in the very old case of *R v Clarence*[15] in which a man who knowingly infected his wife with gonorrhoea was found, on judicial consideration of the case, to be not guilty of inflicting grievous bodily harm and also not guilty of an assault occasioning actual bodily harm.[16] The decision in *Clarence*, however, depended in large measure on the then current interpretation of consent to intramarital intercourse. This has now been reversed (see p 33 et seq) and it is at least doubtful whether *Clarence* would be followed today. Moreover, alternative

14 See, for example, Public Health (Proclaimed Diseases) Amendment Act 1985, s 50 (NSW); Public Health Act 1991, s 13 (NSW) ; Crimes Act 1900, s 36 (NSW) as amended by Crimes (Injury) Amendment Act 1990. In South Australia, an HIV-infected person commits an offence if he fails to take all reasonable precautions to prevent transmission of the infection (Public and Environmental Health Act 1987, s 37(1) (S Aust)). See also A Jesperson 'Aids Law in the USA' (1990) 140 NLJ 125. A very useful precis of the law on AIDS in the USA is to be found in H L Hirsh 'Human Immunodeficiency Virus Infection Confronts the Law, Ethics and Society' (1993) 22 Ann Acad Med Singapore 69.
15 (1888) 22 QBD 23, [1886-90] All ER Rep 133, CCR.
16 Contrary to Offences Against the Person Act 1861, ss 20 and 47 respectively.

charges – for example, of administering a 'destructive or . . . noxious thing'[17] – might succeed. The case does, however, demonstrate the difficulty of applying statute law in the criminal courts[18] and the wider terms of criminal codes[19] or an appeal to common law principles might achieve a more equitable result.

As to principle, the mens rea involved may be that of intent or of recklessness as to the outcome – and there is little doubt that the versatility of Scots law could sustain a charge of recklessly endangering the life of a person.[20] Such a charge – indeed, any criminal charge – would, however, be subject to a consideration of consent. This is well exemplified in two German cases, both of which concerned men knowing they were HIV positive indulging in unprotected sexual connection in either a homosexual or heterosexual relationship. In the first case, a charge of *Totschlag* (roughly equivalent to attempted homicide) was dropped but, nevertheless, the accused was convicted and imprisoned for inflicting serious bodily harm. In the second case, the court was unwilling to convict. The only essential difference in the two cases was that in the latter case the woman concerned was aware of her partner's HIV status.[1] While this may seem the correct pragmatic decision, the fact that manslaughter was considered is sufficient to raise the question of whether it is legally possible to consent to something which is likely to result in severe injury – and it is relatively certain that one cannot do so in England.[2] Logically, it would follow that consent would not vitiate a charge of inflicting serious harm and that *any* sexual connection by an HIV positive person could constitute an offence. It is clear, however, that the courts would be unlikely to follow such reasoning. For example, while it was accepted by the judge of preliminary inquiry in *Ssenyonga*,[3] it was later rejected by the trial judge. Indeed, there are those who would hold that the criminal law has no

17 Offences Against the Person Act 1861, s 24. S H Bronitt 'Spreading Disease and the Criminal Law' [1994] Crim LR 21 discusses the introduction of an offence of 'causing serious injury' which would encompass transmission of significant diseases.
18 This is well demonstrated in K J M Smith 'Sexual Etiquette, Public Interest and the Criminal Law' (1991) 42 NILQ 309.
19 Two Canadian cases involving the 'commission of a common nuisance' by potentially transmitting the HIV virus illustrate the difficulty. In *Thorburn v R* (1991) Ont CA Lexis 126, an attempt to transmit the virus through donation of contaminated blood resulted in conviction. It was held that there was no 'public nuisance' case to answer in a similar prosecution involving sexual intercourse (*R v Ssenyonga* (1992) 73 CCC (3d) 216). This case is, however, continuing on charges of aggravated sexual assault and criminal negligence causing bodily harm. See M R Eastwood and M McKelvey 'HIV Transmission Comes to Court in Canada' (1993) 341 Lancet 1653; C Johnston 'Controversial AIDS-transmission Case Sent to Trial by Ontario Judge' (1992) 147 Can Med Assoc J 522. See also *R v Lee* (1991) 3 OR (3d) 726: in this case the accused was acquitted of a charge of aggravated assault when the court found no distinction to be made between consent to sexual acts and consent to sexual acts with a person who was, unknowingly, HIV-positive.
20 For a discussion of this point, see G T Laurie 'Aids and Criminal Liability under Scots Law' (1991) 36 J Law Soc Scot 312. A man has been imprisoned for 18 months in Denmark on just such a charge although 23 women were involved: C Csillag 'Prison Sentence for Exposing Women to risk of HIV Infection' (1993) 341 Lancet 751.
1 Decision of 16.11.1987, Landgericht Nürnberg-Fürth, 1988 NJW 2311; Decision of 1.7.1988, Amtsgericht Kempten, 1988 NJW 2313.
2 *A-Gs Reference (No 6 of 1980)* [1981] QB 715; [1981] 2 All ER 1057. See also *R v Brown (Anthony)* [1993] 2 All ER 75, [1993] 2 WLR 556.
3 *R v Ssenyonga* (1992) 73 CCC (3d) 216.

place in the control of the spread of AIDS[4] and, to an extent, we would concur in that view. Even so, there is an intuitive feeling that the person who is unwittingly infected with HIV (or, for that matter, any sexually transmitted disease) is entitled to some redress and, for this, it may be necessary to turn to the civil law.

Of the several heads beneath which a claim for damages might lie,[5] negligence seems to be the most appropriate for discussion. This would be based on failure to conform to the standards of reasonable conduct or on flawed consent as a result of being given inadequate information as to the risks involved.[6] In any event, an action would depend upon there being a duty of care owed to each partner in the course of sexual connection. Such a duty is established in the United States[7] but, surprisingly, the issue is by no means settled in the United Kingdom. The nearest 'authority' we can find is an extra-judicial opinion given by Lord Brandon to the effect that such a duty does exist[8] – and we feel confident that the courts would follow such a line. That being so, negligence would be the correct route both to compensation in civil law and to the creation of criminal liability in the event that the negligence be considered gross. This appears to be the route currently adopted in Canada where the Supreme Court has confirmed an 11-year prision sentence on a man who knowingly spread the HIV by having unprotected sexual intercourse; he pleaded guilty to two charges of criminal negligence causing bodily harm.[9] Even so, the plaintiff who brought a civil action would face many hurdles, perhaps the most difficult of these being establishing causation – particularly in the case of AIDS with its long incubation period and the shadowy nature of exposure to the virus. A defence of ex turpi causa non oritur actio would be unlikely to be upheld in the modern moral climate but one of volenti non fit injuria would stand or fall on whether or not an obvious risk was present and accepted. Thus, the nature of the consent would be fundamental to the outcome and could find expression by way of contributory negligence – a concept which could be used to redress the balance of responsibility for transmission of any infectious disease.[10] Certainly, the difficulties faced by a person deliberately infected by sexual contact would be great and, for this reason, there might be a case for retaining a criminal sanction. The indications are, however, that this would require specific legislation in England – and probably also in Scotland. It is open to question whether this would accord with the now generally accepted policies of AIDS containment. There is unlikely to be much support for any such demands in the present political climate.[11]

---

4   R Porter 'History Says No to the Policeman's Response to AIDS' (1986) 293 Brit Med J 1589;
     P Old and J Montgomerey 'Law, Coercion and the Public Health' (1992) 304 Brit Med J 891. Not
     all would agree with this – eg S H Bronitt 'Criminal Liability for the Transmission of HIV/AIDS'
     (1992) 16 Crim L J 85.
5   See J Taitz 'Legal Liability for Transmitting AIDS' (1989) 57 Med-leg J 216.
6   'Informed consent' is discussed in detail at p 237 below.
7   Eg *Long v Adams* 333 SE 2d 852 (Ga, 1985). A short news item indicates that damages of $18
     million have been awarded in Florida to a man who was infected with HIV by his fiancée: (1993)
     Financial Times, 27 August, p 1.
8   K Litton and R James 'Civil Liability for Communication of AIDS – A Moot Point' (1987) 137 NLJ
     755.
9   'Prison Term Upheld for Man Dying of AIDS' (1994) Vancouver Sun, 25 February. A similar
     apprroach could be followed in England following *R v Sullman* [1993] 3 WLR 927.
10 See Old and Montgomerey, fn 4, above.
11 C M Tomkins 'HIV Transmission and the Law' (1992) 340 Lancet 543.

3 The management of infertility and childlessness

The title of this chapter draws attention to a distinction which we believe to be of practical, as well as semantic, importance. Primary infertility is a problem of the production of gametes or of implantation of the embryo. This may be susceptible to hormone therapy – a matter which we only touch on here. Ovum or sperm donation then becomes a secondary treatment of childlessness due to unsuccessful treatment of the primary condition. Similarly, the basic in vitro fertilisation (IVF) technique is most commonly used as a treatment of childlessness due to blockage of the fallopian tubes which is resistant to recanalisation therapy. The distinction appears to be narrow but it may be significant in relation to resource allocation. Thus, it could be held that, whereas the treatment of infertility is clearly a medical matter, childlessness can be seen as a social problem which should be funded from a different source. While we cannot fully subscribe to this theory, it might serve to justify the relative scarcity of the latter facilities in the NHS.[1]

Some 10% of marriages are said to be infertile and the couple desire children in a high proportion of these.[2] In addition, there are couples who should not have children for genetic reasons, either because one may carry a dominant deleterious gene or because both are known to bear recessive characteristics (see ch 6, below). Again, a couple may be able to conceive a child but the woman is unable to carry it for medical reasons. Opportunities for adoption are now meagre and attention has focused on the elaboration of methods designed to substitute the gametes of one or other person or to bypass the natural process in other ways.

There has been intensive consideration of the legal and moral issues involved at governmental level in many countries.[3] Overall, it is remarkable how similar have been the conclusions of the various committees of inquiry which have reported throughout the English-speaking world.

---

1 Only three out of the 50 centres approved in 1990 were wholly funded by the National Health Service; 19 others made some use of NHS facilities: *Sixth Report of the Interim Licensing Authority for Human In Vitro Fertilisation and Embryology* (1991). The *First Annual Report of the Human Fertilisation and Embryology Authority* (1992) (see p 64) indicates that there are now 68 centres offering IVF treatments under transitional licensing arrangements but these are not broken down as to funding.

2 G Douglas *Law, Fertility and Reproduction* (1991) quotes comparable figures (at p 105). Recent studies, however, indicate that the true figure may be less than this: A Templeton, C Fraser and B Thompson 'The Epidemiology of Infertility in Aberdeen' (1990) 301 BMJ 148.

3 For a modern and wide-ranging review of international developments, see S A M McLean (ed) *Law Reform and Human Reproduction* (1992).

Artificial insemination

Artificial insemination by donor (AID)[4] may provide a solution where there is male infertility, a condition which accounts for roughly 50% of cases of involuntary failure to conceive. In this procedure, semen obtained from a donor is injected into the woman and this results in conception in a high proportion of cases. The husband's semen may similarly be introduced into the uterus by artificial means (AIH) – a need which might arise from impotence or from inadequate formation of spermatozoa, in which case treated semen would be used. Many couples who have recourse to AID are loath to abandon all hope of husband/wife offspring. In such circumstances, the semen of the apparently infertile husband is mixed with that of the donor so that the couple can still believe that the ovum may have been fertilised by the husband's sperm. This form of artificial insemination is known as AIHD.

Artificial insemination by the husband

AIH, as ordinarily practised, gives rise to no major ethical problems. All that is entailed is that the woman conceives by a method other than that of normal sexual intercourse and the procedure will only be regarded as questionable if there is objection to *any* interference with nature in this area. The use of AIH as a preliminary to sex selection of the conceptus is, however, discussed as a separate matter.

Before the advent of sex selection, the major issue raised concerned the possibility of 'sperm banking' for use by a wife after her husband's death. There are obviously times when the wife of a member of a high risk profession might wish to undertake this, while semen may be available from 'banking' prior to testicular ablation, say, during treatment of malignant disease. The process has a moral relevance particularly as to the effect on the child born into a single parent family[5] – the subject is considered more fully at p 54. Legally, it could lead to intolerable problems in relation to probate and succession. The dilemma has now been only partially resolved by the Human Fertilisation and Embryology Act 1990, s 28(6)(*b*) which states baldly that where the sperm of a man, or any embryo the creation of which was brought about with his sperm, is used after his death, he is not to be treated as the father of the child. It is to be noted that the process is not prohibited – indeed, Sch 3, para 2(2) allows for the relevant consent. However, the original government White Paper[6] made it clear that it was to be discouraged and, no doubt, the statutory authority (see p 64 below) will take this into account in any cases that come within its ambit. The section leaves open the related questions of the man who is reported missing but is, in fact, dead and of the wife who reasonably believes her dead husband to be alive. We think it is likely that legal paternity could be established in either case.

---

4 There is a movement to replace this acronym by DI (donor insemination) because of confusion with HIV infection. We will, however, continue with the established term, which is widely understood.
5 It is reported that the French Centre for the Study and Conservation of Human Sperm opposed posthumous AID on these grounds – but the husband could have been HIV positive at the time of 'banking': D Geddes 'Life, Death, and the Seeds of Judicial Controversy' (1991) Scotsman, 20 February, p 7. The court subsequently overruled a contrary precedent and refused the widow's request (J Y Nau 'Le Sperme Defunt' (1991) Le Monde, 28 March).
6 Human Fertilisation and Embryology: A Framework for Legislation (Cm 259, 1987).

A second legal problem could arise were nullity of the marriage to be mooted – as it could well be in circumstances calling for the use of AIH. A decree of nullity can still be obtained if a woman conceives in this way and the marriage has not been consummated. Then, any children would still be regarded as legitimate on the grounds that the parents were married at the time of conception. Approbation might, however, exclude such a decree.[7]

A somewhat bizarre application of AIH relates to long-term prisoners whose wives may wish, or need, to conceive before their release. We have access only to a news item[8] in which the Home Office is quoted as saying that facilities for artificial insemination are not normally made available to prisoners but could be allowed in exceptional circumstances at the discretion of the minister. The rationale of this apparently purely retributive restraint is uncertain – particularly as conjugal prison visits are commonplace in many jurisdictions. The fact that there are apparently no reports of any appeal suggests that the concession was granted in the case in point – one which related to the wife's age.

Primary sex selection

As this edition is being prepared, public concern has been roused by the entry into the market place of preconception sex selection of children. Most methods claiming scientific respectability depend upon altering the proportion of male- and female-bearing spermatozoa in the ejaculate and artificial insemination with the processed specimen. Opinions differ as to whether such methods are efficient and, if so, to what extent they can be relied upon. This, however, is not our main concern. What calls for analysis is the ethical position given that a fully efficient method of sex selection at conception became available.[9] Discussion is then at two levels: the practical and the deontological. The fact that both are highly culture-dependent – with a very evident East/West divide – deserves emphasis. Thus, at the practical level, it is probably fair to say that preconception sex selection would have, at most, a negligible effect on the distribution and status of the sexes in the United Kingdom. But this is essentially a Western view and one which might well not be true of countries in the Far East.[10]   Indeed, the Government of India is introducing legislation designed to criminalise an already widely available post-conception sex determination service.[11] On the ethical plane, very few, it is supposed, would oppose primary sex selection for the prophylaxis of X-linked disease (p 123). Similarly, even those concerned to minimise fetal rights would see it as preferable to embryo selection or abortion for this purpose.

Beyond this, sex selection for non-medical or social reasons has been classed as anything from 'playing God' to offering an acceptable new dimension to family planning. The latter view cannot be rejected out of hand – it is difficult to see why family design should not be refined in this way when so much family planning of other sorts is practised and encouraged. This, however, presupposes that the method

7 *REL v EL* [1949] P 211, [1949] 1 All ER 141 (see also *G v G* 1961 SLT 324).
8 D Fernand 'Prisoner Calls for Right to Father a Child' (1989) The Sunday Times, 5 March, p A9.
9 The Lancet 'Jack or Jill?' (1993) 341 Lancet 727.
10 T Marteau 'Sex Selection' (1993) 306 BMJ 1704.
11 G Nandan 'India to Ban Prenatal Sex Determination' (1993) 306 BMJ 353.

is perfected. At present, it seems that, at best, only some 70% of choices will be effected. Couples who have been to considerable expense and discomfort to select the sex of their child will be bitterly disappointed when their wishes are unfulfilled. Thus, we foresee a possibly disastrous outcome for 30% of children currently born using this technique. For this reason alone, we would advocate a legal limitation of 'gender clinics' to those licensed to undertake the practice. The potential consequences for individual children – and, perhaps, for society via a 'eugenic wedge'[12] – are too serious for the process to be left unsupervised.[13]

Artificial insemination by donor

There are those who object strongly to AID on the grounds that the basis of the marriage bond is compromised by the wife's pregnancy through another man. It is supposed that the privity of marriage is invaded and that, in this respect, AID is little different from adultery.

AID and the marital bond

The question of whether AID constitutes adultery in legal terms was debated in the Scottish case of *MacLennan v MacLennan*[14] where it was determined that adultery could not be held to have taken place because there was no sexual contact between the woman and the donor. This approach to the question would probably be acceptable now throughout the Commonwealth. AID without the consent of the husband may, however, be taken as constituting unreasonable behaviour for divorce purposes.

However, given the consent of both parties, the acceptance of AID can be seen as the fulfilment of the perfectly legitimate desire to have a child. The very fact of agreement to the process testifies to the strength of the bond between the parties – and this is confirmed by the comparatively low incidence of divorce in couples who have chosen AID. The marital bond is disturbed by the procedure only in a highly metaphysical sense and this disturbance is, in any event, actively sought by the couple.

This is not to recommend that AID be undertaken lightly. Several jurisdictions have introduced legislation to control the extensive use of donor insemination in the United States where its provision has been of variable quality.[15] In the United Kingdom, it is now illegal to perform AID without a licence unless it is a mutual treatment between the woman and the man,[16] and counselling as to its psychological

---

12 A phrase borrowed from L T Marteau 'Sex Selection' (1993) 306 BMJ 1704.

13 Currently, the Human Fertilisation and Embryology Authority (HFEA) (see p 64) has no control unless the semen comes from a donor or in vitro fertilisation is involved. At the time of writing, the HFEA has expedited publication of a consultation document which clearly allows for such an extension of its remit. See V Choo 'Sex Selection' (1993) 341 Lancet 298.

14 1958 SC 105.

15 See, for example, R M Greenblatt et al 'Screening Therapeutic Insemination Donors for Sexually Transmitted Diseases: Overview and Recommendations' (1986) 46 Fertil Steril 351. The possibility of transmission of disease, including infection by HIV, is recognised everywhere: C L R Barratt and I D Cooke 'Risks of Donor Insemination' (1989) 299 BMJ 1178.

16 Human Fertilisation and Embryology Act 1990 (hereafter referred to as 'the 1990 Act'), s 4.

and legal implications is an integral part of the process. Donor insemination is, however, very widely needed. It is important that regulation does not become merely restrictive and that it is accompanied by its corollary – the unfettered provision of a service through the National Health Service.

Major ethical problems

Major ethical problems do not, therefore, arise within the standard husband and wife situation. But it may be that a single woman or an unmarried couple request AID or the request may come from a lesbian couple. Since there is no legal regulation of the matter, a doctor will have to decide on ethical grounds alone whether or not to proceed in these circumstances.

The Royal College of Obstetricians and Gynaecologists gives some answer to this in the guidelines it has laid down for its members. These recommend that AID be performed only on a married woman and, then, with the consent of her husband in writing. Some would say that this is excessively conservative; a single woman may feel precisely the same desire for a child as a married woman and has the same right to a child as her married counterpart. The same argument may be put forward on behalf of the homosexual woman whether she is living by herself or with a partner. Should the experience of giving birth and raising a child be denied in either case because of the absence of a husband? Why should society exclude the possibility of conception in this way when it allows such women to conceive by natural means and permits them to keep their children as a normal right of parenthood?[17]

Artificial insemination is not, however, a natural process and, legally speaking, it must involve the medical profession. In participating in the process of procreation, the doctor is performing an act which is not morally colourless. Even if the principal objective of AID is to satisfy the desire for a child, thought has to be given to the child who is the end result. Many would hold that the child's interests should be considered paramount – and that this holds throughout the spectrum of assisted reproduction.[18] The doctor must, therefore, question whether he should play a part in the deliberate creation of a child who could be disadvantaged as compared with his peers who have fathers. Whether or not such disadvantage – including any disadvantages of lesbian parenthood – is real or imaginary is, currently, undecided[19] and is, perhaps, indeterminable – for there are probably proportionately as many good and bad homes that are regularised by church or state as are occupied by single parent families.

Section 13(5) of the 1990 Act emphasises the importance of this particular problem by specifying consideration of 'the need of the child for a father' as one of the welfare principles to be satisfied before treatment is given under licence (see also

17 Inevitably, much of the literature in this area is partisan. A good review from the feminist viewpoint is provided by M McGuire and N J Alexander 'Artificial Insemination of Single Women' (1985) 43 Fertil Steril 1982. Others have cast doubt on the motivation of single women seeking AID: see, for example, S Jennings 'Virgin Birth Syndrome' (1991) 337 Lancet 559. For discussion of a typical incident, see S McLean 'Charting Virgin Territory' (1991) The Scotsman, 15 March, p 11.

18 D Giesen 'Developing Ethical Public Policy on Reproduction and Prenatal Research: Whose Interests Deserve What Protection?' (1989) 8 Med Law 553.

19 For a review, see S Golombok and J Rust 'The Warnock Report and Single Women: What About the Children?' (1986) 12 J Med Ethics 182.

p 61). The onus on the doctor is, therefore, considerable. We, ourselves, would fall back on the distinction we have already made between social and medical treatments. It is open to a fertile single woman, whether hetero- or homosexual, to have a child by natural means. Professional intervention in such circumstances is unarguably a matter of social, rather than medical, expedience. We doubt if a doctor ought to confuse his role as a therapist with that of a social worker or political economist – the decision and its solution should be left to the woman herself.[20] On the other side of the coin, s 38 of the 1990 Act now relieves the doctor who conscientiously objects to such procedures of a duty to act. The discussion is, however, more germane to those forms of assisted reproduction which depend wholly upon medical expertise (p 60 below). The Warnock Committee[1] was unable to conclude any more firmly than that it is, as a general rule, better for children to be born into a two-parent family. We suspect that this restrictive attitude will carry considerable weight as AID becomes subject to an official code of practice.

Legal considerations

The legal position of the child born as a result of AID has been established in the United States and in many parts of the Commonwealth for some time.[2] Legislation was delayed in the United Kingdom until the passage of the Family Law Reform Act 1987, s 27. This partial solution to the problem has now been extended in the 1990 Act, ss 27-30 which also resolve the anomalies previously extant between England and Wales and Scotland. Section 28(2) covers the case of the married woman and it is to be noted that, although s 28(3) allows for the common law marriage, there are no provisions for single women. In essence, the rule is that the husband of a woman who has been inseminated with the sperm of another man by a person licensed to do so will be treated as the father of the child provided he has consented to the process; s 28(4) emphasises that, in these circumstances, no other person is to be treated as the father of the child. The s 28(2) rule is voided if the husband can show that he did not, in fact, consent to the procedure. The frankly confusing terms of s 28(5) do, however, retain the common law principle of *pater est quem nuptiae demonstrant*; thus, it seems that the husband who does not consent to AID may still have to rebut that presumption by way of accepted methods of paternity testing. Section 29(4) preserves the somewhat archaic exclusion of hereditary titles, honours and the like from the general principles attaching to the AID child – although where the onus of proof or disproof of patrilinearity then lies or, indeed, how it can be discharged, is a matter for speculation. An exception of greater practical importance is that, by

---

20 This is clearly the situation in the United States. There was apparently no difficulty in recruiting 26 single women without partners who were willing to undergo a definite research project involving pregnancy by AID: see A J Peters, B Hecht, A C Wentz and R Jeyendram 'Comparison of the Methods of Artificial Insemination and the Incidence of Conception in Single Unmarried Women' (1993) 59 Fertil Steril 121.

1 See para 2.11 of the report of the Committee of Inquiry into Human Fertilisation and Embryology (Dame Mary Warnock, Chairman) (Cmnd 9314, 1984) referred to hereafter as Warnock.

2 Eg, see Artificial Conception Act 1985 (W Australia), Status of Children (Amendment) Act 1984 (Vict), and Artificial Conception Act 1984 (NSW). See also Children's Status Act 1987 (RSA); Uniform Parentage Act (1973) (USA). For full discussion, see D J Cusine *New Reproductive Techniques: A Legal Perspective* (1988) chs 7 and 8.

virtue of Sch 4, para 8, ss 27-29 of the 1990 Act do not apply for the purposes of restricting live organ transplants between persons not genetically related (Human Organ Transplants Act 1989, s 2).

It will be seen, therefore, that the problem of the legitimacy of the AID child born in wedlock no longer arises. It cannot be denied that, despite the now negligible consequences of illegitimacy,[3] this is to the advantage of the child – and it was this principle that dominated the Parliamentary debate on the legal consequences of insemination by donor. Much of this concerned the registration of the birth of the child, particularly as to its father. Again, this now appears to be clarified, s 29(1) stating that the treatment in law of a woman's husband as the father of a child resulting from consensual donor insemination is 'for all purposes' – and this must include the registration of births and marriages. While this is very convenient, we tend to share Lord Denning's doubts as to the propriety of statute law abetting perjury.[4] There is, in fact, some opposition to the statutory provisions on genealogical grounds, particularly in Scotland.[5]

The donor's anonymity and freedom from parental responsibility are essential to the success of any donor insemination programme.[6] The latter is ensured by s 28(6)(a) of the 1990 Act which specifically excludes the donor from paternity. The former is now subject to the licensing authority keeping a register (as provided for by s 31(2) of the Act) of identifiable individuals who have been treated, whose gametes have been stored or used and who were, or may have been, born as a result of treatment services. As a corollary to this, a person over the age of 18 years, or a person over 16 years old and intending to marry, may now require the authority to establish whether he or she might have been born as a result of treatment services and, if so, to provide such information as to parentage as is required by regulation. The regulations cannot require the Authority to give any information as to the identity of a person whose gametes have been used and that prohibition will have retrospective force should it be revoked.[7] We imagine that the type of available information will be similar to that recommended by Warnock (at para 4.21) – that is, information as to the donor's ethnic type and genetic health.

Thus, on paper, anonymity seems to be adequately protected. Nevertheless, we have reservations as to the retention of names on the register. Apart from the fact that clandestine breach of confidentiality now seems to be an accepted feature of public administration, the mere fact that a list of names exists may be a source of inspiration to zealots in the cause of freedom of information. From the more specific aspect, a nominal register is held to be important to guard against the possibility of incest or of marriage within the prohibited degrees in later generations. Warnock (at para

---

3 By reason of the Family Law Reform Act 1987 and the Law Reform (Parent and Child) (Scotland) Act 1986.
4 482 HL Official Report (5th series) col 1282, 11 December 1986.
5 D Whyte 'Human Fertilisation and Embryology' (1989) Scot Geneal 88.
6 Cm 259, 1987 Human Fertilisation and Embryology: A Framework for Legislation.
7 See s 31(5). Personal data relating to treatments under the 1990 Act are exempt from the subject access provisions of the Data Protection Act 1984 except so far as their disclosure is made in accordance with s 31. Disclosure can, however, be ordered by the courts in the interests of justice (s 34) and in the case of proceedings under the Congenital Disabilities (Civil Liability) Act 1976 or of comparable actions for damages in Scotland (s 35).

4.26) recommended, on arbitrary grounds, that there should be a limit of ten children who should be fathered by one donor. The dangers, both real and imaginary, of such matings as a result of AID may be overstated. The disclosure provisions in the event of marriage are theoretically sound but may be an example of using a sledgehammer as a nutcracker. Outwith the marriage factor, claims are made that children have a right to know their true parentage and also that they have a strong psychological urge to do so.[8] Much of the evidence for such a desire is, however, anecdotal and no comparable study of children born by way of adultery has been, nor probably can be, made. If there *is* such pressure, the compromise of allowing access to limited information can only lead to frustration. The frequently drawn analogy with adoption – in which there is a statutory right to discover a true genetic relationship[9] – is flawed. In adoption, some bonding with the true parents may have occurred. There is, at least in the 'stranger' process, no necessary genetic affiliation with either adopting parent and, pragmatically, disclosure of status is almost certain once the child requires to see his or her birth certificate. The *need* for the AID child to have the same discovery rights as the adoptee is, therefore, by no means self-evident.

Very few of us ever question our paternity and still fewer will doubt their maternity – for the same regulations apply to ovum donation (see p 59 below) as to sperm donation. It seems to us that the almost inevitable result of regulating for a few to question their parentage will be to encourage the majority to do so. It is doubtful if the statutory creation of children anxiously awaiting their eighteenth birthday in order to exorcise an implanted suspicion can be to the overall benefit of family relationships. Occasionally, and particularly in the event of the reason for AID lying in a genetic abnormality in a woman's husband, disclosure of true parentage may be highly desirable. Such situations are better met by good counselling within a responsible family environment.

The infertile or childless woman

Although we appreciate that treatment for childlessness is available to unmarried women – and is clearly envisaged under the Code of Practice[10] – the majority of requests for appropriate treatment are likely to come from married couples. It is in this sense that we refer to 'husband and wife' in what follows.

Childlessness due to abnormalities in the man is, as we have seen, largely a matter of the defective formation of spermatozoa. A woman may also suffer from primary infertility but, in addition, she may be beset by anatomical problems which prevent her having children by natural means – of which, blockage of the fallopian tubes is the most important. The proportion of cases due to anatomical abnormality and to infertility resulting from faulty ovum production is about equal. We do not, here,

---

8 See, for example, G D Mitchell 'In-vitro Fertilisation: The Major Issues – a Comment' (1983) 9 J Med Ethics 196. From Australia, L Waller 'The Law and Infertility – The Victorian Experience' in S McLean (ed) *Law Reform and Human Reproduction* (1991). A modern full review is K O'Donovan 'A Right to Know One's Parentage?' (1988) 2 Int J Law & Fam 27.

9 Adoption Act 1976, s 51; Adoption (Scotland) Act 1978, s 45(5).

10 Human Fertilisation and Embryology Authority *Code of Practice* (revised 1993), para 3.16 refers to 'husband or partner (if any)'.

discuss the purely medical treatment of the latter and its incidental legal and ethical significance is noted briefly at p 66. When hormonal treatment has failed, however, the anovular woman is in the same position as the azoospermic man and may be able to parent a child by way of gamete replacement and, despite the fact that ova are far more scarce and are more difficult to handle than are spermatozoa, ovum donation is now a practical routine procedure. Even so, it is, perhaps fortunately, still impossible to develop a full-term fetus in a laboratory environment. Ovum donation is, therefore, pointless without, at the same time, providing a womb. Both may be contributed by the same woman or they may be available independently. These are the bases of the legal and moral problems complicating the treatment of the infertile woman.

In vitro fertilisation (IVF)

Many modern reproductive techniques involve the fertilisation of the ovum in laboratory – or in vitro – conditions and the subsequent transfer of the embryo (ET)[11] from the petri dish to the uterus. Strictly speaking, therefore, IVF and ET are technical terms. Nevertheless, popular usage equates IVF with the standard treatment for childlessness due to blockage of the fallopian tubes and ET with the implantation of an embryo which has no genetic relationship either to the recipient or to her husband. This apparently semantic distinction is, we believe, of practical importance. If damage is to be done to the embryo, one would anticipate it being most likely during handling in transit and as such this is a matter of general technique rather than of a specific therapy.[12]

Standard IVF treatment involves collection of ova from the wife's abdomen, fertilisation of these with her husband's sperm in the laboratory and transfer of the resulting embryo to her uterus. The treatment is, therefore, essentially one designed to by-pass diseased fallopian tubes. The actual collection of ova is now relatively simple through a laparoscope; the treatment cycle does, however, involve complex hormonal priming to ensure superovulation. This is important to the process as success is affected by the number of embryos implanted. The mean live birth rate depends to an extent on the size and expertise of the treatment centre but is currently in the order of 12.5% of treatment cycles; pregnancy rates vary from 7% when one embryo is transferred to 27% when three are implanted[13] – and it is only recently that there has been a significant improvement. Thus, while IVF may well

---

11 The First Report of the Voluntary Licensing Authority for Human In Vitro Fertilisation and Embryology (1986), p 8, recommended the use of the term pre-embryo to distinguish the organism before differentiation into fetal and placental cells has occurred. There is, thus, physiological justification for this. We, however, prefer not to use the term as, despite protestations to the contrary, it smacks of an attempt to make a moral distinction between the pre-embryo and the embryo – which we suggest is spurious and unnecessary (see also the Australian Report of a Senate Select Committee on the Human Embryo Experimentation Bill 1985 (1986)).

12 D J Cusine *New Reproductive Techniques: A Legal Perspective* (1988) p 141, prefers the therapeutic distinction, referring to the 'transfer' in IVF as 'embryo replacement'.

13 *First Report of the Human Fertilisation and Embryology Authority* (1992). Strangely, the rate actually drops when more than three embryos are implanted and the Authority believes that there are no longer any circumstances in which there is clinical justification for implanting more than three. Indeed, they are clearly considering reducing the number to two.

be the optional treatment for one of the commonest female causes of childlessness, the expectations of success are relatively low – an important point to be made when counselling childless couples.

The rationale of the process corresponds closely to that of AIH and, as such, presents no legal problems. The genetic and natural parentage of the resulting infant are not disputed. All that has occurred is that a technique has been substituted for a natural process and if any would protest that this is in some way immoral, they would, at the same time, have to contend that the surgical treatment of any disease is similarly immoral.

There is, of course, no technical reason why the sperm must be those of the husband and, in the event of combined male infertility and an impassable female genital tract, donor semen could be used in the same way. In such circumstances, the legal problems would be those of AID which have already been discussed.

Ovum donation

An alternative situation is that the ovum is donated by another woman. The need might arise as being the only way in which a woman with, say, abdominal adhesions could have children and it might be desirable in the event of a potential mother carrying an X-linked genetic disease (see ch 6). About 1% of childlessness for female reasons is due to ovarian failure of uncertain origin and the ovaries may be destroyed during, say, treatment for cancer. The scenario is now that the donated egg is fertilised by the husband's semen and the embryo then transferred to the wife's womb. The process can, therefore, be looked upon as the female variant of AID.

The practical difference is that, whereas spermatozoa are plentiful and easily harvested, ova are scarce and their recovery involves some discomfort and inconvenience to the donor. Thus, the donor must be stimulated hormonally in order to coincide with the recipient's optimal menstrual state and, in many cases, a laparoscopy will be required. Ova may be obtained from women in the course of other surgery – in particular, during sterilisation. There is, however, some concern lest their consent may be flawed in that a measure of coercion is used in the latter case.[14] Nevertheless, centres may offer free sterilisation in return for donated eggs provided that very strict criteria as to counselling, management and consent are met.[15] The difficulties, then, of ovum donation lie not only in the technique but, also, in finding the donors[16] – a difficulty which is compounded by the fact that, unlike spermatozoa and early embryos, ova cannot, at present, be cryopreserved without significant risk of induced chromosomal abnormality.[17] We advert briefly to the possibility of using fetal ovarian tissue as a source of ova in chapter 14 (see p 312)

Once achieved, however, the natural (though not the genetic) parentage will be reasonably clear. We submit that the act of carrying a fetus from implantation to full term confers true motherhood on a woman who has been seeking that state actively.

---

14 'The GMC and Medical Ethics' (1989) 298 BMJ 1380.
15 Human Fertilisation and Embryology Authority *Code of Practice* (1991).
16 P Bromwich 'Oocyte Donation' (1990) 300 BMJ 1671.
17 A Trounson 'Preservation of Human Eggs and Embryos' (1986) 46 Fertil Steril 1; K Dawson 'In Vitro Fertilisation: Legislation and Problems of Research' (1987) 295 BMJ 1184.

It is difficult to see any circumstances in which parenthood would be challenged[18] and, in a patrilineal society, there are fewer objections to an admixture of ovum-derived genes in the family than to those which arise as a result of AID. The matter is now put beyond legal doubt in that s 27(1) of the 1990 Act follows earlier Australian legislation[19] in holding that a woman who carries a child as a result of the placing in her of an embryo or of sperm and eggs, and no other woman, is to be treated as the mother of the child.

But what of the similar wife with an infertile husband? Although such a combination might be regarded as too rare for consideration, it could, theoretically, arise in perhaps one in every 1,000 marriages seeking children. Such a state can be managed by embryo donation whereby an embryo performed from donated ovum and donated sperm is implanted in the sterile woman. The resultant complications then lie somewhere between those of in vitro fertilisation and those surrounding surrogate motherhood and are best discussed under that heading below. Even so, it is emotionally, morally and legally important to distinguish unrelated embryo transfer of this type from surrogate motherhood – the intense relationship between mother and fetus occurs in both but, despite the absence of genetic affiliation, it is only in the former that this progresses naturally to the bond between mother and child.

Once again, the 1990 Act has cleared the legal air. By virtue of ss 27 and 28, the child born of embryo transfer is, for all purposes, the child of the carrying mother and her consenting husband.

The availability of IVF

We have discussed some of the moral issues surrounding assisted reproduction under the heading of artificial insemination. Very much the same principles apply in the case of the infertile wife. There is, however, one major difference: while AID is a relatively simple process, IVF and its counterparts are both cost and manpower intensive. Problems of resource allocation are, thus, superimposed on those of ethical practice.

The response to the question of whether the effort applied to the alleviation of childlessness is well or mis-directed is such a personal matter that specific discussion would be invidious; the general principles of resource allocation are outlined in chapter 11. Whether IVF, in its broad sense, should be available to fertile couples depends upon the motivation.[20] There may be good medical reasons, mainly in relation to the carriage of abnormal recessive genes, which fully justify intervention in any appropriate form on behalf of otherwise fertile couples. Indeed, when combined with embryo biopsy – whereby the genetic status of embryos can be

---

18 See *The Ampthill Peerage* [1977] AC 547, HL, per Lord Simon at 577.
19 Status of Children (Amendment) Act 1984 (Vict). See also the Artificial Conception Act 1985 (W Aust), ss 5(1) and 7(1).
20 K Dawson and P Singer 'Should Fertile People Have Access to In Vitro Fertilisation?' (1990) 300 BMJ 167. Infertility is likely to be a prerequisite to treatment in France: see A Dorozynski 'France Has Another Go at Compiling an Ethics Law' (1993) 307 BMJ 1445. For a very controversial and critical review of the cost-effectiveness of the IVF programme, see M G Wagner and P A St Clair 'Are In Vitro Fertilisation and Embryo Transfer of Benefit to All?' (1989) 2 Lancet 1027.

established before implantation – IVF may offer their currently *correct* management. Non-medical reasons would include the early removal of ova for use in later life, thus circumventing the increased risk of chromosomal abnormalities in the child, and, second, the wholly hedonistic use of 'womb-leasing' for social reasons (which is discussed at p 75). As to the early removal of ova, there would be no legal objections in the United Kingdom to preserving embryos in the same way as sperm and a case can be made out on grounds of social utility for women delaying their pregnancies. There are, however, practical difficulties. In the first place, s 14(4) of the 1990 Act limits embryo storage to five years and second, the pregnancy rate following embryo transfer deteriorates with age. In these circumstances, it is doubtful if the process would gain general approval.

There are, above all, considerations as to the effect on the resultant child and, as in AID, this leads to the question of the potential mother's status – single, lesbian or of doubtful suitability. At the time of writing, the age of the woman has become a burning issue – particularly in relation to the impregnation of one who is post-menopausal. Here, in contrast to the AID situation, medical involvement in the procedure, if it is to be undertaken, is essential in both practical and legal terms; it follows that the doctor cannot opt out of judgments which involve purely social values. It is for this reason that the current guidelines for assisted reproductive treatment centres include the obligatory establishment, and use, of an ethical committee which has a wide remit regarding the management of individual cases. No legally enforceable principles as to selection of candidates for the limited resource have been laid down. It has, however, been determined, in the only apposite case so far reported, that, provided the committee does not behave quite unreasonably, its decision is not subject to judicial review.[1]

Nor is there, in our opinion, a great deal of help to be obtained from the 1990 Act, s 13(5). This, as noted above under AID, states that a woman shall not be provided with treatment services unless account has been taken of the welfare of any child born as a result of the treatment and of any other child who may be affected by the birth. Not only is this condition extremely wide – *any* child within the extended family might be said to be affected – but it is imprecise as to the quality and depth of account to be taken other than subtly indicating a covert disapproval of treatment outside the 'married' state.[2] Moreover, it seems to us to have its own dangers. 'Taking account' of does not imply reaching the same conclusion; it is not too far-fetched to envisage 'shopping expeditions' on the part of unconventional would-be mothers to identify the most 'liberal' clinic as a source of treatment. One would hope not to see a repetition of the early days of legal abortion.

The legal position of the donor
The theoretical hazard which is common to all procedures involving in vitro embryo transfer is that the embryo will be damaged during manipulation and that an

1 *R v Ethical Committee of St Mary's Hospital, ex p Harriott* [1988] 1 FLR 512, [1988] Fam Law 165. The case was somewhat clouded by allegations of deceit.
2 For analysis of the 1990 Act see D Morgan and R G Lee *Blackstone's Guide to the Human Fertilisation and Embryology Act 1990* (1991); G Douglas 'The Human Fertilisation and Embryology Act' (1991) 21 Fam Law 110; P A Wiewiorka 'The Human Fertilisation and Embryology Act 1990' 1991 SLT 65.

abnormal fetus will result. Animal experiments indicate that there is no higher incidence of abnormalities in live born neonates resulting from reimplantation than in those which are conceived normally and, so far as is known, no appreciable excess of human cases beyond the probability of chance has occurred. The number of congenital abnormalities reported in children conceived through IVF in the United Kingdom in 1989 showed a significant increase over the previous year; the figures were not, however, comparable as treatments by gamete intra-fallopian transfer (GIFT), which may not be subject to licensing, were included in 1989.[3] The likely outcome of litigation following such a misfortune would depend very largely on proof of causation. However, the ground rules are clear. Section 44 of the 1990 Act applies the Congenital Disabilities (Civil Liability) Act 1976, s 1, to infertility treatments in that, if a child resulting from embryo transfer, GIFT or AID is born disabled and the disability results from an act or omission in the course of the selection, or the keeping or use outside the body, of the embryo or the gametes used by a person answerable to the child, then the child's disabilities are to be regarded as damage resulting from the wrongful act of that person and actionable at the suit of the child. This does not apply if one or both parents knew of the risk of their child being born disabled. Particular importance is, therefore, likely to attach to the effectiveness of their consent in respect of the information given.

Official bodies in both the United Kingdom and the United States have found concerns regarding the moral status of the embryo and the potential long-range consequences of research on embryos to be among the most difficult to confront them. These issues converge in the treatment of the surplus embryo.

The surplus embryo
It is inevitable that surplus ova and surplus embryos will be produced whether IVF (in which we include GIFT) or ovum donation is being attempted. The status and disposal of such embryos have significance which is independent of the problems of successful implantation.

The criminal law can be considered only to be dismissed. The Offences Against the Person Act 1861, s 58 defines abortion as procuring a miscarriage, while the Abortion Act 1967 refers to terminating pregnancy. The process of disposal is, thus, clearly not abortion and, equally clearly, it is not murder since the embryo can in no way be considered to have achieved a separate existence in a legal sense. Should the 'Brave New World' come upon us and it be possible to develop laboratory embryos to term, it may be necessary to invent an offence of feticide but, in view of the current legal approach to death and the non-viable fetus (discussed at p 107), even that would be problematical. In the absence of any specific legislation on the matter, it is difficult to see that any criminal offence is committed by the simple disposal of unimplanted embryos.

That being so, the problem can be seen as being ethical in nature and devolving on the nature of the embryo. Dr Walters, of the Kennedy Institute of Ethics, is quoted

3 *Sixth Report of the Interim Licensing Authority for Human In Vitro Fertilisation and Embryology* (1991) p 19. The Australian experience, however, is less reassuring. See, for example, N Swan 'IVF Legislation in Australia' (1989) 299 BMJ 1241 quoting P A Lancaster 'Congenital Malformations after In Vitro Fertilisation' (1987) 2 Lancet 1392.

as defining the moral status of the human embryo conceived in vitro as being 'more than that of a mouse embryo but less than that of a full human fetus'.[4] The US Ethics Advisory Board agreed that the 'human embryo is entitled to profound respect' but qualified this: 'but this respect does not necessarily encompass the full legal and moral rights attributable to persons'. Similarly, the Warnock Committee (at para 11.17) recommended only that the embryo of the human species should be afforded *some* protection in law. Such general prevarication indicates the measure of the moral difficulties involved but is, at the same time, unhelpful. In the end, one must come to a decision – either the embryo is a full human being within the rigid, mainly Roman Catholic, theological doctrine or it is a laboratory artefact.

We have argued in our earlier editions that humanity depends upon the establishment of a natural human environment and, from this, have extrapolated that ensoulment – which we equate with humanity – is not established until implantation.[5] Such reasoning is not universally acceptable in an increasingly secular society and it fails to define a soul. An alternative approach, which achieves much the same end, is to regard the process of becoming a human person as 'a progression through a series of linked developmental stages'[6] and to attribute rights to the embryo because it is a phase in the whole human form. The authors go on to base this moral value on the human capacity to react with others – a capacity which exists in modified form from implantation to death. We find this approach helpful, if only in a negative way, because, despite the authors' disclaimer, none of this perfectly valid analysis applies to the in vitro embryo. In the absence of implantation, there is no continuum and there is no human interaction. Moreover, no moral value can be attributed to the embryo by virtue of its potential for personhood – for no such potential exists in the medium of the petri dish.

It therefore seems acceptable – and both kinder and more practical – to liken the in vitro embryo to a culture of fibroblasts – which also have 46 chromosomes in their nuclei. If one accepts this premise, one simultaneously solves one's moral problem as to embryonic research which, when done well, must be valuable to the community as a whole. The concept of 'acquired humanity' also serves to differentiate research on embryos from research on fetuses which is discussed as a separate issue in chapter 17.

Nevertheless, this conclusion cannot be accepted without qualification – at the very least, the embryo must be accorded the respect due to any living human tissue. It has been argued that, in logic, there is no need to control laboratory interference with a research object that one believes has no moral status; but there *is* public disquiet over scientific involvement in the reproductive process and, on these grounds alone, it must be contained within a controlling framework.[7] Most importantly, the argument rests upon the limitations of technology. Currently, it is doubtful if the most dedicated research worker in the field would wish to maintain an embryonic culture for longer than a very few weeks and, equally, it is technically

---

4 B J Culliton and W K Waterfall 'Flowering of American Bioethics' (1978) 2 BMJ 1270.
5 This is argued more fully in J K Mason *Human Life and Medical Practice* (1988). The proposition has received some support – eg, M C Shea 'Ensoulment and IVF Embryos' (1987) 13 J Med Ethics 95. See also N M Ford *When Did I Begin?* (1988).
6 N Poplawski and G Gillett 'Ethics and Embryos' (1991) 17 J Med Ethics 62.
7 H Barnett 'Biotechnology – Can the Law Cope?' (1986) 15 Anglo Amer L Rev 149.

impossible to do so. It is, however, clear that our formula would be inadequate should technology advance to the state of being able to 'grow' fetuses to full term in vitro as we would then be confronted with non-humanised human beings, which would be intolerable.

The control of assisted reproduction

It was against such a possible background that the 1990 legislation was enacted. The main thrust of the Act is to establish (by s 5) a Human Fertilisation and Embryology Authority (HFEA) which is mandated to supervise and provide information and advice to the Secretary of State about embryos and about treatment services governed by the Act. The Authority maintains a Licence Committee and assisted reproductive treatments which involve gamete donation or the creation of embryos outside the body are subject to the possession of a licence by the treatment centre.[8] Thus, in some contrast to the prototype Infertility (Medical Procedures) Act 1984 of Victoria – which, together with its amendments of 1987, sets out the limits of treatment relatively precisely – the 1990 Act allows for a flexible development of the art under the control of peer and lay review.[9] Sections 3 and 4, however, define activities which *cannot* be licensed. These include placing in a woman any live gametes or embryos other than those of human origin, placing a human embryo in any animal, replacement of an embryonic nucleus by a nucleus from any other person or embryo and, of particular significance, keeping or using an embryo after the appearance of the primitive streak – by definition, later than 14 days from the date the gametes were mixed but excluding any time for which the embryo was stored. The spectre of in vitro fetal development is, thus, allayed although critics of the legislation will inevitably ask – 'for how long?' The specific time limit has been attacked by purists mainly on the grounds that a 13-day embryo is no less alive than is one of 15 days' gestation and that it is entitled to the same respect.[10] The counter-argument is that controlled embryonic research is essential if the attack on genetic disease – which may well be the most important single factor dictating morbidity in humans – is to be carried on in a scientifically acceptable way.

The fate of the undeveloped in vitro embryo presents a continuing dilemma which exists in two distinct parts. The first is that of the use and, indeed, the

---

8 It will be noted that intra-fallopian transfer of gametes or zygotes between partners is not subject to licensing. Even so, HFEA is maintaining a watchful eye on the processes.

9 The chairman of HFEA may not be a registered medical practitioner or directly associated with the provision of treatment services. Such persons must, however, constitute at least one third but not more than one half the total membership (Sch 1, para 4). The current chairman is an academic lawyer and the first membership includes appointments from such varied professions as the religious ministry, banking, television production and the stage. Misgivings as to definitive legislation in the medical field are expressed by G Dworkin 'Law and Medical Experimentation: Of Embryos, Children and Others with Limited Legal Capacity' (1987) 13 Monash Univ LR 189.

10 T Inglesias 'In vitro Fertilisation: The Major Issues' (1984) 10 J Med Ethics 32. The same issue contains a contrary view from a moralist: G R Dunstan 'The Moral Status of the Human Embryo: A Tradition Recalled' (1984) 10 J Med Ethics 38. See also M Lockwood (ed) *Moral Dilemmas in Modern Medicine* (1985) ch 1 and the philosophical argument in A Holland 'A Fortnight of My Life is Missing' (1990) 7 J Appl Philosoph 25. See also D Giesen 'Developing Ethical Public Policy on Reproduction and Prenatal Research: Whose Interests Deserve What Protection?' (1989) 8 Med Law 553.

production of embryos for research purposes; this highly emotive issue is discussed in chapter 17. The second relates to the practical problems surrounding the disposal of embryos that are surplus to immediate therapeutic needs. As already mentioned, overproduction of embryos is inseparable from the treatment of infertility by IVF – it is impossible to guarantee receptive wombs for those which remain unused in the individual case and, in many instances involving defective embryos, it could be wrong to attempt to do so. It follows that any new legislation that attempted to criminalise the bona fide destruction of embryos would, at the same time, effectively shut the door on this form of treatment. It has been suggested[11] that the Victorian legislation may do just that in stating in s 6(5) that:

> a person shall not cause or permit [ova obtained from the body of a woman] to be fertilised outside the body of the woman except for the purposes of the implantation of embryos . . . in the womb of that woman or another woman.

Waller, however, maintains that this is not so[12] and that the section merely prohibits the production of embryos for the express purpose of non-therapeutic experimentation. Such a procedure would not necessarily be prohibited by the current United Kingdom legislation under which the disposal of gametes and embryos depends heavily on the consent of those donating the gametes. It follows that whether or not an embryo can be used for treatment or research or whether it is to be destroyed at a certain time or in certain circumstances (eg on the death of the donor) depends upon the agreed consent of two persons (Sch 3, para 6 of the 1990 Act). The 1990 Act, however, makes no provision for the condition most likely to cause difficulty – namely, when there is disagreement between the two parties concerned.

The need for some form of legislation is exemplified in two quite recent causes celèbres. In the first of these, an Australian case,[13] embryos were stored against future use by a couple (one of whom was the genetic mother) but both were killed before the embryos were implanted. There was such public outcry at the thought of their being destroyed that they were retained in storage pending the passage of legislation. Our understanding is that they were not implanted later into volunteer women as had been intended and that, partly for technical reasons, they never will be. An example of disagreement was provided in Tennessee in 1989. Here, a married couple who had provided stored embryos were divorced before the latter could be used. The father asked that they be destroyed while the mother wished to become pregnant by them. The judge at first instance ruled that the embryos were human beings – with all the rights attending that status – and that their fate should, therefore, be decided on the principle of their best interests. This meant that they should be implanted. This decision was reversed by the State Supreme Court which held that

---

11 For example, A Trounson as quoted in the Institute of Medical Ethics Bulletin 19, October 1986, p 14, October 1986.

12 L Waller 'The Law and Infertility – The Victorian Experience' in S McLean (ed) *Law Reform and Human Reproduction* (1991) at 25.

13 The details of the case are hard to come by. Our authority is G F Smith 'Australia's Frozen "Orphan" Embryos: A Medical, Legal and Ethical Dilemma' (1985/86) 24 J Fam Law 27; B Steinbeck *Life Before Birth* (1992) p 212. An American case concerning custody of stored embryos, *Del Zio v Manhattan Columbia Presbyterian Medical Center* 74 Civ 3588 (SDNY, 1976), occurred too early in the development of the procedures to be of precedental value.

the man's interest in not reproducing outweighed those of his spouse in procreating.[14] A rather similar case has been fought in Australia.[15] Our feeling is that similar problems will result from the British legislation[16] and that it would be better for 'consent to disposal' to be vested in the person for whom the embryos were intended – that is, the proposed woman recipient. Parliament's remarkable concern for the embryo in the face of some 180,000 abortions performed annually in Great Britain is difficult to understand. Our preferred solution to embryo disposal would, at least, remove the anomaly which gives powers of disposal to the father of an embryo but allows the father of a fetus no rights as to the survival of his progeny (see ch 5) – while this is explicable on the grounds that the equality of parental interest has altered in the transition, it seems unnecessary to have introduced a complication. In practice, the power of both gamete donors to decide the fate of the embryo is limited by statute – stored gametes must be destroyed at the end of ten years and embryos must be allowed to perish after five years' preservation (s 14(3) and (4)). This, at least, sets a limit to the difficulties in estate planning and the like that are inherent within a permitted policy of indefinite preservation of embryos.[17]

Uterine lavage represents a somewhat unusual extension of the technique of IVF through embryo transfer. In this process, a fertile woman is impregnated with semen and the resultant embryo is washed out of the uterus before implantation and is transferred to the infertile patient. While such a process might be seen as constituting an abortion, it is improbable that it would be considered so in the United Kingdom for reasons discussed below (ch 5). The Warnock Committee looked at the matter from the point of view of the donor and concluded (para 7.5) that the risks were such that the technique of embryo donation by lavage should not be used at the present time. The method seems to us to be so comparable to the practice of animal husbandry that there are good policy reasons for its proscription. Nevertheless, the current UK legislation (namely Sch 3, para 7 of the 1990 Act) clearly allows for the use of embryos formed in vivo.

The surplus fetus

The management of both infertility and childlessness due to abnormalities in the female provokes the particular problem of multiple pregnancies. Hormone treatment of primary infertility can be over-successful and result in pregnancies involving

---

14 *Davis v Davis* 842 SW 2d 588 (Tenn Sup Ct, 1992). The case was, however, clouded by the fact that Mrs Davis now only wanted to donate the embryos. The court recognised that the issue would have been closer had she still wanted to become pregnant.

15 R Cockburn 'Parents Contest Embryo Access' (1989) The Times, 31 October, p 12. This case seems to have been settled out of court. For discussion of it and *Davis*, see C Corns 'Deciding the Fate of Frozen Embryos' (1990) 64 L Inst J 273.

16 This concern for the future is evident also in Australia; see L Waller 'Let IVF Pregnancy Survive Marital Breakup' (1989) Sunday Age, 1 October. In this country, G Douglas 'Human Fertilisation and Embryology Act' (1991) Fam Law 110 agrees with our analysis of the current legislation at p 127.

17 For a very full and helpful review of the many legal problems introduced by artificial reproductive methods, see H Brown, M Dent, L M Dyer et al 'Legal Rights and Issues Surrounding Conception, Pregnancy, and Birth' (1986) 39 Vand LR 597. The relatively academic problems of succession of 'twin embryos' that are implanted at different times are settled by the elimination of 'storage time' from the age of an embryo (1990 Act, s 3(4)). For a specific instance, see C Seton 'Couple Tell of Their Joy as Test-tube Baby Goes Home' (1987) The Times, 24 April, p 3.

anything up to sextuplets – and, occasionally, beyond. As to childlessness, the chances of in vitro fertilisation ending in a live birth are improved by the insertion of two to four embryos and more than one of these then implants in about a quarter of those transfers that result in pregnancy.[18] Few people can afford to bring up several children at the same time. Moreover, the common scenario of very high order pregnancies which lead to live birth is that the infants are of very low birthweight. Accordingly, they occupy the facilities of a neonatal intensive care unit to a disproportionate extent and the parents face the spectre of their children dying one by one over a period of weeks. It is largely in order to circumvent this prospect that the current United Kingdom code of practice now decrees that no more than three eggs or embryos are to be transferred in any one cycle in any circumstances. Nevertheless, even triplets – which will originate from some 1.3% of all triple transfers – may be an unwelcome result of a successful treatment and there is evidence that more eggs, with a multiple pregnancy rate of over 40%, are being used in the GIFT process.[19] Moreover, the superfetation of hormone therapy is hard to control. Thus, the clinician may well be faced with the option of pregnancy reduction in utero.

This process, which is carried out at or earlier than the twelfth week of pregnancy, is generally known as selective reduction of pregnancy but it has been pointed out that, as the individual fetal characteristics are unknown at the time, there is no 'selection' other than that dictated by operative convenience. We prefer the suggested, although rather more cumbersome, alternative of reduction of multifetal pregnancy[20] – a description which serves to distinguish the process from the truly selective termination that may be used, say, when one fetus of twins is found to be defective. The legality of the practice depends upon additions to the Abortion Act 1967 arising from the Human Fertilisation and Embryology Act 1990, s 37(5); its morality is inseparable from that of abortion and we return to the subject at p 122.

Surrogate motherhood

Surrogate motherhood requires the active co-operation of an otherwise uninvolved woman in the process of pregnancy and birth. It thus introduces a third party into what has been, up till now, essentially a doctor/patient relationship. The fact that the third party may have a financial interest in a medical treatment has led to a general antipathy to the procedure in the United Kingdom. Commercialism is, however, accepted in American medical practice (for example, blood is bought and resold) and there does seem to be considerable activity in this field in the United States.

At its simplest, the infertile woman and her husband arrange with another woman that she will carry a child conceived by artificial insemination with the husband's semen and will surrender it to its genetic father after birth. The alternative, which also concludes with the return of the infant to its genetic parents, is that an embryo is created in vitro from the gametes of a husband and wife and is then implanted in the uterus of a 'surrogate'. There are several reasons for separating the two processes

---

18 HFEA Annual Report for 1992, Table 6.
19 *Sixth Report of the Interim Licensing Authority* (1991) p 15.
20 R L Berkowitz and L Lynch 'Selective Reduction: An Unfortunate Misnomer' (1990) 75 Obst Gynecol 873.

which are often described as partial or complete surrogacy; we prefer to refer to the latter technique more descriptively as 'womb-leasing'. We return to this subject at p 75 below but, for the present, we limit discussion to the easily achieved objective of impregnating a fertile woman. That process, as defined, is akin to a pre-emptive adoption with the advantage that the 'adopted' baby shares at least half its genes with its 'adopting' parents. Since the practical possibility of following the normal process of adoption is decreasing steadily, there is much to be said, theoretically, in favour of surrogate motherhood as a treatment for the wholly infertile wife. Yet the great majority of commentators and, possibly, the medical profession as a whole, shy away from accepting it as a means of satisfying an urge to parenthood – although the question should be asked – why?[1] The reason was summarised some time ago by Winslade:[2]

> The practice has a potential for economic exploitation, moral confusion and psychological harm to the surrogate mothers, the prospective adoptive parents and the children.

This view crystallises the debate which has surrounded surrogacy for more than a decade.

The legal issues
The possibility of exploitation is exemplified in the analogy between surrogate motherhood and adoption. The purchase of babies is expressly forbidden by the Adoption Act 1976, s 57, and all American states have laws prohibiting 'baby selling' or private placement of infants. Thus, even before the recent upsurge in interest, there was a real possibility that surrogate motherhood (particularly that which involved some form of commercial transaction) was already illegal.[3] There is, however, much to be said for the view that surrogate motherhood and adoption are distinct, albeit closely linked, processes.[4] In the first place, the surrogate mother is not pregnant at the time the proposition is put to her. She is under no economic pressure to support a child who is already affecting her financial position and a main reason for prohibiting a trade in babies is, therefore, absent. Against this, it has been pointed out[5] that 40% of volunteer surrogate mothers in the United States are unemployed or are in receipt of welfare;[6] an economic incentive may be present but the element of urgent need is still lacking. The nature of the payment is also different in the two cases. In one it is a simple matter of the purchase of a commodity for sale;

1   An opposing view is expressed by I Craft 'Surrogacy' (1992) 47 Brit J Hosp Med 728.
2   W J Winslade 'Surrogate Mothers: Private Right or Public Wrong?' (1981) 7 J Med Ethics 153.
3   In the first American test, the court agreed on the fundamental right to include a third party in a pregnancy arrangement but excluded the right to carry a child for payment: *Doe v Kelly* 307 NW 2d 438 (Mich, 1981).
4   I M Mady 'Surrogate Mothers: The Legal Issues' (1981) 7 Amer J Law Med 323; I Davies 'Contracts to Bear Children' (1985) 11 J Med Ethics 61.
5   P Parker 'Motivation of Surrogate Mothers: Initial Findings' (1983) 140 Amer J Psychiat 117.
6   M Freeman, in a powerful exposure of the 'exploitation' theory, points out that a similar result would probably obtain were a matched sample of applications for a factory job to be considered: 'Is Surrogacy Exploitative?' in S A M McLean (ed) *Legal Issues in Human Reproduction* (1989) ch 7.

in the other it is a matter of expenses coupled with payment for services rendered[7] – not totally unlike a man paying for the support of the mother of his illegitimate child and supplementing this with a generous present on her bringing it to them. Subject to specific legislation, the legality of surrogacy associated with exchange of money depends upon the validity of this distinction which has, in fact, been accepted both in the United States[8] and in the United Kingdom.[9] Thus, there seems to be no intrinsic objection to adoption following receipt of a reasonable stipend by the surrogate. Some formula must be evolved if the commissioning couple is to receive the child. For the surrogate, at least in the United Kingdom, is clearly its mother irrespective of whether or not it is the product of her own ovum and, if she is married and conception was via consensual donor insemination, her husband is its father (s 28 of the 1990 Act). Moreover, neither can simply surrender their parental duties.[10] Adoption could provide the solution but the procedure is often tedious and the issue of an adoption order cannot be guaranteed.[11] Section 30 of the 1990 Act now offers an alternative by which the court may make an order providing for a child carried by a surrogate to be treated in law as the child of the commissioning couple, provided that the gametes of one or both have been involved and that they are adult and married. This is subject to the consent of the surrogate and, where applicable, her husband and the genetic father – provided that they can be found. Further, the agreement is ineffective if made less than six weeks after the child's birth and the application must be made within six months of the birth. Section 30 is not in force at the time of writing but the draft regulations are available for consultation.[12] Nevertheless, twins resulting from womb-leasing have already been so treated and remain wards of court until the official commencement order is promulgated.[13]

The question of consent leads inevitably to consideration of the validity of any contract made between a commissioning couple and the surrogate. The position in the United Kingdom is now clear – no surrogacy arrangement is enforceable by or against any of the persons making it.[14] In so legislating, the Parliament has followed the majority trend of those countries that have addressed the subject; whether it is the correct approach is open to argument. Undoubtedly, it is the nature of the contract which poses the greatest complications for surrogate motherhood. Non-commercial

---

7 R Macklin 'Is There Anything Wrong With Surrogate Motherhood? An Ethical Analysis' (1988) 16 Law Med Hlth Care 57. For a strongly opposing view, see B Cohen 'Surrogate Mothers: Whose Baby Is It?' (1984) 10 Amer J Law Med 243.

8 *Surrogate Parenting Associates Inc v Commonwealth of Kentucky* 704 SW 2d 209 (Ky, 1986). Kentucky legislation has since been altered.

9 *Re an adoption application (surrogacy)* [1987] Fam 81, [1987] 2 All ER 826.

10 Children Act 1989, s 2(9).

11 S M Cretney and J M Masson *Principles of Family Law* (5th edn, 1990), p. 712 regard these cases as 'in family' – though the concept seems to involve an uneasy mix of genetic, legal and social relationships.

12 Department of Health, *Parental Orders for Gamete Donors Regulations* (1993).

13 *Re W (minors)(surrogacy)* [1991] 1 FLR 385. Scott Baker J considered that the court's primary concern 'should be to facilitate any steps that cement [a relationship with the genetic parents]' (see [1991] 1 FLR 385 at 387). Section 30 has been criticised in that it does not overtly provide the same protection for the interests of the child as do the adoption regulations: J G Hogg 'Surrogacy – Nobody's Child' (1991) 21 Fam Law 276. No doubt, however, such problems will be ironed out in the consultation procedure.

14 Surrogacy Arrangements Act 1985, s 1A inserted by Human Fertilisation and Embryology Act 1990, s 36.

surrogacy is not illegal in the United Kingdom (see p 72 below) and is not, therefore, a practice which is fundamentally against public policy. To introduce the uncertainties of a breakable agreement deliberately seems to do little more than reflect an ambivalence in a Parliament which, while unable to follow the German model in outlawing the practice,[15] is determined to avoid any signs of approval – surrogacy is to be seen as a form of legal liberty. A surrogate arrangement is clearly a difficult contract to draw up – it must allow for changes of heart on either side, illness in the surrogate, abnormalities in the resultant child and other imponderables, some of which, such as an abortion within the terms of the Abortion Act 1967, can be seen as basic rights. Nevertheless, it can be done. Indeed, the judicial decision at first instance in the celebrated American case of *Re Baby M*[16] was based very largely on the law of contract. Rather than, in effect, hiding the issues, we feel it would be better to grasp the nettle and lay down what a surrogacy arrangement could *not* include – for example, a contract to pay an unreasonable sum of money, an undertaking not to accept a therapeutic abortion and the like. The rights and wrongs of an individual case should be subject to more than individual judicial interpretations – a point which was taken up by the judge in *Re an adoption application (surrogacy)*.[17] It is to be noted that attitudes in the United States – a jurisdiction which is probably unique in allowing commercial surrogacy – may be polarising in the opposite direction. A Californian court has recently held that it is the intentions of the parties which determines who the mother of a child born by surrogacy should be and, as a consequence, a surrogate who wished to keep her baby was held to her contract – the surrogate had, in the words of the court, done no more than 'facilitate' the procreation of the commissioning couple's child. This decision has been criticised as fundamentally misunderstanding the biological realities of the surrogate's contribution.[18]

Opinions may similarly differ as to the general morality of surrogate motherhood. Outside the United States, however, there appears to be a consensus which condemns the blatant commercialisation of child-bearing by way of intermediate, profit-making agencies. This aspect has been the subject of legislation in many jurisdictions[19] – it is to be found in the Surrogacy Arrangements Act 1985 in the United Kingdom. The main purpose of the 1985 Act is to prohibit the making of a surrogacy arrangement on a commercial basis.[20] The principals involved are expressly excused from criminal liability (s 2(2)). Moreover, payments made to or for the benefit of the surrogate are not regarded as being made on a commercial basis (s 2(3)). On the face

15 Embryonenschutzgesetz (Embryo Protection Act) 1990, s 1(1)(vii).
16 525 A 2d 1128 (NJ, 1987).
17 [1987] Fam 81, [1987] 2 All ER 826. per Latey J at [1987] Fam 81 at 85, [1987] 2 All ER 826 at 829.
18 *Johnson v Calvert* 851 P 2d 776 (1993) discussed by R B Oxman 'California's Experiment in Surrogacy' (1993) 31 Lancet 1468. See also G J Annas 'Using Genes to Define Motherhood: The California Solution' (1992) 326 New Engl J Med 417 discussing the decision in the lower court. Others may, however, feel as strongly as to the importance of the genetic affiliation: D R Bromham 'Surrogacy: The Evolution of Opinion' (1992) 47 Brit J Hosp Med 767.
19 In Australia, see Infertility (Medical Procedures) Act 1984, s 30 (Vict); Family Relationships Act Amendment Act 1988, s 6 (S Aust). For the situation in the United States, see R A Charo 'Legislative Approaches to Surrogate Motherhood' (1989) 16 Law Med Hlth Care 96.
20 Advertising by way of newspapers, periodicals and telecommunications is proscribed in s 3, the criminal liability resting on the proprietor, editor, and publisher, etc.

of it, this hurried and somewhat ill-prepared measure is broadly acceptable, other than to any existing agencies. It has, however, confused the position of professionals, such as doctors and lawyers, whose services in any arrangement are clearly desirable but who would obviously expect some remuneration – indeed, the doctor working in the NHS can scarcely avoid 'payment'. Theoretically, they could give general advice but would be unable to be paid for intervention on behalf of any of the principals without contravening s 2.[1] One potential effect of the 1985 Act is, therefore, to discourage counselling in and supervision of surrogate motherhood – the precise situation that legislation should be seeking to avoid. The matter has not been tested and we feel that, in practice, the courts would be unlikely to take such a rigid view. The courts generally sympathetic attitude to surrogacy can, in fact, be traced through a progressive series of decisions.

The British cases

The earliest example, *A v C*,[2] arose some time before 'assisted reproduction' became widely acceptable. It was not fully reported but the basic facts were that an unmarried couple arranged for a prostitute's friend to be inseminated on the understanding that the resultant child was returned to them; a fee of £3,000 was involved. The mother changed her mind and the father applied for access which was granted in the child's best interests. Nevertheless, the judge described the agreement as 'pernicious and void'[3] and, for reasons which are unrecorded, the Court of Appeal unanimously reversed the decision and decreed that the applicant should not be allowed to see his son.

Re C (a minor)[4] was the first case to be fully covered but was, essentially, a matter of wardship. An American couple arranged a surrogacy in England through a commercial agency. As soon as the child was born, the local authority obtained a place of safety order under the Children and Young Persons Act 1969, s 28 in the belief that it would be abandoned by its mother. The father then initiated wardship proceedings. Latey J refused to discuss the rights and wrongs of surrogacy; he concentrated solely on the welfare of the child and held that how she had been born was irrelevant. On these grounds, he considered that no-one was better equipped than the commissioning couple to care for her and, accordingly, he gave them care and control while, at the same time, continuing the wardship. Nevertheless, permission was given for the baby to live outside the jurisdiction. For present purposes, the most important aspect of the case is that the judge rejected suggestions that the commissioning couple were unfit parents because they had entertained a commercial surrogacy arrangement.

Surrogacy itself, and particularly the relationship between that process and adoption, was more directly considered in *Re an adoption application (surrogacy)*.[5]

---

1 S Sloman 'Surrogacy Arrangements Act 1985' (1985) 135 NLJ 978. A further minor difficulty as to confidentiality has been eradicated in the Human Fertilisation and Embryology (Amendment) Act 1992.
2 (1978) 8 Fam Law 170. Commentators at the time see the case as of interest from the AID aspect only.
3 From a report by D C Parker 'Legal Aspects of Artificial Insemination and Embryo Transfer' (1982) 12 Fam Law 103.
4 [1985] FLR 846.
5 [1987] Fam 81, [1987] 2 All ER 826.

By contrast, this was a remarkably amateurish affair. The principals met casually, the surrogate being motivated by a desire to help a childless couple, and she was impregnated naturally. A fee of £10,000 was agreed but half of this was returned by the surrogate on the grounds that she had obtained money from the sale of her story. All the principals, the judge said later, were supremely happy. They were also inexperienced and it was not for a further two and a half years that the 'parents' applied for an adoption. The issue was thus whether or not such 'payment or reward' as would invalidate an adoption had been made.[6] In summary, Latey J held that a surrogacy arrangement would not contravene the Adoption Act 1976 so long as the payments made did not constitute an element of profit or financial reward; he thought that the payments in the instant case did no more than compensate for the inconveniences of pregnancy. More significantly, he showed his faith in the commissioning parents by stating that, if necessary, he would apply his powers to allow some profit and reward[7] retrospectively in the interests of the child. An adoption order was made.

Re P (minors)[8] was heard contemporaneously with the adoption case. In this instance, the surrogate declined to hand over the twins she had conceived by a married professional man. The children were made wards of court and were allowed to stay with their natural mother; the court action was essentially a matter of custody. The judge was strongly influenced by the degree of maternal bonding that had already arisen and found:

> nothing to outweigh the advantages to these children of preserving the link to the mother to whom they are bonded, and who has exercised a satisfactory degree of maternal care.

Once again, it is to be noted that there was no criticism of either the commissioning parents or of the surrogate for having entered into a surrogacy agreement. It cannot, however, have been a happy arrangement – the natural mother sought a maintenance order.[9]

Only one other case has been reported – *Re W(minors)(surrogacy)*[10] – when, as noted above, the judge was prepared to pre-empt the law in order to ensure bonding of 'womb-leased' twins with their genetic parents. One wonders at this dearth of new cases. It may be that instances are now no longer regarded as meriting report unless there are special circumstances. An alternative explanation, however, is that clinics are less inclined to become involved now that the techniques of AID and embryo transfer are subject to licensing and to the fairly rigorous code of practice of the Human Fertilisation and Embryology Authority.[11]

---

6 Adoption Act 1976, s 57(1).
7 Adoption Act 1976, s 57(3).
8 *Re P (minors)* [1987] 2 FLR 421. See also C Seton 'Natural Mother Is Given Custody of Surrogacy Twins' (1987) The Times, 13 March, p 1.
9 D Brahams 'Surrogacy, Adoption and Custody' (1987) 1 Lancet 817. For further discussion of the British cases see J Montgomery 'Constructing a Family – After a Surrogate Birth' (1986) 49 MLR 635; S P de Cruz 'Surrogacy, Adoption and Custody: A Case Study' (1988) 18 Fam Law 100.
10 [1991] 1 FLR 385.
11 See fn 7, p 76 below. But this is also doubtful – at least one clinic is said to be specifically expanding its surrogacy service: A Ballantyne 'Agency Will Offer Babies without Birth' (1990) The Sunday Times, 19 August, p 15.

The American Scene

It would be impossible in a book of this size to take a comprehensive view of similar situations in the United States. We simply note a report that, by 1988, some 600 children had been born via surrogacy in the United States.[12] It is clear that the great majority of arrangements proceed smoothly; only when there is conflict do cases come to public notice and it may well be that this is a major underlying reason for the general antipathy to the procedure. The rather different attitude to publicity which pertains in the United States may also contribute to its image as projected across the Atlantic. Nonetheless, there are lessons to be learnt from some of the more notorious cases – in particular, perhaps, that of *Re Baby M*.[13]

In that case, the surrogate, who had agreed to a fee of $10,000 refused to relinquish her child and, in fact, absconded with it contrary to a court order. When the matter came to trial, the judge was concerned to limit the issues to those of strict law and, in this respect, he rejected any relevance of the adoption laws. He concluded, on the one hand, that a valid contract had been made and broken and, on the other, that the state's interest in the welfare of its children dictated that the child be adopted by the commissioning couple. The Supreme Court of New Jersey, however, had no hesitation in overturning this decision – and did so in strong terms.[14] The surrogacy contract was found to be against public policy and, as such, invalid. Both the termination of the mother's parental rights and the adoption order were therefore void. Nonetheless, the Supreme Court could find nothing in law against voluntary, non-commercial surrogacy provided that the arrangement did not include any clause binding on the surrogate to surrender her baby. The court unfortunately clouded the 'best interests' issue by awarding custody to the commissioning parents but did, at the same time, establish visiting rights for the surrogate, who had later appealed by the child's guardian ad litem.[15]

The cases assessed

The UK cases indicate that, having come through the technological upheavals of the 1980s, the public, as represented by the judiciary, will be sympathetic to surrogate motherhood – an attitude which probably derives more from the fait accompli nature of the proceedings than from any basic empathy with the practice. It can, we consider, be taken that no decisions will be based on antagonism.

It is, however, clear that much depends on the attitudes of the principals and, in particular, that of the surrogate. A woman who is anxious to surrender her baby is probably unlikely to be an outstanding mother and the best interests of the child are thus secured by the child's placement within a loving, stable relationship. The mere fact that a husband and wife are prepared to endure the difficulties and uncertainties

---

12 R A Charo 'Legislative Approaches to Surrogate Motherhood' (1989) 16 Law Med Hlth Care 96. Others quote lower figures: see, for example, D R Bromham 'Surrogacy: The Evolution of Opinion' (1992) 47 Brit J Hosp Med 767.

13 525 A 2d 1128 (NJ, 1987).

14 537 A 2d 1227 (NJ Sup Ct, 1988).

15 See G P Smith 'The Case of Baby M: Love's Labor Lost' (1988) 16 Law Med Hlth Care 121. The contrast between *Re Baby M* and *Johnson v Calvert* 851 P 2d 776 (1993) (see fn 18, p 70 above) is very marked. We wonder if this really indicates a change of direction in the United States or whether it does no more than reflect a difference between Eastern and Western cultures in that country.

of a surrogate arrangement implies a certain dedication to family life. There is, consequently, no necessary difficulty in those cases in which the principals agree – even though the law may be stretched in achieving the desired result.[16] When, however, the parties disagree, it is evident that the courts will support the rights of the natural or carrying mother – and this even in the face of an economic anomaly in that the commissioning couple are inherently likely to be able to provide a better financial environment. The lifestyle of C in *A v C*[17] seems unlikely to have been ideal while the surrogate in *Re P (minors)*[18] was subsisting on social security. The importance of maternal/filial bonding is such that a child's well-being would have to be threatened in statutory terms[19] before the ties would be cut – maternal conditions in the American *Baby M* case may well have so influenced the State Supreme Court.

We surmise, although there is no precedent, that physical and psychological bonding would still be regarded as more important than genetic incompatibility in a disputed case of womb-leasing. There is no indication of what would result if the commissioning couple were to refuse to accept the infant. The precise details of each case would be all-important but it is difficult to see, in general, an alternative to intervention by the local authority by way of care proceedings. The position of the surrogate's husband under the provisions of s 28(2) of the 1990 Act would then be extremely difficult – indeed, the effect of the new legislation on the relationship between surrogacy and the surrogate's husband seems to have been left open.

The morality of surrogate motherhood

What, then, is so special about the morality of surrogacy that it provokes emergency legislation while the control of in vitro fertilisation takes five years to establish? Clearly, the most important difference lies in the inclusion of a third party to procreation – and in such a way as to provoke not only serious moral but also important socio-political questions. Further, since the surrogate is, by definition, a woman, the latter questions are gender-based. Reduced to its essentials, surrogacy can be viewed from this perspective as being one way of exploiting women for the benefit of men[20] – a matter to which we have alluded above. The alternative is to see the prohibition of the practice as outright paternalism which denies a woman a chance to use her body as she pleases. It seems fair to say that the feminist movement is divided in its approach,[1] but the argument is one which we will not take further here save to note the difficulties that arise from generalising in personal and individual affairs.

The second major objection lies in the suggestion that surrogacy is 'baby-selling'. We find this emotive argument hard to accept since a baby is 'sold' if

---

16 Freeman, for example, applauds but, at the same time, questions the decision in *Re an adoption application (surrogacy)* [1987] Fam 81, [1987] 2 All ER 826 – reported by C Dyer 'Babies in the Courts' (1987) The Times, 13 March, p 15.
17 (1978) 8 Fam Law 170.
18 [1987] 2 FLR 421
19 Children and Young Persons Act 1969, s 1(2); Social Work (Scotland) Act 1968, s 32(2).
20 G J Annas 'Fairy Tales Surrogate Mothers Tell' (1988) 16 Law Med Hlth Care 27.
 1 L B Andrews 'Surrogate Motherhood: The Challenge for Feminists' (1988) 16 Law Med Hlth Care 72. A further example of the debate is to be found in S Dodds and K Jones 'Surrogacy and Autonomy' (1989) 3 Bioethics 18.

persons with no genetic association purchase an infant that is already in being. It seems more logical to regard any monetary transaction as payment for gestational expertise and, as the British cases indicate, the critical distinction lies between reasonable recompense and inducement to gestate. The great majority of assisted reproduction is centred on private health care and, even within a public health service, there is indirect payment for obstetric expertise. Looked at in this way, either both surrogacy and embryo transfer are 'baby purchasing' or neither is – and there is no suggestion that sophisticated reproductive techniques are immoral on this score. Thirdly, it is widely believed that surrogacy must have an ill-effect on children in general or on the individual resultant child. The former, represented by a fear that children may become 'objects for barter', is valid only so long as surrogacy itself is categorised as objectionable. The premise disappears once it is regarded as a legitimate treatment for childlessness. Any effect on the individual child by way of confusion as to parentage is comparable to that which we have discussed in relation to artificial insemination. Whether or not there is a detriment seems to us to be unproven but if there is, it should not be insurmountable – certainly no more than in other examples of the unconventional family. Even so, there is little doubt that the provisions of the 1990 Act, s 13(5) (discussed at p 61 above) are likely to discourage professional implication in surrogacy.

In favour of surrogacy, it must be remembered that it *is* a treatment for some forms of childlessness. Such cases may be rare, yet to encourage treatment by way of ovum donation for the woman who is childless because of ovarian inadequacy and, at the same time, to forbid surrogacy for the one who has no uterus, smacks of unfair discrimination.[2]

Surrogacy could, however, be used for purely selfish reasons – for example, a desire to have a child without interference with a career. Such hedonistic womb-leasing is so comparable to nineteenth century wet-nursing that the process as a whole has become suspect. This is unfortunate because there are, in fact, far more conditions in which womb-leasing would be the preferred treatment of childlessness than there are those in which standard surrogacy would be indicated. Loss, or abnormality, of the uterus is more common than loss of both uterus and ovaries and womb-leasing is the logical answer to an inability to carry, rather than to conceive, a baby for example, by virtue of heart disease, diabetes, or repetitive miscarriages. The other important difference is that, in womb-leasing, the commissioning couple are the genetic parents. This factor might serve to reduce the surrogate's psychological trauma on surrendering the child. Since the receiving parents are in a similar end position as natural coital parents, the child should suffer no 'genetic insecurity', although, of course, the absence of a true 'birth experience' for the parents may have an effect. Certainly, womb-leasing involves the use of high-grade technology – but even this serves to remove some of the intuitive distaste provoked by standard surrogacy. Neither the Warnock Committee nor the resultant legislation distinguish between partial and full surrogacy, but we feel that the better argument lies in favour of clearly separating the two.

---

2   I Davies 'Contracts to Bear Children' (1985) 11 J Med Ethics 61; D R Bromham 'Surrogacy: The Evolution of Opinion' (1992) 47 Brit J Hosp Med 767.

There is, however, one aspect of womb-leasing that merits special attention – that is, the use of intrafamilial surrogates.[3]   Not only does this seriously disturb relationships but the procedure opens the door to emotional coercion. It appears to be a practice which should be made unlawful and, to that end, forbidden womb-leasing relationships could be based on the law of incest by proscribing those involving direct ascent and descent and siblings.

The future

The Government has decided not to bring non-commercial surrogacy services within the framework of the law but, rather, to invite the Human Fertilisation and Embryology Authority to keep the subject under review. In so far as the procedure involves, at least, artificial insemination, the Authority may have indirect control of the practice. Uncertainty arises from the wording of the 1990 Act. Thus, under s 4, a licence is required by any person who carried out artificial insemination 'in the course of providing treatment services for any woman . . . unless the services are being provided for the woman and the man together'. Treatment services are defined (s 2) as meaning '. . . services provided to the public or a section of the public for the purpose of assisting women to carry children'. Is a doctor artificially inseminating a surrogate with the sperm of a commissioning father providing treatment services for the woman and the man together? If so, he does not require a licence. If, however, one interprets treatment for a woman and a man together as being treatment for a couple who are consulting the doctor for a shared problem – that is, intra-familial childlessness – then AID in the context of surrogacy is lawful only under cover of a licence. The solution of the problem is central to the control of surrogacy. We agree with the minority of the Warnock Committee[4] that it should remain available as a treatment option. This view is now widely shared;[5] so far as we know, in the English-speaking world, only Queensland has criminalised the procedure in all its forms.[6] Nevertheless, we also believe that it must be controlled and that this is probably best done by way of statute.

To this end, we suggest, first, that the procedure should be subject to criminal sanctions unless it is undertaken for a bona fide medical reason, other options having been considered and properly rejected.[7] As a corollary, the current doubts as to the legality of active, paid intervention by health carers and lawyers should be dispelled

3   Well-publicised cases have occurred in Australia and South Africa: R Milliken 'Woman Conceives a Problem' (1987) The Independent, 15 April, p 12; R Kennedy 'Early Triplets for First Surrogate Grandmother' (1987) The Times, 2 October, p 9.
4   Cmnd 9314, 1984, Expression of Dissent A – see fn 1, p 55 above.
5   J Sherman 'Doctors Lift Ban on Helping with Surrogate Births' (1990) The Times, 27 June, p 3; N Swan 'Australian Ethics Committee Approves Surrogacy' (1990) 301 BMJ 254; Bromham 'Surrogacy: The Evolution of Opinion' (1992) 47 Brit J Hosp Med 767.
6   Surrogate Parenthood Act 1988 (Qd). Moreover, a doctor who arranged adoptions prior to the births of children has been charged and found guilty under the Act: F Kennedy 'Doctor on Surrogacy Charge' (1993) The Australian, 29 September, p 3; 30 September, p 3.
7   The Human Fertilisation and Embryology Authority's *Code of Practice* (revised 1993) states: 'The application of assisted conception techniques to initiate a surrogate pregnancy should only be considered where it is physically impossible or highly undesirable for medical reasons for the commissioning mother to carry the child.'

by their specific exclusion from the terms of the Surrogacy Arrangements Act 1985 (see p 71); the possibility of unaided, amateurish attempts should be positively averted. Second, the parties should be adequately counselled.[8] Third, as discussed above, we see no advantage in merely declaring surrogate contracts unenforceable; it would not be difficult to specify such contractual clauses as would be against the public interest. Finally, we recommend the availability of competently staffed, non-profitmaking agencies whose accumulated expertise could be invaluable to the process – such an agency could, with advantage, be established as a committee of the Human Fertilisation and Embryology Authority. A case could be made that professionalism and efficiency go hand in hand when a service is being provided; unfortunately, as Macklin[9] has put it – 'there is sufficient evidence of greed, corruption and duplicity of others in the public and private sectors to make us wary of allowing commercial practices to invade and dominate the delivery of health care'. Surrogacy has been likened by its opponents to prostitution. We reject this analogy; nevertheless, the two conditions share the common ground that it is the profitmaking intermediary, not the principal, who is criminalised.

8 A particularly blatant example of inadequate preparation of the principals has been reported: G McBride 'US Battles over Surrogacy' (1990) 301 BMJ 1062. This point is, of course, covered under the Human Fertilisation and Embryology Act 1990, s 13(6); Sch 3, para 3(1)(*a*) and by the *Code of Practice*, Part 6 provided that the procedure is subject to license.
9 R Macklin 'Is there Anything Wrong With Surrogate Motherhood?' (1988) 16 Law Med Hlth Care 57.

4 The control of fertility

Sterilisation

The aim of sterilisation is to end the patient's ability to reproduce. A number of surgical procedures may be used to achieve this. In males, the most common method is vasectomy, in which the vas deferens is cut and tied. Sterilisation in females is usually achieved by division or clipping of the fallopian tubes which carry the ova between the ovary and the womb. An important feature of the operation from the legal and ethical standpoint is that it is generally intended to be irreversible; although it may be possible to repair the operation, prospective attempts to allow for reversibility are likely to result in procedures which fail in their primary purpose. Modern microsurgery has improved on this position – a development which may account for some of the apparently disparate court decisions that have been taken (see p 79ff, below). Nevertheless, it is generally held that sterilisation will, or at least may well, bring a basic human function to an end.[1]

Ethical objections to sterilisation usually focus on this aspect of irreversible interference with the ability to reproduce. Those who object on these grounds would argue that such interference is unjustified in that the individual may later undergo a change of mind and may wish to return to a position which is probably now closed. They would also stress that the decision to sterilise is one which is taken in the midst of subtle social and personal pressures; the likelihood of the decision being entirely free is thereby diminished, yet it is one that cannot easily be retracted. The objection of the Catholic Church is more direct. In Catholic teaching, sterilisation is a mutilation of the body which leads to the deprivation of a natural function and which must, therefore, be rejected. Sterilisation can only be accepted if it is carried out for therapeutic purposes – that is, where it is necessary for the physical health of the patient. The performance of hysterectomy in the treatment of menorrhagia, for example, is admissible.[2] The secular counterpart lies in the concept of maim although, historically, this refers to injuries which limit a man's capacity for military service. For example, the courts might well take exception to castration on

---

1   Current methods also now allow for reversal of vasectomy - a success rate of up to 40% successful pregnancies is claimed. See A K Banergee and A Simpson 'Reversing Vasectomy' (1992) 304 BMJ 1130.
2   For a sensitive view from a Catholic clinician of this and other dilemmas, see J Poole *The Cross of Unknowing* (1989); 'Time for the Vatican to Bend' (1992) 339 Lancet 1340. On a world scale, the attitude of orthodox Islam is just as rigid: D A R Verkuyl 'Two World Religions and Family Planning' (1993) 342 Lancet 473.

non-therapeutic grounds.[3] In so far as it is possible to identify a lay consensus on the matter, it is that sterilisation is an acceptable method of contraception provided that the person undergoing the operation is adequately informed of the implications. Very strong objections may be voiced, however, when there is any question as to the reality of the patient's consent and we return to the subject at p 83 below.

The legality of contraceptive sterilisation in the United Kingdom is now beyond doubt and only a small minority of other countries continue either to forbid the process altogether or to allow it only in narrowly defined circumstances. Not infrequently, there is a minimum age below which sterilisation on request will not be available. For example, in the United States it is 21 years, while in Denmark it is 25.[4] Some jurisdictions require spousal consent (Japan being an example) but there is general resistance to this on the grounds that the decision is an individual matter to be decided by the individual. There is no doubt that this is the case in the United Kingdom. The Medical Defence Union (MDU) emphasises that the doctor owes a duty of care to the patient and not to his or her spouse[5] and the courts would never grant an injunction to stop sterilisation or vasectomy.[6] On the other hand, the very term 'family planning' implies a shared responsibility and we regard it as good medical practice to involve the spouse so long as the patient has given permission to do so.[7] On purely practical grounds, the surgeon may wish to avoid involvement in divorce proceedings and the like. *Bravery v Bravery*[8] is a doubtful modern authority but Lord Evershed MR may still be regarded as correct in saying:

> It would not be difficult . . . to construct in imagination a case of grave cruelty on a wife founded on the progressive hurt to her health caused by an operation for sterilization undergone by her husband in disregard of, or contrary to, the wife's wishes or natural instincts

– and the alternative proposition would apply with equal force.

Liability for a failed sterilisation
Liability for failed sterilisation will not be imposed unless it can be established that the failure to achieve contraception was due to medical negligence or to breach of contract rather than to the inherent possibility that conception might still occur after the operation purely due to the vagaries of nature. There are a number of important UK, Commonwealth and United States decisions which deal with the question.

The first problem to be identified in such circumstances is that of causation and this has, in turn, hinged upon the performance of the operator and, latterly, on the

---

3   A similar legislative attitude is to be found in the Prohibition of Female Circumcision Act 1985. This raises the general question of self-inflicted injury, for which, see *R v Brown* et al discussed at p 219.
4   For a useful comparative survey, see J M Paxman *Law and Planned Parenthood* (1980) p 28.
5   (1987) 3 J Med Def Union (3) 24.
6   *Paton v British Pregnancy Advisory Service Trustees* [1979] QB 276 at 280, [1978] 2 All ER 987 at 990 per Sir George Baker P.
7   See also Confidentiality at p 178 below.
8   [1954] 3 All ER 59 at 62, [1954] 1 WLR 1169 at 1173, CA.

anterior advice given to the plaintiff. The question of competence is exemplified in the Canadian case of *Doiron v Orr*[9] in which the operation agreed upon was one which was more remediable than was the conventional tubal ligation; the judge accepted that, in these conditions, the surgeon concerned had no liability for the subsequent pregnancy. By contrast, the court agreed that there had been technical negligence in the case of *Cataford v Moreau*[10] in which there were no such extenuating circumstances. The courts in the UK show no evidence of bias against the plaintiff following negligently performed operations. Thus, in *Emeh v Kensington and Chelsea and Westminster Area Health Authority*,[11] substantial damages were awarded for the birth of a child following sterilisation despite the fact that abortion was an available option; in *Benarr v Kettering Health Authority*,[12] the court went so far as to include damages to cover the private education of the resultant child; and many cases are undoubtedly settled out of court. Even so, the *Bolam*[13] principle also operates here. A gynaecologist who accepted the patient's word that she could not be pregnant at the time of the operation was held to be not negligent on the grounds that others would have omitted a precautionary curettage in the circumstances.[14]

Far more interest centres on those actions in negligence and in contract which have been based on the grounds of inadequate information and there has been a steady evolution of such cases in the UK. Often, the supposed deficit has proved to be no more than a matter of communication between doctor and patient. Thus, in the interesting case of *Thake v Maurice*,[15] the issue turned eventually on the definition of the word 'irreversible' – the defendant claiming that it implied no more than that the procedure could not be reversed by surgery while the plaintiff contended that it represented a contract to provide absolute sterility which was beyond recall by natural processes. After something of a volte face between the trial court and the Court of Appeal as to breach of contract, it was held that the surgeon had been negligent in his failure to warn of the possibility of natural reversal of vasectomy. A rather similar case turned on the interpretation of the words on the form signifying consent to operation which stated 'We understand that this means we can have no children' and which the plaintiffs contended amounted to a representation that the operation was foolproof. The trial judge, however, held that the words merely acknowledged that the intended effect of the operation was that the couple should not have more children and found for the defendants.[16] Such semantic difficulties had been foreseen in the important Australian case of *F v R*[17] when King CJ specifically drew attention to the need not only to warn of the possible complications of surgery

9   (1978) 86 DLR (3d) 719.
10 (1978) 114 DLR (3d) 585. Discussed by R P Kouri 'Comment' (1979) 57 Can BR 89.
11 [1985] QB 1012, [1984] 3 All ER 1044, CA.
12 [1988] NLJR 179.
13 *Bolam v Friern Hospital Management Committee* [1957] 2 All ER 118, [1957] 1 WLR 582. The case is further discussed at p 200 below.
14 *Venner v North East Essex Area Health Authority* (1987) Times, 21 February. We wonder if this would apply now. In a more recent, although virtually identical case – *Allen v Bloomsbury Health Authority* [1993] 1 All ER 651, (1993) 13 BMLR 47 – the defendant authority admitted liability and the only matter in issue was the quantum of damages.
15 [1984] 2 All ER 513, [1985] 2 WLR 215; revsd [1986] QB 644, [1986] 1 All ER 497. It was later said of the trial stage of this case: 'I, for my part, think that . . . the less we say about that decision, the better' (per Slade LJ in *Eyre v Measday* [1986] 1 All ER 488, CA at 492).
16 *Worster v City and Hackney Health Authority* (1987) Times, 22 June.
17 (1983) 33 SASR 189, SC.

but also of the risk of failure as to the intended end result. There have been further English cases involving much the same issues[18] but these are better discussed under the heading of consent (see p 239).

A further major problem which the courts and commentators have identified in this area is that of the award of damages for the unexpected birth of a healthy child following breach of contract or negligent surgery. Objection to any award in such a context has been based on the view that a child is a blessing and that this constitutes a policy ground for the antipathy. The question was first fully addressed in *Doiron v Orr*, where the judge stated that he would have been prepared to award damages for mental anguish caused to the plaintiff, but was adamant in his refusal to accept that in such a case there could be liability for the cost of bringing up an unwanted child:

I find this approach to a matter of this kind which deals with human life, the happiness of the child, the effect upon its thinking, upon its mind when it realised that there has been a case of this kind, that it is an unwanted mistake and that its rearing is being paid for by someone other than its parents, is just simply grotesque.[19]

Such rejection concentrates on the effect which an award might have on the child whereas in other cases the focus has been more on the entitlement of the parents to damages. American courts have not taken a uniform approach to the problem but there are certainly several cases in which such redress has been refused. The view has, again, been that parents cannot be held to have been damaged by the blessing of children.[20] Elsewhere, a middle view has prevailed, the assumption being that it is illogical to suppose that a benefit – that of parenthood – can derive from failure to provide proper medical care.[1] In still other instances, damages have been awarded not only in respect of the pain and suffering involved in an unwanted pregnancy but also to offset the cost of rearing the child to maturity.[2]

The first comparable English case is that of *Scuriaga v Powell*.[3] The case was concerned with abortion rather than with sterilisation but nonetheless provides some authority. Here the plaintiff consulted a doctor who agreed to perform a legal abortion on her. A healthy child was born by Caesarian section subsequent to a failure to terminate pregnancy. The court held that there was no public policy reason preventing a claim against the doctor in such a case and damages were awarded in respect of the diminution of the plaintiff's marriage prospects, pain and suffering,

---

18 For example, *Eyre v Measday* [1986] 1 All ER 488, CA; *Gold v Haringey Health Authority* [1986] 1 FLR 125; revsd [1988] QB 481, [1987] 2 All ER 888.
19 (1978) 86 DLR (3d) 719 at 722 per Garrett J.
20 For example, *Terrell v Garcia* 496 SW 2d 124 (Tx, 1973); *Sutkin v Beck* 629 SW 2d 131 (Tx, 1982). It has been agreed, however, that damages are recoverable for the birth of a defective child.
1 *Kingsbury v Smith* 422 A 2d 1003 (NH, 1982); *Ochs v Borelli* 445 A 2d 883 (Conn, 1982).
2 *Troppi v Scarf* 186 NW 2d 511 (Mich, 1971) where an obligation to abort or offer for adoption was rejected. The unfairness of a 'balancing' approach was explained in *Public Health Trust v Brown* 388 So 2d 1084 (Fla, 1980). For discussion, see A B Horowitz 'Torts II " The Wrongful Birth Cause of Action" ' [1983] Ann Surv Amer Law 675; J H Scheid 'Benefits vs. Burdens: The Limitation of Damages in Wrongful Birth' (1984-5) 23 J Fam Law 57.
3 (1979) 123 SJ 406.

and anxiety and distress. There was no claim for damages in respect of the child's upbringing but the trial judge, Watkins J, foreshadowed future developments in saying:

> Surely no one in these days would argue [that damages were irrecoverable] if the child was born defective or diseased. The fact that the child born is healthy cannot give rise to a different conclusion save as to a measure of damages.

This view was supported in the Court of Appeal.

The validity of the 'wrongful pregnancy' action was upheld in *Udale v Bloomsbury Area Health Authority*[4] in which damages were given for pain and suffering along with loss of earnings following a negligently performed operation. An award in respect of the cost of bringing up the child was, however, firmly rejected. In his judgment, Jupp J reiterated that the joy of having the child and the benefits it brought in terms of love should be set off against the inconvenience and financial disadvantages resulting from its birth. 'It is an assumption of our culture', he suggested, 'that the coming of a child into the world is an occasion for rejoicing.'

This view was criticised in the later negligence case of *Emeh v Kensington and Chelsea and Westminster Area Health Authority*[5] in which, in addition, there was a strong rejection of the trial judge's view that the plaintiff's refusal of abortion was so unreasonable as to eclipse the defendant's wrongdoing.[6] More significantly, however, the Court of Appeal awarded damages for the cost of rearing the child and rejected the policy objections voiced in *Udale*. This decision, taken with that voiced in at trial in *Thake v Maurice*[7], laid to rest the distinction between entitlement to damages for pain and suffering and that in respect of the cost of the child's upbringing.

The legal position in English law is now clear: unwanted children are potential grounds for compensation. Scottish policy has evolved in its own way. Earlier reports are, for the most part, concerned with procedural matters and do not deal with the arguments or the outcomes in the cases.[8] Two cases have attracted the attention of the media[9] both of which were based on lack of warning of the risk of failure rather

---

4   [1983] 2 All ER 522, [1983] 1 WLR 1098. Similar sentiments were expressed in an unreported negligence case *Jones v Berkshire Area Health Authority* quoted in *Gold v Haringey Health Authority* [1986] 1 FLR 125; revsd [1988] QB 481, [1987] 2 All ER 888 – although damages were allowed.

5   (1983) Times, 3 January; revsd [1985] QB 1012, [1984] 3 All ER 1044, CA.

6   The possibility that refusal of an *early* abortion might be regarded as unreasonable still remains open. For a discussion of the relationship between abortion and wrongful pregnancy, see K McK Norrie 'Damages for the Birth of a Child' 1985 SLT 69; A Grubb 'Damages for "Wrongful Conception"' (1985) 44 CLJ 30; A Mullis 'Wrongful Conception Unravelled' (1993) 1 Med L Rev 320.

7   [1984] 2 All ER 513, [1985] 2 WLR 215; revsd [1986] QB 644, [1986] 1 All ER 497. For discussion of *Scuriaga, Udale* and *Emeh*, see D Brahams 'Damages for Unplanned Babies – A Trend to be Discouraged' (1983) 133 NLJ 643.

8   *Smith, Petitioner* 1985 SLT 461; *Jones v Lanarkshire Health Board* 1990 SLT 19, 1989 SCLR 542; *Teece v Ayrshire and Arran Health Board* 1990 SLT 512.

9   *Pollock v Lanarkshire Health Board* (1987) The Times, 6 January, p 3; *Lindsay v Greater Glasgow Health Board* (1990) Scotsman, 14 March, p 8.

than on operative negligence. Both were settled out of court; the offer of the substantial sum of £50,000 in *Lindsay v Greater Glasgow Health Board*[10] suggested that the Scottish courts might follow those of England in recognising the birth of a healthy child as a suitable matter for 'damages'. This has now been settled. In *Allen v Greater Glasgow Heath Board*,[11] the court explicitly accepted that there were no grounds – of principle or of policy – to prevent an award of damages for the upbringing of a child born in these circumstances. There is, of course, much force in the argument that such compensation amounts to a rejection of a fundamental value in our society – that of family love. On the other hand, it is implicit that the patient undergoing consensual, non-therapeutic sterilisation does not want any more children and that this may be for economic reasons. That being so, it is hard to refute the words of Peter Pain J: 'Every baby has a belly to be filled and a body to be clothed'.[12] There is, in fact, evidence that a wrongful pregnancy action will now be equally successful on both sides of the Atlantic.[13]

As a coda to this section on failed sterilisation, we note what must be the ultimate in negligence actions backed by support from the legal aid fund.[14] The plaintiffs, who became parents eight years after the husband's vasectomy, are said to be suing the Department of Health for failure to publicise information about the risk to them and to others in their situation. The research on which they depend indicates a risk of recanalisation of the vas of 0.04% – which figure would seem to lay a heavy burden on the public bodies concerned. There is, as yet, no information that the case has reached the courts and we doubt it will result in judgment in favour of the plaintiff.

Non-consensual sterilisation

If consensual sterilisation raises certain ethical misgivings, then non-consensual sterilisation is a minefield of powerful objection. This form of sterilisation has been carried out in some countries as an official or unofficial part of programmes of eugenic improvement or birth control. In the United States, for example, the enthusiasm for eugenics which was the feature of the earlier part of this century led to legislative measures in a number of states providing for the sterilisation of mental defectives, those suffering from certain forms of genetically transmissible diseases and, in some cases, criminal recidivists.[15] Such laws were declared unconstitutional

---

10 (1990) Scotsman, 14 March, p 8.
11 (25 November 1993, unreported) Court of Session, Outer House. The court found, however, that there had been no negligence in the case. Similarly, in *Cameron v Greater Glasgow Health Board* 1993 GWD 6-433 (Lexis transcript available), the pursuers failed for want of proof; but, had they succeeded, agreed damages of £40,000 would have been awarded
12 *Thake v Maurice* [1984] 2 All ER 513 at 526, [1985] 2 WLR 215 at 230.
13 In *Lovelace Medical Center v Mendez* 805 P 2d 603 (NM, 1991) the parents were able to recover for economic loss, including the costs of raising a normal child from birth to adulthood, as well as for emotional and physical pain and suffering; they were not required to mitigate damages by way of adoption or abortion. For commentary, see A Grubb 'Damages for the Birth of a Healthy Child' [1993] 1 Med L Rev 249.
14 *Danns v Department of Health* (1992, unreported) quoted by C Dyer 'Department of Health Sued after Husband's Vasectomy' (1992) 305 BMJ 912.
15 D W Meyers *The Human Body and the Law* (1970) p 28 et seq; P R Reilly 'Eugenic Sterilization in the United States' in A Milunsky and G Annas (eds) *Genetics and the Law - III* (1985) ch 17; J K Mason *Medico-legal Aspects of Reproduction and Parenthood* (1990) ch 4. For wide-ranging discussion, see K McK Norrie *Family Planning Practice and the Law* (1991), p 123.

in some states and, in others, the number of operations carried out was small. Nevertheless, compulsory sterilisation measures remain on the statute books in a number of jurisdictions. Interest now centres on the management of individual cases and here, despite some inevitable inconsistencies, a consensus is evolving in favour of non-consensual sterilisation given very specific criteria of justification. The seminal case is *Re Grady*,[16] where the power of the court to exercise jurisdiction as to the sterilisation of an incompetent minor in the absence of statute was firmly upheld. The problem in all such cases is to strike a balance between the individual's right to bodily integrity and the right to choose an operation which, in the case of the mentally handicapped, may carry with it greater freedom of access to community life and relationships.[17]   To make such a choice in surrogate fashion, however, is to invoke a 'substituted judgment' test. The great majority of courts have recognised the near impossibility of doing this in the face of congenital mental illness and have, accordingly, opted for a 'best interests' test which is also central to the welfare principle on which the English wardship jurisdiction is founded.[18] A most important United States case in this respect is that of *Re Hayes*[19] in which it was laid down that the courts could authorise sterilisation in the absence of consent so long as, inter alia, the subject was incapable of forming a judgment, was physically capable of procreation, was likely to engage in sexual activity and there was no reasonable alternative to sterilisation.

The root problem of non-consensual sterilisation, overshadowed as it is by the ghost of the eugenic movement, lies in the fact that it raises starkly the subject of what has been named the basic human right to reproduce – to which we return for general discussion at p 87. The phrase seems to have originated in the American case of *Skinner v Oklahoma*[20] (which, in fact, concerned the punitive sterilisation of a man) and has, since, come into common usage throughout the English-speaking world. In the United Kingdom, the concept was prominent in the very significant case *Re D (a minor) (wardship: sterilisation)*.[1] The minor in this case was an 11 year old girl who suffered from a rare condition known as Sotos' syndrome. Her IQ was roughly 80, a rating which need not necessarily make it impossible for the person in question to cope reasonably well in everyday life and even to marry and raise a child. There was medical evidence to the effect that her condition showed some signs of improvement and that this improvement could continue.

In her judgment in this case, Heilbron J was strongly swayed by the medical evidence given to the court to the effect that sterilisation was not always appropriate in such cases and that such a decision was not within the scope of the clinical judgment of a single doctor dealing with the case. Also to be taken into account was the irreversibility of the operation and the significance of carrying it out on so young a person:

> A review of the whole of the evidence leads me to the conclusion that in a case of a child of 11 years of age, where the evidence shows that her mental and physical condition and attainments have already improved, and where her future prospects are as yet unpredictable,

16 405 A 2d 851 (Md, 1979).
17 In the US, see *Conservatorship of Valerie N* 707 P 2d 760 (Cal, 1985).
18 Established in statute in Guardianship of Minors Act 1971, s 1.
19 *Re Hayes* 608 P 2d 635 (Wash, 1980).
20 316 US 535 (1942).
 1 [1976] Fam 185, [1976] 1 All ER 326.

where the evidence also shows that she is unable as yet to understand and appreciate the implications of this operation and could not give valid or informed consent, that the likelihood is that in later years she will be able to make her own choice, where, I believe, the frustration and resentment of realising (as she would one day) what happened could be devastating, an operation of this nature is, in my view contra-indicated.[2]

The judge in *Re D* has been criticised for not having addressed the general issues involved.[3] She did, however, refer to the 'basic human right of a woman to reproduce' and concluded that it would be a violation of that right if a girl were sterilised without her consent for non-therapeutic reasons. *Re D* remained the English authority for more than a decade and was quoted with approval in the Canadian case of *Re Eve*.[4] *Re Eve* is an important case because, among other reasons, the Supreme Court of Canada took several years to deliberate and, in so doing, canvassed a large number of opinions. Moreover, by the time the trial had gone through all its stages, virtually every variant opinion had been supported in the judgments.

Eve was the mentally retarded adult daughter of a mother who asked that she be sterilised, a major plank supporting the request being that, in the event of Eve becoming pregnant, neither she nor her mother would be able to care for the baby. The Supreme Court was in no doubts as to its having a parens patriae jurisdiction through which to authorise sterilisation should the need arise. That power was, however, limited by the principle of its being exercised in the best interests of the girl. In the light of this, the judgment was concerned to distinguish between therapeutic and non-therapeutic reasons for sterilisation; La Forest J concluded:

The grave intrusion on a person's rights and the certain physical damage that ensues from non-therapeutic sterilization without consent . . . have persuaded me that it can never safely be determined that such a procedure is in the best interests of that person . . . [I conclude that non-therapeutic sterilization] should never be authorised . . . under the *parens patriae* jurisdiction.[5]

He appreciated that there could be difficulty in drawing a line between a therapeutic and a non-therapeutic operation, but was content to emphasise that: 'the utmost caution must be exercised commensurate with the severity of the procedure'.[6] In essence, it was this problem which provoked the apparent conflict between the court in *Re Eve* and that involved in the comparable English case of *Re B (a minor) (wardship: sterilisation)*[7] which was the first of its kind to reach the House of Lords.

---

2 [1976] Fam 185 at 196.
3 A Bainham 'Handicapped Girls and Judicial Parents' (1987) 103 LQR 334.
4 (1986) 31 DLR (4th) 1.
5 (1986) 31 DLR (4th) 1 at 32.
6 The extant case at the time, *Re K and Public Trustee* (1985) 19 DLR (4th) 255, in which the main therapeutic ground for sterilisation was a phobic aversion to blood which would be accentuated with the onset of the menses, was regarded as 'at best, dangerously close to the limits of the permissible' – this despite the fact that an Appeal Court judge in *Re K* thought that the case should never have come to the courts: per Anderson JA at 277.
7 [1988] AC 199, [1987] 2 All ER 206, HL.

Having been reported at much the same time, it is inevitable that the approaches in *Re Eve* and *Re B* have been contrasted. It is unfortunate that the English case concerned a girl aged 17 – she would, therefore, shortly have passed out of the English wardship jurisdiction and it was considered that there was no such parens patriae authority on which to fall back in the case of an adult as was available to the Canadian courts. A speedy decision was, thus, dictated, and there is no doubt that Lord Hailsham LC, on it being suggested that the girl's progress could well be observed for a year, laid open his defences when he said: 'We shall be no wiser in twelve months than we are now.'[8] A massive literature has built up around the case and we are able to refer here only to those aspects that we regard as essential to its understanding.

B was a mentally handicapped epileptic with a mental age of 5-6 years. She had never conceived and was not pregnant but, absent being fully institutionalised, she was in danger of becoming so. Medical opinion – which, in contrast to that given in *Re D*,[9] was scarcely challenged – was that she would either have to be maintained on hormonal contraceptives for the rest of her reproductive life or her fallopian tubes could be occluded. The court recognised this as being an irreversible procedure. It was common ground that any pregnancy that occurred would have to be terminated.

In authorising sterilisation, the House of Lords upheld the decisions of both the court of first instance and the Court of Appeal. The basic principle involved was the welfare of the girl. Lord Oliver, in particular, emphasised that there was no question of a eugenic motive, no consideration was paid to the convenience of those caring for the ward and no general principle of public policy was involved. Lord Hailsham LC made some specific comments aimed, in the main, at explaining any apparent variances from other relevant decisions. With particular reference to *Re Eve*, he said:

> [The] conclusion that the procedure of sterilisation should 'never be considered for non-therapeutic purposes' is totally unconvincing and in startling contradiction to the welfare principle . . . [The] distinction [drawn] between 'therapeutic' and 'non-therapeutic' purposes of this operation in relation to the facts of the present case . . . [is] irrelevant . . . [10]

Lord Oliver also found, in effect, that there was no logic in excluding preventive medicine from therapy directed to the ward's interest and we would certainly agree with this. It is, however, possible to argue that 'non-therapeutic' in terms of La Forest J's judgment in *Re Eve* referred only to treatment designed for the benefit of others. If this be so, *Re Eve* and *Re B* are not greatly in conflict.[11]

The *Re B* decision has been widely criticised in the British academic literature.[12] We wonder, however, how much the *medical* aspects of the case have been taken into

8 [1988] AC 199 at 203, [1987] 2 All ER 206 at 212, per Lord Hailsham LC.
9 *Re D (a minor) (wardship: sterilisation)* [1976] Fam 185, [1976] 1 All ER 326.
10 [1988] AC 199 at 203, [1987] 2 All ER 206 at 213.
11 K McK Norrie 'Sterilisation of the Mentally Disabled in English and Canadian Law' (1989) 38 ICLQ 387.
12 See, for example, M Freeman 'For Her Own Good' (1987) 84 LS Gaz 949; S P de Cruz 'Sterilization, Wardship and Human Rights' (1988) 18 Fam Law 6; R Lee and D Morgan 'Sterilisation and Mental Handicap: Sapping the Strength of the State?' (1988) 15 J Law & Soc 229; J Montgomery 'Rhetoric and "Welfare"' (1989) 9 Oxford J Leg Stud 395 – a particularly trenchant attack. It is fair to remark that the decision in *Eve* has not been applauded everywhere in Canada – see M A Shone 'Mental Health - Sterilization of Mentally Retarded Persons' (1987) 66 Can BR 635.

account. The speed with which the decision was taken has been questioned;[13] but this is, we suspect, no more than a reflection of the unanimity of professional opinion – there can be no doubt that pregnancy *is* contraindicated in some patients with mental handicap and that B was one of them. Medically speaking, *Re B*[14] and *Re D*[15] are poles apart. Norrie, for example, is among those who felt that the former was a case that should never have occupied the courts' time; sterilisation was always legal by way of the doctrine of necessity – or, simply, it was necessary.[16] We suggest that the major conceptual difference between *Re Eve* and *Re B* is that the former attempts to generalise on principles whereas the latter is determined to particularise on the facts – and we see no objection to the latter line of thinking.

Lord Hailsham, however, also addressed the question of rights and it is this issue that has so occupied the commentators. He said:

> The right [of a woman to reproduce] is only such when reproduction is the result of informed choice of which the ward in the present case is incapable.[17]

and, again:

> To talk of the 'basic right' to reproduce of an individual who is not capable of knowing the causal connection between intercourse and childbirth . . . [or who] is unable to form any maternal instincts or to care for a child, appears to me wholly to part company with reality.[18]

The concept of the right to reproduce is one which deserves discussion in depth but which we cannot provide in the space available. Suffice it to say that the existence of an absolute right is by no means certain. Simplistically, it is difficult to envisage a right that requires the co-operation of another person who is under no obligation to provide it. Moreover, an absolute right to reproduce would arguably entail access by right to all means of assisted reproduction including surrogate motherhood and womb-leasing – and this is clearly untenable. Grubb and Pearl[19] have argued very convincingly that the only such right currently recognised in English law is the right to choose whether or not to reproduce – this being grounded in the principle of individual autonomy. If this be so, given the inability of a subject to make a rational choice, there can be no objection to the courts assuming this right on the person's behalf.

13 I Kennedy and S Lee 'This Rush to Judgement' (1987) The Times, 1 April, p 12.
14 *Re B (a minor) (wardship: sterilisation)* [1988] AC 199, [1987] 2 All ER 206, HL.
15 *Re D (a minor) (wardship: sterilisation)* [1976] Fam 185, [1976] 1 All ER 326.
16 K McK Norrie 'Sterilisation of the Mentally Disabled in English and Candian Law' (1989) 38 ICLQ
    387. But this definition of necessity would not always be agreed – see J E S Fortin 'Sterilisation,
    the Mentally Ill and Consent to Treatment' (1986) 51 MLR 634. For assistance, see the opinion of
    Neill LJ in *Re F (mental patient: sterilisation)* [1990] 2 AC 1 at 32, [1989] 2 WLR 1025 at 1053.
17 *Re B (a minor) (wardship: sterilisation)* [1988] AC 199 at 203, [1987] 2 All ER 206 at 212.
18 [1988] AC 199 at 204, [1987] 2 All ER 206 at 213.
19 A Grubb and D Pearl 'Sterilisation and the Courts' (1987) 46 CLJ 439. See also Nicholson CJ in
    the Australian case *Re Jane* [1989] FLC 92-007. The reasoning in this case was very similar to that
    in *Re B*. For a brief overview of Australian cases, see J Goldhar 'The Right to Reproduce' (1989)
    63 Law Inst J 708.

An alternative approach is to regard the 'right' as one to retain the capacity to reproduce.[20] While this is still subject to the individual's ability to choose, it does, at first sight, make the justification for court's interference with that right more difficult. In our view, the resolution of the dilemma rests upon the definition of reproduction which, surely, cannot be limited and impersonalised to the single aspect of giving birth – it must include an element of after-care.[1] Some mentally handicapped persons may not be able to supply this, although, of course, some can. It is, again, a question of degree and a matter of the individual's medical status.[2] Moreover, the significance of this relative right disappears when, as in *Re B*, it is acknowledged that any pregnancy would have to be subject to therapeutic abortion.

A final comment on decisions such as *Re B* relates to criticism that they are sex discriminatory – 'Would the court', asks Freeman,[3] 'have sterilised a boy of 17?' The answer is certainly 'no' but this only proves the rule. Unfair it may be, but it is a fact of life that reproduction can have no immediately adverse physical effect on a man. The only bases for intentional, non-consensual, non-therapeutic sterilisation of a man would be punitive or eugenic, which is what all would agree should be avoided; the fact that decisions such as *Re B* are gender-based actually contributes to their justification.

Two very similar wardship cases have been reported since *Re B*.[4] In both, sterilisation was approved at first instance and neither was appealed. Medical evidence was given at both hearings to the effect that the proposed operation was reversible[5] – in up to 75% of cases said the gynaecologists in *Re M* who, in disclaiming the emotive overtones of 'sterilisation', preferred to regard the operation as contraceptive in nature. We suspect that this greatly influenced the judges because the evidence in favour of early sterilisation was less than fully agreed in both cases – indeed, a change of mind on the part of one medical expert had to be specifically explained as not having been made for eugenic reasons. The most interesting feature of both *Re M* and *Re P* is that they can well be seen as sterilisations which were authorised on social grounds for the benefit of the wards – a matter of protecting their lifestyles. Unless the House of Lords' interpretation of *Re Eve*[6] is flawed, such decisions might well be excluded were that judgment to be followed.

Almost parenthetically, note should be taken of a more recent case which indicates how rapidly judicial opinion has crystallised in this area. The ward in *Re HG (specific issue order: sterilisation)*[7] was an epileptic who suffered from an unspecified chromosomal abnormality. There was no dispute that pregnancy would

20 S A M McLean and T D Campbell 'Sterilization' in S A M McLean (ed) *Legal Issues in Medicine* (1981).
 1 For full (and prophetic) discussion, see J A Robertson 'Procreative Liberty and the Control of Conception, Pregnancy, and Childbirth' (1983) 69 Vand LR 405; A Thomas 'For Her Own Good - A Reply' (1987) 84 LS Gaz 1196.
 2 For a relatively recent appraisal, see L Appleby and C Dickens 'Mothering Skills of Women with Mental Illness' (1993) 306 BMJ 348.
 3 M Freeman 'For Her Own Good' (1987) 84 LS Gaz 949.
 4 *Re M (a minor)(wardship: sterilization)* [1988] 2 FLR 497, (1988) 18 Fam Law 434; *Re P (a minor)(wardship: sterilization)* [1989] 1 FLR 182, (1989) 19 Fam Law 102.
 5 It was said, in *Re P* in somewhat unusual phraseology: 'The situation to-day is that the operation is not irreversible although it is the current *ethical* practice to tell the patients that it is an irreversible operation' [our emphasis] [1989] 1 FLR 182 at 189 per Eastham J.
 6 (1986) 31 DLR (4th) 1.
 7 [1993] 1 FLR 587.

be disastrous for her and that long-term hormonal contraception was contraindicated. In making the order, the deputy judge said:

> [My conclusion is that] a sufficiently overwhelming case has been established to justify interference with the fundamental right of a woman to bear a child. I am certainly satisfied that it would be cruel to expose T to an unacceptable risk of pregnancy and that that should be obviated by sterilisation in her interests.[8]

Times have certainly moved on but, nevertheless, it is still considered that virtually all cases require the sanction of a High Court Judge. Applications may be made under the Children Act 1989, s 8(1) or under the inherent jurisdiction of the court – the latter being the preferred route.[9] Recourse to the court is, however, unnecessary when sterilisation is an incidental result of medical or surgical treatment. This has been made quite clear in two very similar, and closely heard, cases where a hysterectomy was indicated for menstrual disorder. In the first of these, *Re E (a minor) (medical treatment)*[10] (which concerned a 17 year-old) Sir Stephen Brown P held that no formal consent of the court was necessary and that the parents were in a position to give a valid consent: 'A clear distinction is to be made between an operation to be performed for a genuine therapeutic reason and one to achieve sterilization'.[11] In the second case *Re GF,*[12] the President declined to grant a declaration of lawfulness on the grounds that it was unnecessary when an operation was designed to improve the health of the patient. He did, however, lay down the conditions under which no application to the court was needed. These were that two doctors agreed, first, that the operation was necessary for therapeutic purposes; second, that it was in the patient's best interests; and, third, that no practicable less intrusive treatment was available. The medical profession must welcome such unequivocal guidance.

Returning, however, to instances of deliberate sterilisation of those unable to consent for themselves, the Practice Note described above also applies to the mentally incompetent adult. This follows decisions in a line of cases which have profoundly influenced English law.

The first of these was *T v T*[13] which involved an adult incompetent who was found to be pregnant. Medical opinion was consistent that the pregnancy should be terminated under the terms of the Abortion Act 1967 and there was an additional application from the subject's mother for leave to sterilise her at the time of the termination. In the course of his determination, Wood J found that the Mental Health Act 1983 provided no solution to non-consensual treatment other than as to that which was aimed directly at the psychiatric condition; that even if the prerogative powers of the Crown as parens patriae in respect of adults still existed, there was no-one who could now exercise it; that to perform an operation without consent and in

---

8 [1993] 1 FLR 587 at 592.
9 *Practice Note (Official Solicitor: Sterilisation)* [1993] 3 All ER 222, (1993) 16 BMLR 60.
10 [1991] 2 FLR 585, (1991) 7 BMLR 117.
11 [1991] 2 FLR 585 at 587, (1991) 7 BMLR 117 at 119.
12 [1992] 1 FLR 293, [1993] 4 Med LR 77.
13 [1988] Fam 52, [1988] 1 All ER 613. Discussed in depth by JES Fortin 'Sterilisation, the Mentally Ill and Consent to Treatment' (1986) 51 MLR 634. See also C Dyer 'Consent and the Mentally Handicapped' (1987) 295 BMJ 257.

the absence of a defence was tortious irrespective of hostile intent;[14] and that it was not possible to rely on implied consent in such a case. The judge was unhappy with the defence of necessity, mainly on account of its ill-defined limits, and preferred to rely on the demands of good medical practice – although this is not, in itself, the most unambiguous yardstick. In the circumstances, he fell back on the expedient of an anticipatory declaration that the performance of the two operations would not be unlawful.[15] This precedent, set in the Family Division, was approved in the House of Lords in the important case *Re F (mental patient: sterilisation)*.[16]

In *Re F*, the boundaries of the courts' discretion were, again, advanced, F being an adult with arrested mental development who was not pregnant. The conditions of *Re B*[17] were, effectively, duplicated save that F was now beyond the protection of wardship. The course of the action was, by now, almost predictable. The trial judge, Scott Baker J, was prepared to see all treatment for physical conditions that was given to mental patients in good faith and in their best interests as lying within the exceptions to the law of battery which had been created so as to allow for the exigencies of everyday life[18] His declaration that the operation would not be unlawful was upheld by the Court of Appeal where Lord Donaldson MR, likewise, saw nothing incongruous in doctors and others who had a caring responsibility being required to act in the interests of an adult who was unable to exercise a right of choice.[19] The Master of the Rolls was, understandably, reluctant to accept that serious medical treatment could be subsumed under the umbrella of actions acceptable in everyday life and preferred the formula of it falling 'within generally acceptable standards'. Neill LJ, approaching the problem from basic principle, concluded that if surgery was necessary, the performance of a serious operation, including an operation for sterilisation, on a patient who could not consent would not be a trespass to the person or otherwise unlawful.[20] The court was, however, unanimous as to the need for approval of the High Court before a sterilisation operation was undertaken.

The correctness of the decision to sterilise was not challenged in the House of Lords which was, rather, concerned with the resolution of questions of law and of legal procedure. The House, inter alia, confirmed that the parens patriae jurisdiction no longer existed in England, and that, if it were to be recreated, it would be for the legislature to do so – something which no doubt the majority of commentators would approve. Their Lordships also ruled that the procedure by way of declaration was appropriate and satisfactory in cases of the kind,[1] the court having no power to consent to the operation. Undoubtedly, however, the most important aspect of the decision for our purposes was that the common law provides that a doctor can

---

14 Cf *Wilson v Pringle* [1987] QB 237, [1986] 2 All ER 440, CA. We doubt if this would be followed in Scotland.
15 Rules of the Supreme Court, Ord 15, r 16.
16 *Re F (mental patient: sterilisation)* [1990] 2 AC 1, sub nom *F v West Berkshire Health Authority* [1989] 2 All ER 545.
17 *Re B (a minor) (wardship: sterilisation)* [1988] AC 199, [1987] 2 All ER 206, HL.
18 *Collins v Wilcock* [1984] 3 All ER 374 at 378, [1984] 1 WLR 1172 at 1177, per Goff LJ.
19 *Re F (mental patient: sterilisation)* [1990] 2 AC 1 at 18, [1989] 2 WLR 1025 at 1040.
20 [1990] 2 AC 1 at 32, [19989] 2 WLR 1025 at 1052.
 1 The procedural guidelines laid down in at the time ([1989] 2 FLR 47 and [1990] 2 FLR 530) have now been amended - see fn 9, p 89 above.

lawfully give surgical or medical treatment to adult patients who are incapable of consenting, provided that the operation or other treatment is in their best interests. It would be in their best interests if, but only if, it was carried out in order to save their lives or to ensure improvement, or prevent deterioration, in their physical or mental health[2] – which this seems a rather curious juxtaposition of the major emergency with mild palliation. The House went even further in indicating that it might be the common law *duty* of the doctor to provide treatment in the case of adults suffering from mental disability who were in the care of a guardian or who were detained in mental hospitals. Lord Brandon argued pragmatically that this must be so – otherwise the workload on the courts would be unbearable. Logically, this authority would also apply to sterilisation but six reasons were given for distinguishing that operation – including its general irreversibility which would almost certainly deprive the woman of: 'what was widely, and rightly, regarded as one of the fundamental rights of a woman, the right to bear a child'.[3] The House considered, however, that the involvement of the court in cases of this kind was not strictly necessary as a matter of law but it was, nevertheless, highly desirable as a matter of good practice.

We see this as an unfortunate result. It provides no *definite* lead for the medical profession and it certainly leaves the public wondering what proportion of cases has been subject to review in the past.[4] It was resolved in the House of Lords[5] that whether the 'best interests' test had been met would be judged on *Bolam*[6] principles. The application of a test for negligence to a question of clinical practice has been criticised.[7] In any event, it seems to us that, having made a bid for judicial supervision, the court, in so stating, effectively handed back control of the decisions to the doctors.[8] It would surely have been better to strike a rule one way or the other and, in fact, this was the only element of dissent in the House of Lords judgment – Lord Griffiths thought that the non-consensual sterilisation of a woman with healthy reproductive organs should be declared an operation that was unlawful without the consent of the High Court.[9] He thus aligned himself with Lord Templeman in his

2 *Re F (mental patient: sterilisation)* [1990] 2 AC 1 at 55, sub nom *F v Berkshire Health Authority* [1989] 2 All ER 545 at 551, per Lord Brandon.
3 *Re F (mental patient: sterilisation)* [1990] 2 AC 1 at 56, sub nom *F v Berkshire Health Authority* [1989] 2 All ER 545 at 552, per Lord Brandon.
4 C Dyer 'Decisions from the House of Lords' (1987) 294 BMJ 1219 indicated that some dozens of mentally disabled minors are being sterilised each year in England and Wales by way of a parent/ physician decision. We know of no figures for adult incompetents but has been said that about 1,000 operations were performed annually in the former West Germany where the doctors' position was less secure: J Shaw 'Sterilisation of Mentally Handicapped People: Judges Rule OK?' (1990) 53 MLR 91.
5 *Re F (mental patient: sterilisation)* [1990] 2 AC 1 at 68, sub nom *F v Berkshire Health Authority* [1989] 2 All ER 545 at 560.
6 *Bolam v Friern Hospital Management Committee* [1957] 2 All ER 118, [1957] 1 WLR 582.
7 D Ogbourne and R Ward 'Sterilization, the Mentally Incompetent and the Courts' (1989) 18 Anglo-Amer L Rev 230. Attempts to undermine *Bolam*, especially as related to a duty to warn, have been increasing. See, in particular, the Australian High Court in *Rogers v Whitaker* (1992) 67 ALJR 47 (discussed in further detail at p 245).
8 We do, however, appreciate that this depends to some extent on whether 'a matter of good practice' refers to good *medical* or good *legal* practice. Our interpretation has been the former but that may be taking a blinkered view.
9 *Re F (mental patient: sterilisation)* [1990] 2 AC 1 at 70, sub nom *F v West Berkshire Health Authority* [1989] 2 All ER 545 at 562.

obiter recommendations as to minors.[10] Even so, we have already noted the difficulty of distinguishing genuine therapeutic reasons with clarity and, while it is probably true that doctors and their health authorities will rarely by-pass the courts for fear of later legal action,[11] such expectation is still a long way from assured uniformity.

Amongst its other reasons for advocating the intervention of the courts in the 'best interests' analysis, the House of Lords (per Lord Brandon) thought that there might otherwise be a greater risk of it being decided wrongly, thus endorsing the Master of the Rolls' analogy of a judicial 'third opinion'. With the best of wills, we cannot see that this follows any more than that it would be desirable for a highly experienced consultant physician to approve a judicial opinion. Far more important are the subsidiary reasons given – that it might otherwise be *thought* to have been decided wrongly and that the doctors should be protected from consequent adverse criticism or claims. We do not share Lord Brandon's fears that, but for the courts, there is a risk of sterilisation being carried out for improper reasons or with improper motives. There is always the General Medical Council – although we might not go so far as Cook J who is reported as having said:

> It is not conceivable to this court that medical advisors would prostitute their Hippocratic Oath to perform unnecessary or ill-advised and untimely operations, particularly of a major kind.[12]

There is little doubt that many people distrust unbridled power of doctors – particularly in the field of social medicine – yet only the doctors in clinical charge of a case can possess all of the facts. The precedent set by *Re F* is that decisions of this nature will continue to be made on a case to case basis and it is because the details of each case differ that we would approve the process. Calls for specific legislation[13] should, we believe, be resisted because it would inevitably lead to generalisation in an area where the individual is paramount. We do, however, question whether the adversarial system provides the ideal milieu for deciding problems in which morality, legality and personal well-being are so intertwined. Is this not an area, par excellence, which would benefit from a medico-legal council approach to problem-

---

10 In *Re B (a minor) (wardship: sterilisation)* [1988] AC 199 at 205, [1987] 2 All ER 206 at 214. The authority of the Australian jurisdiction must be recognised in this area, as in many others, of medical jurisprudence. In *Department of Health & Community Services (NT) v J W B and S M B* (1992) 66 ALJR 300, the High Court concluded that an order of the court was always needed before sterilisation of a female who was unable to consent for herself; the overall Australian attitude to non-consensual sterilisation seems to lie somewhere between those of England and Canada. For discussion, see N Cica 'Sterilising the Intellectually Disabled: The Approach of the High Court of Australia in *Department of Health v J W B and S M B*' (1993) 1 Med L Rev 186.

11 C Dyer 'Ruling on Consent: Protection for Patients and Doctors' (1989) 298 BMJ 348.

12 In an Australian case *Re A Teenager* [1989] FLC 92-006. See J Goldhar 'The Right to Reproduce' (1989) 63 Law Inst J 708.

13 In the US, see *Re Guardianship of Joan I Eberhardy* 307 NW 2d 881 (Wis, 1981); in Canada, *Re Eve* (1986) 31 DLR (4th) 1; in the UK, J Shaw 'Sterilisation of Mentally Handicapped People: Judges Rule OK?' (1990) 53 MLR 91; J E S Fortin 'Sterilisation, the Mentally Ill and Consent to Treatment' (1986) 51 MLR 634; A Bainham 'Handicapped Girls and Judicial Parents' (1987) 103 LQR 334.

solving?[14] The concluding words of Lord Jauncey in *Re F* provide a suitable finale to this discussion:

> I should like only to reiterate the importance of not erecting such legal barriers against the provision of medical treatment for incompetents that they are deprived of treatment which competent persons could expect to receive in similar circumstances.[15]

Other forms of contraception

It may well be thought that many of the problems posed in the foregoing discussion of sterilisation – and particularly those of non-consensual sterilisation – could be obviated by the use of an alternative form of contraception. Few long-term contraceptive methods can, however, be applied without some risk – and the risk may be serious. Oral hormonally based contraception has been greatly refined over the years but there is no doubt that compounds with a high oestrogen content will predispose to intravascular thrombosis,[16] progestogens increase the liability to cardiovascular disease when combined with smoking, 'depot' preparations may cause menstrual disturbances,[17] and a possible association between contraceptive therapy and an increased incidence of carcinoma of the breast or cervix is still debated.[18] The very effective interceptive methods are also suspect in that, although any association is certainly not a simple one, they may cause pelvic inflammation and permanent infertility – fear of litigation would now deter many physicians in the United States from fitting an intrauterine device.[19] These are, however, mainly aspects of clinical medicine and they are introduced here only to emphasise that non-surgical contraception also has its pitfalls and cannot be imposed without forethought. The main legal and ethical issues relate to the provision of contraceptives for minors and, although this was once a burning issue, it has now lost some of its urgency and

14 J K Mason 'A Comparison of Medico-legal Systems in Scotland and Scandinavia' (1978) 23 JR 198. D Ogbourne and R Ward 'Sterilisation, the Mentally Incompetent and the Courts' (1989) 18 Anglo-Amer L Rev 230, for example, have suggested a useful set of guidelines which could be given great authority by such a council.

15 *Re F (mental patient: sterilisation)* [1990] 2 AC 1 at 83, sub nom *F v West Berkshire Health Authority* [1989] 2 All ER 545 at 571.

16 Relatively recent reviews include J Bonnar 'Coagulation Effects of Oral Contraceptives' (1987) 157 Amer J Obstet Gynecol 1042; J Guillebaud 'Surgery and the Pill' (1985) 291 BMJ 498 (but see also H Sue-Ling and L E Hughes 'Should the Pill Be Stopped Preoperatively?' (1988) 296 BMJ 447).

17 *Blyth v Bloomsbury Health Authority* [1993] 4 Med LR 151, discussed at p 244.

18 J O Drife 'The Contraceptive Pill and Breast Cancer in Young Women' (1989) 298 BMJ 1269. For a succinct analysis of the whole field, see A Szarewski and J Guillebaud 'Contraception' (1991) 302 BMJ 1224.

19 G R Thornton 'Intrauterine Devices: Malpractice and Product Liability' (1986) 14 Law Med Hlth Care 4 provides a good overview. But see N C Lee, G L Rubin, H W Ory and R T Burkman 'The Intrauterine Device and Pelvic Inflammatory Disease: New Results from the Women's Health Study' (1988) 72 Obst Gynecol 1.

the historic case of *Gillick v West Norfolk and Wisbech Area Health Authority*[1] is probably best discussed under 'Consent' (see p 224). Nevertheless, the dilemma confronting the doctor who is consulted by a female minor requesting contraceptive advice and treatment still merits consideration.

The problem is essentially that of deciding whether he should do anything which might facilitate her engaging in sexual activity. If his patient is, say, 14 or 15, he may well be of the view, that that is too young an age for sexual intercourse. This need not be on grounds of disapproval of sexual intercourse outside marriage; the disapproval is more likely to be based on the view that sexual activity at such an age may lead to emotional trauma and a risk of disease – including iatrogenic disease – which is best avoided. On the other hand, a refusal to prescribe contraceptives may ultimately be more damaging to the patient in that sexual activity may result in pregnancy – and giving birth to a child or having an abortion at such an age are likely to be severely disruptive of the patient's life.

The ethical dilemma by no means disappears once the decision is taken to provide contraception. The doctor then has to make the difficult decision whether or not to inform the patient's parents. This is really an issue of medical confidentiality which is discussed in detail in chapter 8, below. The decision in each case might, however, depend on the circumstances. A doctor who informed parents of the fact that their 13-year-old daughter had taken to prostitution could surely claim that it was in the best interests of the child to do so; this may not be the case when a 15-year-old girl is doing no more than engaging in occasional sexual activity with one partner. Two distinct legal issues are raised in this connection. The first is the general question as to whether a doctor can properly treat a minor without consent of the parents and, more specifically, whether he may give advice and treatment as to birth control. The second raises the possibility that, in so doing, he may attract criminal liability as being a party to the offence committed by the man who has sexual intercourse with his female minor patient. Both these issues were partially resolved by the decision in *Gillick*.

This controversial case resulted from the publication of a circular by the Department of Health stating that practitioners could, in strictly limited circumstances, discuss and apply family planning measures to minors without the express consent of their parents. Mrs Gillick sought, inter alia, to have the instruction declared unlawful. In the absence of any binding authority, the trial judge relied heavily on the common law and on the Canadian case of *Johnston v Wellesley Hospital*.[2] While distinguishing between physical or surgical and medical treatment, he concluded that a person below the age of 16 was capable of consent to contraceptive therapy provided she was of sufficient mental maturity to understand the implications. The Court of Appeal, however, concentrated on the duties and rights of parents which they considered inseparable. The trial judge's decision was overturned unanimously and the defendant authority, strongly backed by the British Medical Association, appealed to the House of Lords. This final court of arbitration reverted to what might

---

1   [1984] QB 581, [1984] 1 All ER 365; on appeal [1986] AC 112, [1985] 1 All ER 830, CA; revsd [1986] AC 112, [1985] 3 All ER 402, HL.
2   (1970) 17 DLR (3d) 139.

be loosely termed the 'mature minor' principle – and has come to be known as '*Gillick*-competence' – and decided against Mrs Gillick by a majority of 3:2.

We return to *Gillick* at p 179, but for the present we can note the overall tenor of the judgment as expressed by Lord Scarman:

> If the law should impose upon the process of growing up fixed limits where nature knew only a continuous process, the price would be artificiality and a lack of realism in an area where the law must be sensitive to human development and social change.[3]

The thrust of the case is, however, to be found in Lord Fraser's speech in which he said that the doctor would be justified in proceeding with contraceptive advice without the parents' consent or even knowledge provided that he was satisfied that:
(i)   the girl would, although under 16, understand his advice;
(ii) he could not persuade her to inform her parents or to allow him to inform the parents that she was seeking contraceptive advice;
(iii) she was very likely to have sexual intercourse with or without contraceptive treatment;
(iv) unless she received contraceptive advice or treatment her physical or mental health or both were likely to suffer; and
(v)   her best interests required him to give her contraceptive advice, treatment or both without parental consent.[4]

Lord Fraser emphasised that the judgment was not to be regarded as a licence for doctors to disregard the wishes of parents whenever they found it convenient to do so and he pointed out that any doctor who behaved in such a way would be failing to discharge his professional responsibilities and would be expected to be disciplined by his own professional body accordingly.

The House also considered the second question posed and, despite a dissenting opinion, ruled that it was unlikely that a doctor giving contraceptive advice to a female minor would be committing an offence under the Sexual Offences Act 1956, s 28. It was pointed out that, were the contrary to be so, an offence would be committed irrespective of parental consent. In essence, only if the doctor actually intended to facilitate unlawful sexual intercourse could he be regarded as abetting an offence under s 6 of the 1956 Act – and this must be a condition which borders on the inconceivable. Moreover, as Woolf J explained in the trial stage of the case, an accessory before the fact must know the material circumstances of the offence, not merely, for example, that sexual intercourse might take place at an unidentified time with an unidentified man.[5]

The medical response to the House of Lords decision in *Gillick* was generally one of relief. Yet it is possible that it is something of a Pyrrhic victory; in the event of a complaint being laid, it may be very much harder for a doctor to show that he

---

3   *Gillick v West Norfolk and Wisbech Area Health Authority* [1986] AC 112 at 186, [1985] 3 All ER 402 at 421, HL.
4   [1986] AC 112 at 174, [1985] 3 All ER 402 at 413, HL.
5   An objective view of the whole case is to be found in J Morgan 'Controlling Minors' Fertility' (1986) 12 Monash Univ LR 161. Another interesting Australian comment is in P Gerber and A Rahemtula 'Who Has the Right to Advise Children on Birth Control?' (1986) 144 Med J Austral 419.

conformed to all five of Lord Fraser's conditions than merely to convince his peers that he was following his reasonable medical judgment. Further, the General Medical Council interpreted the decision unusually. The doctor undoubtedly has a difficult task in assessing whether or not his young patient has sufficient understanding and intelligence for him to treat her with equanimity; the GMC's guidelines, however, go further and indicate that, should the doctor decide that she has *not* those attributes, then he may tell the parents about the consultation.[6] The rather unsatisfactory position thus seems to have been reached that the patient has to prove her maturity before being assured of confidentiality – and this cannot improve the professional relationship. The matter is discussed further in chapter 8.

The narrowness of the decision in *Gillick* cannot be overlooked. It is noteworthy that, on a simple head count, more judges supported the plaintiff than opposed her. It is certainly true that the consequences of a medical refusal of contraception would probably be worse for the girls in question than would be the circumvention of parental control. But the case was about bigger issues than the limited question of avoiding unwanted pregnancies. In a significant sense, it represented an attempt to use the law to establish a moral, rather than a legal, point about sexual conduct – and the law is a bad instrument for this purpose. Yet the warnings of those who supported Mrs Gillick should not be summarily dismissed as the protests of a latter-day Mrs Grundy; there is an undoubted tendency at present to undermine the concept of the innocence of childhood.[7] There are many pressures which increasingly encourage the young to seek the status of miniature adults and a readiness for sexual activity is essential to this identity. To quote Lord Templeman: 'There are many things which a girl under 16 needs to practise, but sex is not one of them'.[8] All of this has an effect on the social and psychological well-being of children and the corresponding medical evidence – particularly of the increase in cervical cancer in those who have shown early sexual promiscuity – should not go unnoticed. Mrs Gillick has now passed from the public eye but perhaps she was less villainous than she was painted at the time.

Post coital contraception

Certain types of contraception are designed to or, in practice, do work after the embryo has formed. These are referred to as interceptive methods – or emergency contraception – of which the intrauterine device and the misnamed 'morning after' pill are prime examples.[9] Such methods are, essentially, abortifacient rather than contraceptive and the question has arisen as to whether they offend against the Abortion Act 1967 (see ch 5). Much of the discussion turns on the interpretation of

---

6   General Medical Council *Professional Conduct and Discipline: Fitness to Practise*, January 1993, para 84.

7   For a survey of this process, see M Winn *Children without Childhood* (1984).

8   *Gillick v West Norfolk and Wisbech Area Health Authority* [1986] AC 112 at 201, [1985] 3 All ER 402 at 432.

9   It has been pointed out that the term 'morning after' implies a spurious sense of urgency; in fact, emergency hormonal contraception need only be instituted within 72 hours of sexual intercourse: F C Reader 'Emergency Contraception' (1991) 302 BMJ 801.

the word 'miscarriage' and whether or not this relates only to the displacement of the implanted embryo. The Attorney General has said that: 'the phrase "to procure a miscarriage" cannot be construed to include the prevention of implantation'.[10] Despite this, an argument can be developed to show that the processes are legally similar.[11] We, however, find it illogical to suggest that there can be miscarriage in the absence of true carriage. In any event, to argue that interceptive methods of contraception are illegal is, in practice, unrewarding. The use of an IUD must be morally preferable to the legal destruction of a recognisable human fetus and we would strongly support any move to put these methods of contraception beyond prosecution.[12] So far as we know, only one apposite prosecution has succeeded; the case did, however, concern the insertion of an IUD into a woman who was certainly pregnant.[13] Moreover, since the Abortion Act 1967 was not in force at the time, it does no more than demonstrate that, in certain circumstances, an IUD could be regarded as an instrument used to procure a miscarriage. Rather more help can be gained from the media in an otherwise unreported case[14] which involved a charge under the Offences Against the Person Act 1861, s 58 against a doctor who fitted a contraceptive coil to his secretary some 11 days after they had had intercourse. The judge, having heard gynaecological evidence that implantation would not have occurred, withdrew the case from the jury on the grounds that the woman could not have been pregnant 'in the true sense of the word'. It is unfortunate that this case was disposed of so summarily as there are certain aspects which give rise to doubt as to its value as a precedent – not the least being an apparent rejection of a charge under the 1861 Act on the grounds that 'the modern techniques of interference [with reproduction] were not [then] available'. Nevertheless, it seems unlikely that any such prosecution would succeed in the future – and this is, pragmatically, a good thing.

A need still remains to distinguish interceptive from displanting methods of contraception – the euphemistically termed 'menstrual extraction' being a common example of the latter. The purpose here is to dislodge a possibly implanted embryo and, as such, it seems to us that it must involve an intended procurement of miscarriage under the terms of the Offences Against the Person Act 1861, s 58[15] and/ or it constitutes a technical offence under the Abortion Regulations 1968.[16] Whatever may be the true situation in England a conviction would be virtually imposible in Scotland where any such common law offence requires proof of pregnancy.

10 41 Official Report (6th series) col *239*, 10 May 1983.
11 I J Keown '"Miscarriage": A Medico-legal Analysis' [1984] Crim LR 604.
12 For an interesting commentary, see D Crystal-Kirk 'Embryo Arrest: The "No-man's Land" between Contraception and Abortion' (1989) 57 Med-leg J 111. The most recent call is for making emergency contraception available from pharmacists without prescription: A Glasier 'Emergency Contraception: Time for Deregulation?' (1993) 100 Brit J Obstet Gynaecol 611; J O Drife 'Deregulating Emergency Contraception' (1993) 307 BMJ 695
13 *R v Price* [1969] 1 QB 541, [1968] 2 All ER 282. The conviction was quashed on the grounds of a misdirection.
14 *R v Dhingra* (1991) Daily Telegraph, 25 January, p 5.
15 A number of jurisdictions define the point at which legal pregnancy begins – usually as at implantation. For details, see K McK Norrie 'Post Coital Anti-pregnancy Techniques and the Law' in A A Templeton and D Cusine (eds) *Reproductive Medicine and the Law* (1990).
16 SI 1968/390. For further brief discussion, see p 110.

5   Abortion

The current interest in legal abortion in Great Britain is not whether it should be allowed; the practice has been with us since the passing of the Abortion Act 1967 and it is here to stay. In our view, the major significance of abortion in the context of medical ethics lies in the effect it has had on the medical ethos. The moment the Act was accepted by doctors was the moment the profession abrogated a main tenet of its Hippocratic conscience. As late as 1968, the Declaration of Geneva, as amended in Sydney, reiterated: 'I will maintain the utmost respect for human life from the time of conception' (Appendix B). By 1970, the Declaration of Oslo, while retaining this moral principle, had changed the tune: 'Diversity of response to this situation [the conflict of vital interests of the mother with vital interests of the child] results from the diversity of attitudes towards the life of the unborn child. This is a matter of individual conviction and conscience' (Appendix E). This ethical watershed has spilled over to influence attitudes of doctors and towards doctors in relation to all aspects of life and death. Modern medicine now shows no embarrassment in courting the concept of the wanted and the unwanted.

This is, however, something of a narrow view. In the wider context, attitudes to abortion depend almost entirely on where the holder stands in respect of, on the one hand, the fetal right to life and, on the other, the woman's right to control her own body and it is this which perpetuates a near intractable moral conflict. The trial of strength has been waged at a relatively low key in Britain; whether this has been due to tolerance or to indifference is a matter for argument. Passion has, however, run high in the United States where the protagonists have not been above resorting to serious crime in order to advance their cause.[1] Moreover, the issue has been debated at an overtly political level. The political importance has, however, been no less important nearer to home in the European Community, where it bid fair to forestall the reunification of Germany. There, it is possible to follow the arguments through the more staid deliberations of the legislature and the courts. We return to these examples later and in the meantime, we look briefly at the development of the law on abortion in the United Kingdom.

The evolution of the law on abortion

The evolution of legislation to decriminalise abortion is so well known as to merit only brief description. The fundamental law in England and Wales lies in the Offences Against the Person Act 1861, ss 58 and 59. The 1861 Act proscribes

---

1   See The Lancet 'This Is a Deadly Game' (1993) 342 Lancet 939. For an excellent study of the conflict in the United States, see L H Tribe *Abortion: The Clash of Absolutes* (1992).

procuring the miscarriage of a woman by a third party, self-induced miscarriage, attempted procurement of miscarriage and supplying the means to do so. Somewhat surprisingly, the word 'abortion' appears only in the marginal note to the sections.[2] The Act makes no distinction between criminal and therapeutic activity and has not been repealed. The proscription was so strong that, in addition to being punished by the courts, a doctor involved in an abortion was extremely likely to have his name erased from the Medical Register. As a result, and because of the attitudes adopted to extra-marital pregnancy, a large number of abortions were performed by persons of varying skill and in varying conditions. The extent of this type of abortion has never been established satisfactorily: suffice it to say that, 40 years ago, it provided an appreciable contribution to forensic pathology.

The first statutory break in this chain of events is to be found in the Infant Life (Preservation) Act 1929 which introduced the offence of child destruction or causing the death of a child capable of being born alive before it has an existence independent of its mother. The offence was not committed, however, if the act was done in good faith for the purpose only of preserving the mother's life. This slight concession to the needs of therapy was, on the face of it, still highly restrictive both as to reason and as to time. It was left to the case of *R v Bourne*[3] to temper the legal influence on medical practice in the field. Mr Bourne performed an abortion, with no attempt at secrecy, on a 15-year-old girl who was pregnant following a particularly unpleasant rape. Although he was indicted under the Offences Against the Person Act 1861, the trial judge, Macnaghten J, took the opportunity to link the 1861 and 1929 statutes and ruled that, in a case brought under the 1861 Act, the burden rested on the Crown to satisfy the jury that the defendant did not procure the miscarriage of the girl in good faith for the purpose only of preserving her life: the word 'unlawful' in the 1861 Act 'imports the meaning expressed by the proviso in s 1(1) of the Infant Life (Preservation) Act 1929'.[4] Mr Bourne was acquitted, the summing-up essentially recognising that a woman's life depended upon her physical and mental health and that an abortion was not illegal if it was performed because these were in jeopardy.[5] The law and the medical profession then lived in harmony for many years. The *Bourne* decision was undoubtedly stretched to the limits of interpretation by many doctors but the law turned a sympathetic eye.

However, it is never a good thing for any section of the public, no matter how well intentioned, to flirt with illegality. Further, there was still no authority for abortion in the event of probable deformation or other handicap of the neonate – a proposition which many would regard as being of the first importance. The situation was resolved when the Abortion Act, which started out, rather more aptly we feel, as the

---

2   The distinction, if any, between 'miscarriage' and 'abortion' is of academic interest in relation to pre-implantation methods of contraception (see pp 96, above and 110, below). Some writers believe the terms to be interchangeable: see, for example, I J Keown '"Miscarriage": a Medico-legal Analysis' [1984] Crim LR 604.

3   [1939] 1 KB 687, [1938] 3 All ER 615.

4   [1939] 1KB 687 at 691.

5   *R v Bourne* [1939] 1 KB 687 at 694, [1938] 3 All ER at 619. The Australian courts have also used the word 'unlawful' as indicating that there must be a 'lawful' reason for termination of pregnancy. See *R v Davidson* [1969] VR 667; *R v Wald* (1971) 3 DCR (NSW) 25.

Medical Termination of Pregnancy Bill,[6] came into effect in 1967. Despite repeated attack, it remained unchanged until 1990.

It is interesting to compare the historic attitudes in England with those prevailing in Scotland where abortion, either self or otherwise induced, has always been a common law offence without being defined by statute. The subject, including a review of the 1967 Act, occupies less than three pages in Gordon.[7] The difference in concern lies in the Scottish emphasis on the evilness of intent in crimes at common law. By and large, doctors are assumed to be acting in good faith and there is little doubt that Mr Bourne would have been unable to provoke a test case in Scotland. It is, in fact, arguable that there was no need to extend the Act to Scotland, its inclusion only being justified in that it removed any doubt as to the limits of therapeutic abortion in that country.[8]

The Abortion Act 1967

The Abortion Act 1967 (hereafter 'the 1967 Act') has been significantly amended by the Human Fertilisation and Embryology Act 1990, s 37 (hereafter called 'the 1990 Act'). In summary, it now states that a person shall not be guilty of an offence under the law of abortion when termination is performed by a registered medical practitioner and two registered medical practitioners have formed the opinion in good faith that the continuance of the pregnancy would involve risk, greater than if the pregnancy were terminated, of injury to the physical or mental health of the pregnant woman or any existing children of her family (s 1(1)(*a*)). These therapeutic and social conditions are subject to the pregnancy not having exceeded its 24th week. The remaining justifications are now free of gestational restriction. These are that there is a risk of grave permanent injury to the physical or mental health of the pregnant woman (s 1(1)*(b)*); that the continuance of the pregnancy would involve risk to the life of the pregnant woman (s 1(1)(*c*)); and, finally, that there is a substantial risk that, if the child were born, it would suffer from such physical or mental abnormalities as to be severely handicapped (s 1(1)(*d*)). Subsections (*b*) and (*c*) are not restricted by requiring the opinion of two registered medical practitioners – a single person may operate on his or her own initiative in such circumstances. Termination under the amended Act may be carried out in NHS hospitals or in places approved for the purpose by the Minister of Health or the Secretary of State (s 1(3)). It is this clause which legalises abortions performed privately and for a fee. The demand for abortion is, however, so great that, since 1981, a compromise position has been achieved whereby the private sector acts as an agency for the NHS. The advent of medical methods for the termination of pregnancy has dictated a change in the location rules which will probably be relaxed for this purpose in forthcoming regulations.[9]

6   The title was changed on the last day of the debate – almost, it seems, in a desperate effort to conclude the proceedings: 751 HC Official Report (5th series) col *1780*.
7   G H Gordon *The Criminal Law of Scotland* (2nd edn, 1978) ch 28.
8   See, for example, D Baird 'Induced Abortion: Epidemiological Aspects' (1975) 1 J Med Ethics 122.
9   Section 1(3A) inserted by the 1990 Act, s 37(3).

The great majority of legal abortions are performed for therapeutic reasons (89% of cases involving residents of England and Wales in 1991) and it is obviously not a simple matter to decide whether the risk of injury from continuance of the pregnancy is greater than if it were terminated.[10] The ethical basis of the Abortion Act 1967 thus depends to a large extent on the words 'in good faith'. If there is any lack of good faith, it is most likely to express itself outside the National Health Service and it is notable that 55% of abortions on residents in England and Wales were performed in approved places in 1991.[11] The feeling persists that this extensive use of the private sector indicates something less than strict adherence to the Act although many would attribute it to no more than a lack of facilities within the NHS. In any event, the medical profession as a whole tends to look on the Act as a success[12] – witness the opposition to change which continued to the last days of the Parliamentary debate on the 1990 Act. Occasionally, however, issues arise which strain the constancy even of the medical establishment and such a relatively novel development is that of abortion on the basis of fetal sex selection. The problem being put to him, Dr John Dawson, spokesman on medical ethics for the British Medical Association at the time, is reported as saying:

> To terminate a pregnancy solely on the grounds of the sex of the foetus is an abuse of medical skills. It is unethical and I believe the GMC should take a serious view . . . [of] a doctor who undertakes that sort of work.[13]

This may well be so but it should be remembered that the issue is of a different dimension from pre-conception selection which we have already discussed (at p 52 above). Nevertheless, the question of the legality of the practice remains open. Section 1(2) of the Act specifically states that, in making a determination as to the risk of injury to the woman's or her existing children's health, 'account may be taken of the pregnant woman's actual or reasonably foreseeable environment'. Given the right ethnic ambience (most particularly within Asian and Moslem cultures) there can be no doubt that the birth of a female child could affect a woman's mental health and possibly even her physical well-being, yet there is nothing in the Act which limits such risks to those directly associated with the condition of pregnancy.[14] Even an Anglo-Saxon may be mentally disturbed by the thought of a further male (or female) child and, while gender abortion may not constitute a major problem in our society, it serves to illustrate how wide the facility is for termination within the wording of the 1967 Act.

The availability of abortion has been further extended by s 37(4) of the 1990 Act which amends s 5(1) of the 1967 Act so as to read:

10 The risks of pregnancy and childbirth are not constant. Overall, they are about equal but the risk of pregnancy increases with age. Conversely, the risks of abortion in young nulliparae are greater than of pregnancy unless the procedure is completed in the first eight weeks of pregnancy (See P R Myerscough (1975) 1 J Med Ethics 310). Abortion methods have become much safer in the last 15 years but the complication rates still alter with gestation.
11 The comparable figure for Scotland was 2.3%.
12 D Munday, C Francome and W Savage 'Twenty-one Years of Legal Abortion' (1989) 298 BMJ 1231.
13 'Babies of Wrong Sex Aborted, Claims Report' (1988) Scotsman, 4 January, p 2. See also J Sherman 'Child's Sex "Sways Mothers"' (1987) The Times 2 February, p 3.
14 Similar views are expressed by D Morgan 'Foetal Sex Identification, Abortion and the Law' (1988) 18 Fam Law 355. For a lay opinion, see B Amiel 'Questions of Right and Wrong' (1988) The Times, 8 January, p 15.

No offence under the Infant Life (Preservation) Act 1929 shall be committed by a registered medical practitioner who terminates a pregnancy in accordance with the provisions of this Act.

The criminal associations with 'viability' of the fetus (which we discuss briefly below at p 112) and the living abortus are, therefore, now almost entirely dispelled and we doubt whether it is currently possible to perform an illegal abortion in Great Britain provided the regulations are observed. We have been able to find only one conviction under the Act[15] and this appears to have arisen mainly because of the way the operation was performed.

There are still some who would regard abortion in Great Britain as being unreasonably restricted as compared with other jurisdictions. Even so, the scope of the Abortion Act 1967 probably exceeds that envisaged by its originators. The number of terminations carried out in England and Wales reached a current peak in 1990 when almost 187,000 abortions were performed. The first fall since 1976 occurred in 1991 when the total number of legal terminations was 179,522, giving a rate for resident women of 15.27/1000 in the age group 15-44.[16] The comparable figures for Scotland in 1991 were 11,752 and 10.4/1000; there, both the number and the rate of abortions have continued to rise.

The number of terminations provided for foreign women in England and Wales in 1991 was 12,146 or 6.8% of the total. This shows a marked decline from the peak in 1973 when 34.7% of terminations were for patients from overseas. Clearly, there have been policy changes in other countries and it is worth considering some of these briefly.

The comparative position
Northern Ireland – We have, thus far, spoken only in terms of Great Britain as far as domestic law is concerned. The close association with the Republic of Ireland, where abortion is illegal and is not universally supported even in the event of risk to the life of the mother,[17] makes the position in Northern Ireland particularly sensitive. As a

15 *R v Smith (John)* [1974] 1 All ER 376, [1973] 1 WLR 1510, CA.
16 This is probably still quite a low rate. (See D Munday, C Francome and W Savage 'Twenty-one Years of Legal Abortion' (1989) 298 BMJ 1231.) For a general comparative view of anglo and francophone experience, see B M Knoppers 'Comparative Abortion Law' in J K Mason (ed) *Paediatric Forensic Medicine and Pathology* (1989).
17 A Murdoch 'Irish Doctors Row over Limited Abortion Rights' (1993) 306 BMJ 675. The law in the Republic of Ireland is in a state of flux with a number of important decisions having been taken recently. The right of the State to prohibit the dissemination of abortion information was upheld in the Court of Justice of the European Communities: *SPUC v Grogan* [1991] 3 CMLR 849, (1991) 9 BMLR 100. But this was overturned in the European Court of Human Rights: *Open Door Counselling Ltd and Dublin Well Woman Centre Ltd v Ireland* (1992) Times, 5 November. In addition, the Supreme Court of Ireland extended the grounds for a legal abortion to include instances when it was probable that there was 'a real and substantial risk to the life of the mother': *A-G v X* [1992] 2 CMLR 277 – while, at the same time, affirming that Irish women had no general right to travel abroad to obtain an abortion. A referendum held in November 1992 confirmed the Irish people's preference for access to information and travel; a proposal to liberalise the basic law was defeated – but mainly for procedural reasons: A Murdoch 'Irish Vote Against Abortion on Their Soil' (1992) 305 BMJ 1383. For a fuller discussion of the Irish (and German, see p106 below) scene, see R Boland 'Abortion Law in Europe in 1991-1992' (1993) 21 J Law Med & Ethics 72. A detailed description of the Irish law may be found in A Sherlock 'The Right to Life of the Unborn and the Irish Constitution' (1989) 24 (NS) Irish Jurist 13.

result, the Abortion Act 1967 does not run there and the law is still governed by the 1861 Act as modified by the various court decisions since 1939.[18] The situation has been criticised as 'being so unclear that it may not count as law at all'.[19] Nonetheless, the Secretary of State is quoted as having said that poll results in favour of following the British lead were:

> Consistent with the long accepted practice in Northern Ireland of carrying out therapeutic termination of pregnancy in the interests of the mother's welfare.

Moreover, it will be seen, below, that the practice in New South Wales, where a very similar situation exists, has resulted in a particularly liberal approach to abortion. It may well be that any differences in attitudes in the component parts of the United Kingdom exist only as a form of words.

The United States – Practice in the United States has been profoundly modified as a result of persistent legal intervention which has been notable by its absence in Great Britain.

Abortion laws in the mid-twentieth century differed in various states. Some, such as New York, were wholly liberal, and some, such as Texas, corresponded roughly to the English Infant Life (Preservation) Act 1929. However, the majority followed variations of the British Abortion Act. Then, in 1973, the Supreme Court altered the whole picture in the historic twin decisions of *Roe v Wade*[20] and *Doe v Bolton*.[1] The effect of these well-known decisions can be summarised as follows. It is an invasion of a woman's constitutional right to privacy to limit her access to abortion by statute. and this applies also to schoolchildren although their parents may still be informed of the circumstances.[2] The expression 'to preserve the life' of a woman is unconstitutionally vague although the expression 'to preserve the life or health' is acceptable. This raises an intriguing conflict. It was suggested at the time of the decision[3] that health is inclusive of convenience and that this effectively allows for abortion on demand; although the Supreme Court specifically stated that there was no such absolute constitutional right, there is no doubt that the result of *Roe* is that abortion during the first trimester is an inalienable prerogative of the American woman and is grounded in the right to individual privacy. To confirm the essential nature of privacy, the Supreme Court also ruled that an appeal on the grounds that wholly liberal laws were invalid because they deprived unborn children of the right to life was not available to an individual. Nevertheless, the court did give some regard to the rights of the developing fetus. In the first trimester, the question of abortion was to be decided solely between the woman and her physician; during the second trimester, the state authorities could intervene by reason of its interest in the

18 The Infant Life (Preservation) Act 1929 is repeated in the Criminal Justice Act (Northern Ireland) 1945, s 25. Conditions as to the latter are unaffected by the Human Fertilisation and Embryology Act 1990, s 37.
19 See S Lee as discussed by S Kingman 'Northern Ireland's Abortion Law Criticised as Unclear' (1993) 307 BMJ 284.
20 93 S Ct 705 (1973).
1 93 S Ct 739 (1973).
2 *HL v Matheson* 101 S Ct 1164 (1981).
3 J H Ely 'The Wages of Crying Wolf: A Comment on *Roe v Wade*' (1973) 82 Yale LJ 920.

health of the mother, although no such interest was vested in the fetus. Interference of this type could include stating where and by whom an abortion could be done. After 'viability', which the court assessed as somewhere between the 24th and 28th week of pregnancy, it was agreed that the state had a compelling interest in the health of the fetus and could, therefore, constitutionally intervene on its behalf excepting when the conditions threatened the life or health of the mother.

The decision in *Roe v Wade*,[4] which has resulted in nearly one-third of pregnancies in the United States being terminated legally, has been a subject of controversy ever since its pronouncement. In the first place, it satisfies virtually no-one; the anti-abortionists have been, inevitably, outraged while the feminist lobby sees the result as being still too restrictive of women's rights. Second, the trimester rule is unreliable in that it rests upon fluctuating medical expertise and medical technology.[5] This was well put by O'Connor J:

> The lines drawn [in *Roe*] have now become 'blurred' . . . The state can no longer rely on a 'bright line' that separates permissible from impermissible regulation . . . Rather, the State must continuously and conscientiously study contemporary medical and scientific literature in order to determine whether the effect of a particular regulation is to 'depart from accepted medical practice'.[6]

There are, however, practical reasons why, very unusually in the field of medical jurisprudence, American attitudes have little influence on British thinking in this area. Fundamentally, and despite the emotions it engenders, abortion in the United States is not so much a philosophical issue as it is one of constitutional law.[7] Moreover, the subject has become highly politicised and the Supreme Court, which interprets the Constitution, is subject to political adjustment. Thus, the Supreme Court firmly repelled a major attack on *Roe* which was mounted in the mid-1980s.[8] However, a change in personnel encouraged the further sally towards the end of the decade in *Webster v Reproductive Health Services*[9] which was rather more successful in that, although the court was unwilling to overturn the principles laid down in *Roe*, it upheld a Missouri statute which certainly limited the availability of abortion. The implication is that other States will be able to introduce similar restrictions. Apart from some considerations as to fetal viability, the central issue in *Webster* turned on the state's right to restrict the reasons for which pregnancies could be terminated at public expense. Indeed, it has been held for some time[10] that federal funding in the

---

4 93 S Ct 705 (1973).

5 N K Rhoden 'Trimesters and Technology: Revamping *Roe v Wade*' (1986) 95 Yale LJ 639.

6 In *Akron v Akron Center for Reproductive Health* 462 US 416 (1983) at 455-456.

7 R Dworkin 'The Great Abortion Case' (1989) *The New York Review*, 29 June, p 49. See also I Loveland 'Abortion and the U.S. Supreme Court' (1992) 142 NLJ 974.

8 *Thornburgh v American College of Obstetricians and Gynecologists* 476 US 747 (1986).

9 109 S Ct 3040 (1989). For extensive and critical discussion, see W Dellinger and G B Sperling 'Abortion and the Supreme Court: The Retreat from *Roe v Wade*' (1989) 138 U Penn LR 83 and related papers. In J Bopp and R E Coleson 'What Does *Webster* Mean' (1989) 138 U Penn LR 157, the authors maintain, inter alia, that 'the trimester scheme may be considered de facto and *sub silentio* overruled'.

10 *Harris v McRae* 100 S Ct 2671 (1980).

form of 'Medicaid' is available for abortions only in limited circumstances, such as preserving the life of the mother or terminating pregnancies resulting from rape or incest; accordingly, individual state health systems need not contribute towards expenses incurred on other grounds.[11]

The struggle, however, continues. In 1992, the Supreme Court was again asked to pronounce on the legality of a state statute – in this case, the Abortion Control Act 1982 of Pennsylvania which created a number of obstacles in the way of abortion 'on demand'. The issue, here, as in many of the US cases, was not so much related to a maternal/fetal conflict as to one involving, on the one hand, the woman's right to bodily privacy and, on the other, the state's interest in the protection of life and a preference for childbirth over abortion.[12] Simplistically, the Supreme Court introduced an 'undue burden' test, which meant that the state was empowered to impose financial, medical or emotional barriers to abortion provided that these did not become a substantial obstacle, or undue burden, to choosing abortion. The basic premise of the woman's liberty of conscience and bodily integrity was, in this way, upheld. Even so, some fetal rights were maintained in that states could restrict abortion of the 'viable' fetus save in relation to a medical emergency threatening the mother. Needless to say, this decision was by the barest of majorities and powerful dissenting opinions were handed down, including a rejection of the whole concept of a fundamental women's liberty to choose abortion. The opinion has been said to please no lobby[13] and there is every indication that the abortion debate will continue in the United States in an atmosphere of increasing acrimony and increasing subservience to political exigency.

The British Commonwealth – Turning to the Commonwealth, the most interesting, and hard fought, abortion battles have been waged in Canada where, until recently, the law has not been outstandingly liberal. Control of legal terminations was vested in hospital abortion committees under the Criminal Code 1971, s 251. In the long-running case of *R v Morgentaler*,[14] however, the Supreme Court held that this section violated the security and liberty of the pregnant woman. Dickson CJ expressed his reasons for this conclusion as follows:

> Forcing a woman, by threat of criminal sanction, to carry a fetus to term unless she meets certain criteria unrelated to her own priorities and aspirations, is a profound interference with a woman's body and thus a violation of security of the person.[15]

In parallel litigation, the Canadian Charter of Rights and Freedom was held to be inapplicable to the fetus.[16] Those opposed to abortion gained a surprise victory in

---

11 The Supreme Court was due to hear another case involving financial pressures – in this instance, a matter of refurbishment of abortion clinics – but the matter was resolved out of court (*Ragsdale v Turnock* 763 F 2d 1532 (1985)).
12 *Planned Parenthood of Southeastern Pennsylvania v Casey* 112 S Ct 2791 (1992). See A Charo 'Undue Burden of Abortion' (1992) 340 Lancet 44.
13 See I Loveland 'Abortion and the U.S. Supreme Court' (1992) 142 NLJ 974.
14 [1988] 1 SCR 30.
15 [1988] 1 SCR 30 at 56. For discussion of this decision, see M L McConnell 'Abortion and Human Rights: An Important Canadian Decision' (1989) 38 ICLQ 905.
16 *Borowski v A-G of Canada* (1987) 39 DLR (4th) 731 (Sask, CA).

Tremblay v Daigle[17] in which a father gained an interlocutory injunction to prevent the abortion of his child. The decision rested on the Provincial Charter of Rights and the case was held under the civil law jurisdiction of Quebec. The situation was, however, short-lived, and the full Supreme Court of Canada reversed the decision unanimously.[18] It is to be noted that neither of the Supreme Courts of the United States or of Canada will allow of a 'trade-off' or balancing act between fetal and maternal rights to life or health – it is the mother's position which is to be safeguarded.

The innate tendency towards liberal abortion law is also demonstrated in Australia where, other than in South Australia and the Northern Territories which have enabling statutes, the basic law corresponds to that in the Offences Against the Person Act 1861. Judicial interpretation of the word 'unlawful' in relation to medical practice has resulted in a very wide availability of terminations in, at least, New South Wales. Despite the fact that therapeutic abortion is widely practised without the benefit of enabling legislation throughout Australia, there have been no prosecutions of doctors since 1971.[19]

The German Experience – The recent history of German legislation is instructive and is of practical importance in the light of current attempts to unify abortion law throughout the European Community. Here, abortion legislation was isolated as the only exception to the general reunification formula that western institutional and legislative experience should be extended to the former East Germany.[20] Broadly, the existing situation was that, whereas abortion during the first 12 weeks of pregnancy was controlled solely by the free choice of the pregnant woman in the former East Germany, abortion was illegal in West Germany save in specific circumstances dependent, in large part, on 'stage of the fetus' provisions – a situation analogous to that in Britain with 'general hardship' substituted for the social clause in the Abortion Act 1967. Approximately 33% of pregnancies were terminated in East Germany but, very interestingly, abortions were at least as frequent in West Germany. Controversy, therefore, rested on a purely ideological base. The conflict was fuelled by a resurgence of activity by both conservative and liberal elements in West Germany but was, at the same time, dampened by an increasingly wide perception of abortion as a potentially dangerous piece of social engineering rather than a woman's right.[1]

The compromise was that the issue would be settled on a free vote in the Bundestag two years after reunification. The federal parliament duly passed a law under which a pregnant woman could choose to have an abortion in the first three months of pregnancy provided she had undergone social counselling at least three days before the termination was carried out.[2] After long deliberation, the Constitutional

---

17 (1989) 59 DLR (4th) 609.
18 (1989) 62 DLR (4th) 634.
19 For judicial decisions, see fn 5, p 99 above.
20 Treaty on German Unity (31 August 1990), art 31 *Family and Women*, para 4, Bundesgesetzblatt (BGbl) II (1990) p 885.
 1 E Kolinsky 'Women in the New Germany' in G Smith et al (eds) *Developments in German Politics* (1992) ch 14.
 2 A Tuffs 'Germany: Abortion, the Woman's Choice' (1992) 340 Lancet 43.

Court declared that the new legislation was contrary to the Basic Law in certain respects. The new law failed to meet the minimum standards for the protection of unborn human life as set out in the Constitution.[3] As an interim measure, procedures were laid down which, if followed, would render consensual abortion within the first three months of pregnancy still illegal but not subject to criminal sanction.[4] The court's decision was founded on the premise that abortion offends against that part of the German constitution which 'guarantees the right to life and freedom from bodily harm' – a right which extends, even if in modified form, to the fetus.

Experience in Britain – and, now, in Germany – indicates that compromise, albeit an imperfect solution, depolarises attitudes and fosters less violent confrontation. In the context of abortion, however, it dictates some acknowledgement of fetal rights and, here again, one senses a wind of change.

The rights of the fetus

Roe v Wade[5] highlights the fundamental ethical issue in abortion – at what point, and in what circumstances, does a fetus become a person, and at what point does that person have rights to an existence?

What constitutes the state of being a person, or personhood, is a matter of moral decision and is not one of scientific fact. The conservative view, as exemplified, particularly by the Roman Catholic Church, lies at one extreme and holds that personhood and the right to protection exist from the moment of conception. We suggest that there are few outside the orthodox Catholic church who would support this decision. There are, in fact, relatively good reasons, based, inter alia, on the totipotential capacity of the early embryonic cells, for regarding the pre-implantation morula as being, also, pre-embryonic. At the other end of the scale, however, there are those who would equate personhood with intellect and with the power to make decisions.[6] We reject such an extreme if for no reason other than that it would deprive even young infants of the rights of a person. Many attempts have been made to define the point at which the fetus is morally entitled to protection within these brackets. The Jewish rabbinical law, for example, sets the time as when pregnancy is recognisable externally,[7] the early Christian moralists were attracted to the evidence of life exhibited by quickening[8] and many modern legal jurisdictions are increasingly inclined to accord the fetus 'rights' at viability, the complications of which as to

---

3 H Karcher 'Abortion Law Diluted Again in Germany' (1993) 306 BMJ 1566; A Tuffs 'Germany: Illegality of Abortion' (1993) 341 Lancet 1467.
4 A form of prevarication which seems to be part of the Continental jurisdictions – cf the Dutch attitude to euthanasia (see p 318). A useful summary is in M Prutzel-Thomas 'The Abortion Issue and the Federal Constitutional Court' (1993) 2 German Politics 467.
5 93 S Ct 705 (1973).
6 M Tooley 'A Defense of Abortion and Infanticide' in J Feinberg (ed) *The Problem of Abortion* (1973) and H Kuhse and P Singer *Should the Baby Live?* (1985), in particular, ch 6.
7 A Steinberg 'Induced Abortion in Jewish Law' (1980) 1 Int J Law Med 187.
8 See G R Dunstan 'The Moral Status of the Human Embryo: A Tradition Recalled' (1984) 10 J Med Ethics 38 for a comprehensive review.

definition are discussed later in this chapter. Here, we would only remark on the now well appreciated fact that the limits of viability in terms of gestation periods will be steadily lowered to their physiological baseline as neonatal medicine improves and becomes more widely available. As O'Connor J put it in *Akron*:[9] 'The [*Roe v Wade*] framework is on a collision course with itself.' It is this inevitable trend that has sustained the many attempts to amend the British Abortion Act. The indications are, therefore, that the conflict between fetal rights and increasingly permissive abortion laws is likely to continue.

As to the law, it is everywhere accepted that, although fetal rights may be established while in utero, or even before conception, they cannot be realised unless the fetus is born alive. Moreover, the legal concept of a separate existence is still further limited in the Congenital Disabilities (Civil Liability) Act 1976 under which the neonate must survive for 48 hours before being able to recover damages in negligence. 'There can be no doubt, in my view', said Sir George Baker,[10] 'that in England and Wales the foetus has no right of action, no right at all, until birth' and the same is almost certainly true in Scotland. From across the Atlantic, we have:

> There is no existing basis in law which justifies a conclusion that foetuses are legal persons.[11]

From which it follows that a stillbirth cannot benefit and that no suit for wrongful fetal death is recognisable in the United Kingdom.[12] This leaves us with an apparent paradox – as Pace[13] has put it: 'Liability is incurred for negligent injury to the foetus but not – or, at least, not necessarily – for its deliberate destruction.' There is, however, some evidence that many jurisdictions are moving towards the recognition of such suits. Thus, in the United States, we read in very similar vein:

> To deny a stillborn recovery for fatal injuries during gestation while allowing such recovery for a child born alive would make it more profitable for the defendant to kill the plaintiff than to scratch him.[14]

The tone in this case, and in others that have both preceded it and followed it, indicates not so much a shift in jurisprudential reasoning as a logical wish for punitive sanctions.against the person who negligently destroys the child in utero and

---

9 *Akron v Akron Center for Reproductive Health* 462 US 416 (1983) at 458.

10 *Paton v British Pregnancy Advisory Service Trustees* [1979] QB 276 at 279, [1978] 2 All ER 987 at 989.

11 *Borowski v A-G of Canada and Minister of Finance of Canada* (1984) 4 DLR (4th) 112, per Matheson J at 131.

12 Damages have been given for a stillbirth resulting from negligent treatment: see *Bagley v North Herts Health Authority* [1986] NLJ Rep 1014. The award was, however, to the mother, although damages in respect of bereavement under the Fatal Accidents Act 1976 were expressly disallowed on the grounds that the negligence had caused the child to die in utero. The court was, however, at pains to ensure adequate compensation notwithstanding that fact. See also *Grieve v Salford Health Authority* [1991] 2 Med LR 295 where only the quantum of damages for negligence leading to stillbirth was considered.

13 P J Pace 'Civil Liability for Pre-natal Injury' (1977) 40 MLR 141.

14 *Amadio v Levin* 501 A 2d 1085 (Pa, 1985).

as such is another form of expression of an intrinsic public concern for the status of the fetus.[15]

There are strong indications that the UK courts are also anxious to invest the fetus with as positive an identity as is possible within current legal constraints. In general terms, we have the Master of the Rolls stressing the right of an adult to refuse life-saving treatment but, at the same time, acknowledging that there might well be an exception to the rule were a viable fetus to be involved.[16] This was an obiter statement that was later put to the test in *Re S*.[17] In England, it has been held that the fetus has common law rights irrespective of the Congenital Disabilities (Civil Liability) Act 1976[18] and, in Australia, this has been extended to an acceptance of a fetal right to sue its mother for negligent injury in utero. The trial judge in this case said:

> I would hold that an injury to an infant suffered during . . . its journey through life between conception and parturition is not injury to a person devoid of personality other than that of the mother-to-be. – [N's] personality was identifiable and recognisable.[19]

A similar trend has been clearly evidenced in Scotland where a fetus has been recognised as a person when criminally injured under the Road Traffic Act 1972,[20] while a similar extension of the statutory 'person' beyond a being 'with legal personality' has been approved under the Damages (Scotland) Act 1976:[1]

> 'It is perfectly common in ordinary speech to refer to a child in the womb as "he", "she", "him" or "her" . . . It was this child who sustained injuries to his person and who died in consequence of personal injuries sustained by him'.[2]

All of these later examples depend upon the fetus being born alive – there is still no action available to the fetus in the United Kingdom for its negligent death.[3] Nevertheless, the cases demonstrate a clear intention to acknowledge (or even create) a persona in the fetus when it is possible to do so.[4]

---

15 It must be said, however, that attitudes are not uniform across the United States – an action for wrongful death was dismissed in *Milton v Cary Medical Center* 538 A 2d 252 (Me, 1988). For further discussion, see B Dickens 'Wrongful Birth and Life, Wrongful Death before Birth, and Wrongful Law' in S A M McLean (ed) *Legal Issues in Human Reproduction* (1989). H Brown et al 'Legal Rights and Issues Surrounding Conception, Pregnancy, and Birth' (1986) 39 Vand LR 597 include an outstanding review of the problem.

16 *Re T (Adult: Refusal of medical treatment)* [1992] 4 All E R 649 at 653, (1992) 9 BMLR 46 at 50.

17 *Re S (Adult: Refusal of medical treatment)* [1992] 4 All E R 671, (1992) 9 BMLR 69.

18 *Burton v Islington Health Authority; de Martell v Merton and Sutton Health Authority* [1992] 3 All ER 833, (1992) 10 BMLR 63.

19 Reported by D Brahams 'Australian Mother Sued by Child Injured in Utero' (1991) 338 Lancet 687. This being a road traffic accident, there seems no reason why such an action should not be available in England under the 1976 Act (see p 136).

20 *McClusky v H M Advocate* 1989 SLT 175.

1 *Hamilton v Fife Health Board* 1993 SLT 624, (1993) 13 BMLR 156.

2 1993 SLT 624 at 629, (1993) 13 BMLR 156 at 165 per Lord McCluskey.

3 A Whitfield 'Common Law Duties to Unborn Children' (1993) 1 Med L Rev 28.

4 But the Canadian courts are still resolute: see the criminal case *R v Sullivan* (1991) 63 CCC (3d) 97.

This movement is fuelled by two developments which are of growing importance. First, the availability of fetal therapy and second, an increasing recognition of risks to the health of the fetus which may be taken by a pregnant woman. Neither affects the abortion issue directly but each may have a profound effect on instinctive reactions to the debate.[5] For the present, we note only that both offend against the extreme view which can be paraphrased as asserting that the fetus is no more than a complex cellular appendage to its mother. There cannot be many who would sustain this strict interpretation – the 'wart on the face' philosophy falls down if only on genetic principles. Life is a constructive continuum from conception to birth and from infancy to adulthood and the moral conflict can be expressed in two quotations:

> The increasing tendency to view the fetus as an independent patient or person occurs at the cost of reducing the woman to the status of little more than a maternal environment.[6]

and

> The developing human life has a great intrinsic value. It cannot be viewed purely as a part of the woman's body.[7]

Some middle view has to be reached if we are not to drift into accepting the principle that the unwanted should be destroyed simply because they are unwanted. Many years ago, Ely[8] remarked, in relation to the right to privacy, that there is not a wide difference between being inconvenienced by a fetus and being inconvenienced by an unwanted infant. There is much to commend the concept of the maternal-fetal unity[9] which forces attention on the individual pregnant woman rather than simply on a woman or on a fetus – a dichotomy which serves only to polarise opinion.

We have already discussed some of the moral and intuitive values that can be attributed to the fetus. The fetal status does, however, have additional important legalistic connotations at the beginning and towards the end of pregnancy. The Abortion Act 1967 deals with the termination of pregnancy but certain procedures, in particular menstrual extraction and post-coital insertion of intra-uterine devices, are performed partly because a pregnancy might exist before any definite diagnosis can be made. In the absence of any relevant amendment of the Act, it is doubtful if menstrual extraction, which deals with a problematical implantation, can be legal

---

5   See the searching article by D Callahan 'How Technology is Reframing the Abortion Debate' (1986) Hastings Center Report, February, p 33. The relevant cases are discussed below at p 136 et seq.
6   J Benschol 'Reasserting Women's Rights; in 'Late Abortion and Technological Advances in Fetal Viability' (1985) 17 Fam Plan Perspect 162.
7   Swedish Government Official Report 'The Pregnant Woman and the Fetus – Two Individuals' SOU 1989.51. The aborted pre-viable fetus which is recognisable as such must now be given a respectful cremation in Sweden. See K Kallenberg, L Forslin and O Westerborn 'The Disposal of the Aborted Fetus – New Guidelines: Ethical Considerations in the Debate in Sweden' (1993) 19 J Med Ethics 32.
8   See J H Ely 'The Wages of Crying Wolf: A Comment on *Roe v Wade*' (1973) 82 Yale LJ 920 at p 932.
9   Originally expressed in R F R Gardner 'A New Ethical Approach to Abortion and its Implications for the Euthanasia Dispute' (1975) 1 J Med Ethics 127.

under the terms of the statute which is concerned with the assessment of an established pregnancy. Nevertheless, interceptive and displanting contraception are forms of 'after the fact' action to prevent the birth of an unwanted baby which are less likely to offend the public conscience than is frank fetal destruction. It seems illogical that they may be uniquely liable to censure under the Offences Against the Person Act 1861, s 58. The acquittal in *R v Dhingra* on just such a charge has been discussed at p 97. In withdrawing the case from the jury, the judge said:

> It is highly unlikely any ovum became implanted and only at the completion of implantation does the embryo become a fetus. At this stage she can be regarded as pregnant.[10]

Whether or not this is a binding statement of the law, it is a policy which we feel should be accepted. We have argued the importance of implantation on general ethical grounds at p 63; we also agree strongly that the ruling in *Dhingra* needs to be followed in order to harmonise the Offences Against the Person Act 1861, the Abortion Act 1967 and the Human Fertilisation and Embryology Act 1990.[11]

Consideration of early termination techniques must now include 'medical' abortion. Whether this will exacerbate the abortion controversy in Britain is uncertain, although there has been little overt opposition. The introduction of mifepristone in France, however, resulted in pressure sufficient to force the manufacturers to withdraw the product until the government, as major shareholders, insisted on the resumption of research and clinical evaluation.[12] Emotional accusations such as 'the launching of chemical warfare against unborn children' have been met by emollient attempts to recategorise the process as 'contragestation' rather than abortion.[13] It is a measure of the intensity of the abortion debate in the United States that the antiprogestin RU 486 is not available there because of the manufacturers' reluctance to become involved.[14] The drug has a limited license in the United Kingdom, where it is known as mifegyne, and it has been used successfully in pilot studies.[15] The treatment is distinguished from post-coital contraception (discussed above at p 96) in that it is clearly abortifacient. It can, therefore, be administered only within the terms of the 1967 Act. Interestingly, a company attempting to patent a similarly acting product was forced to include a disclaimer to this effect over a decade ago.[16] This development again highlights the

10 *R v Dhingra* (unreported): But see T Shaw 'GP Cleared of Procuring His Secretary's Miscarriage' (1991) Daily Telegraph, 25 January, p 5. In the absence of a full report of this case, it is difficult to see why, even so, there was no offence insofar as an offence is created by s 58 'whether [the woman] be or be not with child'.
11 A Grubb 'The New Law of Abortion: Clarification or Ambiguity?' [1991] Crim LR 659.
12 A Dorozynski 'Tempest in a Pill Box' (1988) 297 BMJ 1291.
13 E-E Baulieu 'RU 486 as an Antiprogesterone Steroid: From Receptor to Contragestion and Beyond' (1989) 262 J Amer Med Ass 1808.
14 R Boland 'RU 486 in France and England: Corporate Ethics and Compulsory Licensing' (1992) 20 Law Med Hlth Care 226. The whole of vol 20, part 3 of this journal was devoted to the subject. Of particular interest is R Macklin 'Antiprogestin Drugs: Ethical Issues' at 215.
15 M W Rodger and D T Baird 'Induction of Therapeutic Abortion in Early Pregnancy with Mifepristone in Combination with Prostaglandin Pessary' [1987] 2 Lancet 1415, See also J Guillebaud 'Medical Termination of Pregnancy' (1990) 301 BMJ 352. The relevant circular is PL/CMO (91) 9 of 5 July 1991.
16 *Upjohn Co (Kirton's) Application* [1976] RPC 324. The way is now cleared for medicinal abortion by the Abortion Act 1967, s 1(3A) (inserted by Human Fertilisation and Embryology Act 1990, s 37(3)) which extends the premises in which a legal abortion can be performed.

essential abortion issue – that is, the validity of the sanctity of life principle. We view the introduction of 'contragestation' therapy with some concern as, in the same way as the 'morning after pill', it will inevitably come to be regarded as a safe form of contraceptive back-up. The result must be to blur the distinction (a distinction which we regard as essential) between contraception and abortion. While the two processes may be comparable in that they both *prevent* new life, it is only abortion that can be seen as *taking* life.

At the other end of fetal life, any criminal liability of doctors for aborting a viable fetus has now been removed.[17] Nonetheless, practical and moral implications still surround the living abortus and a brief consideration of 'viability' is still apposite. Viability is something of a legal fiction, originating in the United States, designed to define some point at which the state accepts a compelling interest to protect the lives of its unborn citizens. Conceptually, therefore, viability is a term of constitutional law and it probably has no place in English law.[18] The attainment of American viability purports to coincide with the gestational age at which the fetus can be presumed to be capable of an existence separate from its mother and, as has been seen, the US Supreme Court in *Webster v Reproductive Health Services*[19] set this as lying between the 24th and 28th weeks of pregnancy. United Kingdom legislation has, however, concentrated on being born alive. Live birth is undefined and has generally been interpreted as the converse of stillbirth; effectively, a certificate of stillbirth cannot be issued if, having fully proceeded from its mother, the neonate breathed or showed any other sign of life. This carries no time limitation and, furthermore, leaves open what are 'other signs of life'. Williams[20] believed that they included a beating heart – in which case, every normally developed fetus delivered after 18 weeks' gestation could be said to be born alive. While we believe that this cannot hold, it is obvious that such a standard requires very little of the neonate – it need only have managed one breath to have been 'born alive'. By contrast, viability is a term of medical art implying an ability to live – at least for a reasonable time. Thus, viability is a product not only of fetal maturity but also of the motivation and resources of any medical attendants at the birth. As the Supreme Court of the United States pointed out in *Webster*, viability cannot be defined legally and is a matter for medical determination.

Considerable confusion existed in England and Wales as a result of the apparently interchangeable use of the words 'born alive' in the Infant Life (Preservation) Act 1929 and 'viable' in the Abortion Act 1967.[1] There are now a number of cases in which the matter has been addressed.

The most widely publicised of these was *C v S*[2] in which it was held that a fetus born following 18-21 weeks' gestation was not capable of being born alive because

---

17 1990 Act, s 37(4).

18 K McK Norrie 'Abortion in Great Britain: One Act, Two Laws' [1985] Crim LR 475.

19 109 S Ct 304 (1989).

20 G Williams *Textbook of Criminal Law* (2nd edn, 1983) p 290. In this, he is supported by the World Health Organisation – see *C v S* [1988] QB 135 at 142 [1987] 1 All ER 1230 at 1236, CA.

1 V Tunkel 'Late Abortions and the Crime of Child Destruction: (1) a Reply' [1985] Crim LR 133; G Wright '(2) a Riposte' [1985] Crim LR 140.

2 [1988] QB 135, [1987] 1 All ER 1230, CA. For a discussion, see S P de Cruz 'Abortion, *C v S* and the Law' (1987) 17 Fam Law 319.

it was incapable of breathing by the use of its own lungs – with or without the use of a ventilator. Live birth and viability were, thus, approximated although the use of the ventilator maintained a medical resource element in the definition. The court avoided addressing the question of viability directly, a manoeuvre which was followed in the case of *Gregory v Pembrokeshire Health Authority*.[3] However, the Court of Appeal, there, was not prepared to reject out of hand the notion that a fetus of 24 weeks' gestation was 'viable'.

A firmer approach was taken at first instance in *Rance v Mid-Downs Health Authority and Storr*[4] which was, like *Gregory*, a 'wrongful birth' case. Here it was held that a child was born alive if, after its birth, it existed as a live child, that is to say was breathing and living through the use of its own lungs alone. Brooke J found that the child in question would certainly have been born alive at 27 weeks' gestation. The judge also believed that the word 'viable' was used in the original Abortion Act 1967, s 5(1) as convenient shorthand for 'capable of being born alive' – an interpretation which appears to us to be too facile but is, nevertheless, one which indicates that the intense academic argument can now be regarded as a storm in a teacup. From the point of view of the criminal law, the meaning of being born alive remains as it was decided more than a century ago[5] and viability has disappeared from the statute book. A further major good to come from these cases is that the confusing phrase 'any other sign of life' is removed from the definition of live birth.

The case of *Rance* demonstrates vividly the unsatisfactory state of the law prior to 1990. In that case, the plaintiff's child was known to be physically abnormal but, by the time the diagnosis was established, the gynaecologists were unable to terminate the pregnancy for fear of transgressing the criminal law. That concern has now been removed. It has, however, been replaced by moral considerations which are, if anything, exaggerated by the 1990 amendments to the 1967 Act.

Those who support the interests of the fetus have always been concerned to avoid the abortion, or feticide, of those capable of a free existence by lowering the fetal age above which termination is impermissible so as to keep pace with medical abilities. They can be said to have succeeded to an extent by having this set at 24 weeks for relatively slight medical and social reasons.[6] The offset is that it may be difficult, particularly in the face of human error, to make a prognosis of serious neonatal handicap within that timescale. Accordingly, the 1990 Act removes the pre-existing 28 weeks' legal limit and imposes no other time restrictions on abortions performed by reason of fetal abnormality. Similar derestriction applies in the event of risk of grave injury to the pregnant woman – and such conditions are likely to arise particularly in late gestation. The *need* for late abortion thus remains and the Act is silent as to what is to be done with a live abortus. It has to be remembered that a living abortus is legally a creature in being; to kill such a being or to allow it to die without good reason may be murder or manslaughter and s 37(4) of the 1990 Act absolves the gynaecologist of child destruction only.

3 [1989] 1 Med LR 81.
4 [1991] 1 QB 587, [1991] 1 All ER 801.
5 *R v Handley* (1874) 13 Cox CC 79. Section 5(1) of the 1967 Act has been substituted by virtue of the 1990 Act, s 37(4).
6 In passing, s 37 of the 1990 Act now brings the law, as well as the practice, of abortion in Scotland into line with that of England.

One practical solution is to ensure that no mature abortus is given the opportunity to live. Not only may this involve the use of feticidal methods which are, at the same time, relatively dangerous to the pregnant woman but such methods may also be repugnant to all associated with the procedure. It is difficult to visualise a process which offends the Hippocratic and intuitive conscience more than the dismemberment of a relatively well-formed fetus.[7] This is precisely the situation the 'pro-life' Parliamentary lobby sought to avoid and a clause designed to ensure that reasonable steps were taken to assist a mature abortus to live was introduced at a late stage in the debate on the 1990 Bill.[8] The motion was defeated in the House of Lords, largely as a result of advice that doctors carrying out terminations after the 24th week of pregnancy 'would make every conceivable effort . . . to make sure the baby was capable of living . . . a normal and independent existence'.[9] Lord Ennals[10] quoted a letter from 20 gynaecologists:

> If the fetus is mature enough to have a reasonable chance of survival with intensive care, all possible steps are taken to optimise the recovery of both mother and fetus. Delivery then is usually by Caesarean section.

Since the avowed purpose of the clause was to control the maverick, it is surprising that the medical profession was so antipathetic to a measure approved by its senior practitioners. Moreover, the stated practice raises some interesting issues. What distinction, if any, is made between the normal and handicapped fetus? Could the doctor be required to use a process which might result in a damaged neonate and possible litigation?[11] Can a woman in such a condition give a valid consent to a serious operation? Is it right to subject a woman to an invasive procedure on behalf of the fetus? This is a matter to which we return in chapter 6. Above all, Parliament gave no indication of how the doctor was to dispose of his new patient.

The gynaecologist is certainly in a difficult position. On the one hand, he has effectively contracted to relieve a woman of her fetus. On the other, he is confronted by an infant who, on any interpretation, is entitled to a birth certificate and, if necessary, a certificate as to the cause of death.[12] Considerations as to the proper use of limited resources must also colour any decision-making. The principles of selective non-treatment of a defective neonate (see chapter 7) might well be applicable but, otherwise, we can see no theoretical objection to the view that failure to attempt to sustain a living infant could result in a charge of homicide.

Legal precedents are slender in Great Britain and, what few there are, are inconsistent. In one case, an area health authority inquiry concluded that allowing an aborted fetus to die was an action which was fully within the law. In another,

---

7   R J Lilford and N Johnson 'Surgical Abortion at Twenty Weeks: Is Mortality Determined Solely by the Outcome?' (1989) 15 J Med Ethics 82.
8   Such a condition has been declared unconstitutional in the United States: See *Colautti v Franklin* 439 US 379 (1979), and *American College of Obstetricians and Gynecologists Pennsylvania Section v Thornburgh* 106 S Ct 2169 (1986).
9   522 HL Official Report (5th series) col 1043, 18 October 1990, per Lord Walton at col 1050.
10 Ibid at col 1052.
11 For discussion, see R P S Jansen 'Unfinished Feticide' (1990) 6 J Med Ethics 61.
12 See 355 HL Official Report (5th series) col 776, 12 December 1974, per Lord Wells-Pestell.

where an infant lived for 36 hours after having been aborted at 23 weeks, the coroner found that death was due to prematurity and that there was no culpability on the part of the medical staff. So far as can be ascertained, only one coroner, faced with such circumstances, has brought in a conclusion of death due to want of attention at birth to a premature infant;[13] and even then no further action seems to have been taken. One prosecution is known to have been mounted by the DPP against a doctor who was alleged to have left a living abortus to die in the sluice-room but the magistrates took the unprecedented step of deciding there was no case to answer.[14] There was a further instance of a supposedly 21 week-old fetus, breathing and with a heart beat, being left to die without assistance for three hours but neither the birth nor the death were registered and the body was incinerated. In the absence of a cadaver, the coroner applied to the Home Office for authority to hold an inquest but this was refused for reasons which were not given publicly.[15] Similar uncertainty has been noted in the United States where one Dr Waddill, who ordered 'oxygen only' for a 26 week delivered fetus, was brought to trial for murder. Two juries failed to agree, whereupon all criminal charges were dismissed.[16]

We find it illogical to distinguish in legal terms between abandonment of the newborn infant and abandonment of the living abortus. The apparently pragmatic attitude of the law seems to be a further example of its reluctance to interfere in medical practice. Morally, it is perhaps hard to divert further from the Hippocratic ethos than to leave a normal infant to die which is crying for the incubator simply on the grounds that it is unwanted.[17]

We admit to some disappointment that the 'pro-abortus' motion in the House of Lords was lost and we deprecate any movement towards equating late abortion with deliberate feticide.[18] There is, in fact, no certainty that all women seeking a termination of pregnancy also seek the destruction of their fetus. Indeed, it could be argued that such right as the woman may have to control her pregnancy does not extend so as to include a right to control the destiny of a 'viable' fetus. McLean, while insisting on the former right throughout pregnancy, has enlarged this concept and has suggested that much of the current rancour could be dispelled if women were given encouragement and the *opportunity* to undergo late, and salvageable, abortions.[19] We still hold to the view that, in general, 'viable' fetuses should be given a chance to live – there is no reason why such as can and do survive should not be regarded

---

13 Inquest on Infant Campbell, Stoke-on-Trent, 19 October 1983, unreported.
14 *R v Hamilton* (1983) The Times, 16 September, p 1.
15 Reported by M Fletcher (1988) The Times, 25 February, p 2. The case was raised in Parliament on a motion for the adjournment: 154 HC Official Report (6th series) col 460, 8 June 1989.
16 B Towers 'The Trials of Dr Waddill' (1979) 5 J Med Ethics 205.
17 Anne Widdicombe MP, a Parliamentary 'pro-life' activist, put the issue as lying between 'I perceive this to be a human being because I want it' and 'I perceive this not to be a human being because I do not want it': 171 HL Official Report (6th series) col 192, 24 April 1990.
18 In fact, it has been government policy since 1975 that abortions beyond the 20th week of pregnancy should be carried out only in hospitals having appropriate facilities including resuscitation equipment: 898 HC Official Report (5th series) col 245, 21 October 1975.
19 S A M McLean 'Women, Rights and Reproduction' in S A M McLean (ed), fn 15, p 109 above; see, by the same author 'Abortion Law: Is Consensual Reform Possible?' (1990) 17 J Law & Soc 106. But would it not be both medically and economically more logical to encourage the woman to carry her fetus to term?

as parentless infants and offered for adoption on that basis. It is unlikely that there would be any shortage of adopting parents – particularly if the process was simplified to accord with the unusual circumstances.

Other people's rights

The great majority of what is written on the subject of abortion is directed to a discussion of the rights of the mother and the fetus – comparatively little attention is given to those who participate as third parties.

Conscientious objection

This unconcern may well spring from the fact that the Abortion Act 1967, s 4 excuses the conscientious objector from participating in treatment by abortion unless that treatment is directed towards the saving of life or of preventing grave permanent injury to the health of the mother. But, while this would seem to be perfectly clear, the doctor's situation is not uncomplicated. The curious provision which stipulates that the English doctor must prove his conscience while his Scottish counterpart's sworn word will, quite properly, be accepted at face value is illogical but is of minor significance. The most important and unfortunate result of the 1967 Act is that some discrimination takes place against doctors, and especially those seeking to become gynaecologists, who are unable to accept its wide terms.[20] It is to be noted that, while a doctor may, in general, refuse to take part in the abortion procedure, he remains under an obligation to advise. Such advice is subject to the normal rules of medical negligence and the conscientious objector's only recourse is, therefore, to refer his patient to another practitioner, a practice which is only marginally compatible with a strong conscience and which must damage the essential bond of trust between doctor and patient. The facts that the woman may well be unaware of her practitioner's attitude and that a second referral inevitably delays the termination provide one of the most powerful arguments put forward by those who would demedicalise early abortion. It is often forgotten that a doctor's objection to abortion may be Hippocratic rather than, say, religious in origin and a logical case can be made, and a major ground for confrontation thereby removed, for delegating abortions which have no immediate therapeutic dimension to trained abortionists.[1] The doctor's conscience does not absolve him from treating a woman when the continuation of the pregnancy is life-threatening and there is, of course, no right to conscience in treating the *results* of a legal abortion. These considerations apply equally to the nursing staff.

The nursing staff and others involved

The role of the nurse in therapy of all sorts is becoming more significant. This is exemplified in the sphere of abortion by the widespread use of prostaglandin

20 J Warden 'Abortion and Conscience' (1990) 301 BMJ 1013.
  1 J K Mason *Human Life and Medical Practice* (1988) p 121.

infusions for induction of premature labour. Nurses have so great a part to play in this process that some doubt was raised as to whether they were, in fact, thus guilty of performing illegal abortions in the sense that they were not 'registered medical practitioners' as required by the 1967 Act. The Royal College of Nursing accordingly sought a declaration to the effect that the advice in a departmental circular[2] stating that, irrespective of the precise action taken, an abortion was legal provided that it was initiated by and was the responsibility of a registered medical practitioner, was wrong in law. The complexities were such that the Royal College lost its case in the High Court, won it in the Court of Appeal and, finally, lost it in the House of Lords.[3] Effectively, therefore, abortion, no matter how it is performed, is a team effort and is no different in this respect from any other form of treatment. It is, nevertheless, interesting that, in total, five out of nine judges involved took the view of the nurses.

It is a very tenable argument that the sensibilities of the nursing staff are inadequately recognised within the abortion debate. The damage that conscientious objection causes to their career prospects is even greater than that sustained by doctors – a doctor does not *have* to practice gynaecology but, as Lord Denning emphasised, nurses are expected to be mobile throughout the hospital system.[4] Moreover, current methods of termination beyond the 12th week of pregnancy involve the nursing staff in an uncompromising way – whether it be in the delivery of what is comparable to a premature birth or in counting the fragmented parts of a formed fetus.[5] There can be no doubts as to their *rights* even if these are not always respected.

Valid conscientious objection within the terms of the Abortion Act 1967, s 4 is, however, limited by a proximity test – that is, that it covers only those involved in the therapeutic team effort. The case of a woman employed as a doctor's receptionist and secretary, who regarded herself as having been unfairly dismissed following her refusal to type a letter referring a patient for termination of pregnancy, was considered so important that it was taken to the House of Lords.[6] In the event, the applicant failed at every step, essentially on the grounds that participation in treatment, as applied to s 4, referred to actually taking part in treatment administered in a hospital or other approved place. The suggestion in the Court of Appeal that the conscience clause applied to activities which would have been criminal but for the 1967 Act was rejected in the House of Lords – and, at any rate, a typist could not be held to be an accessory in the criminal sense. The applicant was clearly well distanced from the actual treatment but one can only guess whether others more closely involved (eg hospital porters) would be similarly excluded. Indeed, the dividing line might be fine. The advent of medical termination raises the unusual position of the conscientiously objecting pharmacist who is asked to supply the necessary prescriptions. In our view, the proximity test would be satisfied although

2 CMO (80) (2).
3 *Royal College of Nursing of the United Kingdom v Department of Health and Social Security* [1981] AC 800, [1981] 1 All ER 545, HL.
4 [1981] AC 800 at 805, [1981] 1 All ER 545 at 555.
5 See R J Lilford and N Johnson, 'Surgical Abortion at Twenty Weeks: Is Mortality Determined Solely by the Outcome?' (1989) 15 J Med Ethics 82. J Glover *Causing Death and Saving Lives* (reprinted 1986) p 142 points to the effects on the health carers as providing a major moral distinction between, say, contraception and abortion.
6 *R v Salford Health Authority, ex p Janaway* [1988] 2 WLR 442, CA; *affd* sub nom *Janaway v Salford Area Health Authority* [1989] AC 537, [1988] 3 All ER 1079, HL.

much depends on how the relationship between the pharmacal and medical professions is viewed.[7]

The father

The anomalous position of the father in the right to life debate also falls to be considered. It is clear from current worldwide decisions that, in so far as abortion is concerned, he has, for practical purposes, *no* rights. It seems incongruous that this should be so irrespective of the reason for the abortion and that it should apply even in cases which do not relate to the health of the mother. A father could not, for example, save the existence of a *potentially* haemophiliac son.

The English position was established in *Paton v British Pregnancy Advisory Service Trustees* where it was clearly laid down that a husband cannot by injunction prevent his wife from undergoing a lawful abortion. The decision was upheld by the European Court of Human Rights; the European Court, however, was clearly worried by the possible complication of fetal 'viability' – the matter was not decided and it remains an area of potential doubt.[8] It was clarified no further in *C v S*[9] in which the unmarried father's locus standi was firmly rejected (and was not appealed) but in which the main thrust of the hearing was to establish that the fetus in question was *not* viable. Occasional arguments are advanced in favour of limited paternal rights. It has been mooted that the fetus, at least in Scotland, might be able to petition through its tutor (ie its father) for interdict of any threatened harm[10] and the interesting suggestion has been made[11] that the father might have a legal footing as part of the actual environment into which his child might or might not be born – the environment being a factor which may be taken into account when assessing the risks of continuing the pregnancy (1967 Act, ss 1(1)(*a*) and 1(2)). Neither proposition seems to have been tested in the long period since they were first mooted and it is very doubtful if either would succeed.

Attitudes elsewhere in the English-speaking world are diverse. The firm English stance would seem to be accepted in New Zealand but the reasoning there is based more on statute than on common law.[12] It is unlikely that an injunction to prevent a maternally-desired abortion would ever be granted in Australia but the position there is, again, complicated – this time by considerations of legality.[13] There is some flexibility in the United States where it has been said that the state courts believe the father to have a real interest in the fate of his fetus but that the woman's interest in her health and her freedom from unwanted pregnancy must prevail.[14] Relevant cases

---

7 For analysis, see B D Weinstein 'Do Pharmacists Have a Right to Refuse to Fill Prescriptions for Abortifacient Drugs?' (1992) 20 Law Med Hlth Care 220. This is from the American view where the matter is not addressed by statute – but the principles remain the same.

8 [1979] QB 276, [1978] 2 All ER 987; *Paton v United Kingdom* (1980) 3 EHRR 408.

9 [1988] QB 135, [1987] 1 All ER 1230, CA. See also p 112 above.

10 D M Yorke 'The Legal Personality of the Unborn Child' 1979 SLT 158.

11 P T O'Neill and I Watson 'The Father and the Unborn Child' (1975) 38 MLR 174.

12 *Wall v Livingston* [1982] 1 NZLR 734 (NZCA). The code of decision-making is laid down in the Contraception, Sterilisation, and Abortion Act (NZ) 1977.

13 *A-G of Queensland (ex rel Kerr) v T* (1983) 46 ALR 275 indicates the difficulties.

14 J L Caldwell 'Abortion: The Father's Lack of Standing' [1988] NZLR 165.

denying paternal rights to veto abortions are very old[15] and the door seems, now, to have been closed in *Planned Parenthood of Southeastern Pennsylvania v Casey*.[16] It is, however, in Canada that the fetus has been the least unsuccessful in obtaining paternal representation. Thus, in *Medhurst v Medhurst*[17] a husband was given standing to seek an injunction against abortion and in *Tremblay v Daigle*[18] it was considered that a potential father had as much right to speak on behalf of the fetus as anyone. Neither of these cases succeeded and they probably represent no more than the general willingness of the Canadian courts to grant a locus standi to interested parties.[19] Caldwell has drawn attention to the increasing erosion of the traditional role of the husband who is steadily undertaking a more caring role in the upbringing of his children. But it is doubtful if this will affect his future control over a pregnancy, for nothing can alter the fact that it is the woman who carries the fetus for nine months and whose health is mainly at risk during that time – and it is probably this factor which explains the difference in legal attitudes to the father's interest in his fetus and in his in vitro embryo.[20]

In our view, while acknowledging that the woman's right to control her body may well take precedence, the interests of the father still deserve more consideration than is currently afforded them. The potential harm or wrong done to the father by the destruction of his unborn child ought not to be ignored.

The nature of the doctor's duty
As yet the nature of the doctor's duties, in relation not only to the mother but also to the fetus itself, is not completely solved – and this is particularly so in the case of the fetus that is known to be defective. It is clear that the doctor then owes a duty of care to the mother under the terms of the Abortion Act 1967, s 1(1)(*b*). It could, however, be argued that he has a similar duty to the fetus in protecting it from a life of pain and suffering or from one which is diminished for other reasons. Actions for the dereliction, if any, of the duty to the fetus are known colloquially as suits for 'wrongful life' which are discussed in greater detail in chapter 6. For the present, it need only be said that the British position is summed up in the words of Stephenson LJ who asked how there could be imposed upon a doctor a duty towards the child to take away life by means of abortion:

> to impose such a duty towards the child would be to make a further inroad – in addition to that created by the Abortion Act 1967 – into the sanctity of human life which would be contrary to public policy.[1]

This view is not easy to accept as, apart from the saving of the mother's life, the 'eugenic' clause of the Abortion Act is probably that part which offends the Hippocratic conscience least.

15 *Coe v Gerstein* 41 L Ed 2d 68 (1973); *Doe v Doe* 314 NE 2d 128 (Mass, 1974); *Planned Parenthood of Missouri v Danforth* 428 US 52 (1976).
16 112 S Ct 2791 (1992).
17 (1984) 9 DLR (4th) 252.
18 (1989) 59 DLR (4th) 609.
19 Footnotes 17 and 18 above. See also *Re Simms and H* (1980) 106 DLR (3rd) 435.
20 See p 66 above.
 1 In *McKay v Essex Area Health Authority* [1982] 2 WLR 890 at 902, CA.

At the same time, Stephenson LJ agreed that there could be a duty to the mother to give her an opportunity to have the life of the fetus terminated. Such an action – for wrongful birth – is of a quality different from the wrongful pregnancy cases which have been discussed under 'Sterilisation' in chapter 4. The cause has been widely upheld in the United States[2] and the near inevitability of success in the event of a negligent failure to give advice or warning probably accounts for the lack of reported cases in the United Kingdom.[3] Such cases as do reach the reports are generally those which fail on the grounds of causation or of public policy.[4] It is in the nature of things that most wrongful birth actions arise from laboratory errors; as a result, the children are more usually damaged mentally than physically and often grow up in a loving environment.

Abortion and the incompetent

We have no reason to believe that termination of pregnancy in minors is to be regarded as different from any other aspect of medical treatment; the principles involved are, therefore, best considered within the whole spectrum of consent which is addressed in chapter 10. In theory, any concerns for the fetus must be added to the equation but, in practice, the courts will always put the interests of the young mother above those of her fetus in the event of conflict.

Specific problems as to confidentiality are, however, likely to arise in the unique context of under-age pregnancy and these merit consideration. These have caused particular concern in the United States where a distinction has been drawn between a duty to inform the parents of an impending procedure[5] and a need to obtain their authority.[6] There have been a number of conflicting decisions[7] but the matter has now probably been put beyond dispute in *Casey*[8] where the need for parental consent was confirmed.

In Britain, the concept of the 'understanding child' has gone unchallenged since it was first mooted by Butler-Sloss J in 1982.[9] There can, however, be no doubt that

---

2   *Curlender v Bio-Science Laboratories* 165 Cal Rptr 477 (1980); *Noccash v Burger* 290 SE 2d 825 (Va, 1982); *Robak v United States* 658 F 2d 471 (1981).

3   In *Salih v Enfield Health Authority* [1990] 1 Med LR 333, for example, only the quantum of damages was in issue.

4   *Scuriaga v Powell* (1979) 123 Sol Jo 406; See also *Rance v Mid-Downs Health Authority and Storr* [1991] 1 QB 587, [1991] 1 All ER 801, *Gregory v Pembrokeshire Health Authority* [1989] 1 Med LR 81.

5   *HL v Matheson* 101 S Ct 1164 (1981).

6   *Hallmark Clinic v North Carolina Department of Human Resources* 519 F 2d 1315 (1975).

7   In *Re T W* 551 So 2d 1186 (Fla, 1989), the court was unable to discern a compelling state interest in overriding a minor's right to privacy only when abortion was concerned. In *Hodgson v Minnesota* 110 S Ct 2926 (1990) and in *Ohio v Akron Center for Reproductive Health* 110 S Ct 2972 (1990) the Supreme Court held that only one parent need be notified. In both cases, however, it was noted that a judicial process to by-pass parental consent was sufficient protection for the minor. For discussion of the early cases, see H L Hirsch 'The Law Protecting Children in the United States' in J K Mason (ed) *Paediatric Forensic Medicine and Pathology* (1989).

8   *Planned Parenthood of Southeastern Pennsylvania v Casey* 112 S Ct 2791 (1992). The importance of the judicial by-pass was re-emphasised.

9   *Re P (A minor)* [1986] 1 FLR 272, 80 LGR 301.

to perform an operation without parental permission on a child too young to understand the issues (and, hence, to give a valid consent) would constitute an assault and, logically, this applies to an abortion. In practice, short of very intense religious views, it would be surprising if the parents of a girl below the age of 16 – and, therefore, below the age of marriage – were to object to the termination of her pregnancy. However, the question still remains – *must* the parents be informed prior to the legal termination of minor's pregnancy? The Abortion Act itself makes no distinction between age groups and, by implication, gives no grounds for supposing that the special conditions of abortion give rise to special rights to privacy. Yet it is hard to believe that all of the considerable number of abortions performed each year on 13-15 year-olds are carried out with parental knowledge. Again, we can turn to practical considerations among which it is reasonable to assume that the majority of children who are old enough to *become* pregnant are also old enough to understand the consequences; the conditions which can be extrapolated from *Gillick*[11] would apply. Thus, although the knowledge and agreement of the parents are clearly desirable, it is likely that a doctor who has made reasonable efforts to induce his patient to confide in her parents and is still faced with an adamant refusal of consent to disclosure and who goes on to terminate a minor's pregnancy would be secure from action in the courts or before the General Medical Council. The trend in medical, legal and social attitudes over the last decade gives added support to this view.

Almost certainly, many abortions have been carried out on the mentally handicapped under the twin cover of good medical practice and legal necessity. Authority for termination of pregnancy has probably also been obtained *in camera* on more than one occasion.[12] The legal uncertainties arising from the abolition of the courts' parens patriae powers to care for adult incompetents have now been largely dispelled in respect of termination of pregnancy. Abortion is to be distinguished from, say, sterilisation in that the former is governed by statute which gives sufficient protection to doctors provided they comply with its terms and a formal declaration of lawfulness by the High Court, is not, therefore, needed.[13] Ethical problems, however, linger on. Thus, although the very wide terms of the 1967 Act would be met in virtually any of the circumstances under consideration, one might, on occasion, question whether the termination was being undertaken for the benefit of society rather than for the genuine good of the pregnant woman – for any 'right to procreate' is violated as well by non-consensual abortion as it is by non-consensual sterilisation.[14] We can only suggest that this is an area where

---

10 For a case in which a mother opposed a termination for her 12 year old daughter, see *Re B (Wardship: Abortion)* [1991] 2 FLR 426.

11 *Gillick v West Norfolk and Wisbech Area Health Authority* [1986] AC 112, [1985] 3 All ER 402, HL. For a full discussion, see p 224 below.

12 F Gibb 'Judge Orders Abortion on Woman, Aged 25' (1987) The Times, 28 May, p 1 records the surprise of a judge when his decision was publicised.

13 *Re SG (Adult mental patient: Abortion)* [1991] 2 FLR 329, *sub nom Re SG (A patient)* (1990) 6 BMLR 95. Superseding *Re X* (1987) Times, 4 June.

14 M J Gunn 'Sex and the Mentally Handicapped: A Lawyer's View' (1986) 5 Med Law 255. The author believed that non-consensual abortion contravenes art 12 of the European Convention on Human Rights (the right to marry and to found a family) – but it seems difficult to apply if the woman concerned is unmarried.

clinical judgment is all important. Given that the Abortion Regulations 1991[15] are followed, we would agree that the routine involvement of the High Court serves no useful purpose.

Reduction of multiple pregnancy and selective reduction

The need for a reduction in the number of fetuses carried at one time has been discussed in chapter 3. Until recently, there has been considerable doubt as to the legality of the process once the conditions have been allowed to develop. Objections have been based mainly on terminological grounds. First, whether the phrase 'termination of pregnancy' in the 1967 Act relates to the pregnancy as a whole and, second, if this strict interpretation is inappropriate, whether individualised feticide in situ can be regarded as an abortion.[16] Whatever the solution of this interesting academic argument may be, the situation has now been resolved in practice – both selective reduction and reduction of multiple pregnancy in utero are legal when the requirements of the Abortion Act 1967, as amended, are fulfilled.[17] Thus, there is now no difficulty in justifying pregnancy reduction on the grounds that continuance of a multiple pregnancy would involve a risk of injury to the mental health of the pregnant woman. It might be equally appropriate to plead risk to the physical or mental health of the existing family – particularly if the intended remaining fetus or fetuses were regarded as 'existing children of the family'. Selective destruction of an abnormal fetus is, of course, justified under the serious handicap clause. Whether there is tort liability in the event of damage to a surviving fetus is arguable but the probability is that the doctor would not be liable in the absence of negligence in the operation.[18]

15 SI 1991/499.
16 For somewhat opposing views, see J Keown 'Selective Reduction of Multiple Pregnancy' (1987) 137 NLJ 1165 and D P T Price 'Selective Reduction and Feticide: The Parameters of Abortion' [1988] Crim LR 199.
17 Human Fertilisation and Embryology Act 1990, s 37(5) amending the Abortion Act 1967, s 5(2).
18 M Brazier 'A Legal Commentary' (1990) 16 J Med Ethics 68 in discussion of Jansen, fn 11, p 114, above.

6 Prenatal screening and wrongful life

The importance of genetically dependent diseases has risen as the control of those due to infection has increased. Currently, the proportion of childhood deaths attributable wholly or partly to genetic factors runs at about 50%.

Types of genetic disease

Genetic diseases are of three main types. The first is chromosomal – the structure or the number of chromosomes is altered and typical disease states arise, many of these being associated with mental illness. The classic example is Down's syndrome or mongolism. Some chromosomal abnormalities increase markedly with maternal age. Approximately 2% of women aged 40, left to uncontrolled pregnancy, will produce a chromosomally defective child, half of these suffering from Down's syndrome. By the age of 45, the risk of a mongol child rises to about 4%. There is some evidence that advanced paternal age may also be a risk factor.

The second group includes those conditions described as unifactorial in origin. Genes are positioned on chromosomes which exist in the cells in pairs, one member of each pair being derived from each parent. Unifactorial disease results from the presence of a specific abnormal gene and, since either of a pair of genes can be donated at random by either parent to their offspring, it is a simple calculation to determine the statistical probability of an infant being so endowed (see Fig 1, p 124, below). The genes may be 'autosomal dominants' – in which case they will express themselves, in this case as a disease, when the pair of genes contains only one which is abnormal. Normal natural selection should lead to the eradication of dangerous dominant genes. They may arise by mutation, or spontaneous change, a process which is greatly augmented by, say, ionising radiation, or the gene may possess some special attribute. Huntington's disease, for example, persists because the symptoms associated with the responsible gene often do not appear until after the age at which procreation usually takes place. Alternatively, the gene may be an 'autosomal recessive' in which case its expression is repressed by its normal dominant partner. Those persons possessing a single abnormal recessive gene will be 'carriers' of the disease with which it is associated. Frank disease will result only if an individual inherits the same two recessive genes – which means that both parents must have been carriers or one was a carrier and the other diseased. This, incidentally, provides the genetic basis for discouraging in-breeding.

Unifactorial disease may also be 'sex-linked' – or, better, 'X-linked'. Simplistically, this implies that the abnormal gene is present on part of the X chromosome which has no counterpart on the Y chromosome, the possession of

FIGURE 1 UNIFACTORIAL DISEASE

Father

Mother	N	N
N	NN	NN
A	AN	AN

(a)

Father

	N	A
N	NN	NA
A	AN	AA

(b)

Father

	X	Y
X	XX	XY
x	xX	xY

(c)

(a) The mother has an abnormal gene (A). If this is dominant, half the children will have the disease; if it is recessive, half the children will be carriers.

(b) Both the mother and the father have one deleterious recessive gene (A); half the children will be carriers and one in four will suffer from the disease.

(c) The mother is a carrier of an abnormal X-linked gene (x). Half the male children will have the disease and half the female children will continue to carry the disease.

which determines maleness. An abnormal recessive X-linked gene will be suppressed in the female by the dominant normal gene on the other X chromosome. It will, however, be free to express itself when coupled in the male XY configuration. Haemophilia is a classic example of such a disease.

The third group of disorders, referred to as multifactorial traits, is believed to be the result of both environmental factors and the effects of one or several genes. The environmental factors may also be of diverse types and interactions and it is, therefore, generally impossible to predict mathematically the occurrence of this commonest type of genetic disorder. Coronary heart disease, for example, is to some extent genetically determined but the occurrence of symptoms will depend upon a number of uncertain features such as the potential patient's job, diet, recreation and smoking habits. Such conditions, however, lie in the unpredictable future. We are, here, concerned with defects which can be demonstrated in utero and, in that respect, neural tube defects (spina bifida and anencephaly) are the most important multifactorial diseases.

Some form of behavioural or surgical treatment is available for those suffering from multifactorial disease and the same is true for a few unifactorial conditions. But there is no curative treatment for most of the more serious genetic disorders, the control of which then depends on prevention. This 'public health' objective is an important function of the genetic counsellor but its relative importance poses one of the major ethical problems of modern medicine – and one which is likely to increase in importance.

Genetic counselling[1]

Assessed as an arm of public health, the task seems easy yet, in practice, it abounds with practical, ethical and, inevitably, legal problems. Modern genetic counselling involves more than merely quoting risks. The ideal is to avoid a directive approach but, rather, to concentrate on the psychological circumstances so that couples can be led to make decisions which are right for them rather than right for the scientists. Almost inevitably, however, the counsellor's opinion will be sought and how this is reached depends particularly on whether the counselling is retrospective or prospective – are parents seeking advice because they already have an abnormal child or is the consultation based on information derived from other sources?

If the latter be the reason, the extent of the ethical difficulty depends on whether the couple are actually seeking advice or whether this is being offered to them. A request for guidance implies foreknowledge and understanding and poses relatively few problems. But what of the 85% of high risk couples who are reported as having no knowledge of their condition? In such circumstances, information must have come to the counsellor in ways which may well raise issues of confidentiality – particularly if those being counselled require to know the source. The problem of confidentiality has been considered by those advocating genetic registers, several of

---

1   This chapter was completed before publication of the important report: Nuffield Council on Bioethics *Genetic Screening: Ethical Issues* (1993). It has proved impossible to incorporate its findings in the text – but we do not think there are any fundamental differences between us.

which are successfully operated and which are approved by the World Health Organisation. Safeguards include that no-one shall be placed on the register without their consent and that security of access is strictly controlled.[2] Inevitably, however, the necessary information can be both better stored and better retrieved by computer; the conditions of the Data Protection Act 1984 provide further assurance that all entries will be accurate and consensual.

Even so, while the prevention of genetic disease may well be seen as admirable community medicine, there are difficulties when the principles are applied to the individual.[3] Should one impose knowledge on someone who has not sought it and who may well, perhaps irrationally, be disturbed as a consequence? At what stage should this knowledge be used? It is arguable that premarital advice is preferable to prenatal warning but such a policy has implications which are scarcely acceptable. On the other hand, has a doctor a moral duty to impose counselling? It might almost be asked if there is a legal duty in so far as an action might be brought were parents to discover after the birth of an abnormal child that relevant information had been available. For our part, we believe that, once the information is available, there is both a moral and a legal duty to use it but that this is determined to some extent by the severity of the condition and by the probability of it being passed on to children. Perhaps illogically, we feel that information and guidance which have not been requested should be given only in the event of pregnancy – many who would resent gratuitous advice that they were, or might be, carriers of a disease would adopt a completely different attitude were it known that a child was involved. The force of the counter-argument is, however, appreciated. In any event, the information should be passed only to the general practitioner of the subject; he alone is able to assess the family situation in the light of all the background knowledge.

A word should be interpolated here on the very specific problems arising from the relationship of genetic testing to life insurance – although those associated with health insurance would be even more pressing in countries lacking a national heath service. In some ways, the dilemmas are similar to those found in testing for HIV infection which we have discussed at p 24. The main practical difference lies in the compulsory disclosure of a family history in all insurance proposals. Since a positive history will, of itself, result in discrimination, there is considerable pressure on the individual to undergo testing in order to indicate the absence of risk – the person with a family history of Huntington's disease provides the classic example. More significant are the cases discovered in the absence of any family indication. The occasions on which this could affect the individual tested are, currently, few but, as discussed below (at p 127), the effect on other family members may be serious. One might ask, in particular, when does a positive test become a family history?

2　For a review of the principles of genetic registers see A E H Emery et al, 'A Report on Genetic Registers' (1978) 15 J Med Genet 435. For later consideration of the issues see J Knox *Clinical Genetic Services in Scotland: Report of a Working Party of the National Medical Consultative Committee* (1987), SHHD.

3　For general discussion of the implications of imparting genetic knowledge, see I Pullen 'Patients, Families and Genetic Information' in E Sutherland and A McCall Smith (eds) *Family Rights* (1990) ch 3. But not everyone would see a contradiction between concern for the genetic health of the population and concern for the problems of the individual family: see, for example, R F Chadwick 'What Counts for Success in Genetic Counselling?' (1993) 19 J Med Ethics 43.

Moreover, the number of significant abnormalities which could be disclosed is increasing and could escalate as the enthusiasm of geneticists grows in parallel with the map of the human genome – reports of varying credibility appear, for example, of the discovery of genetic markers for homosexuality[4] and of a propensity to heart disease. The Association of British Insurers has said that 'it does not intend to ask proposers for life insurance to undergo screening for genetic information within the foreseeable future, but where individuals have had a specific test as part of their medical assessment these tests will fall into the same category as other medical tests and must be declared on proposal forms'.[5] Under the common law, fortified by the Access to Medical Reports Act 1988, disclosure of test results is entirely at the discretion of the individual. The importance of a genuinely 'informed' consent to the original test is, thereby, underlined. It has been suggested by Harper that insurers should not be allowed to require disclosure of genetic test results within the ordinary run of life insurance policies. Whether it is right that the increased costs of such a scheme should be passed on to the 'normal' population is probably a matter for Parliament to decide. We take the view that it would be a small price to pay for a gesture of support for those who, through no fault of their own, are likely to find themselves increasingly disadvantaged.

But to return to the mainstream. In the great majority of cases, the genetic counsellor will be consulted retrospectively because an abnormal child has been born and his opinion is asked as to the advisability of further pregnancy. The solution of the problem is still difficult but, with one exception, the goal is reasonably clear. The exceptional difficulty arises, again, in connection with other members of the family, especially the siblings of the unfortunate parents. Given the fact that the doctor or his specialist adviser now knows that they are in the high risk category, should he so inform them? Clearly, this cannot be done without the consent of the affected couple but, even when this is given, the problems of providing unsought, and perhaps unwanted, information are revived. There are, in our opinion, unassailable reasons why the relatives should not be informed directly but there seems little doubt that their practitioners should be advised of the position. The practitioner's decision must, in turn, depend upon the severity of the disease and the likelihood of its reappearing. As in the case of the propositus family, he or she must also be influenced by the family circumstances as a whole.

As to the couple's immediate problem, the counsellor can virtually never make a firm statement as to having or not having a further child. He can take extraneous circumstances – eg religious or financial status – into consideration but, in the end, he is down to speaking about probabilities. In the case of unifactorial disease, he can give accurate figures – ie if both the mother and father carry recessive deleterious genes, the chance of an overtly affected child is one in four pregnancies.

---

4   Caution is recommended by M Baron 'Genetic Linkage and Male Homosexual Orientation' (1993) 307 BMJ 337.
5   Quoted in the invaluable paper: P S Harper 'Insurance and Genetic Testing' (1993) 341 Lancet 224. The author points to the doubt as to whether genetic counselling can be seen as part of a 'medical assessment'. The majority approach would seem to be much the same in the United States: B R Furrow 'Cystic Fibrosis and DNA Tests' (Book review) (1993) 19 Amer J Law Med 177. For experience elsewhere, see S Gevers 'Use of Genetic Data, Employment and Insurance: An International Perspective' (1993) 7 Bioethics 126.

The position as to chromosomal disease is rather more complicated. In the usual circumstance, the condition is due to trisomy in which three similar chromosomes are present in the cells rather than a pair; this is a chance occurrence which cannot be predicted mathematically. Males with trisomy-21 or Down's syndrome are sterile but there is the theoretical risk that half the children of a female sufferer will also have the chromosomal defect. In practice, not only is such a pregnancy unlikely but, also, more than half of any affected fetuses will miscarry naturally. However, rather under 5% of Down's syndrome patients are not trisomic but, instead, demonstrate a chromosomal abnormality known as translocation – parts of chromosome-21 are exchanged for those of another.[6] This may also occur sporadically but, once it has done so, a carrier state can develop and affect one in three children. Passage to later generations is, thus, possible and its occurrence will be independent of maternal age. The counsellor must, therefore, consider each sub-type of chromosomal disorder separately.[7] In the event of a multifactorial condition, the probabilities can only be derived in an empirical fashion. Even then, the prospects are subject to interpretation. Thus, presented with a child with spina bifida, one can say there is a 10% chance that the couple will have a further child with developmental abnormality; it will sound quite different when expressed as a 90% chance of a normal infant. Moreover, 9 to 1 are acceptable odds to many; others might regard anything less than 99 to 1 as an unacceptable risk. In the end, the choice rests with the couple and this choice is a product of their ability to understand and the skill of the counsellor.

Which is, perhaps, an easy enough thing to say but is, at the same time, a statement fraught with underlying ethical difficulty. One has to ask, first, whether the goal of an free patient choice is possible, given the fact that, once genetic counselling has been offered and accepted, a likely chain of events has already been set up in the minds of all those involved.[8] Clarke also asks whether the objective is, itself, morally defensible – or have we, for fear of being labelled eugenists, 'fled so far from medical paternalism that we deny ethical responsibility for our professional activities?' Moreover, the whole concept of genetic counselling can be questioned insofar as it increasingly involves the systematic selection of fetuses and, hence approaches children as consumer objects subject to quality control.[9] The increasing 'need' for genetic counselling can be seen as being based on the increasing number of disorders which can be diagnosed and, as Lippman has said, before long, the definition of fetal imperfection will come to mean any condition which can be diagnosed in utero. The social and economic pressures on a woman to terminate a pregnancy once an abnormality is discovered in her fetus are such that her autonomous choice is severely prejudiced. These pressures would escalate were the somewhat bizarre

6   Some readers may require a more detailed explanation than we have space for. A readable description is to be found in A E H Emery *Elements of Medical Genetics* (6th edn, 1983), ch 4.
7   The risk is 1:3 rather than the anticipated unifactorial 1:4 because a quarter of the conceptuses will be monosomic and will die in utero. The significance of translocation disease was noted in *Gregory v Pembrokeshire Health Authority* [1989] 1 Med LR 81.
8   See, particularly, A Clarke 'Is Non-directive Genetic Counselling Possible?' (1991) 338 Lancet 998.
9   Much of this discussion is founded on A Lippman 'Prenatal Genetic Testing and Screening: Constructing Needs and Reinforcing Inequities' (1991) 17 Amer J Law Med 15.

suggestion adopted that the cost-efficiency of a genetic counselling service could be gauged by the number of abortions performed.[10]

One thing is certain, no woman can be forced to destroy her fetus. There is no legislative basis for such a suggestion which has strong overtones of positive eugenics.[11] However, in advising, the counsellor has several options: he can dismiss the risks, he can advise sterilisation of either partner, he can put the options of artificial insemination by donor or of ovum donation, or he can arrange for a suitably controlled pregnancy coupled with the alternatives of live birth or abortion as conditions indicate.

Controlled pregnancy

The counsellor may have advised a pregnancy or he may be presented for the first time with a couple in whom the wife is already pregnant. In either event, should he feel that a risk exists, he now has at his disposal a considerable technical armamentarium to help in closing the gap between probability and certainty. His methods may be non-invasive or invasive.

Non-invasive techniques

X-rays of the fetus are contra-indicated save in an emergency. The modern alternative is visualisation by means of ultrasound. This is accepted as being innocuous as far as the fetus and mother are concerned and is widely used in obstetric management – so much so that testing may well be considered to be governed by implied consent alone;[12] moreover, its use in locating the placenta is an essential prerequisite to amniocentesis, chorionic villus sampling and fetoscopy.[13] Ever-increasing technical and interpretative skills have transformed ultrasonography from a fairly crude diagnostic tool to one which is capable of demonstrating not only major external abnormalities, such as spina bifida or anencephaly, but also congenital disease of the internal organs and minor defects such as cleft lip – not to mention the sex of the baby. The processes of obstetric management and genetic counselling are, therefore, irrevocably entwined and it is important that the woman is aware of the implications, which are similar to those we discuss below under amniocentesis. The clinician who discovers a fetal abnormality as a by-product of management can scarcely conceal his knowledge while the woman, for her part, may be ill-prepared to receive it. The case for what is commonly known as informed consent (see p 237) to ultrasonography is strong. It is an interesting psychological side-effect of the process that many parents regard the sonogram as their first 'baby-picture' –

---

10 For discussion, and rejection, see A Clarke 'Genetics, Ethics, and Audit' (1990) 335 Lancet 1145; R F Chadwick 'What Counts for Success in Genetic Counselling?' (1993) 19 J Med Ethics 43.

11 A V Campbell 'Ethical Issues in Prenatal Diagnosis' (1984) 288 BMJ 1633. See also *Emeh v Kensington and Chelsea and Westminster Area Health Authority* [1985] QB 1012 at 1024, [1984] 3 All ER 1044 per Slade LJ at 1053, CA.

12 See A Lippman, 'Prenatal Genetic Testing and Screening: Constructing Needs and Reinforcing Inequities' (1991) 17 Amer J Law Med 15. It is difficult to know how seriously we should take suggestions such as ultrasound predisposing to, say, left-handedness: K A Salvesen, L J Vatten, S H Eik-Nes et al 'Routine ultrasonography in utero and subsequent handedness and neurological development' (1993) 307 BMJ 159 – perhaps they should serve as gentle reminders.

13 See below at p 131.

something which tends to endow the fetus with a recognisable personality. This, in itself, has some influence on the management decision.[14]

Maternal invasion

Fetuses with neural tube defects – spina bifida or anencephaly – secrete an excess of the protein α-fetoprotein into the amniotic fluid and some of this is transferred to the maternal circulation. Testing the maternal serum thus offers a simple and risk-free method of diagnosing abnormality in the fetus and is very acceptable to mothers. While 80-90% of neural tube defective fetuses can be diagnosed in this way, the test is best regarded as a major indication of the need for amniocentesis.[15] Conversely, it is now recognised that a low maternal concentration of α-fetoprotein is associated with Down's syndrome in the fetus.[16] Other maternal serum constituents – eg unconjugated oestriol and human chorionic gonadotrophin – are also influenced; a very effective rate of diagnosis of Down's syndrome can be achieved by combining such analyses with consideration of the mother's age[17] and the number of appropriate markers is likely to increase. Most practitioners, however, probably would still wish to offer amniocentesis or chorionic villus sampling to women aged over 35 years and at, generally, higher risk. Nonetheless, the introduction of a relatively cheap and effective test raises the possibility of extending routine testing to all pregnant women rather than to the older group alone. Here, however, we enter the realm of resource allocation – a subject dealt with in detail in chapter 11. For the present, we only draw attention to the conflict which arises between those who would hold to the assumption that 'because a test is possible, testing should be implemented as a service' and[18] those who emphasise the importance of cost-effectiveness before a new policy is established – in itself, often a source of contention.[19] The potential dangers of the former policy are shown by the mounting of an action for negligence in not disclosing the merits of the improved test at a time when it was scarcely beyond the development stage.[20]

Serum tests are best performed at about 16 weeks' gestation; reliance on maternal serum for diagnosis thus leads to late terminations when they are indicated whereas the current emphasis is on identifying chromosomal abnormalities in early pregnancy (see p 131 below).

---

14 D Callahan 'How Technology is Reframing the Abortion Debate' (1986) Hastings Center Report, February, p 33.
15 D J H Brock 'Impact of Maternal Serum Alpha-fetoprotein Screening on Ante-natal Diagnosis' (1982) 285 BMJ 365.
16 H S Cuckle, N J Wald and R H Lindenbaum 'Maternal Serum Alpha-fetoprotein Measurements: A Screening Test for Down's Syndrome' (1984) 1 Lancet 926.
17 N J Wald, A Kennard, J W Densem et al 'Antenatal Maternal Serum Screening for Down's Syndrome: Results of a Demonstration Project' (1992) 305 BMJ 391.
18 Editorial Comment 'Screening for Fetal Malformations' (1992) 340 Lancet 1006
19 See, for example, M Connor 'Biochemical Screening for Down's Syndrome' (1993) 306 BMJ 1705. The original article sparked a massive correspondence, most of which was doubtful of the justification for extended screening; see correspondence columns (1992) 305 BMJ 768 et seq.
20 A Ballantyne 'Mother Sues over Lack of Down's Test' (1992) The Sunday Times, 23 August, p C5. The outcome of the case is not known; it may, in fact, have lapsed for want of legal aid.

Uterine invasion

The commonest invasive techniques for prenatal diagnosis which involve the fetus or its environment are amniocentesis and chorionic villus sampling. The former is technically easier and carries a lesser risk to the pregnancy. Despite the theoretical advantages of the latter, amniocentesis is still probably the most popular method of direct investigation in the United Kingdom.

More than 1% of British mothers undergo amniocentesis. The process consists of needling the sac surrounding the fetus and withdrawing fluid which contains excretions and metabolites of the fetus together with representative cells. The cells can then be grown in culture for chromosomal studies and to detect certain metabolic diseases; the fluid can also be used for biochemical testing.

Biochemical tests can be made rapidly and can directly diagnose some rare diseases of defective metabolism of the gargoylism type. The onset of 'rhesus disease' can also be detected. But by far the most important test is for α-fetoprotein by means of which an efficient laboratory can now diagnose all neural tube lesions. Cell culture can indicate the presence of chromosomal disorder in some 10–20 days. In expert hands, the presence of what are termed 'inborn errors of metabolism' can be detected after some six weeks' culture.

On the face of things, therefore, amniocentesis provides very powerful means of preventing genetic disease but, at the same time, it presents both technical and ethical problems. First, the number of centres practising amniocentesis is limited. A 'defensive' policy of amniocentesis for all would offer little or no benefit in terms of the proportion of positive results and would impose considerable strain on manpower resources. In practice, some selection has to be imposed and it has been suggested that routine amniocentesis should be offered only to mothers with a raised serum α-fetoprotein, those who already have a child with neural tube defect or in whom there is such a family history, those with a family history of chromosomal abnormality and mothers over the age of 35.[1] Even in the best hands, an adequate amount of fluid can only be obtained after about the 14th week of pregnancy, although the use of sophisticated ultrasonography may reduce this to 12 weeks. No fluid is obtained in some 5–10% of cases and the test must then be repeated. Add to these factors the time required for effective cell culture and it will be seen that one is close to producing a viable infant – and a consequently more hazardous operation in the event that termination of pregnancy is indicated.[2]

These concerns can, however, be reduced by the use of chorionic villus sampling – or removal and study of the early placental cells; used in conjunction with recombinant DNA techniques, it may revolutionise the diagnosis and management of genetic disease.[3] Chorionic villus sampling suffers in being of no value in the identification of neural tube defects; the incidence of doubtful chromosomal analyses is some four times greater than that following amniocentesis; it is more expensive, and, currently, the risk of miscarriage following the procedure is certainly greater – possibly up to four times that associated with amniocentesis. Against this, chorionic

---

1 For a full analysis of screening methods for fetal abnormality see J G Evans (Chairman) 'King's Fund Forum Consensus Statement: Screening for Fetal and Genetic Abnormality' reported in (1987) 295 BMJ 1551. See also H M Kingston 'Prenatal Diagnosis' (1989) 298 BMJ 1368.

2 The Human Fertilisation and Embryology Act 1990, s 37(4) has eliminated the legal concern here; the aesthetic distaste for, and the comparative danger of, late abortions remains.

3 For a good account of the latter, see A E H Emery *An Introduction to Recombinant DNA* (1984).

villus sampling provides a good source of fetal DNA. Perhaps the most important practical consideration lies in the fear that early villus sampling may result in facial or limb abnormalities in an otherwise normal fetus.[4] For all these reasons, the early enthusiasm with which the procedure was greeted has waned somewhat. It should probably be reserved for those women who are at greatest risk – and, therefore, most likely to seek an early termination – or for cases where there is a single gene defect likely to require diagnosis.[5]

Amniocentesis itself is said to carry a fetal mortality rate of up to 0.5%. Slight though this may be, it is still not inconsiderable and, again, indicates the need for case selection – particularly if fertility is already low. It, too, cannot be used in a 'blanket' fashion – only specific diseases can be sought and discovered. Moreover, irrespective of negligence, some false positive or false negative tests are inevitable and will increase with the complexity of the tests undertaken. For all these reasons, research and, indeed, paediatric opinion are now directed towards primary prevention – for example, towards identifying the underlying environmental causes in multifactorial disease.

Limitations of technique give rise to ethical, as well as practical, problems. Although modern techniques of gene marking have reduced the toll,[6] a proportion of normal male children at risk of X-linked disease are still legally aborted. Again, a raised α-fetoprotein level does not give a clear indication of the degree of neural tube defect.[7] The routine abortion of fetuses with any detectable spinal abnormality will, therefore, result in the destruction of some salvageable children. On the other hand, 10–20% of 'missed' cases will have a severe defect and will require much corrective surgery. Similarly, the presence of the typical chromosomal abnormality does not indicate the likely severity of Down's syndrome. There are other problems of interpretation. For example, given a chromosomal abnormality, what does it mean? Certain arrangements are well known to be associated with severe disease but in others (notably the 'XYY syndrome') the evidence is by no means clear.[8] XYY boys are said to be prone to vicious behaviour but 'prone' is a very relative concept. Should doctors, on the one hand, seek to abort all such fetuses as a precaution or, on the other, inform the parents of the risk, allow the pregnancy to run naturally and, thereby, possibly tarnish the parent/child relationship irrevocably? What is one to do when one of the other common aberrations of the sex chromosomes (eg Klinefelter's (XXY) or Turner's (XO) syndrome) is discovered?[9] Such abnormalities are often, but not always, associated with a degree of infertility or mental dysfunction. The variations are so many that it is impossible to generalise. The essential point is

4 H V Firth, P A Boyd, P Chamberlain et al 'Severe Limb Abnormalities after Chorionic Villus Sampling at 56-66 Days' Gestation' (1991) 337 Lancet 762.
5 R J Lilford 'The Rise and Fall of Chorionic Villus Sampling' (1991) 303 BMJ 936.
6 For example, markers are already available for cystic fibrosis, Duchenne muscular dystrophy and Huntington's disease.
7 This situation may be improved by combining α-fetoprotein analyses with high quality ultrasonography: M J Seller 'Is Antenatal Selection for Spina Bifida Possible?' (1990) 301 BMJ 251.
8 See L Taylor 'Genetically Influenced Antisocial Behaviour and the Criminal Justice System' (1982) 33 NILQ 215.
9 J M Connor 'Prenatal Diagnosis of the Turner Syndrome: What to Tell the Parents' (1986) 293 BMJ 711.

that patients who request or consent to antenatal diagnoses of this type must fully understand the extent of their consent and must be aware of the potential consequent decisions to be made.[10] Some might wish to be informed of every item of information which has come to light while others might require to know only of conditions which have a fully understood and significant prognosis. Much subsequent searching of conscience can be avoided by preparatory discussion of the issues.

At the same time, as we have already intimated, the doctor's own motivation, prejudices and failings cannot be discounted. Much will depend upon whether, and to what extent, he sees himself as a community rather than a personal physician – and how much that is personal to the woman or to her progeny. We have already concluded that it is well-nigh impossible to perform an illegal therapeutic abortion in Great Britain but the clinician is still confronted with the moral problems inherent in the interpretation of 'severe handicap' in the Abortion Act 1967, s 1(1)(*d*). It is, for example, possible to construct an argument which casts doubt on the ethical justification for abortion even in such a serious condition as Huntington's disease.[11] What may seem, at first sight, to be an uncomplicated and desirable procedure presents, in the end, as a Pandora's box of moral uncertainties.

Some of the difficulties can be overcome by more modern techniques. Fetoscopy, for example, allows for direct inspection of the fetus and, thence, an assessment of the degree of abnormality. At the same time, fetoscopy carries with it a fetal mortality of about 1%. Fetal blood sampling, originally developed for the diagnosis, inter alia, of the haemophilias has had a relatively short life as the need for such relatively dangerous investigations recedes with the availability of recombinant DNA techniques.[12] Mention must also be made of the potential for embryo biopsy as an answer to the very high risk pregnancy. This technique combines in vitro fertilisation with removal and genetic analysis of single cells from eight cell embryos followed by selection of those found to be normal for implantation. This immediately raises the question of the status of the surplus embryo which we discuss in detail at p 62. Here, it need only be noted that many would argue that embryocide is preferable to – or, perhaps, less reprobate than – feticide. The procedure also carries the many difficulties associated with in vitro fertilisation of itself (see chapter 3) and we would align ourselves with those who doubt whether its benefits outweigh the imposed emotional and financial costs.[13]

But increasing sophistication to some extent only serves to underline the fundamental moral issue of prenatal screening which is – how far is one to go in defining abnormality? Is the 'perfect baby' to be encouraged?[14] The concept of parents obtaining a termination on the grounds of, say, the sex of the child may seem

---

10 An interesting survey is reported by H Statham and J Green 'Serum Screening for Down's Syndrome: Some Women's Experiences' (1993) 307 BMJ 174.
11 S G Post 'Huntington's Disease: Prenatal Screening for Late Onset Disease' (1992) 18 J Med Ethics 75.
12 N M Fisk and S Bower ' Fetal Blood Sampling in Retreat' (1993) 307 BMJ 143.
13 A very good discussion is to be found in M Michael and S Buckle 'Screening for Genetic Disorders: Therapeutic Abortion and IVF' (1990) 16 J Med Ethics 43.
14 R F Chadwick 'The Perfect Baby: An Introduction' in R F Chadwick (ed) *Ethics, Reproduction and Genetic Control* (1987) p 93. See also E Yoxen *Unnatural Selection* (1986).

frivolous – or unprincipled – to many, but, as we discuss at p 101, it may be medically defensible and, by extension, legal. One can foresee more generally applicable dilemmas of conscience. Cases of Down's syndrome or of spina bifida which have not been discovered through prenatal screening are already candidates for neonaticide or local authority care. Is such disposal to run parallel with an increasing prenatal diagnostic capability when, as a result, more parents reject what will be regarded as imperfect children on increasingly demanding criteria? It is for such reasons that we argue later in favour of legislation which ensures that, whatever may be the legal situation of the fetus, the interests of the neonate are paramount.

On the other side of the coin, it seems clear that genetic counsellors should not overemphasise the interests of the state in reducing the incidence of genetic disease and, as clinicians, should not join with the scientists in welcoming the genetic issue as 'unstoppable'.[15] Rather, the aim should be to concentrate on the particular circumstances and interests of the parents in wanting a child. An elderly couple, for example, might see a pregnancy as their last possibility and might prefer to take their chance in the ignorant way of natural parenthood – and they should be allowed to do so. Similarly, a woman who has managed to conceive by assisted means may rightly refuse to take the risks involved in chorionic villus sampling or amniocentesis. Actions for wrongful life and for wrongful birth, which are, essentially, actions for negligence brought over genetic counselling, must be viewed in the light of this complex and, sometimes, conflicting moral background.

Counselling and negligence

If a genetic counsellor or doctor fails either to advise prospective parents of the risk of genetic illness, or to carry out and interpret correctly appropriate diagnostic procedures which would disclose abnormality in the fetus, the parents of an afflicted child may choose to raise an action against him in respect of his negligence. The counsellor or doctor owes them a duty of care in which he has failed; the parents may contend that, as a result, they have been deprived of the opportunity to terminate the pregnancy and are now burdened with a sick or handicapped child. Such an action, brought by and on behalf of the parents, is generally known as one for wrongful birth. Damages may be sought in respect of the distress occasioned the parents by the existence of the defect in their child and in respect of the extra costs which are entailed in bringing up the child.

The courts in the United States were at first divided in their attitudes to such actions but have steadily become more amenable to recognising damages for the birth of a handicapped child as a legitimate claim. In *Becker v Schwartz*,[16] the New York Court of Appeals allowed a parental claim for damages in respect of the cost of the institutional care of a child suffering from Down's syndrome. The negligence in question was the failure of the doctor to recommend amniocentesis to a 37-year-old mother who, by virtue of her age, had a relatively high risk of bearing a

15 Editorial Comment 'Ethics and the Human Genome' (1991) 351 Nature, (Lond) 591 quoted by
  A Clarke 'Is Non-directive Genetic Counselling Possible?' (1991) 338 Lancet 998.
16 386 NE 2d 807 (NY, 1978).

handicapped child. The courts have, however, found difficulty, in the resultant conflict of interests. On the one hand, there is the question of public policy which should, in theory at least, favour birth over abortion.[17] On the other hand, the woman's prerogative to control her own body, and the consequent acceptability of abortion, are being increasingly recognised. The rule which is apparently emerging is that, while wrongful life actions (see p 140 below) will fail, the corresponding claim for wrongful birth will succeed.[18] Even so, the causation problem remains. It is, for example, still up to the plaintiff to convince the court that, given the information, she would have undergone a termination.[19] The causation issue also arises in damages. In *Noccash v Burger*,[20] for example, widely-based damages were awarded for the birth of an infant with Tay-Sachs disease but costs concerned with the child's funeral were disallowed on the grounds that the fatality was the result of hereditary factors rather than of the defendant's negligence. Other difficulties relate to the fact that pregnancy has been actually sought in these cases. Should the damages awarded then reflect the full costs of rearing a defective child or should they be limited to the difference in financial burden posed by a normal and a handicapped infant? Should they extend to compensation for emotional distress? These questions seem to be very finely balanced in the American courts.[1]

Comparable cases are rare in the United Kingdom but the limited reports indicate that the courts are wrestling with very similar problems. There is no doubt that damages will be awarded in respect of negligent counselling; in other words, a wrongful birth action is available in the United Kingdom and we suspect that most cases are settled out of court.[2] The case of *Salih v Enfield Health Authority*[3] is interesting as it was specifically concerned with quantum. It was held at first instance that the parents were entitled to claim for the basic cost of bringing up the child, not just the difference between normality and abnormality. The parents wanted a child but the cost of maintaining a handicapped child was something they did not want. The only other apposite report we have found is that of *Gregory v Pembrokeshire Health Authority*.[4] In this somewhat unusual case, the trial judge found that the doctors' neglect to inform of the failure of an amniocentesis was a breach of the duty of care. The action failed, however, on grounds of causation, the plaintiff having failed to convince the trial court, or the Court of Appeal, that she

---

17 See, for example, *Azzolino v Dingfelder* 337 SE 2d 528 (NC, 1985) and *Siemieniec v Lutheran General Hospital* 512 NE 2d 691 (Ill, 1987).
18 *Smith v Cote* 513 A 2d 341 (NH, 1986); *Proffitt v Bartolo* 412 NW 2d 232 (Mich, 1987) – where the inconsistency of dissociating the two types of action was vented.
19 *Dumer v St Michael's Hospital* 233 NW 2d 372 (Wis, 1975) – cf the English case of *Gregory* fn 4 below.
20 290 SE 2d 825 (Va, 1982).
1 See G G Sarno 'Recoverability of Compensatory Damages for Mental Anguish or Emotional Distress for Tortiously Causing Another's Birth' (1989) 74 ALR 4th 798.
2 *Rawnsley v Leeds Area Health Authority* (1981) The Times, 17 November, p 2 is an example of an unreported case. For general discussion of the liability of genetic counsellors, see M L Lupton 'The Impact of Genetics on Society: The Law's Response' (1991) 10 Med Law 55.
3 [1990] 1 Med LR 333. The ruling was overturned on appeal but this was by reason of the special circumstances of the case: [1991] 2 Med LR 235, (1991) 7 BMLR 1.
4 [1989] 1 Med LR 81.

would have had a second investigation had she been offered one. Once again, the courts seem to be being particularly protective of the medical profession.

The rights of the fetus

The basis of a parental claim may be clear enough, but what is the juristic nature of a claim brought on behalf of the child itself? The status of the child in utero is legally established – the fetus has a general right not to be injured by the wrongful act of a third party. This right was recognised at common law in Canada and in Australia respectively in two important decisions, *Duval v Seguin*[5] and *Watt v Rama*.[6] Similar recognition is afforded to the fetus by the common law in Scotland and has been held retrospectively to have existed in England prior to the Congenital Disabilities (Civil Liability) Act 1976.[7]

The most important aspect of these rights in the present context relates to the responsibilities of the mother to her fetus. The Law Commission considered this question and decided that an action against its mother in respect of damage resulting from her negligence during pregnancy should not be available to a child. It was felt that a claim of this type would compromise the parent/child relationship and might also be used as a weapon in matrimonial disputes. Accordingly, the English legislation excludes claims by a child against its mother except as to injuries sustained during traffic accidents. Here, special policy grounds and the availability of insurance were held to justify the admissibility of such claims.[8] The matter remains open in Scotland because there is no legislation on the subject and there is no reason in law to exclude a claim by a child against its mother in respect of prenatal injuries. It is possible, however, that the courts may be unsympathetic to such claims on policy grounds.

It is also difficult to determine the extent to which the mother's duty of care towards her unborn child might be held to limit her freedom of action during pregnancy. Interest in this aspect of the fetal/maternal relationship escalated in the past decade.[9] The fetus has emerged as a patient in its own right and major attention has been directed to the use of alcohol and other drugs, including tobacco, on fetal morbidity and mortality – and it is almost certain that the last word on the subject has not yet been said. A few years ago, it was easy to hold that social smoking and drinking of alcohol could hardly be viewed in law as negligence. Yet there is virtually irrefutable evidence of their harmful effect on the fetus and, at least in the former context, negligent injury to other parties has been successfully litigated or

5   (1973) 40 DLR (3d) 666.
6   [1972] VR 353.
7   See *Burton v Islington Health Authority*; *de Martell v Merton and Sutton Health Authority* [1992] 3 All ER 833, (1992) 10 BMLR 63.
8   An apposite case, possibly the prototype, has been reported by C Dyer 'Boy Wins Damages after Injury in Utero' (1992) 304 BMJ 1400.
9   See, for example, E W Keiserlingck 'A Right of the Unborn Child to Pre-natal Care – the Civil Law Perspective' (1982) 13 Rev de Droit 49; P L Hallisey 'The Fetal Patient and the Unwilling Mother: A Standard for Judicial Intervention' (1983) 14 Pac LJ 1065; J L Lenow 'The Fetus as a Patient: Emerging Rights as a Person' (1983) 9 Amer J Law Med 1.

settled out of court.[10] It seems only a matter of time before the neonate – who could not even protest at the passive smoking to which he was subjected in utero – can sue for the damage done although, admittedly, success would be difficult if not impossible in England by virtue of the Congenital Disabilities (Civil Liability) Act 1976, s 1(1).

The problem of parental neglect in the form of refusal of treatment in the fetal interest is becoming more controversial as the opportunities become ever more feasible. This has had comparatively little impact in Britain. We suspect that the great majority of women who have carried a fetus long enough for it to be available for treatment are anxious that it should survive to childhood. Most fetal treatments, or other interventions in the pregnancy on behalf of the fetus, are carried out in a consensual medical environment. The greater publicity attracted in the United States may reflect no more than a stiffer polarisation of attitudes and this leads to more conflicts of conscience which can be resolved only in the public courtroom.[11] There are a number of precedents where a mother has been ordered to undergo treatment, including Caesarian section, on behalf of the fetus[12] and, occasionally, such directions end disastrously. The exemplar case is *Re A C*[13] where a Caesarian section was ordered against the wishes of a moribund woman suffering from malignant disease in an attempt to salvage a 26-week-old fetus – the mother survived only long enough to see her baby die in a matter of hours. Brahams noted that the case should sound a warning bell to all interventionists in Britain. The majority of commentators adopted a similarly cautious approach to the subject on the grounds, among others, that it is nearly impossible to balance the benefits to the fetus against the reasonableness of withheld consent,[14] that unwanted intervention must injure the maternal doctor/patient relationship and that the standards of enforcement would be uneven. Although it is clear that, in general, we support the notion of fetal rights, we would align

10 D Brahams 'Tobacco Litigation (USA, UK and Australia)' (1992) 340 Lancet 230; 'Passive Smoking' (1993) 341 Lancet 552. *Bland v Stockport Metropolitan Borough Council* unreported – discussed by C Dyer 'UK Woman Wins First Settlement for Passive Smoking' (1993) 306 BMJ 351. See also S Chapman and S Woodward 'Australian Court Decision on Passive Smoking Upheld on Appeal' (1993) 306 BMJ 120 for the Australian courts' view of passive smoking.
11 There is some disagreement as to how often this occurs. L J Nelson and N Milliken 'Compelled Medical Treatment of Pregnant Women: Life, Liberty and Law in Conflict (1988) 259 J Amer Med Ass 1060 is at some odds with V E B Colder, J Gallagher and M T Parsons 'Court-ordered Obstetrical Interventions' (1987) 316 New Engl J Med 1192. See also N Rhoden 'The Judge in the Delivery Room: The Emergence of Court-ordered Cesarians' (1986) 74 Calif LR 1951. For a contrary view, see E-H W Kluge 'When Caesarian Operations Imposed by a Court are Justified' (1988) 14 J Med Ethics 206.
12 For example, *Raleigh Fitkin-Paul Morgan Memorial Hospital v Anderson* 201 A 2d 537 (NJ, 1964); *Jefferson v Griffin Spalding County Hospital Authority* 274 SE 2d 457 (Ga, 1981).
13 533 A 2d 611 (DC, 1987). For discussion, see D Brahams 'A Baby's Life or a Mother's Liberty: A United States Case' (1988) 56 Med-leg J 156; M A Field 'Controlling the Woman to Protect the Fetus' (1989) 17 Law Med Hlth Care 114.
14 There is, nonetheless, a tide in favour of some sort of balancing act. Thus, in *Taft v Taft* 446 NE 2d 395 (Mass, 1983), the court refused surgical intervention but might have been prepared to accept medical treatment of the fetus. See F A Chervenak and L B McCullough 'Perinatal Ethics: A Practical Analysis of Obligations to Mother and Fetus' (1985) 66 Obst Gynecol 442. The views of F H Miller 'Maternal-Fetal Ethical Dilemmas: A Guideline for Physicians' (1991) 10 Seminars Anaesth 157 are particularly attractive.

ourselves with this view in the special circumstances of *Re A C* – a view which has now been vindicated by the District of Columbia Appeal Court. There, the court vacated the judgment in *Re A C* and, by a 7:1 majority, held that the right to informed consent encompassed a right to informed refusal of treatment and that a fetus cannot have rights in this respect superior to those of a person who has already been born. Even so, the door was not quite shut:

> We do not quite foreclose the possibility that a conflicting State interest may be so compelling that the patient's interest must yield but we anticipate that such cases will be extremely rare and truly exceptional[15]

One such case has arisen in England and has provoked a similar discussion. In *Re S*,[16] a woman who had been in labour for several days with the fetus impacted in a transverse lie steadfastly refused to undergo Caesarian section due to her strongly held religious belief. The clinicians appealed to the court and a declaration was granted to the effect that, the operation being in the vital interests of the patient and the unborn child , it could be performed lawfully despite the woman's refusal to give consent. Apparently paradoxically, we support this decision – *Re A C* and *Re S* provide perfect examples of circumstances altering the case. While Sir Stephen Brown P emphasised that the life of the unborn child was at risk (to the extent that it could only be born alive by Caesarian section), there was also no question but that the mother would die in great pain in the absence of surgical intervention; by contrast, there was no way in which maternal death could be avoided in *Re A C*. The case is, however, better discussed under 'Consent' (see ch 10).

But, whatever compromise is reached by the lawyers, the doctor's dilemma persists whenever, and in whatever context, he seeks to protect the fetus from its mother. Once he agrees to intervene on behalf of the fetus – or, more contextually, to treat it individually – he has both a moral and a legal duty to treat it with all due care. The problem, therefore, lies in the original acceptance of the unborn as a patient. We suggest that prudence should dictate a very cautious approach to fetal therapy which could, in the great majority of instances, be properly withheld until birth.

Scrutiny of the interplay of fetal rights and maternal lifestyle has been nowhere more intense than in the United States where well over 6,000 children are born each year suffering from the fetal alcohol syndrome and where the occurrence of drug withdrawal symptoms in neonates increased by 450% from 1984 to 1986.[17] There, the state has not only a right but also a duty to protect its children under the parens patriae jurisdiction and there is little doubt that this extends to an interest in the well-

---

15 Per Terry J in *Re A C* 573 A 2d 1235 (DC, 1990).   See D Brahams 'Enforced Caesarian Section: A US Appeal' (1990) 58 Med-leg J 164.

16 *Re S (Adult: Refusal of medical treatment)* [1992] 4 All ER 671, (1992) 9 BMLR 69.

17 For recent data, see E J Larson 'The Effects of Maternal Substance Abuse on the Placenta and Fetus' in G B Reed (ed) *Diseases of the Fetus and Newborn* (2nd ed, 1994); W A Vega, B Kolody, J Hwang, and A Noble 'Prevalence and Magnitude of Perinatal Substance Exposures in California' (1993) 329 New Engl J Med 850.

being of the 'viable' fetus.[18] Cases of fetal neglect that have come before the courts have been assessed both under the common law and through the federal and state legislation prohibiting child abuse and neglect. As might be expected, the outcomes have not been entirely consistent. The most extreme example that we have noted concerned a mother whose infant was born brain damaged and was found to have ingested amphetamines and cannabis. The mother was charged in the criminal court with omitting to furnish necessary medical attendance or other remedial care but the case was dismissed on the grounds that there was no statutory basis for the charge.[19] Such instances are often reported only anecdotally but a number of civil actions have been officially reported. These suggest that the fetus enjoys an enhanced standing in such courts and, having been born, may be able to sue on its own behalf.[20]

The courts in Canada have also appreciated the concept of intra-uterine child abuse and have immediately placed in care and protection neonates who have been subjected seriously to drugs or alcohol during pregnancy.[1]

Just such an eventuality arose in England in *D (a minor) v Berkshire County Council*[2] when the House of Lords upheld a decision to make a care order in respect of a child born prematurely and suffering from drug dependency. The House held that the words: '[The child's] proper development is being avoidably prevented or neglected' in the Children and Young Persons Act 1969, s 1(2)(*a*), referred to a continuing, rather than an instant, situation. So long as there was a genuine continuum, conditions both before birth and in the hypothetical future could be taken into account when assessing a neonate's need for care and control. The decision caused considerable concern: first, on the grounds that its application to family law might be extended to the criminal field and, second, because it denied the drug addicted mother the right to prove her capacity for motherhood. For ourselves, we see *D v Berkshire CC* as yet another case that was decided on its own facts. There is no reason to suppose that a similar decision would be taken in every instance – only that the remedy is there should it be needed in serious cases.[3]

D v Berkshire CC is an example of fetal 'rights' maturing at birth but the English courts have not, however, gone so far as to extend such rights to existence in utero. In *Re F (in utero)*,[4] the local authority sought to make the fetus a ward of court so that it could be protected from its mother who was leading a nomadic existence and who, shortly before the child was due, went missing as she had done on previous occasions. The application was refused both at first instance and in the Court of Appeal on the grounds that, until the child was actually born, there would be an inherent incompatibility between any projected exercise of the wardship jurisdiction

---

18 For an early exhaustive review of the US scene, see J E B Myers 'Abuse and Neglect of the Unborn: Can the State Intervene?' (1984) 23 Duquesne LR 1. A recent note, written from an interesting feminist perspective, is to be found in R I Solomon 'Future Fear: Prenatal Duties Imposed by Private Parties' (1991) 17 Amer J Law Med 411.

19 For this and similar cases, see Solomon, footnote 18 above.

20 *Grodin v Grodin* 301 NW 2d 869 (Mich, 1981). See also *Re Vanessa F* 351 NYS 2d 337 (1974).

1 *Re Children's Aid Society of Kenora and JL* (1982) 134 DLR (3d) 249; *Re Superintendent of Family and Child Service and McDonald* (1982) 135 DLR (3d) 330.

2 [1987] AC 317, [1987] 1 All ER 20, HL.

3 The court will certainly use its power. In *Re P (a minor) (child abuse: evidence)* [1987] 2 FLR 467, CA a place of safety order was granted on the day of a child's birth into a family which had a history of sexual abuse.

4 [1988] Fam 122, [1988] 2 All ER 193. The Canadian courts have also followed *Re F*: see *Re Baby R* (1989) 53 DLR (4th) 69.

and the rights and welfare of the mother. Relying heavily on *Paton v British Pregnancy Advisory Service Trustees*,[5] the Court of Appeal first concluded that the fetus had no individual personality and that, therefore, there could be no jurisdiction in wardship and, second, it made it clear that, in practice, it would be impossible to follow the principle of the paramountcy in wardship of the child's welfare if that conflicted with the liberty and legal interests of the mother.

The reasons for seeking fetal protection in *Re F* were, we feel, far less pressing than were those in, say, *D v Berkshire CC*; the nature of any maternal improbity differed and it is possible to explain the two decisions in that simple light.[6] Nonetheless, *Re F* is the more significant in that it lays down a principle which is likely to be followed in the absence of Parliamentary intervention. Any rights vested in the fetus are strictly circumscribed and, as we have previously seen under the terms of the Congenital Disabilities (Civil Liability) Act 1976, s 1(1), there can be no action against the mother for negligent injury inflicted in utero. Whether or not one agrees with such a loading of the odds, there is little doubt that it has to be accepted on pragmatic grounds. There is simply no practical way in which the criminal law could be invoked so as to control a pregnant woman's smoking, eating or sexual habits, nor is it desirable – amongst other ill-effects, doctors would be turned into police informers. We can also foresee great difficulty in proof of causation; teratogenic effects are maximal in the first trimester of pregnancy and the further in time that the cause is removed from the visible effect, the more difficult it becomes to associate the two. The whole subject is intimately related to any supposed neonatal right to be born healthy – which leads to a consideration of the 'wrongful life' suit.

Diminished or wrongful life actions

Apart from the straightforward case of an injury to the fetus in utero, a child born with an abnormality may argue that some other sort of wrong has been done to it. First, he or she may claim that there was negligence prior to its conception, and that this negligence has resulted in its being born with certain abnormalities. An example of such a claim is provided by the American case of *Yeager v Bloomington Obstetrics and Gynaecology Inc*.[7] This concerned a child born suffering from brain damage due to haemolytic disease of the newborn which occurred because the hospital negligently failed to treat rhesus immunisation of the mother during a previous pregnancy. The court held it to be reasonably foreseeable that subsequent children would be injured as a result. Such a claim would also be competent in English law provided that, at the time of conception, the parents were not aware of the risk that their child would be born disabled. This exemption does not apply if, in an action by the child against its father, it is established that the father knew of the risk while the mother did not.[8]

---

5   [1979] QB 276, [1978] 2 All ER 987.
6   It is noteworthy that the Court of Appeal was unable to see any logical difference between the early and the 'viable' fetus as regards a need for protection (per Balcombe LJ, [1988] Fam 122 at 142, [1988] 2 All ER 193 at 199).
7   585 NE 2d 696 (Ind, 1992). For earlier examples, see *Lazevnick v General Hospital of Monro County Inc* 499 F Supp 146 (Md, 1980); *Jorgensen v Meade-Johnson Laboratories* 483 F 2d 237 (1973); *Renslow v Mennonite Hospital* 367 NE 2d 1250 (Ill, 1977).
8   Congenital Disabilities (Civil Liability) Act 1976, s 1(4).

The child may also bring a claim in respect of its 'wrongful life'. The basis of this claim is that, through the negligence of the defendant, the child's parents were not afforded the opportunity to abort the fetus and as a result, the child seeks damages for the impaired existence he or she is now being forced unwillingly to lead. The negligence in question may occur either before the child's conception – as, for example, in a case of negligent genetic counselling – or after conception – as when a doctor fails to detect an abnormality in the fetus. A high proportion of such cases result from laboratory errors which are, in general, clearly recognisable as negligent.

The history of the wrongful life action can be traced through the US courts. Attempts to extend the cause of action to merely being born have, not unnaturally, received short shrift.[9] Suits brought by defective children, however, pose difficulties with which the American legal system has been struggling for many years. In *Gleitman v Cosgrove*,[10] the plaintiff was born deaf, mute and nearly blind as a result of his mother's exposure to German measles during pregnancy. The Supreme Court of New Jersey dismissed the plaintiff's claim for damages against the doctors who were alleged to have told the mother that there was no risk of German measles harming her child. The basis for dismissal was that its acceptance would amount to a statement that it was better not to be born at all than to be born handicapped. It was logically impossible, the Court felt, to weigh the value of a handicapped life against non-existence. As it was expressed:

> It is basic to the human condition to seek life and to hold on to it however heavily burdened. If Jeffrey [the plaintiff] could have been asked as to whether his life should be snuffed out before his full term of gestation could run its course, our felt intuition of human nature tells us he would almost surely choose life with defects against no life at all. For the living there is hope, but for the dead there is none . . .

A year later, the claim of a child similarly damaged by its mother's illness was rejected on the grounds that to allow a claim based on failure to abort the plaintiff would be the antithesis of the principles of the law of tort which is directed towards the protection of the plaintiff against wrongs. The greatest wrong, it was pointed out by the court, is to cause another person's death.[11] In other cases, the courts have chosen to reject the claims of handicapped children on the grounds that it is impossible to assess the child's damages.[12]

There is no indication that the courts, in refusing the children's claims, have intended to limit compensation for this type of negligence. Actions by the parents for emotional shock, expenses incurred in rearing a defective child and the like have been successful and the trend has been, as explained in *Robak v United States*,[13] to focus on the family as the true object of the claim. This was emphasised in *Prokanik*

9 *Beardsley v Wierdsma* 650 P 2d 288 (Wyo, 1982).
10 296 NYS 2d 687 (1967).
11 *Stewart v Long Island College Hospital* 296 NYS 2d 41 (1968).
12 For example, *Dumer v St Michael's Hospital* 233 NW 2d 372 (Wis, 1975); *Blake v Cruz* 698 P 2d 315 (Idaho, 1984); *Smith v Cote* 513 A 2d 341 (NH, 1986); *Cowe v Forum Group Inc* 575 NE 2d 630 (Ind, 1991).
13 658 F 2d 471 (1981).

v Cillo,[14] which was a rare instance of a wrongful life action being accepted. The main reason for so doing was that the parents were time barred and could not sue on their own behalf. In line with other common law jurisdictions, the American courts will, where it is possible, allow the neonate a suit for pre-natal injury while denying one for wrongful life.[15]

We have found only one straightforward instance of a wrongful life action being allowed in full.[16] This case was effectively overturned by the Supreme Court of California in *Turpin*[17] when it adopted the principle of allowing the suit to proceed and accepting a claim to special damages (ie those incurred as a result of the congenital defects) but not to general damages. The basis for the restriction on general damages lay in the still insoluble problem of comparing an impaired existence with not being born at all. The movement towards acceptance of the suit has, however, been arrested and there is now a definite trend in favour of rejecting such claims in toto.[18] The plaintiff in *Bruggeman v Schimke*[19] averred that actions for wrongful life were being increasingly recognised but the court replied that this was simply not true and that any theory sustaining a legal right to be dead rather than to be alive with deficiencies was one completely contrary to the laws of the state. In practical terms, children are unlikely to be disadvantaged when an action for wrongful life fails. Since the courts allow the parents to recover the medical expenses in rearing a defective child, the child's separate claim will apply only to expenses incurred after reaching majority. In most cases, the defect will be so serious that the damaged child will never achieve that age. Even so, both the US courts and the state legislatures appear increasingly concerned to express their preference for birth over abortion – and this to the extent that not only wrongful life but also wrongful birth actions may be rejected.[20]

A similar judicial antipathy to abortion is to be seen in the only apposite English case – *McKay v Essex Area Health Authority*.[1] Prior to this Court of Appeal decision, the Law Commission had considered the merits of the wrongful life action in its Report on Injuries to Unborn Children[2] and had come to the conclusion that it should not be allowed. The gravamen of this recommendation lies in the belief that to allow such actions would place 'an almost intolerable burden on medical advisors' who might be under 'subconscious pressures' to advise abortions in doubtful cases. As a result of these recommendations, the Congenital Disabilities (Civil Liability) Act

---

14 478 A 2d 755 (NJ, 1984). A similar option has been left open more recently: *Viccaro v Milunsky* 551 NE 2d 8 (Mass, 1990).
15 Eg, *Cowe v Forum Group Inc* 575 NE 2d 630 (Ind, 1991).
16 *Curlender v Bio-Science Laboratories* 165 Cal Rptr 477 (1980).
17 *Turpin v Sortini* 182 Cal Rptr 377 (1982). Also followed in *Harbeson v Parke-Davis Inc* 656 P 2d 483 (Wash, 1983).
18 See, for example *Ellis v Sherman* 515 A 2d 1327 (Pa, 1986); *Proffitt v Bartolo* 412 NW 2d 232 (Mich, 1987); *Cowe*, fn 15 above.
19 718 P 2d 635 (Kan, 1986).
20 *Azzolino v Dingfelder* 337 SE 2d 528 (NC, 1985). For major reviews, see E H Morreim 'The Concept of Harm Reconceived: A Different Look at Wrongful Life' (1988) 7 Law & Philos 3; B R Furrow 'Actions for Wrongful Life' in J K Mason (ed) *Paediatric Forensic Medicine and Pathology* (1989) ch 26.
1 [1982] QB 1166, [1982] 2 All ER 771, CA.
2 Law Com no 60.

1976, s 1(2)(*b*) appears to exclude the right of a child to sue in such circumstances.[3] The infant plaintiff in *McKay* was, however, born before 22 July 1976 and, therefore, did not come within the ambit of the Act; the issue of wrongful life was, therefore, open to the Court.

In this case, the mother of the handicapped child had been in contact with the virus producing German measles and had consulted her doctor. A blood sample was taken but this was mislaid. A second sample of blood was taken and the mother was duly informed that neither she nor the infant had been infected with rubella. However, the infant girl was found to be severely handicapped when she was born. The plaintiffs alleged that there was negligence on the part of the defendants in that they either failed to carry out the necessary tests on the blood samples or failed to interpret them correctly. A number of claims were made as a result of this alleged negligence, including a claim by the child for damages in respect of entry into a life of distress and suffering.

The court discussed the major issues of legal policy to which this case gave rise in an extensive judgment. While recognising that there was no reason why a mother in such circumstances may not be able to claim in respect of the negligent failure to advise her of her right to choose abortion, the court was not prepared to recognise any claim by a child to damages for wrongful life. The grounds on which this decision was reached are similar to those which have appeared in the American cases.

The initial analysis is in terms of the duty of the doctor. The doctor clearly owes to the fetus a duty not to do anything to injure it, but what duty is owed to a fetus which has been damaged by some agency for which the doctor can bear no responsibility – in this case by the rubella virus? The only duty which the court could see would be an alleged duty to abort the fetus and the question then to be considered was whether this could ever be legal.[4] As to 'wrongful life', it was held that an *obligation* to abort:

> would mean regarding the life of a handicapped child as not only less valuable than the life of a normal child, but so much less valuable that it was not worth preserving, and it would even mean that a doctor would be obliged to pay damages to a child infected with rubella before birth who was in fact born with some mercifully trivial abnormality. These are the consequences of the necessary basic assumption that a child has a right to be born whole or not at all, not to be born unless it can be born perfect or 'normal', whatever that may mean.[5]

Having declined to find a duty basis of the claim, the court also cavilled at the difficulties of assessing damages in such a case. Here the impossibility of comparison argument was seen as a strong one: how could a court compare the value of a flawed life with non-existence or, indeed, with any 'after life' which an aborted child was experiencing? The Court declined to undertake any judgment on the conflicting views of theologians and philosophers on the latter aspect. Even faced with this

---

3 A good argument can, in fact, be made out that wrongful life actions are not excluded: J E S Fortin 'Is the "Wrongful Life" Action Really Dead?' [1987] JSWL 306. See also the commentary on *Cowe v Forum Group Inc*: A Grubb [1993] 1 Med LR 262.

4 This attitude, particularly as related to rubella immunisation, is challenged by Morreim, fn 20, p 142 above.

5 Per Stephenson LJ [1982] QB 1166 at 1180, [1982] 2 All ER 777 at 781.

conceptual difficulty, Stephenson LJ was of the opinion that it was better to be born maimed than not to be born at all except, possibly, in the most extreme cases of mental and physical disability – which provokes the questions: 'what is extremity?' and 'by what right do the courts take the view that existence is always to be preferred to non-existence?' The decision is, surely, one which should be left to the handicapped child by way of substituted judgment.

The doubtful aspect of the wrongful life action lies in the fact that it requires that the court should say to the plaintiff: 'Yes, it would be better had you not been born'. This judgment, however sympathetic to the motives behind it, would seriously compromise the value of human life which the courts are more usually called upon to endorse. The disabled should be helped and, if possible, compensated for the suffering which their lives may entail but the moral basis for such compensation should be the desire to make life more comfortable and bearable – not the notion that they should not be in existence at all.

In line with this argument, we believe that the conceptual difficulties would largely disappear if, first, the Abortion Act 1967, s 1(1)(*d*) (the 'eugenic clause') were accepted as having been drafted in the fetal, rather than the maternal, interest.[6] The right of the handicapped fetus to abortion is then comparable to the defective neonate's right to refuse treatment (see ch 7 below). Failure to respond to the interests of either, albeit necessarily expressed by proxy, then falls into the ambit of consent-based negligence (see ch 10). In effect, the fetus is saying: 'but for the negligent advice given to me through my parents, I would not have chosen a disadvantaged condition; I now have to be disadvantaged and, therefore, I am entitled to compensation'. Second, we favour abandoning the principle of 'wrongful life' in favour of 'diminished life'. The comparison, then, is not the stark choice between non-existence and current existence but, rather, that between current existence and normality – at least the courts could not then claim that they had no yardstick on which to judge.[7]

There are, we admit, philosophical objections to this approach – especially that, in the majority of instances, the particular neonate had no opportunity to lead a normal life. Nonetheless, the practical counter-arguments that it is a proposition that the courts can understand and that it allows for distinction to be made between serious and slight defect seem to us to have greater force. Recently, Lord Donaldson MR, in a comment on *McKay*, has explained that the child also claimed that, if her mother had received appropriate treatment, her disabilities would have been less. She therefore, sought damages based on the difference between her quality of life as it was and the quality of life which she would have enjoyed if her mother had been treated – and this claim was allowed to proceed.[8] This is very close to an action for diminished life and is an aspect of *McKay* which merits closer study – though there seem to be no reports of the action.

Powerful legal and philosophical arguments can be adduced in favour of rejecting the wrongful life action, yet intuition urges that justice is, thereby,

---

6   For discussion, see J K Mason *Medico-Legal Aspects of Reproduction and Parenthood* (1990) p 132.

7   The case for the child's action was well put by T K Foutz '"Wrongful Life": The Right Not to be Born' (1980) 54 Tul LR 480.

8   *Re J (a minor) (wardship: medical treatment)* [1990] 3 All ER 930 at 935, (1990) 6 BMLR 25 at 31, CA.

thwarted.[9] It is interesting that at least one jurisdiction has accepted the infant plaintiff's cause when confronted with the problem de novo.[10]

Gene therapy

Advances in screening are only one aspect of the progress which has been made in human genetics over recent decades. Perhaps more significantly from the scientific point of view, possibilities have opened up for manipulation of the genes of existing and future individuals. This is best known as gene therapy, or, in some contexts, as genetic engineering. Inevitably, it has given rise to considerable bioethical debate.[11]

Gene therapy may be of two types – somatic or germ-line. Somatic gene therapy is directed towards the remedying of a defect within the patient and involves the insertion of genetic material which will perform some function which the patient's own genetic material is failing to do. Germ-line gene therapy can be visualised in two ways – the insertion of genetic material into the pre-embryo, which is pre-emptive treatment of the future being and his or her progeny, or as the insertion of a gene into the germ cells of an individual. The latter therapy has no direct bearing on the individual but is intended to ensure that any subsequent children are born with or without certain characteristics. Although the scientific techniques involved are in their infancy, both forms of manipulation have already spawned considerable and emotional debate. Indeed, genetic engineering is one of the few modern medical technologies in which study of the moral aspects has preceded the practical realities.

The ethical implications of somatic gene therapy were considered by the Committee on the Ethics of Gene Therapy (the Clothier Committee) which reported in 1992.[12] The Committee thought that this form of treatment was uncontroversial, if novel, and felt that it gave rise to no new ethical challenges. We can accept this assessment; the goals of somatic gene therapy are identical to the goals of other forms of treatment and, provided that it does not involve undue risk to the patient or to others, it is ethically as acceptable as is drug therapy or surgical intervention. There may be a need for caution if somatic gene therapy is developed so as to combat behavioural disorders but, even then the ethical considerations will be similar to those which already arise from the use of psychotropic drugs or psychosurgery and which are discussed in greater detail in chapter 18.

The controversial nature of germ-line gene therapy, whether directed to the pre-embryo or to an individual's germ cells, rests on its capacity to change future people. Some such changes will, in themselves, be unobjectionable. It is difficult, for example, to find grounds for objection to preventive medicine which will ensure that the bearers of a serious genetically transmissible disease will not pass the condition

---

9   M Slade 'The Death of Wrongful Life: A Case for Resuscitation?' (1982) 132 NLJ 874; G E Jones and C Perry 'Can Claims for "Wrongful Life" Be Justified?' (1983) 9 J Med Ethics 162; B Dickens 'Wrongful Birth and Life, Wrongful Death Before Birth, and Wrongful Law' in S A M McLean (ed) *Legal Issues in Human Reproduction* (1989) ch 4.
10 J Levi 'Wrongful Life Decision in Israel' (1987) 6 Med Law 373.
11 See, for example, P Wheale and P McNally *Genetic Engineering: Catastrophe or Utopia?* (1988).
12 *Report of the Committee on the Ethics of Gene Therapy* (1992).

on to their children. Such medical practice is no different from other, long-accepted, efforts to eradicate disease within the human population and which, arguably, interfere with the natural order to a comparable degree.

The difficulty that some have with any form of germ-line therapy is that of the 'slippery slope' which is encountered at a number of points in medical jurisprudence.[13] If we allow germ-line therapy in relation to, say, a seriously debilitating disease, then how are we to prevent its use to eliminate characteristics which we would not, currently, label as a defect but which may be considered undesirable? Rifkin has put the question as follows:

> Once we decide to begin the process of human genetic engineering, there is really no logical place to stop. If diabetes, sickle cell anaemia, and cancer are to be cured by altering the genetic make-up of an individual, why not proceed to other 'disorders': myopia, colour-blindness, left-handedness? Indeed, what is to preclude a society from deciding that a certain skin colour is a disorder?[14]

This represents a bleak view of scientific ambitions but the concern that it expresses for possible abuse has been potent enough to mean that a number of governmental or other official bodies have taken the step of forbidding germ-line gene therapy. The Council of Europe was, initially, sufficiently suspicious to recommend a complete prohibition on such practice on the grounds of its insult to human dignity but, later, modified this view to allow germ cell manipulation for therapeutic purposes.[15] In Germany, the total outlawing of germ-line therapy has been recommended and this view was endorsed in a statement from the medical research councils of eleven European states in 1988.[16]

However, germ-line gene therapy is not without its supporters. As Harris has asked: is there anything really wrong in wanting to have a fine child?[17] The real difficulty lies in distinguishing between eugenically-motivated, or enhancement, germ-line manipulation on the one hand and truly therapeutic intervention on the other. It should be necessary to forbid *all* work in this area only if it is felt that the demarcation line can never be held . Unfortunately, science's bad record in keeping to a narrow, acceptable track lends some force to the arguments of those who would prevent such meddling altogether. It certainly seems to us to be one of those subjects which should only be acceptable following wide and informed public discussion.

13 N Holtug 'Human Gene Therapy: Down the Slippery Slope' (1993) 7 Bioethics 402.

14 J Rifkin *Algeny* (1983) p 232, quoted by Holtug, fn 13 above at p 405.

15 Council of Europe *Recommendation 934 on Genetic Engineering* (1982); *Recommendation 1100 on the Use of Human Embryos and Foetuses in Scientific Research* (1989).

16 M A M de Wachter 'Ethical Aspects of Human Germ-line Gene Therapy' (1993) 7 Bioethics 166. The tone of the Declaration of Inuyama and Report of a Working Group on Human Gene Therapy is cautious but not prescriptive. It is reproduced and discussed in J C Fletcher and W F Anderson 'Germ-line Gene Therapy: A New Stage of Debate' (1992) 20 Law Med Hlth Care 26.

17 J Harris 'Is Gene Therapy a Form of Eugenics?' (1993) 7 Bioethics 178.

7 The defective neonate

When the first edition of this book was written, selective non-treatment of the newborn and, most particularly, withholding the means of survival from mentally handicapped infants were burning issues. The legal and ethical standards in this area are, however, now relatively stabilised. Nonetheless, the principles established and the practices condemned in the management of the defective neonate have provided a template for similar decisions which are now being made as a routine throughout life. Much as we predicted originally, selective non-treatment of the newborn has progressed to the selective non-treatment of the defective child while 'nursing care only' for the infant is now mirrored in withdrawal of sustenance from the severely brain-damaged adult – it is somewhat ironic that the long and careful deliberations of the House of Lords in *Airedale National Health Service Trust v Bland*[1] can trace their origins to the thoroughly unsatisfactory case of *R v Arthur*.[2] It is also only logical that discussion of the defective neonate should follow discussion of wrongful birth and wrongful life. For all these reasons, we have decided to retain this chapter as a separate entity while emphasising that it deals with what is no more than the first act in the wider drama of euthanasia.

Even so, selective non-treatment of the newborn[3] retains its unique features. It concerns human beings who are at the most vulnerable period of their lives – human beings, moreover, who cannot express their feelings for the present or the future. As such, it poses different ethical problems from those associated with euthanasia at the end of life and it may well be that the two states demand different legal rules. Also, it is intimately bound up with the subject of abortion.

Several methods, which we have discussed in some detail in chapter 6, are available for the diagnosis of chromosomal, genetic and physical disorders in the fetus. Many can be detected early in pregnancy when probably the majority would support a prophylactic termination. But what of those which come to full term undiagnosed? Where does public opinion and the law stand between the opposite extremes, on the one hand, of an absolute right to life and, on the other, of a positive policy of elimination of the imperfect? There has to be a middle road but, in contrast to the abortion issue, we must now find it without the aid of statute.

---

1 [1993] 1 All ER 821, (1993) 12 BMLR 64, HL.
2 (1981) The Times, 6 November, pp 1, 12, (1981) 12 BMLR 1.
3 We have retained this expression because it is well established. Paediatricians will, however, point out that it covers a period of care which demands particular clinical and nursing skills. Everyone should read I Laing 'Withdrawing from Invasive Neonatal Intensive Care' in J K Mason (ed) *Paediatric Forensic Medicine and Pathology* (1989).

Sanctity or quality of life?

The doctors' dilemma is self-evident – are they practising truly 'good' medicine in keeping alive a neonate who will be unable to take a place in society or who will be subject to pain and suffering throughout life? In short, is one to sacrifice the Hippocratic, and theological, concept of the sanctity of life and adopt, instead, a standard related to the quality of life?[4] The situation gives rise to a catalogue of almost unanswerable questions. Who is to determine the minimum quality of life? Whose life are we considering – the infant's or are we also taking into account that of the parents or, indeed, the well-being of society? Do we, in fact, *want* a society in which the right to life depends upon achieving a norm which is largely measured in material terms? Should the abnormal infant who resolutely refuses to die be helped on its way – and, if so, is this help to be a matter of omission or should positive steps be taken to end life? In the discussion of euthanasia which follows in chapter 15, stress is laid on the relationship between the quality of life and the proportionate or disproportionate treatment which is needed to maintain that quality. But the quality of the therapeutic environment at the beginning of life is very hard to assess. Not only can the patient express no opinion but, were it possible, he or she has no yardstick by which to judge; as put by the Canadian McKenzie J:

> . . . he would not compare his life with that of a person enjoying normal advantages. He would know nothing of a normal person's life having never experienced it.[5]

As an inevitable result, parents must be invited to make 'life or death' decisions on behalf of their abnormal offspring and they will be guided by the doctor whose advice is likely to be on the lines that consideration for the preservation of life is secondary to that of preventing suffering. Medical leadership has supported this parental responsibility – 'in the absence of a clear code to which society adheres, there is no justification for the courts usurping the parents' rights'[6] – and it has been backed by influential academic legal thought – 'the criminal law should stay its hand. The decision of the parents should prevail'.[7] All of which may be good medico-social economics but it is far from certain that it is good ethics.

The rights of the neonate

In our view, the newly born baby has the same rights to self-ownership of the body as has every human being. This proposition is, however, increasingly under attack as the definition of personhood in terms of intellect is developed. We have already observed that, if it is valid to treat the fetus as a non-person, it is also valid to use the same parameters by which to deny personhood to the neonate. There are, indeed,

---

4　A very full review of the whole question is to be found in L Gostin 'A Moment in Human Development: Legal Protection, Ethical Standards and Social Policy in the Selective Non-treatment of Handicapped Neonates' (1985) 11 Amer J Law Med 31.
5　*Re Superintendent of Family and Child Service and Dawson* (1983) 145 DLR (3d) 610 at 621.
6　Editorial Comment 'The Right to Live and the Right to Die' (1981) 283 BMJ 569.
7　G Williams 'Life of a Child' (1981) correspondence, The Times, 13 August.

those who are prepared to equate the status of 'infanticide' with that of 'feticide'[8] – or even of contraception. Certainly, it may well be that the obligation to maintain human life is not absolute[9] which, presumably, justifies Dr Dunn's evidence at the trial of Dr Arthur (see p 151 below):

> no paediatrician takes life but we do accept that allowing babies to die is in the baby's interest at times[10]

– and the wealth of distinguished supporting evidence showed that this is clearly acceptable paediatric practice.

This expert opinion embodies a number of assumptions:

(a) that there is an essential difference between activity and passivity when the same end – death – is realised by either and, arising from this, that passivity does not conflict with the doctor's duty to 'maintain life from the time of conception';[11] moreover, passivity is clinically preferable from the patient's viewpoint;

(b) that there is a point at which death is preferable to life; and

(c) that someone can decide that point in surrogate fashion and that it is right and proper for someone to act on that judgment.

The legal position

Yet this seems to come perilously close to breaking the law. To kill a living human being deliberately is murder and, except in relation to the specific crime of infanticide,[12] the age of the victim has no relevance. Killing a child by omission could be prosecuted under the Children and Young Persons Act 1933, s 1; it is more likely to be charged as manslaughter although it could be murder[13] – the paramount considerations being whether or not there is a duty of care and, if there is, what is the extent of that duty.[14] It is difficult to see how the consultant in charge of the paediatric ward does not have a duty of care to his patients. Yet, anything up to 30% of deaths in a neonatal intensive care unit follow the deliberate withdrawal of life support[15] and we have Farquharson J charging the jury in the leading apposite criminal case:

8 See in particular H Kuhse and P Singer *Should the Baby Live?* (1985) ch 6. Other more recent observations along the same lines include J G Bissenden 'Ethical Aspects of Neonatal Care' (1986) 61 Arch Dis Childh 693; C Wells 'Whose Baby Is It?' (1988) 5 J Law & Soc 323.

9 As argued by G Williams 'Down's Syndrome and the Doctor's Responsibility' (1981) 131 NLJ 1040.

10 *R v Arthur* (1981) The Times, 6 November, pp 1, 12, (1981) 12 BMLR 1 at 18. Dr Dunn would now consider withholding life saving treatment from only three groups of neonate: those with severe malformations, those with severe hypoxic/traumatic brain damage and those of extreme prematurity with major problems such as brain haemorrhage – P M Dunn 'Appropriate Care of the Newborn: Ethical Dilemmas' (1993) 19 J Med Ethics 82.

11 Declaration of Geneva (see appendix B).

12 Infanticide Act 1938.

13 *R v Gibbins and Proctor* (1918) 13 Cr App Rep 134, CCA.

14 *R v Stone; R v Dobinson* [1977] QB 354, [1977] 2 All ER 341, CA.

15 A Whitelaw 'Death as an Option in Neonatal Intensive Care' [1986] 2 Lancet 328; C H M Walker '. . . Officiously to Keep Alive' (1988) 63 Arch Dis Childh 560.

I imagine that you will think long and hard before concluding that doctors, of the eminence we have heard, . . . have evolved standards that amount to committing a crime.[16]

Case law

The law in this area has been clarified in the present decade. Nonetheless, we must look at the early cases because they demonstrate vividly the dilemmas involved and they form the base from which the modern position has evolved. This is particularly so of *Re B (a minor) (wardship: medical treatment)*,[17] the judgment in which has been said to represent the law in this particular field.[18]

The circumstances leading up to the Court of Appeal hearing in *Re B* could be described as bizarre and typified the medical and legal uncertainties at the time concerning parental power to veto life-saving treatment for a neonate. In essence, B was an infant suffering from Down's syndrome complicated by intestinal obstruction of a type which would be fatal per se but which was amenable to surgical treatment. The parents took the view that the kindest thing in the interests of the child would be for her not to have the operation and for her to die – in passing, a decision which was later described by Dunn LJ as 'an entirely responsible one'. The infant was made a ward of court and, in the face of judicial indecision and medical disagreement, the question 'to treat or not to treat?' came before the Court of Appeal.

Templeman LJ , adhering to the general principles relating to the affairs of minors,[19] concluded that the judge of first instance, in refusing to authorise the operation, had been too much concerned with the wishes of the parents; the duty of the court was to decide the matter in the interests of the child. In coming to the conclusion that these interests were best served by treatment, he said:

> . . . it devolves on this court . . . to decide whether the life of this child is demonstrably going to be so awful that in effect the child must be condemned to die or whether the life of this child is still so imponderable that it would be wrong for her to be condemned to die . . . Faced with [the] choice, I have no doubt that it is the duty of this court to decide that the child must live.[20]

and it was this that led Lord Donaldson to look upon *Re B* as close to a binding authority for the proposition that there is a balancing exercise to be performed in assessing the course to be adopted in the best interests of such children.

Templeman LJ did, however, clearly leave the door open for an alternative decision in saying:

16 *R v Arthur* (1981) The Times, 6 November, pp 1, 12, (1981) 12 BMLR 1 at 22.
17 (1981) [1990] 3 All ER 927, [1981] 1 WLR 1421, CA.
18 *Re J (a minor)(wardship: medical treatment)* [1990] 3 All ER 930, (1990) 6 BMLR 25, CA paraphrasing Lord Donaldson MR at [1990] 3 All ER 930 at 938; (1990) 6 BMLR 25 at 34.
19 Guardianship of Minors Act 1971, s 1.
20 (1981) [1990] 3 All ER 927 at 929, [1981] 1 WLR 1421 at 1424, CA. The case is well discussed by D D Raphael 'Handicapped Infants: Medical Ethics and the Law' (1988) 14 J Med Ethics 5.

There may be cases . . . of severe proved damage where the future is so certain and where the life of the child is so bound to be full of pain and suffering that the court might be driven to a different conclusion.

This is important for, only a few weeks later, the Director of Public Prosecutions decided that no action would be taken against a doctor who had allegedly refused to sustain a baby, Stephen Quinn, who was suffering from spina bifida.[1] The two decisions can, therefore, be seen as compatible once it is accepted that baby Quinn would have been not only handicapped but, almost certainly, would have been in great pain. It might, however, be said that they are contradictory in that *Re B*[2] and the Quinn case demonstrate a contrast in legal readiness or reluctance to override the rights of parents, or to 'interfere' in the traditional doctor/patient relationship.

Then came *R v Arthur*,[3] the salient features of which are: a baby was born with apparently uncomplicated Down's syndrome and was rejected by his parents. The defendant, a paediatrician of high repute and impeccable professional integrity, wrote in the notes 'Parents do not wish it to survive. Nursing care only'. The baby died 69 hours later and Dr Arthur was charged with murder but during the course of the trial, the charge was reduced to one of attempted murder. Dr Arthur was acquitted.

It has been said that there are surprisingly few substantive issues in medical ethics that *Arthur* does not raise[4] and, for this reason, it remains an important landmark. Legally speaking, however, we believe it has negligible precedental value in that it does little more than demonstrate the understandable reluctance of a British jury to interpret such an action as murder – a strong suspicion remains that the verdict would have been different had the defendant been charged with a lesser offence.[5]

The legal vacuum

Even so, the medical profession was now left in a cleft stick. *Re B* and *Arthur* are virtually impossible to reconcile – and *Re B* was not referred to in the criminal trial. All interested parties were, therefore, left unsure of their ground. Even the leaders of the medical profession failed to appreciate that there is a world of difference between withholding treatment from a dying patient and refusing sustenance to one who shows firm evidence of a will to live.[6] Morally, it is difficult to introduce the proportionate/disproportionate therapeutic form of argument in a physically uncomplicated case. No matter what the surrounding circumstances, it is stretching sophistry to its limits to characterise feeding as extraordinary means of treatment.[7]

---

1 The Times, 6 October 1981, p 1.
2 *Re B (a minor) (wardship: medical treatment)* (1981) [1990] 3 All ER 927, [1981] 1 WLR 1421, CA.
3 (1981) The Times, 6 November, pp 1, 12, (1981) 12 BMLR 1.
4 R Gillon 'An Introduction to Philosophical Medical Ethics: The Arthur Case' (1985) 290 BMJ 1117.
5 This view is not supported by all academics at the time: see, for example, M J Gunn and J C Smith 'Arthur's Case and the Right to Life of a Down's Syndrome Child' [1985] Crim LR 705. However, D Brahams 'Putting Arthur's Case in Perspective' [1986] Crim LR 387 reached much the same assessment as we do.
6 See for example, Editorial Comment 'Paediatricians and the Law' (1981) 283 BMJ 1280.
7 See D Poole 'Arthur's Case (1) A Comment' [1986] Crim LR 383 and the follow-up comment M J Gunn and J C Smith [1986] Crim LR 390.

Legally speaking, it is difficult to see why the parents' wishes as to the death of their offspring should be overruled when major surgery is involved yet be regarded as ultimately decisive when it is not and, in a clarification which seems only to add to the confusion, the Attorney General said shortly after the trial:

> I am satisfied that the law relating to murder and to attempted murder is the same now as it was before the trial; that it is the same irrespective of the age of the victim; and that it is the same irrespective of the wishes of the parents or of any other person having a duty of care to the victim. I am also satisfied that a person who has a duty of care may be guilty of murder or attempted murder by omitting to fulfil that duty, as much as by committing any positive act.[8]

This unsatisfactory situation persisted for almost a decade but has now been clarified in the companion cases of *Re C (a minor) (wardship: medical treatment)*[9] and *Re J (a minor) (wardship: medical treatment)*.[10] Strictly speaking, the decisions in these cases do not relate to treatment of the newborn, the children being between four and five months old at the time of the hearing. Both, however, were concerned with physical damage sustained at birth and the findings are entirely appropriate to the present context.

Re C concerned a moribund child and the essence of the decision was that the hospital were given authority to treat her so as to allow her life to come to an end peacefully and with dignity. Such treatment as would relieve her from pain, suffering and distress would be given but it was specifically said to be unnecessary to use antibiotics or to set up intravenous infusions or nasogastric feeding regimes. It was emphasised that the decision was based on the paramountcy of her welfare, well-being and interests. *Re B* and *Re C* provide the extreme examples of neonatal care and, in retrospect, were not difficult to decide.

Baby J was, however, not dying and the case illustrates more closely the real dilemma in the neonatal ward – for non-treatment in these circumstances cannot be dressed in such euphemisms as 'allowing a peaceful and dignified death'. In this case the brain-damaged child suffered from repetitive fits and periods of cessation of breathing for which he required ventilation; the question before the court was what was to be done if he sustained a further collapse. The Court of Appeal had little difficulty in agreeing with the judge of first instance that:

> it would not be in J's best interest to reventilate him [by machine] in the event of his stopping breathing unless to do so seemed appropriate to the doctors treating him given the prevailing clinical situation.

In the course of his judgment, the Master of the Rolls made several observations that are of particular importance in relation to our analysis which follows later. In the first place, he stressed that, while there was a strong presumption in favour of a course of action that will prolong life, nevertheless, the person who makes the decision must

---

8 19 HC Official Report (6th Series) written answers col 349, 8 March 1982.
9 [1990] Fam 26, [1989] 2 All ER 782.
10 [1990] 3 All ER 930, (1990) 6 BMLR 25.

look at it from the assumed view of the patient. Second, consideration must be given to the prognosis in terms of pain and suffering – including the distress caused by any treatment of itself; in this case, the quality of life, even without the added effect of further hypoxic episodes, was extremely low. Third, the court held that decision making was a co-operative effort between the doctors and the parents – or, in the case of wardship, between the doctors and the court with the views of the parents being taken into consideration. Any choice must be made solely on behalf of the child in what was believed to be his best interests. Finally (and this we see as especially significant) it was emphasised that any decision taken was one which would affect death by way of a side-effect; the debate was not about terminating life but solely about whether to withhold treatment designed to prevent death from natural causes:

> The court never sanctions steps to terminate life. That would be unlawful. There is no question of approving, even in a case of the most horrendous disability, a course aimed at terminating life or accelerating death. The court is concerned only with the circumstances in which steps should not be taken to prolong life.[11]

The intention of the words is crystal clear.[12] Taken in conjunction with the tone of the rest of the opinion, this seems to indicate firmly that the treatment regime adopted in *Arthur*[13] would not, now, be lawful. Legally, *Arthur* can be relegated to something best forgotten. It is to be hoped that this can also be applied medically – not least for its effect on other parties. Few involved in this debate appear to have considered the effect of the decisions on, particularly, the nurses.[14] The doctors may make the decisions but it is the nurses who have to carry them out and their increasing involvement in treatment policies is to be welcomed.

Comparative common law experience
The American experience in this field demonstrates a somewhat turbulent history. Three cases in the late 1970s indicate that there was, at that time, a strong legal bias in favour of the infant's right to a sanctity of life approach. Opinions were handed down such as: 'If there is any life-saving treatment available, it must be given regardless of the quality of life that will result'[15] or 'Children are not property whose disposition is left to parental decision without hindrance'[16] and, in general, extensive surgery was ordered so long as it was feasible. However, a change appeared in the next decade. In *Weber v Stony Brook Hospital,*[17] the Court of Appeal in New York would not overturn a judgment to the effect that, in refusing permission for surgery, the parents had 'elected a treatment which was within accepted medical standards'; 'to allow [a guardian]' it was said 'to bypass the statutory requirements would

11 [1990] 3 All ER 930 at 943, (1990) 6 BMLR 25 at 40, per Taylor LJ.
12 In *Re C*, the Court of Appeal would not even tolerate the expression 'treat to die'.
13 *R v Arthur* (1981) Times, 6 November, pp 1, 12, (1981) 12 BMLR 1.
14 The nurses were, however, singled out for praise in the Court of Appeal in *Re C*.
15 *Re McNulty* No 1960 Probate Court (Mass, 1980) following *Maine Medical Center v Houle* No 74-45, Sup Ct (Me, 1974).
16 *Re Cicero* 421 NYS 2d 965 (1979).
17 456 NE 2d 1186 (NY, 1983).

catapult him into the very heart of a family circle to challenge the parents' responsibility to care for their children'. The decision in *Re Infant Doe*[18] was that the value of parental autonomy outweighed the infant's right to live when 'a minimally adequate quality of life was non-existent' – this despite the fact that the anatomic abnormality present in association with Down's syndrome was amenable to relatively routine surgery. Moreover, the case arose in Indiana which was, at the time, the only state in which the life of the newborn was protected by statute. It has been described as a case: 'in which a baby whose life could almost certainly have been saved was starved to death under color of law'.[19]

The Canadian courts have also addressed the problem. In the most influential case,[20] it was held that parental refusal to allow replacement of a shunt for the alleviation of hydrocephalus might result in increasing disability and pain for the child and the operation was ordered. In discussion of this case, Dickens[1] has suggested that the courts are concentrating on the brain, and particularly its capacity to experience pain, as the central focus of human personality.

An apposite case to come before the Australian courts is *Re F*.[2] In his judgment, Vincent J put it:

> No parent, no doctor, no court, has any power to determine that the life of any child, however disabled that child may be, will be deliberately taken from it . . . [the law] does not permit decisions to be made concerning the quality of life, nor does it enable any assessment to be made as to the value of any human being.

The judge was addressing himself to the specific problem of feeding, but, nevertheless, it would seem to state clearly the law as it stands in Australia.

Neonaticide as a separate issue

As we have already indicated, there are at least two good reasons for isolating the issues in the perinatal period from those which are essentially perimortal. In the first place, decisions in this situation rest on prognosis which is another way of expressing an informed guess as to the future. This may, in any event, be difficult and, while we know that we are dealing with only short-term survival at the end of life, this is not the case at birth – we may be confident of what will be the state of affairs next week but we cannot say the same about the next decade. Moreover, the neonate is not passing from a settled norm into a progressively less satisfactory condition; he is developing in a milieu which is his norm. Can one say with any certainty that the

18 (1982) GU 8204-004 A (Monroe County Cir, April 12), cert denied 52 USLW 3369 (US, 1983). See G P Smith 'Defective Newborns and Government Intermeddling' (1985) 25 Med, Sci Law 44.
19 N Lund 'Infanticide, Physicians and the Law' (1985) 11 Amer J Law Med 1.
20 *Re Superintendent of Family and Child Service and Dawson* (1983) 145 DLR (3d) 610. The case was quoted with particular approval in *Re J (a minor) (wardship: medical treatment)* [1990] 3 All ER 930, (1990) 6 BMLR 25.
 1 B M Dickens 'Withholding Paediatric Medical Care' (1984) Can BR 196.
 2 *Re F, F v F* (2 July 1986, unreported), Supreme Court of Victoria.

person with Down's syndrome, who has never known anything different, is dissatisfied with his existence within himself? Thus, we would take issue with the reasoning of Professor Williams who has said: 'If a wicked fairy told me she was about to transform me into a Down's baby and would I prefer to die I should certainly answer yes'[3] because this is not the question being asked of the infant. The better view is that of Lord Donaldson – that the starting point in analysing the defective's condition is not what might have been but what is.[4]

The second major distinction between life and death decisions at the extremes of life is that, while the adult sufferer is likely to be able to express an opinion or, save in a few cases, to have previously intimated his wishes, there is no way in which the neonate can consent to treatment, suffering or death. Consent must be parental and one then asks where, in fact, do the parents' rights lie that it is feared will be usurped by the courts? Have they any more right to reject a child than to abandon it? If it can be criminal to disbar an older child from treatment[5] why is it less culpable to fail or to connive at failure to provide the minimum of neonatal treatment – infant feeding? How do these rights differ when exercised in the light of medical advice rather than by way of simple intuition in the privacy of the home? Is it likely that a blind eye would be turned on parents who, on their own initiative, decided to abandon their defective child? And can the parents who are, in addition to their emotional involvement, economically and socially concerned, make a truly objective decision on behalf of the child?

Re C and *Re J* have gone some way to taking the urgency out of these questions but they dealt with cases in which there was no conflict either of ideals or as to the practical approach. Who holds the moral and legal high ground in the event of disagreement? As one discussant of *Arthur* put it – the parents' wishes should be disregarded in the interests of the child. The law, it was suggested, is either out of step or has evolved double standards in favour of the doctors.[6] Others[7] have looked at the concepts of omission and commission as they affect the case and have concluded that, while no-one can say that a surgeon who refuses to operate on a mongol child suffering from duodenal atresia and who allows it to die commits murder or manslaughter, it is, nevertheless, beyond doubt that a parent who refuses to feed a child may be guilty of homicide if the child dies as a result and that the doctor who concurs in this action should be equally guilty. The English cases have demonstrated that there is no such thing as an absolute obligation to preserve the life of a physically abnormal baby. The decision of the parents in *Re B*[8] seems to have

---

3 G Williams 'Down's Syndrome and the Duty to Preserve Life' (1981) 131 NLJ 1020.
4 In *Re J (a minor) (wardship: medical treatment)* [1990] 3 All ER 930 at 936, (1990) 6 BMLR 25 at 32, paraphrasing McKenzie J.
5 *R v Senior* [1899] 1 QB 283, CCR. The accrual of rights with age is discussed by C Wells 'Whose Baby Is It?' (1988) 5 J Law & Soc 323.
6 D Brahams and M Brahams '*R v Arthur* - is Legislation Appropriate ?' (1981) 78 LS Gaz 1342. The doubtful basis of the parental autonomy doctrine is further argued in D Brahams 'Acquittal of Paediatrician Charged after Death of Infant with Down's Syndrome' [1981] 2 Lancet 1101. For discussion in depth see M A Crossley 'Selective Non-treatment of Handicapped Newborns: An Analysis' (1987) 6 Med Law 499.
7 Gunn and Smith (in their following comment to D Poole 'Arthur's Case (1) A Comment' [1986] Crim LR 383), at [1986] Crim LR 390.
8 *Re B (a minor) (wardship: medical treatment)* (1981) [1990] 3 All ER 927, [1981] 1 WLR 1421, CA.

been one which they could take without, thereby, acting unlawfully but it is clear that they could not have done so in the case of a normal child. Campbell,[9] writing on severely brain damaged children, believed that anything, including feeding, that prolongs such non-human or artificial life is 'wrong for the child, wrong for the family and wrong for society'. This may well be an expression of the current state of the law. We suggest, however, that decision makers in this field should be wary of extending the bounds of *Re J*[10] with impunity – life clearly carried great weight in Lord Donaldson's balance pan and there is no certainty that his successors will be so ready to decide in favour of the clinician.

The American position became even more turbulent in the wake of *Re Infant Doe*.[11] This case provoked Presidential reaction on the grounds that selective non-treatment contravened federal laws protecting the handicapped. Hospitals receiving federal aid were reminded that they were prohibited from withholding life-saving medical or surgical treatment from handicapped infants. Particular attention was paid to the provision of nourishment, fluids and routine nursing care – items which were not considered options for medical judgment: 'no health care provider should take it upon itself to cause death by starvation or dehydration'.[12] Nevertheless, the United States District Court for the District of Columbia rapidly invalidated these rules by declaring, inter alia, that the Rehabilitation Act 1973, s 504, which protects the rights of the handicapped, 'could never be applied blindly and without any consideration of the burdens and intrusions which might result'.[13] The federal regulations were, therefore, revised but were again struck down.[14] Several states then introduced legislation designed to protect the neonate – this being based, in general, on existing child care law but much of the confusion has now been eliminated by Congressional action which is discussed further at p 161 below.

United States' opinion appears to be unanimous on one fundamental point – the uncomplicated Down's syndrome baby is excluded from discussion. Denying treatment to a mongol child would be a social, not medical, judgment and such a denial, it has been said, should not be permitted in the American society.[15] The severely defective newborn is defined as one who is not likely to survive without medical intervention;[16] this clearly excludes the uncomplicated Down's case. Indeed, mortal inactivity with respect to non-dying but defective infants is probably illegal in the United States.

We take the view that the greater part of the confusion surrounding the subject of neonaticide and selective non-treatment of the newborn stems from just such a failure to distinguish between, on the one hand, infants with pure mental defects and, at the other extreme, those with severe physical incapacity resulting, say, from neural

9 A G M Campbell 'Children in a Persistent Vegetative State' (1984) 289 BMJ 1022.
10 *Re J (a minor) (wardship: medical treatment)* [1990] 3 All ER 930; (1990) 6 BMLR 25.
11 (1982) GV 8204 - 004 A (Monroe County Cir, April 12), cert denied 52 USLW 3369 (US, 1983).
12 48 Fed Reg 9630 (1983) superseded by 48 Fed Reg 30, 846 (1983).
13 *American Academy of Pediatrics v Heckler* 561 F Supp 395 (DDC, 1983).
14 *American Hospital Association v Heckler* 105 S Ct 3475 (1985). The death knell was sounded in *Bowen v American Hospital Association* 106 S Ct 2101 (1986).
15 J J Paris and A B Fletcher 'Infant Doe Regulations and the Absolute Requirement to Use Nourishment and Fluids for the Dying Infant' (1983) 11 Law Med Hlth Care 210.
16 R S Shapiro 'Medical Treatment of Defective Newborns: An Answer to the "Baby Doe" Dilemma' (1983) 20 Harvard J Legis 137.

tube defects. Treatment of the latter is a matter of careful medical management which must incorporate an element of selection.[17] Many such handicapped children will inevitably die and many should be allowed to do so; the principle of 'allowing nature to take its course' on the basis of a shared decision between doctor and parents is acceptable in both a moral and a legal sense provided that the decision is taken in the best interests of the child.[18] By contrast, if the mentally handicapped child is not to live, it must be encouraged and guided towards death. We agree wholeheartedly with many of the observations of Gunn and Smith.[19] Withholding food may be an omission but giving instructions to do so must be a commission. Even more so, the prescribing of a drug to inhibit appetite during starvation can only be regarded as a positive act. There is no non-treatment for the anatomically normal Down's baby because it needs no treatment. The problems of physical and mental defects are both practically and ethically distinct and failure to feed in the latter instance can only be categorised as neonaticide – ie *killing* of the neonate.

Kuhse[20] has argued most persuasively that there is no moral or legal distinction to be drawn between activity and passivity in this area of medical practice. As Gillon[1] put it:

> While there may be some social benefit in distinguishing between actively 'allowing to die' and painlessly killing such infants, there is, I believe, no other moral difference and doctors who accept such 'allowing to die' of severely handicapped newborn infants should not deceive themselves into believing that there is such a difference.

Elsewhere, the same author emphasised that, while there is no *necessary* moral difference between killing and letting die, it does not follow that there is a moral equivalence.[2] Were this so, we would have to approve the spectre of the paediatrician armed with a lethal syringe – and the concept is quite unacceptable. It is hard to assail the logic which says that a quick death is preferable to one which depends upon the vagaries of nature; nevertheless, we believe that natural death is the only acceptable concomitant of a decision not to treat a severely physically defective infant – and we also believe that food and water should be provided for any child which is capable of taking nourishment by mouth. In so saying, we admit to being guided, to a very considerable extent, by moral intuition alone. As a well-respected medical philosopher has put it:

17 Lorber's early work is summarised in J Lorber and S A W Salfield 'Result of Selective Treatment of Spina Bifida Cystica' (1981) 56 Arch Dis Childh 822. For a philosophical assessment, see J Harris 'Ethical Problems in the Management of Some Severely Handicapped Children' (1981) 7 J Med Ethics 117. More recent results are reported in A Whitelaw, 'Death as an Option in Neonatal Intensive Care' [1986] 2 Lancet 328.
18 DD Raphael 'Handicapped Infants: Medical Ethics and the Law' (1988) 14 J Med Ethics 5 points to the conceptual difficulty in attributing any *interest* in death - 'the most you can say is that someone would prefer to die'.
19 See their follow-up comment to D Poole 'Arthur's Case (1) A Comment' [1986] Crim LR 383, at [1986] Crim LR 3900.
20 H Kuhse 'A Modern Myth. That Letting Die is not the Intentional Causation of Death: Some Reflections on the Trial and Acquittal of Dr Leonard Arthur' (1984) 1 J Appl Philosophy 21. The same point is made by Harris, fn 17 above.
 1 R Gillon 'Conclusion. The *Arthur* Case Revisited' (1986) 292 BMJ 543.
 2 R Gillon 'Euthanasia. Withholding Life-Prolonging Treatment and Moral Differences between Killing and Letting Die' (1988) 14 J Med Ethics 115.

> We are, here, noting a deep human inhibition which it might be unwise to tamper with in the name of logic[3]

Clinicians are similarly beset by the illogic of intuition:

> There is a powerful psychological distinction [between 'killing' and 'allowing to die'] which is important to the staff of intensive care units. To them, there is a big difference between not using a respirator to keep an infant of 600 g alive and giving a lethal injection, although the end result is the same.[4]

And, whatever logic may tell us, *Re J*[5] spells out clearly what the law is. The situation is one in which the most acceptable course is not, unhappily, the kindest.

Advances in modern medicine have, at the same time, brought their own problems to the neonatal period. It is increasingly possible to maintain and rear premature infants of low birth weight and evidence is accumulating that a number of such children are disadvantaged to an extent which is inversely proportionate to their birthweight – thus, some 12-19% of extremely low birthweight babies (less than 1 kg) who have survived will be severely handicapped.[6] The discussion of selective non-treatment is, accordingly, being extended to include attitudes to intensive care of the premature infant. It is trite medicine to say that premature births should be prevented by improved ante-natal care. The fact remains that they will continue and their numbers will be augmented not so much due to poor maternal care as by the improved medical management of high risk pregnancies. It has been said: 'we obstetricians and neonatologists are caught in a trap of our own design'.[7] In these circumstances, we can see little alternative but to agree with those who believe that, since an accurate prognosis is generally impossible, such infants should always be offered treatment until such time as it is clearly ineffective – the test for treatment is, on these terms, one of feasibility. The difficulty of such a rule is that, while resuscitation may be successful, the end result may be a severely handicapped survivor. Quite apart from the individual clinical result, there may also be a serious problem of resource distribution:

> The ability to preserve the lives of these infants must be weighed against the resultant increase in the numbers of impaired children, the distress and suffering caused by lengthy

3   R S Downie 'Modern Paediatric Practice: An Ethical Overview' (1989) in J K Mason (ed) *Paediatric Forensic Medicine and Pathology* (1989) ch 31.
4   A G M Campbell 'Ethical Issues in Child Health and Disease' in J O Forfar (ed) *Child Health in a Changing Society* (1988).
5   *Re J (a minor) (wardship: medical treatment)* [1990] 3 All ER 930; (1990) 6 BMLR 25.
6   V Yu 'The Extremely Low Birthweight Infant: Ethical Issues in Treatment' (1987) 23 Austral Paediatric J 97; L W Doyle, L J Murton and W H Kitchen 'Increasing the Survival of Extremely-immature (24-28 weeks' gestation) Infants – At what Cost ?' (1989) 150 Med J Austral 558.
7   M T Stahlman 'Medical Complications in Premature Infants – Is Treatment Enough ?' (1989) 320 New Engl J Med 1551.

treatment and hospitalisation, their eventual expected quality of life, and the socio-economic consequences for society as a whole.[8]

Even so, were an alternative approach to be adopted, there is little doubt that it would be accepted by the courts if it was one that would be approved by a responsible body of medical opinion.[9] In the only apposite case that we have noted (a Scottish fatal accident inquiry) the decision not to resuscitate an extremely premature infant was regarded as a reasonable medical option – legal intervention resulted only from a failure in communication between physicians and parents.[10]

A need for legislation?

While we do not wish to extend discussion of selective non-treatment or neonaticide unduly, there are several more uncomfortable aspects which have to be addressed. First, once the premises of the Abortion Act 1967 have been accepted, there are, like it or not, logical grounds for approving active neonaticide. Depending on the severity of the abnormality, a positive policy of neonaticide will obviate a deal of suffering or hardship to the child or to its parents while, as we have touched on above, the pressures imposed on the social services or on the NHS force one to consider the rational deployment of scarce resources in some cases (see ch 11). There are more subtle and logical arguments in its favour which stem directly from the provisions of the 1967 Act. As previously mentioned (see ch 6), it may be difficult, even with the aid of both amniocentesis and ultrasonography, to assess the likely *degree* of handicap when chromosomal or physical abnormality is diagnosed in utero. Why, then, it may be asked, terminate the pregnancy rather than wait until birth and have a look? Why, if we have failed to detect an abnormality in utero should we not recoup the situation after birth? Or there is the other side of the picture: suppose a pregnant woman says that her psychic health will be damaged if she has her baby – why not give her the chance to change her mind when it has been born? In short, a powerful argument can be developed to the effect that, in simple brutal logic, neonaticide is scientifically preferable to abortion. Yet, in practice, such a concept is abhorrent and intolerable – as the former President of the British Paediatric Association once put it: '. . . we are guilty of inconsistency but not of infanticide.'[11]

Secondly, as we have already argued, there are some infants who *ought* not to be assisted to live by invasive methods. The incapacitated child has as much right to die in peace as has his grandfather and there are times when it is clear that that right should be exercised. Moreover, it is now clear that a responsible clinician who believes that to be the right course cannot be compelled to provide treatment with

---

8 J Griffin quoted by L Hunt 'Cost "Dilemma" Posed by Premature Babies' (1993) Independent, 20 January, p 6 in discussion of Office of Health Economics *Born Too Soon* (1993).

9 The English courts have had no difficulty in applying the *Bolam* principle (see *Bolam v Friern Hospital Management Committee* [1957] 2 All ER 118, QBD) to treatment decisions – see, for example, *Re F (mental patient: sterilisation)* [1990] 2 AC 1, [1989] 2 All ER 545, HL; *Re C (a minor) (wardship: medical treatment)* [1990] Fam 26, [1989] 2 All ER 782.

10 D Brahams 'No Obligation to Resuscitate a Non-viable Infant' (1988) 1 Lancet 1176.

11 P Tizard and T L Chambers 'Human Embryos' (1984) The Times, 1 June, p 13.

which he disagrees.[12]   Nevertheless, there remains a need to provide the clinician with relief from the threat of an accusation of homicide in such circumstances. With this aim in view, there are, in essence, three routes available – through the medium of hospital ethical committees, by acceptance of officially approved codes of conduct and/or by way of direct legislative intervention. The first has been particularly popularised in the United States where the role of ethics committees is being increasingly promoted by the courts themselves – at least in respect of treatment decisions in adults (see ch 15). 'Ethics committees' have, however, developed differently on either side of the Atlantic – the United Kingdom variant is designed to oversee research projects and has not yet ventured into the field of clinical choice. Thus, while a strong case can be made for the use of the hospital committee as a way of attaining emotional stability and consistency,[13] it is unlikely to be adopted as such in the United Kingdom. Recent United Kingdom legislation has, in fact, shown an increasing predilection for the 'Code of Conduct' – sometimes mandatory, sometimes relatively unofficial but, in general, serving as a model against which to measure negligence or bad faith. A recent example in this field has come from The Netherlands where the Dutch Paediatric Association have produced a code which they feel should be widely available for both the health care staff and parents. Under this code, treatment decisions are founded on prognosis which they present in functional terms:

- what communicative abilities will the child have later?

- will he or she be able to lead an independent life?

- will the child be continuously dependent on medical care?

- will he or she suffer, mentally or physically?

- how long is the life expectancy?

As a result, four options are regarded as being available – to continue intensive care and extend if necessary, to maintain the status quo (which can only be a temporary measure), to stop the most intensive treatment or to stop all life-prolonging measures.[14] The code stresses the importance of the parents' wishes and of the involvement of the whole health care team. Such a code of practice would be generally acceptable and the principles are no doubt being followed widely even if not 'codified'. The majority of decisions are, often, not difficult to make but there

---

12 *Re J (a minor)(wardship : medical treatment)* [1992] 2 FLR 165, (1992) 9 BMLR 10. Interestingly, one of the reasons given was that to do so might require the health authority to use intensive care resources and, thereby, to deny them to someone who might derive greater benefit (per Balcombe LJ [1992] 2 FLR 165 at 176, (1992) 9 BMLR 10 at 20). The implication is that the courts see a difference between not starting a life-saving treatment and withdrawing it.

13 See L-J Greenstein 'Withholding Life-sustaining Treatment from Severely Defective Newborns: Who Should Decide?' (1987) 6 Med Law 487.   A critical review of US institutional ethics committees is to be found in R F Weir 'Pediatric Ethics Committees: Ethical Advisers or Legal Watchdogs?' (1987) 15 Law Med Hlth Care 99.

14 Working Group of the Dutch Paediatric Association (C Versluys, chairman) *To Do or Not to Do? Boundaries for Medical Action in Neonatology* (1992).   See C Versluys 'Ethics of Neonatal Care' (1993) 341 Lancet 794.

is always the core of problem cases where a severely disabled infant is able to survive without intensive therapy. The Dutch solution, here, might well be active euthanasia.[15] This, however, would currently be unacceptable in the United Kingdom and judicial opinion voiced in *Bland*[16] is clearly of the view that the legality of euthanasia – including by way of withdrawal of sustenance – should be a matter of legislation.[17]

The call for legislation has been strong in the United States and has ultimately been met by the Child Abuse Amendments of 1984 which amend the Federal Child Abuse Prevention and Treatment Act 1974.[18] The essential thrust is that, having defined medical neglect, the amendments lay down the circumstances in which withholding medically indicated treatment would not be so described. These include the presence of irreversible coma, when treatment would merely prolong dying and when treatment would be futile or inhumane – but the correction of a simple complication of Down's syndrome is not included as an exception.

The question arises as to whether similar legislation is needed in the United Kingdom in the light of the expression of the current law in *Re J*.[19] It is not difficult to argue that there are still good reasons why the doctor's position should be settled as unambiguous. It has, for example, been stated that a pregnancy in a mentally handicapped woman can be terminated without a declaration from the court *because* [our emphasis] the Abortion Act 1967 provides fully adequate safeguards for the doctors involved.[20] The same principle might well be applied in other legally 'grey' areas in medicine. Legislation can also anticipate and forestall the 'domino effect'. It does not need much imagination, for example, to envisage parental rejection of the newborn as being justified by a club foot or even unattractive features. The possibility of a change of mind in favour of rejection after a few months must be considered. If mental handicap at birth is to justify extinction, is it more than a short step to concluding that a similar handicap following a fall at the age of one year merits a similar fate?[1] Neonaticide is disturbingly close to feticide by abortion; the application of the Abortion Act has escalated and the practice of neonaticide must not be encouraged to do the same.

In our view, the case for legislation lies in the need to emphasise that, after parturition, the 'interests' involved shift from being those of the mother to being those of the neonate. If there were to be legislation, it should not create new offences but should do no more than lay down the conditions under which a doctor commits no offence. Furthermore, since legislation is always difficult to adapt to changing circumstances, it should be relatively non-specific and should allow for the free

15 See ch 15 for a discussion of the Dutch approach to ending life.
16 *Airedale National Health Service Trust v Bland* [1993] 1 All ER 821, (1993) 12 BMLR 64, HL.
17 The Report of the House of Lords Select Committee on Medical Ethics (HL Paper 21, 1994) comes down firmly against any change in the law to permit euthanasia. The Committee also saw little ethical difference between withdrawing a treatment and not starting it.
18 The onus of monitoring and enforcing the Act remains with the individual states.
19 *Re J (a minor) (wardship: medical treatment)* [1990] 3 All ER 930, (1990) 6 BMLR 25.
20 *Re SG (Adult mental patient: Abortion)* [1991] 2 FLR 329; (1990) 6 BMLR 95.
1 The scenario is well developed by G J Fairburn 'Kuhse, Singer and Slippery Slopes' (1988) 14 J Med Ethics 132.

exercise of clinical decision-making in individual cases. We anticipate some form of legislation following the House of Lords special report[2] and, should this arise, would suggest the inclusion of a clause to the effect:

> In the event of positive treatment being necessary for a neonate's survival, it will not be an offence to withhold such treatment if two doctors, one of whom is a consultant paediatrician, acting in good faith and with the consent of both parents if available, decide against treatment in the light of a reasonably clear medical prognosis which indicates that the infant's further life would be intolerable by virtue of pain or suffering or because of severe cerebral incompetence.

We believe that, on the one hand, this emphasises the interests of the infant while, on the other, it clarifies and protects the legal position of paediatricians who are forced into making particularly stressful clinical decisions. Open legislation is best backed by guidelines for decision-making and we have attempted to evolve a consensus view.[3] Essentially, this proposes that positive treatment which is needed for the infant's survival may be withheld when: (a) there is corroborated opinion that the decision is medically proper; (b) there is adequate written explanation of the decision; (c) the parents have been enabled to give, or refuse, an information-based consent; and (d) the decision is made with the interests of the child providing the guiding principle. We also suggest that any treatment of the newborn which has been instituted may be abandoned if death is highly probable regardless of treatment, or if there is no reasonable possibility that the infant will be able to participate in normal human relationships, or if the treatment cannot alleviate a level of chronic pain which makes continued life-preserving therapy inhumane.[4] None of these codes really address the critical dilemma of the infant who satisfies all the requirements but still survives without treatment. We find it difficult, if not impossible, to disagree with those who hold that normal feeding, not involving medical intervention, should be continued whenever the infant is capable of taking nourishment by mouth – yet we have to acknowledge that there are times when this does not seem to be in the neonate's best interests in terms of suffering. The status of normal feeding is, however, a similar problem at all ages and is better discussed under the heading of euthanasia.

The interests of others

It is possible to see the problems attaching to selective non-treatment and neonaticide as concurrent with, at one extreme, abortion and, at the other, with euthanasia in the aged. In either case, no practical solutions can be applied without giving thought to those who must participate in any process.

2   Report of the House of Lords Select Committee on Medical Ethics (HL Paper 21, 1994). There has been no governmental reaction at the time of writing.
3   J K Mason and D W Meyers 'Parental Choice and Selective Non-treatment of Defective Newborns: A View from Mid-Atlantic' (1986) 12 J Med Ethics 67.
4   Although reached independently, these conclusions are very similar to those found in the amendments to the US Child Abuse Prevention and Treatment Act 1974 (see above) and to those set out by the Canadian Paediatric Society; they are also compatible with the teaching of the Roman Catholic Church – *Care of the Handicapped Newborn: Parental Responsibility and Medical Responsibility* (1986).

The most important of such considerations lies in conscientious objection to the procedures. Subject to certain conditions (see ch 5, above), s 4 of the Abortion Act 1967 excuses the conscientious objector from participating in treatment by abortion. It is clear that any legislation which legalises neonaticide in specified circumstances must include a similar clause. We would draw particular attention to the role of the nursing staff and to the importance of safeguarding their position both now and in the event of legislation. It is the nurses, not the doctors, who will bear the brunt of selective non-treatment; not only must they be spared responsibility for carrying out instructions but, also, their sensitivities must be fully respected. We strongly commend the increasingly accepted principle of a team approach to neonatal intensive care.[5]

The anomalous position of the father in the debate must also be considered. In so far as abortion is concerned, he has no rights but, once the baby is born, he seems, in current practice, to have a voice equal to the mother's as to the disposal of an abnormal infant. He could, presumably, override his wife's rejection of the baby even if he would be unlikely to undertake much of the burden of caring. However, this point has not been openly decided. In practice, common attitudes to the disposal of abnormal infants are based on the assumption of marital harmony in that they relate so firmly to the wishes of 'the parents'. The decision in *Re B*[6] was surprisingly badly received by the medical and legal professions because of a belief in so-called parental rights.[7] The significance of possible clashes of interests would be minimised if the absolute importance of the infant's rights were defined by law.

While the birth of a defective child may uncover qualities of goodness in the parents that are beyond expectation, there can be no doubt that an opposite reaction can be provoked.[8] We are, therefore, on the horns of a dilemma which is an inexorable result of the Abortion Act 1967 – given that we acknowledge a woman's right to terminate her pregnancy because she feels unable to accept her defective fetus, by what reason should we insist that the roles are reversed and that the interests of the defective neonate outweigh those of its main potential carer? Raphael[9] concluded that the current medical perspective in this field differs markedly from that of the common law. It is essential that the medical and legal professions – as well as society at large – should make sure of the lines they intend to draw in this area of potential conflict.

5   The point was well taken in the judgment in *Re C* [1990] Fam 26, [1989] 2 All ER 782.
6   *Re B (a minor) (wardship: medical treatment)* (1981) [1990] 3 All ER 927, [1981] 1 WLR 1421, CA.
7   The decision was, however, firmly defended by M D A Freeman 'Using Wardship to Save a Baby from its Parents' (1982) 12 Fam law 73.
8   See B Shepperdson 'Abortion and Euthanasia of Down's Syndrome Children - The Parents' View' (1983) 9 J Med Ethics 152. And, for an interesting debate - 'Informed Dissent': M Simms 'The Views of Some Mothers of Severely Mentally Handicapped Young Adults'; A Davis 'The View of a Disabled Woman' (1986) 12 J Med Ethics 72, at 75.
9   D D Raphel 'Handicapped Infants: Medical Ethics and the Law' (1988) 14 J Med Ethics 5.

Medical practice

8 Medical confidentiality

In the absence of a specific contract to that effect, a general common law duty is imposed on a doctor to respect the confidences of his patients.[1] The nature of this obligation, which applies to all confidential information and not only to medical material, was discussed by the Court of Appeal in *A-G v Guardian Newspapers Ltd (No 2)*[2] in which it was affirmed that there was a public interest in a legally enforceable protection of confidences received under notice of confidentiality. There are three elements required to establish a breach of the obligation. First, the information divulged must have the necessary quality of confidence about it; second, that information must have been imparted in circumstances importing an obligation of confidence; and, third, there must be an unauthorised use of that information to the detriment of the party communicating it.[3] All these criteria would apply in a medical context where the duty of discretion has been endorsed judicially. Thus, in *Hunter v Mann*[4] the court accepted that:

> . . . the doctor is under a duty not to [voluntarily] disclose, without the consent of the patient, information which he, the doctor, has gained in his professional capacity.

More recently, in the very significant case of *W v Egdell*,[5] which we discuss in greater detail at p 171 below, the court accepted the existence of an obligation of confidentiality between a psychiatrist and his subject, an obligation which counsel submitted was based not only on equitable grounds but also on implied contract.

Whatever may be the legal basis for the duty, its moral content is considerable. Indeed, in the context of medical law in particular, it is difficult to dissociate the two disciplines – thus, we have Lord Coleridge CJ: 'A legal common law duty is nothing else than the enforcing by law of that which is a moral obligation without legal enforcement'.[6] We can, therefore, look not only at what the patient feels is his legal entitlement but also at the ethical requirements of the medical profession itself. Here

---

1 The doctor/patient and priest/penitent relationships were accepted a being among those in which an implied obligation of confidence existed in *Stephens v Avery* [1988] Ch 449 at 455, [1988] 2 All ER 477 at 482.
2 [1990] 1 AC 109, [1988] 3 All ER 545.
3 Per Megarry J in *Coco v A N Clark (Engineers) Ltd* [1969] RPC 41 at 47 quoted in *Stephens v Avery*, fn 1, above. The need for an element of detriment is, however, not universally accepted. See Rose J in *X v Y* [1988] 2 All ER 648 at 657, (1987) 3 BMLR 1 at 12.
4 [1974] QB 767, [1974] 2 All ER 414, per Boreham J at QB 772, All ER 417. For a general discussion of the duty of confidentiality in the medical context, see G Parker and M Spencer 'Confidentiality – Medical Reports' in M J Powers and N H Harris (eds) *Medical Negligence* (1990) p 69.
5 [1990] Ch 359, [1990] 1 All ER 835.
6 In *R v Instan* [1893] 1 QB 450 at 453.

there are a number of sources from which the doctor can seek guidance. The Hippocratic Oath (Appendix A) makes several demands which can scarcely be regarded as binding on the modern doctor; nonetheless, its stipulations as to professional confidentiality are still firmly endorsed. The translation cited in the sponsio academica at graduation ceremonials in the University of Edinburgh runs:

> Whatever things seen or heard in the course of medical practice ought not to be spoken of, I will not, save for weighty reasons, divulge.

The Declaration of Geneva (amended at Sydney) (Appendix B) imposes much the same obligation on the doctor, requiring him to 'respect the secrets which are confided in me, even after the patient has died'.

The great majority of commentators on medical ethics endorse a continued adherence to a strict principle[7] although some doubt the efficacy of an absolute rule and prefer a form of contractual obligation which, it is thought, would promote the individual patient's autonomy.[8] Most critics, however, see the concept as being something of a pretence in that bureaucracy, fired by modern administrative technology, is increasingly invasive of the principle. Certainly, patients' records must circulate fairly widely – and among professionals who are less deeply indoctrinated as to confidentiality than are their medical colleagues. As a result, it has been suggested that institutions should take over custodianship of confidences and, thus, impose an overall standard of duty on all who work in, say, the hospital.[9]

Even so, the special position of the doctor is unlikely to change in the foreseeable future and he is currently bound by the authority of, and is subject to the discipline of, the General Medical Council. Subject to certain exceptions which we discuss further below, the Council imposes a strict duty on registered medical practitioners to refrain from disclosing voluntarily to any third party information about a patient which he has learnt directly or indirectly in his professional capacity.[10] A breach of this duty will be a serious matter, exposing the doctor to a wide range of potential professional penalties. It is to be noted, however, that sanctions of this nature are purely intra-professional and it has long been questioned whether they give adequate protection to the aggrieved patient. Thus, the Law Commission has suggested that the common law position should be strengthened by establishing a statutory offence of breach of confidence which would include those arising between doctor and patient.[11] It may well be that additional regulation will be forced upon the United

---

7 See, for example, J M Jacob 'Confidentiality: The Dangers of Anything Weaker than the Medical Ethic' (1982) 8 J Med Ethics 18; M H Kottow 'Medical Confidentiality: An Intransigent and Absolute Obligation' (1986) 12 J Med Ethics 117.

8 S J Warwick 'A Vote for No Confidence' (1989) 15 J Med Ethics 183.

9 D L Kenny 'Confidentiality: The Confusion Continues' (1982) 8 J Med Ethics 9; M Siegler 'Confidentiality in Medicine: A Decrepit Concept' (1982) 307 New Engl J Med 1518. See also D F H Pheby 'Changing Practice on Confidentiality: A Cause for Concern' (1982) 8 J Med Ethics 12; A W Macara ' "Confidentiality" A Decrepit Concept?' (1984) 77 J R Soc Med 577.

10 *Professional Conduct and Discipline: Fitness to Practise* ('The Blue Book'), (1993) para 76. The advice of the British Medical Association has no disciplinary authority but provides invaluable background to the GMC's instructions: see *Philosophy and Practice of Medical Ethics* (1988) ch 3 and *Rights and Responsibilities of Doctors* (1988) ch 2.

11 *Breach of Confidence* (Cmnd 8388), para 6.1.

Kingdom. Medical confidentiality in France and Belgium is absolute and is protected in the criminal code.[12] With the unrestricted interchange of doctors between the countries of the European Community it may well be that other Member States will pressurise the UK into taking steps to limit erosion of what they regard as a fundamental principle.

Relaxation of the rule

Nevertheless, all the classic codes of practice imply some qualification of an absolute duty of professional secrecy. Thus, the Hippocratic Oath has it: 'All that may come to my knowledge . . . which ought not to be spread abroad, I will keep secret', which clearly indicates that there are some things which *may* be published. The Declaration of Geneva modifies this prohibition to: 'I will respect the secrets which are confided in me' and the word 'respect' is open to interpretation. The General Medical Council, while always emphasising its strong views as to the rule dictating professional secrecy, still lists eight specific possible exceptions to the rule which provide a sound basis for discussion.

Consent to publish

The first, and most easily recognisable exception is when the patient or his legal adviser consents to a relaxation of secrecy. The situation is simple when viewed from the positive angle: a positive consent to release of information elides any obligation to secrecy owed by the person receiving that consent.[13]   Equally, an explicit request that information should not be disclosed is binding on the doctor save in the most exceptional circumstances – a matter which is of major concern in relation to communicable disease (see p 174 below).

Looked at from the negative aspect, however, the position is not so clear and may be frankly unsatisfactory. How many patients know whether the person standing with the consultant beside the hospital bedside is another doctor, a social worker or just an interested spectator? Would they have consented to their presence if they had been informed? The consultant may be responsible if, as a result, there is a breach of confidence – but this is small consolation to the patient who feels his rights have been infringed. What patient at a teaching hospital out-patient department is likely to refuse when the consultant asks 'You don't mind these young doctors being present, do you?' – the pressures are virtually irresistible and truly autonomous consent is impossible, yet the confidential doctor/patient relationship which began with his general practitioner has, effectively, been broken.

In practice, it is obvious that such technical breaches must be, and generally are, accepted – a modern hospital cannot function except as a team effort and new doctors have to be trained, the return for a technical loss of patient autonomy being access

---

12 France: Penal Code, art 378; Belgium: Penal Code, art 458. Attention is also drawn to the Evidence Amendment Act 1980 in New Zealand where, subject to minor reservations, privilege is accorded to medical confidence (ss 32 and 33); the rights of the dead are specifically covered as is, incidentally, the religious confessional (s 31).

13 *C v C* [1946] 1 All ER 562.

to the best diagnostic and therapeutic aids available. The GMC recognises this in permitting the sharing of information with other practitioners who assume responsibility for clinical management of the patient and, to the extent that the doctor deems it necessary for the performance of their particular duties, with other health care professionals who are collaborating with the doctor in his patients' management.[14] The exception notes that it is the doctor's responsibility to ensure that such individuals appreciate that the information is being imparted in strict professional confidence. The doctor's duty is, thereby, restricted in a reasonable way; it is difficult to see how he can be expected to carry the onus for any subsequent actions by his associates. Any such infringement might be the basis of a complaint to the Health Service Commissioner.[15]

The patient's interests
The next exception – that it is ethical to break confidentiality without a patient's consent when it is in his own interests to do so and when it is undesirable on medical grounds to seek such consent[16] – is acceptable save to those who are fanatically opposed to so-called professional paternalism. The recipient of the information may be a close relative, or, in rare circumstances, an unrelated third party – but it remains the doctor's duty to make every reasonable effort to persuade the patient to allow the information to be given. Such instances must be rare in these days of public medical instruction through the news media. When they occur, decisions rest, by definition, on clinical judgment – a properly considered clinical decision cannot be *unethical* whether it proves right or wrong and, in the event of action being taken on the basis of breach of confidence, the fact that it was a justifiable breach would offer a complete defence both in the civil courts and in the Professional Conduct Committee of the General Medical Council. The Council does, however, stress the need for caution when the patient has insufficient understanding, by reason of immaturity, of what the treatment or advice being sought involves. We return to this aspect later in the chapter.

The doctor in society
The doctor's overriding duty to society represents what is arguably the most controversial permissible exception to the rule of confidentiality in so far as it rests on subjective definitions. Society is not homogeneous but consists of groups amenable to almost infinite classification – regional, political, economic, by age and so on. It follows that what one man regards as a duty to society may be anathema to another. Individual doctors are bound to weigh the scales differently in any particular instance while, in general, all relative weighting must change from case

14 *Professional Conduct and Discipline: Fitness to Practise* (Blue Book) (1993) para 79.
15 National Health Service Act 1977, Pt V, as amended by Parliamentary and Health Service Commissioners Act 1987. An investigation by the Health Service Commissioner will not be precluded by the Hospital Complaints Procedure Act 1985 which enforces a duty to deal with complaints and to publicise the arrangements made for so doing.
16 Blue Book, para 82.

to case. There is, for example, a great deal of difference in respect of confidentiality between a bee sting and venereal disease. While it is clear that no rules can be laid down, some aspects of this societal conflict are of sufficiently wide importance to merit individual consideration.

The most dramatic dilemma is posed by the possibility of violent crime. What is the doctor to do if he knows his patient has just committed rape – particularly if there is evidence that this is but one of a series of attacks on women? Perhaps even more disconcertingly, what if it becomes apparent that his patient is about to commit such an offence? Statute law is helpful here only in a negative sense – misprision of felony, other than as related to treason, is no longer an offence.[17] There is case law to the effect that the doctor need not even assist the police by answering their questions concerning his patients although he must not give false or misleading information.[18] The obligation on the prosecution to disclose to the defence all unused material which might have some bearing on the offences charged has caused some difficulty for police surgeons. Generally speaking, an accused gives consent to disclosure of specific information only. Other information may, however, come to light during the course of the examination and once this is in the police notes, the police may feel it their duty to include it in their 'disclosure' despite the fact that there is no consent to their so doing. The police surgeon may, therefore, feel it his ethical imperative to conceal his knowledge – but the decision must, at times, be difficult to make.[19]

In the early part of the century, both medical and legal opinion was divided on the issue of disclosure of serious crime. Discussion was, however, based largely on the subject of illegal abortion which has emotional overtones of its own. Nevertheless, it was in that context that Avory J made his well-known observation:

> There are cases where the desire to preserve [the confidential relation which exists between the medical man and his patient] must be subordinated to the duty which is cast on every good citizen to assist in the investigation of serious crime . . .[20]

This probably represents the foundation of the doctrine of the public interest as applied to medicine. This doctrine crystallised in the case of *W v Egdell*.[1]

In this case, a prisoner in a secure hospital sought a review of his case with a view to transfer to a regional secure unit. His legal representatives secured a report from an independent consultant psychiatrist which was, in the event, unfavourable to W. As a result, the application for transfer was aborted. W was, however, due for routine review of his detention and the psychiatrist, becoming aware that his report would not be included in the patient's notes, feared that decisions would be taken on

---

17 Criminal Law Act 1967, s 5(5).
18 *Rice v Connolly* [1966] 2 QB 414, [1966] 2 All ER 649. See also P Schutte 'Medical Confidentiality and a Police Murder Inquiry' (1989) 5 J Med Def Union (Spring) 21.
19 For discussion, see P Schutte 'Medical Confidentiality and the Police' (1993) 9 J Med Def Union 63.
20 Birmingham Assizes, 1 December 1914. Reported in (1914) 78 JP 604. The judge referred to a possible moral duty in the event that the patient was not dying; his views as to strict moral duty were mainly concerned with the loss of evidence in failing to take a dying declaration from a moribund patient.
1 [1990] Ch 359, [1990] 1 All ER 835.

inadequate information with consequent danger to the public. He therefore sent a copy of his report to the medical director of the hospital and a further copy reached the Home Office; W brought an action in contract and in equity alleging breach of a duty of confidence. The trial judge, Scott J, considered that, in the circumstances:

> The question in the present case is not whether Dr Egdell was under a duty of confidence; he plainly was. The question is as to the breadth of that duty.[2]

Attention was drawn to the advice of the General Medical Council as to the circumstances in which exception to the rule of confidentiality is permitted. The new Blue Book para 79 states that:

> Most doctors in hospital and general practice are working in health care teams, some of whose members may need access to information, given or obtained in confidence about individuals, in order to perform their duties. It is for doctors who lead such teams to judge when it is appropriate for information to be disclosed for that purpose.

This new paragraph is certainly more restrictive than was its counterpart at the time of the trial but it would still, probably, justify the disclosure to the hospital authorities. The new para 86 is, however, similar – albeit, again, rather less open-ended – to the version extant at the time in saying:

> Rarely, cases may arise in which disclosure in the public interest may be justified, for example, a situation in which the failure to disclose appropriate information would expose the patient, or someone else, to a risk of death or serious harm.

Scott J based his conclusions on broad considerations – that a doctor in similar circumstances has a duty not only to the patient but also to the public and that the latter would require him to disclose the results of his examination to the proper authorities if, in his opinion, the public interest so required. This would be independent of the patient's instructions on the point.

The Court of Appeal unanimously confirmed the trial judge's decision to dismiss the action but did so with rather more reservation – particularly as expressed in the judgment of Bingham LJ. The concept of a private interest competing with a public interest was rejected in favour of there being a *public* interest in maintaining professional duties of confidence; the 'balancing' of interests thus fell to be carried out in circumstances of unusual difficulty. Doubts, which we share, were cast on the applicability of para 79 (then para 78(b)) to a doctor acting in the role of an independent consultant. Disclosure would have to be justified under para 86 (then para 78(g)) and, here, it was for the court, not the doctor, to decide whether such a disclosure was or was not a breach of contract. Moreover, there was no doubt that the Mental Health Act 1983, s 76, showed a clear Parliamentary intention that a restricted patient should be free to seek advice and evidence for specific purposes which was confidential in respect of the authorities. Only the most compelling

---

2   Ibid [1990] Ch 359 at 389, [1989] 1 All ER 1089 at 1102.

circumstances could justify a doctor acting contrary to the patient's perceived interests in the absence of consent. Nevertheless, in the instant case, the fear of a real risk to public safety entitled a doctor to take reasonable steps to communicate the grounds of his concern to the appropriate authorities.

Looked at superficially, it is easy to view *W v Egdell* as a serious intrusion into the relationship of confidential trust between doctor and patient. It is equally possible to perceive the principle as emerging relatively unscathed. W's case was clearly regarded as extreme and, although we cannot exclude some concern, there is no evidence in the judgment that the courts would condone a breach of confidence on less urgent grounds. The 'danger area' seems to be better deliminated by way of independent activity on the part of doctors – as anticipated by Bingham LJ in *Egdell* above. In *R v Crozier*,[3] a psychiatrist called by the accused, concerned that his opinion should be available to the court, apparently handed his report to counsel for the Crown. The now sentenced accused appealed on the grounds that the breach of confidentiality between doctor and patient had denied him the opportunity of deciding whether medical evidence would be tendered. The Court of Appeal again thought that there was a stronger public interest in the disclosure of the psychiatrist's views than in the confidence he owed to the appellant. The psychiatrist was found to have acted responsibly and reasonably in a very difficult situation. But what if a doctor acts *un*reasonably in such circumstances? The damage to the patient is done and he will get little satisfaction from the fact that the doctor is censured; it is surely a thoroughly paternalistic practice that should be carefully restrained.

On a more mundane note, the importance of disease in drivers has increased and presents a major dilemma to the conscientious doctor. The urgency of decisions is maximised by the facts that driving licences are now issued for the lifetime up to the age of 70 and that responsibility for reporting health deficiencies is placed firmly on the licence holder. Heart disease is always thought of as being paramount in this context but, in practice, very few car accidents that result in serious personal injury are caused by cardiac conditions. Moreover, the majority of cardiac patients are mature and conscious of their responsibilities. Epilepsy is a far more apposite example. Nearly half the instances of unconsciousness at the wheel of a car are epileptic in origin and the condition is found to have been undisclosed in over three quarters of these – the public need seems clear but what is the doctor to do? The standard answer is that he should either persuade the patient to report the disability or obtain the patient's consent to disclosure but this does not help when, as is likely, both courses are rejected. It has been suggested[4] that a doctor who knew that an unsafe patient of his was continuing to drive and who then failed to take any action on the point might be liable in damages for negligence to anyone harmed by his patient on the road. This seems unlikely to happen in the United Kingdom context and has been rejected even in the United States.[5] We conclude that doctors are not only protected against any action for breach of confidence by qualified privilege but also that they have a positive moral duty to inform the medical authorities at the

---

3 (1990) 8 BMLR 128.

4 Legal Correspondent 'Doctors, Drivers and Confidentiality' (1974) 1 BMJ 399.

5 In *Crosby v Sultz* 592 A 2d 1337 (Pa, 1991) a suit against a doctor who allowed a diabetic patient to drive was rejected on the grounds that injuries inflicted on a person who could not be notified of the driver's condition were not foreseeable.

vehicle licensing centre of patients who are a danger on the road by virtue of their medical condition. In the unlikely event of it being needed, *Egdell* would almost certainly be applied.

An interesting example of the problems posed has been reported from New Zealand. There, a bus driver underwent a triple coronary by-pass operation and was, subsequently, certified as fit to drive by his surgeon. His general practitioner, however, asked that his licence to drive be withdrawn and, furthermore, warned his passengers of their supposed danger. The practitioner's activities resulted in a report to the Medical Practitioners' Disciplinary Committee and a finding of: 'guilty of professional misconduct in that he breached professional confidence in informing lay people of his patient's personal medical history'. Dr Duncan sought judicial review of this decision. The High Court accepted the propriety of breaching medical confidentiality in cases of clear public interest but refused the application on grounds which can be summed up:

> I think a doctor who has decided to communicate should discriminate and ensure the recipient is a responsible authority.[6]

Seldom can there have been a case which demonstrates the 'need to know' principle so forcibly.

Confidentiality and HIV infection

The spread of the human immunodeficiency virus has given rise to a host of problems related to confidentiality. Sexually transmitted diseases are not new to the medico-legal arena but what sets AIDS apart is the current absence of a proven treatment of a condition which, in its full-blown state, appears to be always fatal. Its relatively specific sexual connotation, together with its serious association with drug addiction, leads to considerable stigmatisation. Those who are found to be HIV positive may be disadvantaged in a number of practical ways which have been discussed in chapter 1 and to which we refer again at p 231; all serve to fuel the concern which many such persons harbour as to the confidentiality of their status.

Such concerns attract great sympathy, yet there are also social interests to be considered. The crucial dilemma here is whether relaxation of the confidentiality rule would lead to failure to seek advice and treatment and, hence, to the spread of the disease or whether the imposition of absolute secrecy improperly denies others the opportunity to avoid the risk of exposure to infection. Should a sexual partner be told of the risk if the patient himself declines to pass on the information? What is the situation if a person known to be infected is employed in circumstances in which he might expose others to the virus? The problem of confidentiality cannot, however, be settled by the balancing of conflicting private interests alone – the public health dimension has to be taken into account. AIDS is not, at present, a notifiable disease[7] – a dispensation which certainly helps to maintain confidentiality. The

6   *Duncan v Medical Practitioners' Disciplinary Committee* [1986] 1 NZLR 513, per Jeffries J at 521.
7   Under the AIDS (Control) Act 1987, health authorities must provide reports to the responsible minister. The Minister can also order the hospitalisation and, if necessary, the detention of sufferers (Public Health (Infectious Diseases) Regulations 1985, SI 1985/434).

rationale given for this is that notifiability would inhibit persons from undergoing testing.[8] While some would doubt the validity of this, any potential public health 'risk' is justified on the grounds that, in the conditions of everyday social contact, HIV is transmitted only with great difficulty – if at all. As a result, it is government policy, supported by the majority of informed opinion, that any departure from the strictest anonymity in respect of HIV-related information must be subject to intense scrutiny.[9]

The English courts have already declared their hand in weighing the balance between a strongly supported public policy in favour of freedom of the press against the need for loyalty and confidentiality with particular reference to AIDS patients' hospital records. In *X v Y*,[10] the names of two doctors being treated in hospital for AIDS were improperly disclosed. The health authority sought, and obtained, an injunction to prevent their publication by a newspaper. While holding that the health authority had not made out a case for forced disclosure of the source of the information, Rose J stated that such luck a second time was highly unlikely and that prison would be the probable consequence if the informer repeated his or her betrayal of confidence:

> The public in general and patients in particular are entitled to expect hospital records to be confidential and it is not for any individual to take it upon himself or herself to breach that confidence whether induced by a journalist or otherwise.[11]

The authority's action was not, as has been suggested, a 'cover-up' operation. The basic reasons underlying absolute confidentiality in AIDS related cases should be applied irrespective of the patient's calling. The decision can be justified medically on the grounds that the risks of a well counselled physician passing the disease to a patient are, at worst, slightly more than negligible.[12] This is, however, an area in which the media are insatiable. We have already noted (at p 22) a rash of recent cases in which the names of infected doctors have been widely publicised in the press and a number of letters from the health boards concerned have testified to the fact that, given that the boards must notify all patient contacts of such practitioners, it is virtually impossible to preserve anonymity.[13] The current policy of the General Medical Council to the effect that:

> Only in the most exceptional circumstances, where the release of a doctor's name is essential for the protection of patients, may a doctor's HIV status be disclosed without his or her consent . . .[14]

is, in practice, unworkable.

8 M W Adler 'HIV, Confidentiality and a "delicate balance"' (1991) 17 J Med Ethics 196.
9 For a general overview of the ethical position, see R Gillon 'AIDS and Medical Confidentiality' (1987) 294 BMJ 1675. A useful review is M Brazier and M Lobjoit 'AIDS, Ethics, and the Respiratory Physician' (1990) 45 Thorax 283.
10 [1988] 2 All ER 648, (1987) 3 BMLR 1.
11 [1988] 2 All ER 648 at 665, (1987) 3 BMLR 1 at 21, per Rose J.
12 It is widely accepted that only one case has been confirmed – and the patient was later found to be an intravenous drug abuser: B Mishu, W Schaffer, J M Horan et al 'A Surgeon with AIDS: Lack of Evidence of Transmission to Patrons' (1990) 264 J Amer Med Ass 467.
13 See D S G Sloan 'Guidelines Must Be Reformed' (1993) 307 BMJ 566 and supporting correspondence.
14 General Medical Council *HIV Infection and AIDS: The Ethical Considerations* (Revised 1993).

Anyone infected with HIV constitutes an undoubted danger to his or her sexual partner although the risk of transmission depends upon the nature of the sexual activity, the frequency and diversity of exposure and the extent to which precautions are taken. Counselling of HIV cases includes such information routinely and patients are advised as to the need to disclose their status to those whom they might have put at risk of infection. It is unsurprising that there will be some patients who are not prepared to do so nor, indeed, to inform their general practitioners. The doctor is then faced with the problem of whether or not he, himself, should inform those with 'a need to know'.

The General Medical Council has advised doctors that patients should be persuaded of the need for their general practitioners to be informed of the diagnosis but states that the patient's wishes should be respected if consent to disclosure is refused.[15] An exception may be made, however, if the doctor believes that a failure to pass on the information may expose other health caring staff to serious risk – but the doctor must still be prepared to justify such action. Passing information to a patient's spouse or other sexual partner in the absence of consent is allowable so long as every effort has been made to persuade the patient to do so and there is a serious and identifiable risk to a specific individual. The GMC emphasises that their paper does not represent a code; the original document has now been clarified in many ways but there are still ambiguities. What is one to make of phraseology such as 'the doctor may consider it a duty to seek to ensure that a sexual partner is informed'? In an interesting discussion of the original guidelines, the Institute of Medical Ethics (IME) has shown that two doctors could react to the issue of confidentiality in diametrically opposed ways, yet each could still be acting within the 'guidelines'.[16] The GMC concludes that the responsibility for any action taken is entirely that of the individual doctor – which tells us nothing as to how to construct that responsibility.

The IME's solution is to rely on a relationship of mutual empowerment based on a balance between, on the one hand, the patient's proper power of decision making and, on the other, the doctor's exercise of clinical skills and, most importantly, of effective communication of information. The ideal is that the person at risk should be able to make an informed choice whether or not to accept the risk and that this choice will be offered by the patient. In the exceptional case where the patient frustrates this policy, the doctor should, in the Institute's view, base his decision as to whether or not to breach confidentiality on the strength of his judgment that, by maintaining confidentiality, he can encourage the infected patient to acknowledge his or her responsibility to respect the interests of others. In this respect, great importance is laid on whether or not the person at risk is also a patient of the doctor – the implication being that, in the former case, disclosure would be justified fairly easily but that confidentiality would be the better choice if he or she were not.

This may be a pragmatic solution but it appears to us to be morally ambivalent. If it is medical beneficence to inform one's *patient* of a risk, it is scarcely justifiable to bask in the safety-net of confidentiality when one's duty of care is no more than

---

15 See the previous note. The British Medical Association is silent on the question in *Philosophy and Practice of Medical Ethics* (1988). See also fn 10, p 168 above.
16 K M Boyd 'HIV Infection and AIDS: The Ethics of Medical Confidentiality' (1992) 18 J Med Ethics 173.

indirect. A discussion based on moral principles, however, takes little account of the legal issues involved and it is arguable that a patient would have a right of action against a doctor who warned his or her spouse or other sexual partner of their potential risk. Despite the prima facie breach of confidence, a court would almost certainly balance the two private interests involved and hold that disclosure was justified by the intention to protect others from a possibly fatal risk. It is difficult to imagine a court awarding damages to such a plaintiff and there has been no decision directly in point taken in the United Kingdom. Conversely, it seems that there is a general common law duty and a statutory duty on the doctor in some parts of the United States and Canada to inform those at risk[17] – and the *Tarasoff* decision[18] which we discuss in chapter 18, could be taken as a pointer. The inference of a duty of care in respect of endangered third parties would, however, be difficult to reconcile with existing notions in the United Kingdom. No duty to warn exists in the absence of a special relationship between the parties and it is difficult to see why the AIDS situation should constitute an exception to the general common law rule, in both England and Scotland, that there is no duty to rescue.[19] It is, however, certainly possible that a doctor would be held to have a duty to warn a third party *who was also his patient* as, in this case, there is a relationship which is sufficiently proximate to give rise to a duty of affirmative action.

It is impossible to leave the subject of confidentiality in HIV infection without mention of the specific problem of prisons – the environment could have been designed for the spread of the condition and the consequences of disclosure of a positive status could be disastrous for the individual. A policy of confidentiality exists but, clearly, it is difficult, if not impossible, to maintain so long as positivity is associated with segregation, provision of personalised eating utensils and the like. There has also been some limited purposeful breaching of confidentiality in respect of a 'need to know' on the part of the staff.[20] Such potentials for disclosure discourage voluntary testing and counselling and serve as barriers to effective public health measures; they have been phased out since 1991. It has been shown that a guarantee of confidentiality results in a marked increase in identified positive subjects.[1] Such evidence tends to support the general national policy on confidentiality and HIV; at the same time, it cannot be denied that more prisoners are infected than are identified – the issue is, indeed, delicately balanced.

---

17 L Gostin and A Ziegler 'Review of AIDS-related Legislative and Regulatory Policy in the United States' (1987) 15 Law Med Hlth Care 5; D I Casswell 'Disclosure by a Physician of AIDS-related Patient Information: An Ethical and Legal Dilemma' (1989) 68 Can BR 225.
18 *Tarasoff v Regents of the University of California* 529 P 2d 55 (Cal, 1974); 551 P 2d 334 (Cal, 1976). Decisions following upon this include the contrasting cases of *Brady v Hopper* 751 F 2d 329 (1984) and *Peterson v State* 671 P 2d 230 (Was, 1983).
19 For further discussion, see A McCall Smith 'The Duty to Rescue and the Common Law' in M Menlowe and A McCall Smith (eds) *The Duty to Rescue* (1993) p 55.
20 T Groves 'Prison Policies on HIV under Review' (1991) 303 BMJ 1354. The vexed question of the police's 'need to know' is discussed in J K Mason 'Recording HIV Status on Police Computers' (1992) 304 BMJ 995.
1 S A M Gore and A G Bird 'No Escape: HIV Transmission in Jail' (1993) 307 BMJ 147.

Confidentiality within the family

A narrower area of societal privilege lies within the family where the doctor may be the first to recognise the signs of violence. The police are, in general, disinclined to interfere in cases of marital violence because of the unsympathetic reception they are likely to get from both sides in so doing. However, this may not always be the case and the doctor cannot be content to watch his patient suffer not only physical injury but also intense mental trauma. In the end, it is clear that an adult woman of sound mind is entitled to her autonomy; she has the opportunity of reporting to the police or, often more usefully, she has access to one of the many voluntary shelters which are now being established. She now has considerable protection under the law.[2] All the doctor can effectively do is to advise and, in this, he may be able to help by arranging for treatment of the offender – 'wife battering' is markedly associated with alcoholism and neurotic symptoms in the husband.

The position is different in the case of child abuse. Here the victim is defenceless and the victim is the patient. Parental autonomy must be forfeited on the grounds of impropriety while the doctor is covered, legally, by the doctrine of necessity – in this case to assume consent to disclosure by one who cannot give consent – and, professionally, by the advice of the General Medical Council:

> [W]here a doctor believes that a patient may be the victim of physical or sexual abuse [and the patient cannot be judged capable of giving or withholding consent to disclosure], the patient's medical interests are paramount and may require the doctor to disclose information to an appropriate person or authority.[3]

It has been suggested that, as a matter of law, such action probably does constitute a technical breach of the duty of confidence[4] but this proposition seems barely tenable. Rather, the doctor faces a clinical dilemma which, although less publicised, is of greater importance. The introduction of registers for infants at risk from violence and the obvious merit in nipping violence in the bud act as servo-mechanisms to one another. The possibility is increasing that truly accidental injuries are being misdiagnosed with a consequent reluctance on the part of parents to seek help for fear of being 'branded',[5] and children may, therefore, actually suffer despite the doctor's concern for their safety. A case misdiagnosed as child abuse will cause considerable distress for those accused,[6] but, equally, a missed case which

---

2   Domestic Violence and Matrimonial Proceedings Act 1976; Matrimonial Homes (Family Protection) (Scotland) Act 1981.
3   Blue Book, para 83. Compulsory reporting of suspected child abuse is statutory in all of the United States, in Canada and in several Australian States.
4   A Samuels 'The Duty of the Doctor to Respect the Confidence of the Patient' (1980) 20 Med, Sci & L 58.
5   D M Wheeler and C J Hobbs 'Mistakes in Diagnosing Non-accidental Injury: 10 Years; Experience' (1988) 296 BMJ 1233. It seems that no action for negligence can be brought in England in such cases: *M v Newham London Borough Council* [1994] NLJR 357.
6   See two 'at-risk register' cases: *R v Norfolk County Council Social Services Department, ex p M* [1989] QB 619, [1989] 2 All ER 359; *R v Harrow London Borough Council, ex p D* [1990] Fam 133, [1990] 3 All ER 12, CA.

ends in murder can bring great recrimination on the doctor. The concern of the profession as to possible actions for defamation was certainly eased by the decision that a recognised caring authority may refuse to disclose the name of an informant.[7] In the end, however, such a right to or privilege of non-disclosure depends not so much on principles of confidentiality as on what lies in the public interest.

Confidentiality between parents and their teenage children becomes further involved. Consent to treatment is discussed in detail in chapter 10 below. In the present context, we are concerned only with confidentiality and, particularly, with the doctor's relationship with the family. There may be other medical conditions which a minor might wish to conceal from his or her parents but, in practice, those related to sexual affairs are likely to prove the most important. Given that young persons of both sexes do have intercourse, so the doctor may be confronted by requests as to contraception or abortion by young girls or for treatment of venereal disease by minors of either sex. It is, therefore, unsurprising that the leading case to address the question of minors' rights to confidentiality – *Gillick*[8] – should concern contraception and has, in fact, been discussed under that head at p 94. The twin issues of consent to treatment and right to privacy in young people are inextricably interwoven and, again, further discussion will be found elsewhere.[9] Here, we will attempt to limit discussion to those issues in the case which are specific to confidentiality.

From this point of view, the background to the *Gillick* decision is relatively simple, yet it represents the core of the case. As we have already suggested, contraception must be seen as sociologically preferable to abortion; even so, only a few young girls are likely to consent to their parents being told they 'are on the pill' and refusal by the doctor to supply is unlikely to deter those who want sexual intercourse. On this basis, the doctor who secretly supplies contraceptives on request to a girl under the age of 16 is performing a duty to society. On the other hand, it is widely agreed that parents have a right to know what is happening to their children and should, ideally, give consent to medical treatment irrespective of the minor's capacity to understand the complexities. It is, therefore, apparent that any entitlement to consent carries with it a simultaneous entitlement to confidentiality and vice versa. The House of Lords' solution of the problem is to be found in Lord Fraser's five criteria which have been recapitulated at p 95 and which can be summarised as granting a right of confidentiality to the mature minor when the exercise of that right is in her best interests. It must, however, be emphasised that, throughout the case, an obligation was firmly imposed on the doctor to attempt to persuade the girl to inform her parents or to allow him to do so and that, in itself, constitutes an important qualification of the normal rules of professional secrecy. Additionally, the General Medical Council has intimated that confidentiality between doctor and minor patient is not absolute in that, should the young girl prove too immature to appreciate the

---

7 *D v National Society for the Prevention of Cruelty to Children* [1978] AC 171, [1977] 1 All ER 589, HL. Protection of the informant is guaranteed by law in places having compulsory reporting (eg Child Welfare Act 1977 (NSW)).
8 *Gillick v West Norfolk and Wisbech Area Health Authority* [1984] QB 581, [1984] 1 All ER 365; on appeal [1986] AC 112, [1985] 1 All ER 533; revsd [1986] AC 112, [1985] 3 All ER 402, HL.
9 See under 'Consent', p 222.

significance of the treatment sought, the doctor would be entitled to inform the parents of the consultation – subject to informing the girl that he was about to do so.[10] Thus, despite the case seeming to represent a victory for the autonomy of youth, the situation remains uneasy for both the doctor and the patient. On the one hand, the patient cannot know the doctor's intentions until after the consultation; on the other, the doctor must be prepared to justify his decision – but to whom and in what circumstances is left unstated.

The longest established family relationship is that of spouses – what are their rights in both the positive and negative aspects of confidentiality? If the treatment is for a medical condition, a married person has the same rights to confidentiality in respect of the spouse as in respect of anyone else and, since the Abortion Act 1967 refers only to medical indications, this must apply to abortion. This can be implied also on legal grounds in that, since the husband has no right of veto either in Great Britain or in the United States,[11] he, similarly, has no right to information, and it is not hard to think of instances where disclosure of an abortion to the spouse could be construed as being malicious.

The conditions are not quite so clear, however, when treatment of an individual is not primarily based on medical considerations but, at the same time, affects the whole family; the issue of sterislisation is a case in point. Lord Denning was in no doubt in an early minority opinion that the surgeon should 'approach the spouse in order to satisfy himself as to consent'.[12] This must certainly be the case when genetic considerations are involved. Either or both parties may be contributing to a multifactorial trait; genetic counselling is impossible unless both husband and wife are involved. There is, however, less certainty when sterilisation is purely a matter of convenient family planning. On the face of it, there ought to be a consensual decision but the twentieth century couple are not certainly going to be together until parted by death, religious differences may prohibit agreement and there must be times when one spouse feels compelled to act for his or her individual reasons. The doctor may rightly refuse to sterilise in the absence of consent to spousal consultation but he would, we believe, be acting correctly both in law and in ethics were he to go ahead without it; adults have a right to privacy and it could probably be left to the Divorce Court, as in *Bravery*, to decide whether such unilateral action rendered marriage intolerable.[13] The matter has been discussed in greater detail in chapter 4. The very particular conditions attaching to genetic counselling are, similarly, addressed in detail in chapter 6.

Other special groups
Finally, there are many special groups which can be conceived of as raising particular problems in relation to medical confidentiality – those which spring to

---

10 Blue Book, para 84.
11 *Paton v British Pregnancy Advisory Service Trustees* [1979] QB 276, [1978] 2 All ER 987; *Planned Parenthood of Missouri v Danforth* 428 US 52 (1976).
12 *Bravery v Bravery* [1954] 3 All ER 59 at 67, [1954] 1 WLR 1169 at 1177, CA.
13 The British Medical Association state that the custom of obtaining consent from the patient's spouse to operation on the reproductive organs is one of courtesy not of legal necessity: *Philosophy and Practice of Medical Ethics* (1988) p 33.

mind most readily are accused persons, prisoners and members of the Armed Forces. Accused persons are legally innocent and therefore have the same rights as any member of the public. The police surgeon must state that the result of his examination will be reported to third parties and cannot proceed if, as a result, consent to examination is refused. In the interests of justice, however, he may make, and transmit the results of, observations which need not be confined to purely visual impressions.[14] The doctor/patient relationship is complicated in respect of prisoners and confidentiality is best considered as part of the whole spectrum (see chapter 1). Much loose talk is often voiced as to the status of medical officers in the armed forces. In reality, their relationship to individual patients is precisely the same as in civilian practice with the proviso that the doctor's duty to society is accentuated when this is formulated as a duty to a fighting unit where, eventually, the lives of many are dependent upon the health of individuals. There is, thus, a wider justification for disclosure than exists in civilian life and the serviceman has tacitly accepted this in enlisting. Nevertheless, the principle of justification remains valid. Similar considerations apply, say, to doctors in medical charge of sports teams; the discussion has come full circle in that, basically, one's ethical standards depend upon one's definition of society.

Doctors employed by companies or other institutions to act as medical advisers on staff health occupy a special position which has been singled out by the General Medical Council. It must now be stated explicitly before carrying out a pre-employment medical examination, or for fitness to work, that the results of that examination may be communicated to the employer and the written consent of the examinee must be obtained in the light of that information. Likewise, in the case of examinations carried out for insurance purposes, the doctor must obtain the positive agreement of the patient to waive the normal obligations of confidentiality within a 'need to know' formula. In the absence of such agreement, it is unlikely that the doctor engaged in industrial or insurance medicine could justify, on either ethical or legal grounds, a breach of a patient's confidence on the grounds that he, the doctor, owed a duty as an employee to his employer.

For the purposes of medical research
Information may be disclosed if necessary for the purposes of a medical research project which has been approved by a recognised ethical committee. The matter is included in the general discussion of medical research in chapter 16, below.

Confidentiality and the legal process
Disclosure of confidential medical information as part of the legal process can be looked at in two main categories – statutory and non-statutory. Statutory disclosure presents no problem to the doctor but it is, nevertheless, showing signs of encroachment on traditional values. Thus, the original requirements for reporting by the doctor of infectious disease[15] or industrial poisoning[16] are clearly directed to the good of

---

14 *Forrester v H M Advocate* 1952 JC 28.
15 Public Health (Infectious Diseases) Regulations 1988, SI 1988/1546.
16 Reporting of Injuries, Diseases and Dangerous Occurrences Regulations 1985, SI 1985/2023.

society. More recently, however, compulsory notification has become required more for statistical purposes[17] or for the protection of individuals by the state.[18] The two latter examples also show an increasing acceptance of some state control of the medical profession itself. Despite occasional protests at 'interference', there can be very little valid objection to such regulations.

It is to be noted that no immunity is granted to the doctor when a statutory duty is imposed on 'any person' to provide information. Few would complain at this in relation to the Prevention of Terrorism (Temporary Provisions) Acts 1974-89, s 18. Opinion is more divided as to the working of the Road Traffic Act 1988 when, by virtue of s 172, the doctor must provide on request any evidence which he has which may lead to the identification of a driver involved in an accident. The patient can scarcely expect the doctor to breach confidentiality, yet the doctor's liability under the law has been confirmed.[19]

There may, of course, be other times when the police would have an interest in access to medical records. This was an issue that was hotly debated during the progress of the Police and Criminal Evidence Act 1984 and, on the whole, those seeking to preserve medical confidentiality gained the day. Police engaged in the investigation of a serious arrestable offence may obtain a warrant to search for material which is likely to be relevant evidence.[20] The magistrates cannot, however, issue a warrant to search for 'excluded material' which includes personal records relating to a person's physical or mental health and which are held in confidence;[1] medical records are, therefore, excluded material. However, a constable may still apply to a circuit judge for an order to obtain such records. Not only must the court be satisfied of the need for access but there must have been some statutory authority passed before the 1984 Act which would have authorised such a search. The Act illustrates some of the difficulties in applying an ethical principle by way of statute. Hospital notes are clearly excluded material and can, therefore, be withheld from the police irrespective of the purpose of their search. Thus, the police cannot obtain them even though their sole purpose is, say, to establish the whereabouts of a potential murderer at a given time, as in *R v Cardiff Crown Court, ex p Kellam*.[2] As Morland J said in that case 'Presumably Parliament considered that the confidentiality of records of identifiable individuals relating to their health should have paramountcy over the prevention and investigation of serious crime' but one wonders if this was really in the contemplation of the legislature or of those who lobbied them so assiduously. Even so, we can see no reason within the statute why a doctor who sees it as a public duty to co-operate with the police should not do so if asked – provided, of course, that he is prepared to justify this later in a court of law or before his peers.

Other than by regulations, courts of law can compel the disclosure of medical material either through the production of documents or during evidence and cross-examination.

---

17 Abortion Regulations 1991, SI 1991/499; Abortion (Scotland) Regulations 1991, SI 1991/460.
18 Misuse of Drugs (Notification and Supply to Addicts) Regulations 1973, SI 1973/799.
19 *Hunter v Mann* footnote 4, p 167 above.
20 Police and Criminal Evidence Act 1984, s 8.
 1 Ibid ss 11,12.
 2 *R v Cardiff Crown Court, ex p Kellam* (1993) 16 BMLR 76. The court set aside the order to produce the documents 'with considerable reluctance'.

Disclosure of documents

Authority for the order to produce documents is to be found in the Administration of Justice Act 1970, ss 31 and 32 and the Administration of Justice (Scotland) Act 1972, s 1. Section 31 of the 1970 Act empowered the court to order disclosure to the applicant of documents related to negligence suits before litigation was started. Section 32 of the 1970 Act extended this, once suit had been filed, to the disclosure to the applicant of any records held by a third party which might be relevant to cases involving personal injury. In so far as they indicated a further breach of medical confidentiality and, consequently, a possible restriction of information given and opinions recorded, these sections – and particularly s 32 – caused some concern in medical circles. To an extent, this was unnecessary as the information sought was bound to come out at trial and the purpose of the Act was simply to ensure fairness to both sides and, at the same time, to forestall any hopeless actions. The question of who should receive the reports has now been resolved in the Supreme Court Act 1981, ss 33 and 34, by which the court is empowered to order disclosure as it sees fit either to the applicant, the applicant's legal advisers or, in the absence of legal advisers, to his medical advisers. Reports and documents must be exchanged with an eye to fairness and saving of litigation time.[3] There is, thus, no justification for hospitals or doctors to employ delaying tactics based on the principle of medical confidentiality – it has, indeed, been suggested that, by so doing, they might risk being ordered to pay the entire costs of a court application.[4]

Court directions may also be made for the disclosure before trial of expert medical reports which it is proposed to bring in evidence. The exception to this policy once lay in cases involving a suggestion of medical negligence – the rationale being that parties should not have to disclose experts' reports which were directed to establishing liability rather than to the prognosis and quantum of damages.[5] Largely as a result of the unsatisfactory trial in *Wilsher v Essex Area Health Authority*,[6] alterations were made to the Rules of the Supreme Court so as to bring medical negligence cases into line with others involving personal injury – prior disclosure was to become the norm rather than the exception. The situation was clarified in the Court of Appeal in *Naylor v Preston Area Health Authority*[7] where it was said that the basic objective of disclosure was the achievement of true justice which 'took account of time, money and the anguish of uncertainty as well as of a just outcome':

> Nowadays, the general rule is that, while a party is entitled to privacy in seeking out the cards for his hand, once he has put his hand together the litigation is to be conducted with all the cards face up on the table. Furthermore, most of the cards have to be put down well before the hearing.[8]

3 This may also apply when the subject is a child. In *Parks v Tayside Regional Council* 1989 SLT 345, the Court of Session ordered the recovery of the medical and social work documents of a child who was said to have infected a foster mother with hepatitis. Social work records also have no absolute immunity from disclosure in England: *Re M (A minor)* [1990] 2 FLR 36, CA.

4 See C Dyer 'Disclosure of Medical Records in Litigation' (1986) 293 BMJ 1298.

5 *Rahman v Kirklees Area Health Authority* [1980] 3 All ER 610, [1980] 1 WLR 1244, CA.

6 [1987] QB 730, [1986] 3 All ER 801, CA.

7 [1987] 2 All ER 353, [1987] 1 WLR 958, CA.

8 Ibid [1987] 2 All ER 353 at 360, [1987] 1 WLR 958 at 967, per Sir John Donaldson MR.

Moreover, *all* the cards must be put down, not just those obviously concerned with the action; the current view is that the court can deal with problems of confidentiality relating to irrelevant conditions – such as a past history of sexually transmitted disease – by limiting disclosure to the other side's medical advisers who must respect medical confidentiality except where litigation is affected.[9] Brahams[10] has suggested that the duty of pre-trial publication may be wider than is generally thought. As things stand, however, the expert is not expected to consider or anticipate every possible form of cross-examination – the need is only to disclose that evidence which he, himself, intends to give at trial.[11]

Disclosure of documents and information is, however, subject to what is commonly known as 'legal professional privilege' – a doctrine designed to allow the client unfettered access to his advisers. The concept is not without difficulties of which the doctor should be aware. First, legal professional privilege is tightly defined and is likely to be overridden, whenever this is possible, in the interests of legal fairness.[12] Thus, disclosure of reports which are designed primarily for accident investigation and prevention and only secondarily for the purpose of seeking legal advice is likely to be ordered. It is clear that this gives rise to a conflict of interests. On the one hand, it could be held that the public good of preventive medicine must take second place to the threat of private litigation;[13] on the other, the imposition of legal professional privilege has, on occasion, been granted only reluctantly in that secrecy is inequitable to the person who suffers medical mishap.[14] Second, while legal professional privilege is there in order to allow the client to be uninhibited when approaching his legal advisers, there is no corresponding privilege to encourage a patient to be equally open in relation to his medical advisers. This was demonstrated forcefully in *W v Egdell*[15] where it was concluded that a clear and important distinction was to be made between, on the one hand, instructions given to an expert and, on the other, the expert's opinion given in response to those instructions. The former was covered by legal professional privilege while the latter was not. We have some difficulty in understanding how a question can be subject to absolute confidentiality while the answer is not; nevertheless, the ruling given at first instance was fully supported in the Court of Appeal. Third, a request for

9 *Dunn v British Coal Corpn* [1993] ICR 591, CA.
10 D Brahams 'Medical Confidentiality and Expert Evidence' (1991) 337 Lancet 1276.
11 *Derby Co Ltd v Weldon (No 9)* (1990) Times, 9 November quoted by Brahams (in previous note) above. Whether this will be so if the recommendations of the Royal Commission on Criminal Justice *Report* (1993) are put into operation remains to be seen. For discussion, see J P Shepherd 'Presenting Expert Evidence in Criminal Proceedings' (1993) 307 BMJ 817.
12 Legal professional privilege is, in a sense, a product of the adversarial system of presenting evidence and is less likely to be upheld when proceedings are more akin to inquisitorial. The classic example of the latter is the case brought under the Children Act 1989 or in wardship proceedings: *Oxfordshire County Council v M* [1994] 1 FLR 175.
13 *Waugh v British Railways Board* [1980] AC 521, [1979] 2 All ER 1169. For discussion, see G Robertson 'Discovery of Hospital Accident Reports' (1983) 133 NLJ 1020 and, with rather different emphasis, 'Hospital Inquiries: Evidence and Privilege' (1982) 284 BMJ 519. The order to disclose may extend to specific accident report forms which might well be thought to be privileged (*Lask v Gloucester Health Authority* (1985) Times, 13 December).
14 *Lee v South West Thames Regional Health Authority* [1985] 2 All ER 385, [1985] 1 WLR 845, discussed also in 'Disclosure of Documents by Doctors' (1985) 290 BMJ 1973.
15 [1990] Ch 359, [1989] 1 All ER 1089.

information from a solicitor is not the same as an order of the court even though the conditions – eg that litigation is in progress – may seem similar. Medical practitioners have been found guilty of serious professional misconduct for making such a mistake in good faith but in ignorance.[16] Finally, it is worth noting that, while the legal representative may, of course, withhold any documents to which the privilege applies, the adversary may have advantage of these if they are disclosed in error and it is not obvious that privilege has not been waived.[17]

The doctor in the witness box has absolute privilege and is protected against any action for breach of confidence. Lord Halsbury LC provides the highest possible authority: the immunity of the witness in court 'is settled in law and cannot be doubted'.[18]

This privilege extends to pre-trial conferences and Scottish precognitions, the exception being that a privileged communication must not be made maliciously.[19] Judges may go to great lengths to protect the witness but, when so ordered, the doctor is bound to answer any question which is put to him.[20] Refusal to answer in the absence of the court's discretion to excuse a conscientious witness must expose the doctor to a charge of contempt and the court will take precedence even when there is a statutory obligation of secrecy.[1] In some European countries, however, the obligation to maintain confidentiality extends to the courtroom.

Patient access to medical records
The right to see one's own medical records has been vigorously asserted by advocates of patients' rights and equally firmly denied by at least a sizeable section of medical opinion. The Council of Europe's Data Protection Convention required the recognition of a right of access to personal data stored in computer banks and this led to the Data Protection Act 1984. The protection of persons about whom computerised information is stored lies in preventing the holding of inaccurate information or of concealing the fact that information is stored at all. Subject to a fee, a patient now has the right to be told by the 'registered data user' – who could be any health caring body holding computerised records – whether any such information is held and to be supplied with a copy of that information (s 21); the patient may, then, ensure its accuracy. There is provision, which is generalised throughout this area of legislation, for doctors to prevent access to information that is 'likely to cause serious harm' – a condition which is left undefined.

16 See 'Medical Confidence and the Law' (1981) 283 BMJ 1062.
17 *Pizzey v Ford Motor Co Ltd* (1993) Times, 8 March, CA.
18 In *Watson v M'Ewan* [1905] AC 480 at 486, HL.
19 *AB v CD* (1904) 7 F 72, per Lord Moncrief. This is the Court of Session stage of *Watson v M'Ewan*. It is the same in other Commonwealth countries. See *Hay v University of Alberta Hospital* (QB, Alberta) [1991] 2 Med LR 204 in which it was held that the plaintiff had no right to withhold consent to pre-trial discussions by the defendants with his medical attendants.
20 The exception to this requirement being disclosure of a source of information for which special rules apply (Contempt of Court Act 1981, s 10). For a robust criticism of the present status of doctors, see J D J Havard 'A Question of Privilege' (1985) 25 Med Sci Law 242 and the same author 'The Responsibility of the Doctor' (1989) 299 BMJ 503.
1 *Garner v Garner* (1920) 36 TLR 196.

The next development in patient access to personal medical information came with the Access to Medical Reports Act 1988. This is not descended linearly from the 1984 Act as the relevant reports are limited to those prepared by a doctor who has clinical charge of the patient for direct supply to the patient's employer, prospective employer or to an insurance company (s 2). Reports by doctors who have had only a casual, non-caring professional association with the patient are excluded. Such reports as are included have always been subject to the patient's consent but the applicant must now positively seek such consent and must inform him of his rights to access (s 3). The patient can see the report before it is sent and, unless he has done so, issue of the report must be delayed for three weeks (s 4). He has the right to ask the doctor to alter anything that he feels is inaccurate; he may add a dissenting statement should the doctor refuse to do so (s 5). Once again, access may be withheld if disclosure would cause serious harm to the patient's physical or mental health – or to that of any other person – but, in those circumstances, the patient may withdraw his consent.

It was clear, however, that public opinion was dissatisfied with the illogical limitation of general access to computerised records only and this gave rise to the Access to Health Records Act 1990. This extends the patient's rights to access to include health records relating to him that have been prepared manually and which are held by a variety of health professionals including doctors, dentists and psychologists. The patient may now see his records and may ask the holder to correct the information contained if he forms the view that it is inaccurate (s 6). A holder who agrees that the information is, indeed, inaccurate may make an appropriate amendment; otherwise, he may make a note in the relevant part of the record setting out the respect in which the patient regards it as inaccurate. There is the standard exemption of records which are likely to cause serious physical or mental harm (s 5). The right of access does not apply to notes made before 1 November 1991 (when the Act came into operation) unless such access is needed for the understanding of a later record. A suggestion that a common law right existed before that date has been rejected.[2]

The right of access extends to children provided that the child is capable of understanding the nature of his or her application for access (s 4). Alternatively, the right may be exercised by a parent or guardian on behalf of the child.

While patients' access to medical records is a subject dear to the hearts of civil libertarians, it has less support in the medical profession – an antipathy which is not entirely derived from professional protectionism. The majority of those giving whole-hearted support work in the field of general practice; by the very nature of primary care, reports compiled and received in that area are largely factual and, most importantly, do not include a deal of varied, and possibly contradictory, opinion. By contrast, hospital notes are fuller, they are contributed to by members of the health care team who will be of differing experience and the several consultative opinions will be written from differing standpoints and with varying emphasis. It is possible that the notes will be limited and their content 'tailored' to the possibility of disclosure; interchange of opinion may be increasingly by way of word of mouth. The disadvantage to the patient is, then, evident – in the event of a change of location,

2 *R v Mid-Glamorgan Family Health Services, ex p Martin* (1993) 16 BMLR 81, QBD.

his accompanying medical documents will be of less value to his new health carers than ought to be the case.[3] There is, however, no hard evidence that the 1990 Act has affected medical practice adversely and such musings may be unduly pessimistic; certainly, an impressive body of research can be quoted which stresses the practical advantages. The Access to Health Records Act 1990 undoubtedly attracts general popular support and there is a movement towards giving patients physical possession of their records.[4] Whether this would be possible is uncertain for the general understanding is that ownership of the notes is vested in ownership of the paper on which they are written; the ownership of intellectual property is a vexed question – the intellectual property in the notes being mainly that of the doctors and only partially that of the patients.

The patient's remedies

The law has been slow to develop a remedy for breach of confidentiality in spite of its clear recognition of such breaches as a proper basis for legal action. The latter has been considerably clarified and its requirements set out in the House of Lords decision in *A-G v Guardian Newspapers (No 2)*.[5] It is likely that a patient would be able to claim damages for improper disclosure of information about his health even if he suffered no financial loss as a result; this is almost implicit from *X v Y*[6] in which it was said that 'No-one has suggested that damages would be an adequate remedy in this case' – the clear implication being that they were there for the taking in the absence of a better solution. They might, of course, be only nominal; on the other hand, they might be considerable were it possible to show effects such as loss of society, severe injury to feelings, job loss, interference with prospects of promotion or the like. However, a distinction has to be made between actions in contract and in tort. Thus, in the trial stage of *W v Egdell*,[7] Scott J discarded the possibility of damages for shock and distress – other than nominal – largely on the particular facts of the case but also because it was based on breach of an implied contractual term.[8] The decision has no relevance to an action in tort.

In Scotland, the matter came before the courts in two similarly named decisions, the *AB v CD* cases. In the earlier *AB v CD*,[9] the Court of Session considered an action for damages brought against a doctor who had disclosed to a church minister that the pursuer's wife had given birth to a full-term child six months after marriage. The court held that there was a duty on the part of the doctor not to reveal confidential information about his patient unless he was required to do so in court or if disclosure

---

3   For a relatively early debate, see A P Bird and M T I Walji 'Our Patients Have Access to Their Medical Records' (1986) 292 BMJ 595; A P Ross 'The Case Against Showing Patients Their Records' (1986) 292 BMJ 578.
4   See M L M Gilhooly and S M McGhee 'Medical Records: Practicalities and Principles of Patient Possession' (1991) 17 J Med Ethics 138.
5   [1990] 1 AC 109, [1988] 3 All ER 545.
6   [1988] 2 All ER 648, (1987) 3 BMLR 1.
7   [1990] Ch 359, [1990] 1 All ER 835.
8   Citing *Bliss v South East Thames Regional Health Authority* [1987] ICR 700.
9   (1851) 14 D 177.

were 'conducive to the ends of science' – but, in that case, identification of the patient would be improper. In the second *AB v CD*,[10] the pursuer was seeking a separation from her husband. Having been examined by the defender at the suggestion of her lawyers, she was later examined by the same doctor who was, then, acting on behalf of her husband. The doctor disclosed to the husband certain information he had obtained in the course of his first examination and the wife argued that this constituted a breach of confidence. Once again, the court accepted that there was a duty on the part of a doctor not to disclose confidential information about his patient but stressed that not every disclosure would be actionable. As Lord Trayner pointed out,[11] some statements may be indiscreet but not actionable; but there might be, for example, an actionable breach if the disclosure revealed that the patient was suffering from a disease which was a consequence of misconduct on his part.[12] In fact, disclosure of the background to the illness may be of greater importance than the disclosure of illness itself.

Reliance on the law of defamation alone provides inadequate protection for the patient. In both English and Scots law, the patient is not being defamed if what the doctor says is true.[13] Moreover, in England, the law of slander (spoken defamation) requires that the plaintiff should be able to prove special damage – which is, essentially, pecuniary damage – except in those limited cases of slander which are actionable per se. The protection provided by the law of defamation in cases where the doctor verbally reveals confidential information to another is, thus, unlikely to be significant.

Qualified privilege should, in the absence of malice or reckless unconcern as to the truth of the statement, be a defence against any action for breach of confidence, as it already is in the law of defamation – qualified privilege in this context being but another expression of the 'need to know' principle. This is the ultimate determinant of ethical disclosure. The profession is not, or should not be, so concerned with the niceties of intra-professional relationships or of communication in good faith with paramedical or other responsible groups; what really matters is irresponsible gossip – and, here, the ultimate deterrent is the Professional Conduct Committee of the General Medical Council. Punitive action against a doctor is unlikely to be of material benefit to a wronged patient but it is still a very effective preventive weapon.

Confidentiality and death
Final reflection might, appositely, be concerned with death. The Declaration of Sydney provides: 'I will respect the secrets which are confided in me, even after the patient has died'. In practice, this is incapable of fulfilment as a death certificate, signed by a doctor, is a public document – albeit, available only on payment of a fee for a copy. Once again, the spectre of AIDS raises its head in so far as confidentiality

10 (1904) 7 F 72.
11 (1904) 7 F 72 at 85.
12 Scots law provides a potential remedy in the form of the *actio iniurarium*. For comments on the possible application of this delict in cases of breach of confidence, see Scottish Law Commission, Memorandum No 40 *Confidential Information* (1977) p 28.
13 The doctor's most likely exposure to defamation is, of course, on an intra-professional basis. For a brief overview, see Legal Correspondent 'Doctors and Defamation' (1985) 290 BMJ 1342.

may, here, be as important to the bereaved family as to the deceased during life. It is certain that death certification in the United Kingdom – and probably elsewhere – is inaccurate but this can only be compounded if doctors take it upon themselves to 'sanitise' the diagnosis so as to spare the relatives distress and, maybe, harm. A government publication[14] suggests that certificates relating to recent deaths should be available only to those who may legitimately want them – but such measures are unlikely to achieve strict confidentiality.[15] The dilemma of conscience for doctors is acute in many types of death which carry a social stigma but, pending an alteration in the law, we find it hard to accept that doctors should be encouraged to falsify facts which are attested to be 'true to the best of my knowledge and belief'. Our major concerns here, however, are first, with conditions discovered after death and second, with the circumstances leading to death. The legal position is that, as the confidence is prima facie a personal matter, the legal duty ends with the death of the patient;[16] the GMC is, however, unequivocal – 'The death of the patient does not absolve the doctor from this obligation [of professional secrecy].' There can be no doubt that a post-mortem report merits the same degree of confidentiality as does the report of the clinical examination; insurance companies and similar institutions have an obvious interest in its content but their right to disclosure is the same as the right to discovery of hospital records, namely that, in the absence of a court order, consent to disclosure from the next of kin of the deceased is essential.

But has the public any rights to details of the medical history of the dead?[17] While the principle remains irrespective of personalities, this is essentially a problem of public figures – and it is remarkable how rapidly professional ethics can be dissipated, say, in describing to the media the wounds of President Kennedy or the psychiatric history of the principals in any cause celèbre. It is easy to say that history will out, so let it be sooner than later but it is less easy to decide at what point revelations become history. The GMC has suggested that whether or not disclosure after death will be improper depends, inter alia, on the nature of the information given, the extent of previous publication and the time elapsed since death – as to the last, the GMC rightly will not specify a number of years, merely remarking that a doctor who discloses such information without the consent of a surviving relative may be required to justify his action. Moreover, a bark in this context carries a bite – no less a person than the editor of the British Medical Journal has been taken to task for reporting information concerning the health of a well-known, albeit controversial, general after his death.[18]

Respect for the privacy of the dead seems reasonable – particularly when children or, especially, spouses are alive.[19] Not only is it difficult to see the logic which accords to death the status of the liberator of conscience but, in turn, publicity may

14 *Registration: A Modern Service* (Cm 531, 1988).
15 M B King 'AIDS on the Death Certificate: The Final Stigma' (1989) 298 BMJ 734.
16 However, any action for breach of confidence before the death of the patient could be transmitted to the executor.
17 See S E Woolman 'Defaming the Dead' 1981 SLT 29.
18 S Lock and J Loudon 'A Question of Confidence' (1984) 288 BMJ 123, 125.
19 The courts are, however, concerned for a balancing of interests between those of the bereaved and of freedom to publish. See *Re X (A minor) (Wardship: Restriction on Publication)* [1975] Fam 47, [1975] 1 All ER 697.

raise questions as to the ethics of non-disclosure. It has, for example, been seriously argued that Lord Moran invited criticism not so much for his disclosures after the death of Winston Churchill[20] as for his failure to draw attention to the physical state of his patient during life. Which brings us back almost to where we started – to the dilemma of the doctor's relationship to his patient vis-à-vis society.

20 Lord Moran *Winston Churchill: The Struggle for Survival, 1944-1965* (1966).

9 Medical negligence

There is no shortage of evidence that claims against doctors in the United Kingdom for professional negligence have increased markedly over the last decade. The cost of this is considerable: in 1990 the NHS spent approximately £45m on such claims, paying damages of over £300,000 in some 35 cases. This rise in the level of litigation, accompanied by a corresponding increase in the size of medical insurance premiums, has raised in some minds the prospect of the development on this side of the Atlantic of a North American-style 'malpractice crisis'. Such a development is expected to bring with it not only a deterioration in doctor/patient relationships, but also the practice of so-called 'defensive medicine' – a form of medical practice which owes more to the protection of the doctor's legal position than to the patient's anticipated benefit. In fact, the very concept of 'defensive medicine' is controversial. In one view it is no more than conservative, cautious practice which does the patient no harm – and may, in fact, do some good; in the alternative, it is time-wasting, expensive, and interferes in the proper exercise of the doctor's clinical judgment.[1] Although some accounts of the practice of defensive medicine are merely anecdotal, there is good evidence that the way in which doctors approach their work may be affected by their understanding of the legal risk.[2] It is also clear that, in countries where private medicine is the norm, patterns of litigation may affect the access that people have to specialist services.[3]

It would be a mistake to think of doctors and hospitals as easy targets for the dissatisfied patient. It is still very difficult to raise an action of medical negligence in Britain; some, such as the Association for the Victims of Medical Accidents, would say that it is unacceptably difficult. Not only are there practical difficulties in linking the plaintiff's injury to medical treatment, but the standard of care in medical negligence cases is still effectively defined by the profession itself. All these factors, together with the sheer expense of bringing a legal action and the denial of legal aid to all but the poorest, operate to inhibit medical litigation in a way in which the American system, with its contingency fees and its sympathetic juries, does not.

It is difficult to single out any one cause for what increase there has been in the volume of medical negligence actions in the United Kingdom. A common explanation is that there are, quite simply, more medical accidents occurring – whether this be due to increased pressure on hospital facilities, to falling standards of professional competence or, more probably, to the ever-increasing complexity of therapeutic and diagnostic methods. This hypothesis is difficult to substantiate, although recent

1 For a sceptical view of defensive medicine, see C Ham et al, *Medical Negligence: Compensation and Accountability* (1988); M A Jones *Medical Negligence* (1991), p 4.
2 B Dickens 'The Effects of Legal Liability on Physicians' Services' (1991) 41 Univ Tor LJ 168.
3 L R Walker, R W Broyles and B R Furrow 'The Effect of Malpractice Litigation on Patient Access to Speciality Physician Services' (1990) 11 J Leg Med 199.

empirical work, undertaken in the United States, paints a frankly alarming picture. According to the Harvard Medical Practice Study of New York,[4] medical misadventure occurs in 3.8% of hospital admissions. If these figures applied in the United Kingdom, about 300,000 patients would experience medical misadventure in hospital each year and such incidents would contribute to the deaths of some 45,000 patients. These figures must be treated with caution. There are great disparities in the standard of care offered by private and public hospitals in the United States; moreover, the definition of medical accident becomes ever more liberal pari passu with increasing litigation.

There are other possible reasons for the increase in claims. One is the existence of a growing 'compensation awareness' in the public mind. It might be that a greater proportion of the population is now aware that the courts can and, on occasion, do provide substantial compensation for personal injury; extensive press coverage of issues such as claims for physician-induced addiction to tranquillisers has undoubtedly served to alert the general public to the possibilities. For many people, the vicissitudes of life, which might previously have been borne with resignation, are a matter of potential financial enrichment. Scientific progress may also have had an impact. Patients are accustomed to a high success rate from modern medicine and any failure to effect a cure may be thought to be the result of medical negligence rather than of the recalcitrance of disease. To an extent, this is part of the culture of blame in which we search for a scapegoat of some sort. Consumerism is now firmly established in medical practice – and this has been encouraged on a wide scale by government in the United Kingdom through the introduction of 'charters'. Complaint is central to this ethos – and the notion that blame must be attributed, and compensated, has a high priority. Another factor which is sometimes suggested as providing an explanation for the increase in actions for negligence is the depersonalisation of the doctor-patient relationship. It is undoubtedly easier to sue a relatively anonymous defendant, such as a hospital consultant, than to sue a family doctor whom one has known for many years – and this is even more true of a hospital authority.

There is no doubt that actions by patients against doctors are unusually time-consuming, expensive and potentially destructive. The professional time involved in the processing of such claims is considerable and the period between injury and compensation can be long. An award which has been made against a hospital will eat into funds which were originally intended for other purposes and the quality of care given to other patients may be correspondingly diminished. The professional reputation of the doctor may be seriously damaged by a single alleged incident of negligence and the effect which this has may be out of all proportion to the seriousness of the fault.

Yet it is impossible for the medical profession to wish out of existence the real damage so caused. A patient who has been injured by an act of medical negligence has suffered in a way which is recognised by the law – and by the public at large – as deserving compensation. This loss may be continuing and what may seem like an unduly large award may be little more than that sum which is required to compensate

---

4   Harvard Medical Practice Study *Patients, Doctors, and Lawyers: Medical Injury, Malpractice Litigation and Patient Compensation in New York* (1990), discussed by R Smith 'The Epidemiology of Malpractice' (1990) 301 BMJ 621.

him for such matters as loss of future earnings and the future cost of medical or nursing care. To deny a legitimate claim or to restrict arbitrarily the size of an award would amount to substantial injustice. After all, there is no difference in legal theory between the plaintiff injured through medical negligence and the plaintiff injured in an industrial or motor accident.

Concern in the United States over the consequences for medical practice of actions by patients has resulted in attempts to make the bringing of a claim less attractive to the potential litigant. This may be achieved by bringing benefits which accrue from collateral sources, such as insurance, into the reckoning of damages. Limiting lawyers' contingency fees also seems to have had some effect on the readiness to file suits. A further, more radical, option involves the interjection of procedural barriers to litigation. In general, these may invoke either arbitration which, although elective, is binding on the parties, or screening which attempts to screen out frivolous claims and to promote the settlement of those which are valid. Such schemes may, however, be open to constitutional objection on the grounds that they inhibit the exercise of legally protected rights.[5] Yet another, and perhaps extreme, resort which, nevertheless, contains an attractive element of poetic justice, is the encouragement of the malpractice countersuit[6] – something which one would hope to be a long way off in the United Kingdom!

A widely canvassed alternative to negligence actions which commands much support is to introduce a system of no-fault compensation which will provide for the making of awards to injured patients irrespective of the requirement of proving fault on the part of medical personnel.[7] Such a scheme has operated in New Zealand since 1974 as part of an overall no-fault compensation scheme and has been shown to work reasonably satisfactorily. In the medical context, however, the claimant must establish that the injury resulted from 'medical or surgical misadventure', a requirement which has caused difficulties in distinguishing between those conditions which result from the physiological progress of a medical condition and those which are genuinely the result of misadventure occurring in the course of treatment. A considerable body of case law is devoted to determining just when a complication following upon a medical procedure is so rare as to amount to a misadventure.[8] It will be seen that such schemes do not do away entirely with all the difficult issues of foreseeability and causation which dog the operation of conventional tort law. It is, perhaps, significant that organisations such as the British Medical Association, whose primary concern is for the interests of the profession, have consistently

5 For discussion of the limitation techniques used in the United States, see G Robinson 'The Medical Malpractice Crisis of the 1970's: A Retrospective' (1986) 49 Law Contemp Probls 5.
6 Discussed in D J Sokol 'The Current Status of Medical Malpractice Countersuits' (1985) 10 Amer J Law Med 439.
7 For a survey of the alternatives to fault-based compensation, see the discussion of New Zealand, Swedish and German schemes in D Giesen *International Medical Malpractice Law* (1988) p 529. The New Zealand scheme is discussed by J Fleming *The Law of Torts* (7th edn, 1987) p 375; see also, S A M McLean 'Liability Without Fault – the New Zealand Experience' [1985] J Soc Welfare Law 125. For the Swedish system, see C Oldertz 'The Swedish Patient Insurance System – 8 Years of Experience' (1984) 52 Med-leg J 43.
8 For example, *Re Lloyd*: Decision No 737 [1982] NZACR 259 – reaction to a cortisone cream was not a misadventure as such reactions were not uncommon. A chance of occurrence of over 1% might elevate an incident out of the category of misadventure: *McDonald v Accident Compensation Corpn* (1985) 5 NZACR 276. These cases are discussed in Giesen at p 533 et seq – see fn 7 above.

supported the introduction of a no-fault based system into the United Kingdom.[9] Under the scheme proposed by the Association, compensation would be available for medically-induced injury but would exclude those injuries which were not avoidable through the exercise of reasonable care. The concept of negligence is therefore effectively preserved, although it would undoubtedly be easier to establish; moreover, there would be no inference of 'fault' of quite the same nature as is inferred in a tort-based system. A no-fault system of compensation is also the preferred option in the report of the Royal College of Physicians on the subject.[10]

For a variety of reasons, predominantly those of cost, the government has not supported the movement and a Private Member's Bill aimed in that direction has been defeated in Parliament.[11] The government's attitude has not, however, been one of total inaction and the Department of Health has encouraged discussion of ways of making compensation more readily available and less costly. The ways in which arbitration might help to reduce the time and expense involved in meeting a claim for medical injury have attracted official attention.[12] A suggested scheme involves a panel of three arbitrators – composed of one doctor nominated by each litigant and a lawyer chairman – which would work entirely on paper and which would, therefore, avoid the cost of court proceedings and witnesses' time. Some objections to this are foreseen; in particular, it might be difficult to avoid the need for the examination of experts in certain cases of special complexity.

The argument in favour of retaining the present system for compensating the victims of medical accident or negligence can be couched in positive as well as negative terms. One is based on the deterrent value of the law of tort, the view being taken that to remove the threat of litigation will affect adversely the care with which doctors treat their patients. There is certainly some evidence that doctors are more cautious when they are aware of the Damoclean possibility of legal action; surveys undertaken in the United States indicate that successful litigation provokes greater care – at least in the realm of diagnosis.[13] Yet there are other ways of deterring carelessness and it may be that a more extensive power of the General Medical Council to deal with doctors who fail to live up to an expected standard of competence could prove a more effective incentive to maintain high standards of practice.[14] The existence of a clear, effective and patient-friendly system of investigating grievances may do more than satisfy those potential litigants whose principal goal is to find out what went wrong and to get an apology; it may also form a valuable element in a system of professional audit.

The deterrence argument is also qualified by the financial realities of the United Kingdom system. In this country, outwith private practice, the doctor has no direct

9 British Medical Association *Report of the BMA No Fault Compensation Working Party* (1987); discussed by C Dyer 'No Fault Compensation' (1988) 297 BMJ 939, (1989) 298 BMJ 143.
10 *Compensation for Adverse Consequences of Medical Intervention* (1990).
11 National Health Service (Compensation) Bill 1991. The case against no-fault compensation is summarised by B Capstick, P Edwards and D Mason 'Compensation for Medical Accidents' (1991) 302 BMJ 230.
12 Department of Health *Arbitration for Medical Negligence in the National Health Service* (Discussion Paper, 1991).
13 P M Danzon *Medical Malpractice* (1985), especially ch 1.
14 For discussion of the deterrent argument in the context of reforms in medical discipline, see M Stacey 'Medical Accountability: A Background Paper' in A Grubb (ed) *Challenges in Medical Care* (1992) p 109.

contract with the patient and medical damages are usually underwritten by the state[15] (see p 197, below). If one adds to these the surrealistic conditions surrounding legal aid – under which it may be economically preferable to settle an action out of court rather than to win a contested action – it becomes possible to raise an argument that the doctor in the United Kingdom is exposed to too little by way of deterrence.

The question of compensation for medical injury in the United Kingdom was discussed as a special issue by the Royal Commission on Compensation for Personal Injury (The Pearson Commission).[16] The commission considered the arguments and concluded that there were not, at this point, sufficient grounds for introducing no-fault compensation schemes. It would seem, then, that the victims of medical negligence will have to continue to seek compensation through a fault-based tort system. In the following sections, we analyse the operation of this system and the rules it has developed for the adjudication of such claims.

The basis of medical liability

Most claims in respect of medical injury are brought in tort – that is, on the basis of a non-contractual civil wrong. The reason for this is that, within the NHS, patients are not in a contractual relationship with the doctor treating them. In the private sector, by contrast, there will be a contractual relationship and it is, therefore, possible to bring an action for damages in contract. In practice, there is very little difference between the two remedies,[17] although the law of contract may provide a remedy for an express or implied warranty given by a doctor.[18] In a Canadian case, *La Fleur v Cornelis*,[19] the court held that a plastic surgeon was bound to an express contractual warranty that he had made to the patient. This warranty arose when he was unwise enough to say: 'There will be no problem. You will be very happy.' This sort of case will be comparatively unusual and, for all practical purposes, any discussion of medical negligence can confine itself to liability under the law of torts, in which the first question to be asked is: whom do we sue?

A medical injury may have been caused to the plaintiff by any one or more of the health care personnel who have treated him. Locating negligence may be simple in some cases but, in others, the patient may have to choose the responsible party from a fairly large group, which may include a general practitioner, a hospital consultant, other hospital doctors and the nursing staff. Locating the specific act of alleged negligence which caused the injury may also involve a degree of disentanglement.

The plaintiff may proceed directly against the doctor in question if an allegation is made of negligence on the part of a general practitioner. The general practitioner

15 Department of Health *Claims of Medical Negligence against NHS Hospital and Community Doctors and Dentists* (1989) HC(89) 34. See J D J Harvard 'Doctors and Medical Negligence' (1990) 300 BMJ 343.

16 Cmnd 7054-1, 1978.

17 For a useful discussion of the distinction between contractual and tortious remedies in this context, see M A Jones *Medical Negligence* (1991) p 15.

18 An issue which arose in *Thake v Maurice* [1984] 2 All ER 513, [1985] 2 WLR 215; revsd [1986] QB 644, [1986] 1 All ER 479.

19 (1979) 28 NBR (2d) 569 (NBSC); discussed by Jones (fn 17 above) at p 18.

in the United Kingdom is solely responsible for the treatment of his patients and there can be no question of responsibility being imposed on a health authority unless the authority has intervened in the practitioner's treatment of his patient – all partners in a practice may, however, be liable for the actions of one of their number. Normally, of course, the general practitioner will be a member of a medical defence society, to whom he will refer any claim against him; the society then advises him and undertakes the defence or settlement of the claim. General practitioners are not covered by the NHS indemnity which applies to hospital doctors (see p 197) unless a claim arises in respect of work undertaken under a health authority contract. A general practitioner will be vicariously liable for the negligence of staff employed by him – nurses, receptionists etc – but not for the acts of a locum tenens or a deputising doctor.[20]

The position is different if the alleged negligence occurs after the general practitioner has referred the patient for further treatment within the NHS. If the negligent act is committed by a health service employee, the patient then has the choice of proceeding either against the individual he feels has been negligent or against the health authority or against both in a joint action. In practice, many actions are brought against the health authority on the grounds of convenience. The liability of the authority may be based on either of two grounds: (1) the duty of a hospital to care for patients, or (2) the vicarious liability of a health authority for the negligence of its employees.

There is some doubt as to whether a hospital owes a non-delegable duty to use skill and care in treating its patients.[1] This has been addressed in some Commonwealth jurisdictions which have a somewhat different form of health care delivery to that existing in the United Kingdom. Thus, in the Australian case of *Ellis v Wallsend District Hospital*,[2] the majority held that there was a non-delegable duty in those cases where patients were permitted to go directly to the hospital for treatment and advice; no such duty would exist where the hospital merely provided services which a doctor could use to treat his own patients.[3] By contrast, the Ontario Court of Appeal has found that the hospital's duty extends no further than employing competent staff.[4] The minority view was, however, that hospitals, to a growing extent, hold out to the public that they provide medical treatment and emergency services – and that the public increasingly relies upon them to do so. Blair JA, in expressing this view, drew upon the evolution of the law in England which he thought supported the view that the hospital itself could be liable for negligent treatment in certain circumstances.[5] The English case of *Wilsher v Essex Area Health Authority*[6] could have provided an

20 There was no vicarious liability for the negligence of a locum tenens in the Canadian case of *Rothwell v Raes* (1988) 54 DLR (4th) 193.

 1 For discussion, see A M Dugdale and K M Stanton *Professional Negligence* (2nd edn, 1989) para 22.21; M A Jones *Medical Negligence* (1991) p 283.

 2 (1989) 17 NSWLR 553 (CA).

 3 The matter was also pronounced upon, obiter, by the High Court of Australia in *Commonwealth v Introvigne* (1982) 56 ALJR 749 and *Kondis v State Transport Authority* (1984) 154 CLR 672, 55 ALR 225.

 4 *Yepremian v Scarborough General Hospital* (1980) 110 DLR (3d) 513.

 5 (1980) 110 DLR(3d) 513 at 579, per Blair JA.

 6 [1987] QB 730, [1986] 3 All ER 801, CA; [1988] AC 1074, [1988] 1 All ER 871, HL.

ideal ground to decide the matter but the issue was not raised by the plaintiffs. Nevertheless, the possibility clearly remains open – it was said that:

> I can see no reason why, in principle, the health authority should not be [directly] liable if its organisation is at fault.[7]

The point seems to be of some importance particularly in respect of the nursing staff who may well be covered themselves by a common insurance policy taken out by the Royal College of Nursing on behalf of its members but who have less than doctors by way of personal representation etc. It could scarcely be denied that a hospital undertakes to provide nursing care for the patients.[8]

The discussion is, however, relatively sterile in the case of hospital doctors, the vast majority of whom are direct employees of the NHS. The health authority is, therefore, liable for their negligence under the principle of vicarious liability. This provides that an employer is liable for his employee's negligent acts, provided that the employee is acting within the scope of his employment. It should be borne in mind that the employer may still be held vicariously liable even if the employee acts in direct contradiction of his employer's instructions or prohibitions.[9] The vicarious liability of hospitals throughout their hierarchy has been clearly established for over 30 years[10] and requires no further discussion.

In the past, an agreement between the Ministry of Health and the Secretary of State for Scotland and the medical defence societies allowed for the costs of any actions to be shared between the two parties.[11] All doctors employed in the NHS were, accordingly, contractually bound to be members of a defence organisation; the membership fees, however, increased so dramatically that they had to be subsidised by the authorities. Crown immunity has been extended to doctors, dentists and community physicians since January 1990[12] and, as a result, the entire costs of negligence litigation are now borne by the NHS. The scheme has not yet been fully assessed, yet it is difficult to see it as an unmitigated blessing as no special financial provisions are available. Health authorities may, as a consequence, feel obliged to settle cases on the grounds that this is the cheapest, if not the fairest, option. Moreover, there is a strong suspicion that compensation for the injured may be bought at the expense of limitations in treatment facilities for the remainder – but this is, perhaps, to take too pessimistic a view. It is to be noted that the scheme applies only to services provided within the NHS; doctors should, therefore, retain cover for any private or 'good Samaritan' work – and, indeed, for medico-legal activity.

---

7 [1987] QB 730 at 778; [1986] 3 All ER 801 at 833, per Browne-Wilkinson V-C.
8 *Gold v Essex County Council* [1942] 2 KB 293 at 299, CA, per Lord Greene.
9 R F V Heuston and R A Buckley (eds) *Salmond and Heuston on the Law of Torts* (20th edn, 1992) p 460.
10 *Roe v Minister of Health; Woolley v Minister of Health* [1954] 2 QB 66; *Hayward v Board of Management of the Royal Infirmary of Edinburgh* and *Macdonald v Glasgow Western Hospitals Board of Management* 1954 SC 453.
11 Ministry of Health circular HM (54) 32.
12 Department of Health *Claims of Medical Negligence against NHS Hospital and Community Doctors and Dentists* (1989) HC (89) 34.

What constitutes negligence?

In determining whether there has been negligence in medical treatment, the courts pursue the same line of enquiry as they pursue in any other similar claim: did the conduct of the defendant amount to a breach of the duty of care which he owed to the injured plaintiff? Expressed somewhat differently, this amounts to asking whether the standard of the treatment given by the defendant fell below the standard expected of him by the law and whether there was, therefore, any fault in the legal sense. Fault remains the theoretical underpinning of the law in this area until such time as strict liability may be imposed.

A major difficulty for any plaintiff will be the onus which falls upon him to prove that the defendant's negligence caused his injury. This is often a difficult obligation to discharge and, indeed, suggestions have been made that the patient attempting to succeed in an action against a doctor should face a heavier burden in establishing his case than that required in any other personal injury litigation. There is an indication that this occurs in practice in so far as payment is made in some 30-40% of medical cases as compared with 86% in the general run;[13] the figures may, however, conceal more than a simple cause and effect phenomenon. The legal foundation for this view, which was put forward by Lawton LJ,[14] may be tenuous and it was, in fact, strongly opposed in *Ashcroft*;[15] nevertheless, it is certainly true that there has been a degree of policy-based judicial reluctance to award damages against doctors. In *Dwyer v Roderick*, May LJ suggested that it would be:

> To shut one's eyes to the obvious if one denied that the burden of achieving something more than the mere balance of probabilities was greater when one was investigating the complicated and sophisticated actions of a qualified and experienced [inter alia] doctor than when one was enquiring into the inattention of the driver in a simple running down action.[16]

At the same time, the courts have not been insensitive to the plaintiff's difficulties in a medical negligence case. The correctives applied have been the occasional invocation of the principle of res ipsa loquitur (see below) or, as in *Clark v MacLennan*,[17] an attempt to shift the burden of proof to the defendant. The observations of Kilner Brown J on this point are revealing:

> When an injury is caused which never should have been caused, common sense and natural justice indicate that some degree of compensation ought to be paid by someone. As the law stands, in order to obtain compensation an injured person is compelled to allege negligence against . . . a person of the highest skill and reputation.[18]

We return to this problem at p 208 below.

---

13 M A Jones 'Medical Negligence – the Burden of Proof' (1984) 134 NLJ 7 quoting the Pearson Report Cmnd 7054-1, 1978.
14 In *Whitehouse v Jordan* [1980] 1 All ER 650 at 659.
15 *Ashcroft v Mersey Regional Health Authority* [1983] 2 All ER 245 at 247, per Kilner Brown J.
16 (1983) 127 SJ 805, CA.
17 [1983] 1 All ER 416.
18 *Ashcroft v Mersey Regional Health Authority* [1983] 2 All ER 245 at 246.

The reasonably skilful doctor

There have been many judicial pronouncements by the courts on the standard of care which is expected of the doctor. As early as 1838 we see Tindall CJ ruling that:

> Every person who enters into a learned profession undertakes to bring to the exercise of it a reasonable degree of care and skill. He does not undertake, if he is an attorney, that at all events you shall gain your case, nor does a surgeon undertake that he will perform a cure; nor does he undertake to use the highest possible degree of skill.[19]

An echo of this is to be found in *R v Bateman*[20] where the court explained that:

> If a person holds himself out as possessing special skill and knowledge, by and on behalf of a patient, he owes a duty to the patient to use due caution in undertaking the treatment ... The jury should not exact the highest, or very high standard, nor should they be content with a very low standard.

The doctor is thus not expected to be a miracle-worker guaranteeing a cure or a man of the very highest skill in his calling. What standard then is he expected to meet? McNair J provides us with an unambiguous answer to this question in *Bolam v Friern Hospital Management Committee*.[1]

> The test is the standard of the ordinary skilled man exercising and professing to have that special skill. A man need not possess the highest expert skill at the risk of being found negligent. It is a well-established law that it is sufficient if he exercises the ordinary skill of an ordinary man exercising that particular art.

Nevertheless, he *is* professing a particular skill and, in the immortal words of McNair J, the test of that skill 'is not the test of the man on the top of the Clapham omnibus because [that man] has not got this special skill'.[2]

The doctor having that degree of competence expected of the ordinary skilful doctor sets the standard. He is the practitioner who follows the standard practice of his profession – or, at least, follows practices that would not be disapproved of by responsible opinion within the profession. He has a reasonably sound grasp of medical techniques and is as informed of new medical developments as the average competent doctor would expect to be. The circumstances in which a doctor treats his patient will also be taken into account. A doctor working in an emergency, with inadequate facilities and under great pressure, will not be expected by the courts to

---

19 *Lanphier v Phipos* (1838) 8 C & P 475 at 478.
20 (1925) 94 LJKB 791 at 794, CCA.
 1 [1957] 2 All ER 118 at 121, [1957] 1 WLR 582 at 586.
 2 A test approved in the Privy Council: *Chin Keow v Government of Malaysia* [1967] 1 WLR 813. The *Bolam* test is applied throughout medical practice – including the providing of information and warnings: *Sidaway v Board of Governors of the Bethlem Royal Hospital and Maudsley Hospital* [1985] AC 871, [1985] 1 All ER 643, HL. See also *Hills v Potter* [1983] 3 All ER 716, [1984] 1 WLR 641.

achieve the same results as a doctor who is working in ideal conditions.[3] This was alluded to by Mustill J in *Wilsher*, where he said that, if a person was forced by an emergency to do too many things at once, then the fact that he does one of them incorrectly 'should not lightly be taken as negligence'.[4]

Usual practice

The 'custom test' – the test whereby a defendant's conduct is tested against the normal usage of his profession or calling – is one that is applied in all areas of negligence law.[5] The courts have given expression to this test in the medical context in a number of decisions. In the important Scottish case of *Hunter v Hanley*,[6] for example, there was a clear endorsement of the custom test in Lord Clyde's dictum:

> To establish liability by a doctor where deviation from normal practice is alleged, three facts require to be established. First of all it must be proved that there is a usual and normal practice; secondly it must be proved that the defender has not adopted that practice; and thirdly (and this is of crucial importance) it must be established that the course the doctor adopted is one which no professional man of ordinary skill would have taken if he had been acting with ordinary care'.[7]

This attractively simple exposition of the law, however, conceals a hurdle at the outset. It may, in many cases, be possible to prove that there is a 'usual and normal practice' but there will obviously be disagreement as to what is the appropriate course to follow in a number of medical areas. In some circumstances, the existence of two schools of thought may result in more than one option being open to a practitioner. If this is so, then what are the liability implications of choosing a course of action which a responsible body of opinion within the profession may well reject? Precisely this question arose in *Bolam*[8] where the plaintiff had suffered fractures as a result of the administration of electro-convulsive therapy without an anaesthetic. At the time, there were two schools of thought on the subject of anaesthesia in such treatment, one holding the view that relaxant drugs should be used, the other being that this only increased the risk. In this case, the judge ruled that a doctor would not be negligent if he acted 'in accordance with the practice accepted by a responsible

---

3   This is in accordance with the general principle in the law of torts that errors of judgmnet are more excusable in an emergency: *The Metagarma* (1927) 138 LT 369 at 370. In the medical context: *Rodych v Krasey* [1971] 4 WWR 358. See also *Wilson v Swanson* (1956) 5 DLR (2d) 113 (emergency removal of suspected cancerous tissue before a firm pathological report was available).
4   *Wilsher v Essex Area Health Authority* [1987] QB 730 at 749, [1986] 3 All ER 801 at 812, CA.
5   J Fleming *The Law of Torts* (7th edn, 1987) 1 p 109; A M Linden 'Custom in Negligence Law' [1968] Can BJ 151; R B M Howie, 'The Standard of Care in Medical Negligence' [1983] Juridical Rev 193; K McK Norrie 'Common Practice and the Standard of Care in Medical Negligence' [1985] Juridical Rev 145.
6   1955 SC 200.
7   1955 SC 200 at 206. The rigid simplicity of Lord Clyde's definition is defended in an anonymous article, 'Medical Negligence: *Hunter v Hanley* 35 Years On' 1990 SLT 325. *Hunter* was specifically approved by Lord Scarman in *Maynard*, fn 9 below. For recent discussion of custom in a medical context, see *E v Australian Red Cross* (1990) 99 ALR 601 at 647 et seq.
8   *Bolam v Friern Hospital Management Committee* [1957] 2 All ER 118, [1957] 1 WLR 582.

body of medical men skilled in that particular art'. Negligence would not be inferred merely because there was a body of opinion which took a contrary view. More recent cases have confirmed this approach. In *Maynard v West Midlands Regional Health Authority*, the trial judge had preferred an alternative medical approach to that which had been chosen by the defendant notwithstanding the fact that this latter course found support in responsible medical opinion; both the Court of Appeal and the House of Lords confirmed that this was an unsatisfactory way of attributing negligence.[9] As a corollary to this, the plaintiff will have failed to discharge the burden of proof if the court is unable to select between two possible explanations.[10] It has, however, been pointed out that a medical practice must be *rightly* regarded as professionally tenable before it is acceptable to the court – and it is for the court to decide on this point.[11] While this has always been true, its reaffirmation by the Master of the Rolls is, perhaps, a straw in the wind as to the future course of medical negligence actions –'the law', he said, 'will not allow the medical profession to play God'. This sentiment has now been firmly endorsed by the High Court of Australia in the controversial consent case *Rogers v Whitaker*[12] in which the Court excluded the purely professional custom test:

> In Australia, it has been accepted that the standard of care to be observed by a person with some special skill or competence is that of the ordinary skilled person exercising and professing that special skill. But that standard is not determined solely or even primarily by reference to the practice followed or supported by a responsible body of opinion in the relevant profession or trade.[13]

Ultimately, then, the courts retain the right to decide whether an established professional practice is acceptable or not. Expert evidence of professional custom will carry the day in the overwhelming majority of cases but this is not something on which a doctor may rely with complete certainty.

The doctor has a duty to keep himself informed of major developments in practice but this duty obviously cannot extend to the requirement that he should know all there is to be known in a particular area of medicine. In the case of *Crawford v Board of Governors of Charing Cross Hospital*,[14] the plaintiff had developed brachial palsy as a result of his arm being kept in a certain position during an operation. Six months prior to the operation an article had appeared in The Lancet pointing to just this danger, but the anaesthetist against whom negligence was being alleged had not read the article in question. The Court of Appeal eventually found in favour of the anaesthetist, Lord Denning stating that —

---

9 [1985] 1 All ER 635, [1984] 1 WLR 634. *Maynard* was followed in *Hughes v Waltham Forest Health Authority* [1991] 2 Med LR 155, in which the court emphasised that the fact that a surgeon's decision was criticised by other surgeons did not amount *in itself* to an indication of negligence.
10 *Harrington v Essex Area Health Authority* (1984) Times, 14 November.
11 *Sidaway v Board of Governors of the Bethlem Royal Hospital and Maudsley Hospital* [1984] QB 493, [1984] 1 All ER 1018, CA. For a rather similar Canadian view of the relationship, see *Reibl v Hughes* (1980) 114 DLR (3d) 1.
12 (1992) 109 ALR 625, [1993] 4 Med LR 79.
13 (1992) 109 ALR 625 at 631, [1993] 4 Med LR 79 at 82.
14 (1953) Times, 8 December, CA.

it would, I think, be putting too high a burden on a medical man to say that he has to read every article appearing in the current medical press; and it would be quite wrong to suggest that a medical man is negligent because he does not at once put into operation the suggestions which some contributor or other might make in a medical journal. The time may come in a particular case when a new recommendation may be so well proved and so well known, and so well accepted that it should be adopted, but that was not so in this case.

Failure to read a single article, it was said, may be excusable, while disregard of a series of warnings in the medical press could well be evidence of negligence. In view of the rapid progress currently being made in many areas of medicine, and in view of the amount of information confronting the average doctor, it is unreasonable to expect a doctor to be aware of every development in his field. At the same time, he must be reasonably up-to-date and must know of major developments. Hindsight is, of course, a harsh judge; yet, in a number of HIV-related cases, the courts have indicated that doctors could not have been expected to have known of a risk at a time when its significance was only just being established.[15] The practice of medicine has, however, become increasingly based on principles of scientific elucidation and report and the pressure on doctors to keep abreast of current developments is now considerable. It is no longer possible for a doctor to coast along on the basis of long experience; as in many professions and callings, such an attitude has been firmly discredited.

Innovative techniques   Resort to an innovative therapeutic technique may be appropriate in certain cases but should be made with caution. Whether or not the use of such a technique could amount to negligence would depend on the extent to which its use was considered justified in the case in question (see also chapter 16, below). In assessing this, a court would consider evidence of previous trials of the treatment and would also, no doubt, take into consideration any dangers which it entailed. It is possible that a court would decline to endorse the use of an untried procedure if the patient was thereby exposed to considerable risk of damage. Other factors which might be taken into account would be the previous response of the patient to more conventional treatment, the seriousness of the patient's condition and the attitude of the patient himself towards the novelty and risk. The standard of care to be applied in such circumstances would be expected of a doctor who is reasonably competent in the provision of *such treatment*. A doctor should not, therefore, undertake procedures which are beyond his capacity.[16]

15 *Dwan v Farquhar* [1988] 1 Qd R 234. In this case the risk of HIV transmission through blood transfusions was discussed in an article published in March 1983; there was no negligence in respect of a transfusion given in May of the same year. See also *H v Royal Alexandra Hospital for Sick Children* [1990] 1 Med LR 297.
16 In *Tomkins v Bexley Area Health Authority* [1993] 4 Med LR 235, the patient's lingual nerve was damaged in the course of an operation for the removal of wisdom teeth. Wilcox J observed: 'When fine movements and fine judgements are the order of the day, with surgery being conducted in the confined space of the mouth, a high degree of care is needed.'

Misdiagnosis

A doctor is expected by the law to use the same degree of care in making a diagnosis that is required of him in all his dealings with his patients. A mistake in diagnosis will not be considered negligent if this standard of care is observed but will be treated as one of the non-culpable and inevitable hazards of practice.[17] Liability may, however, be imposed when a mistake in diagnosis is made because the doctor failed to take a proper medical history,[18] failed to conduct tests which a competent practitioner would have considered appropriate, or simply failed to diagnose a condition which would have been spotted by a competent practitioner. As a minimum, the doctor must examine his patient and pay adequate attention to the patient's medical notes and to what the patient tries to tell him.[19] Telephone diagnosis is hazardous, especially if the facts as related by the patient are such as to raise in the doctor's mind a suspicion that can only be allayed by proper clinical examination.[20]

One of the problems in determining whether there has been a mistake in diagnosis turns on deciding what investigative techniques need to be used in a particular case. Ordinary laboratory tests must be used if symptoms suggest their use[1] but elaborate and expensive investigative procedures would not be expected other than in complicated or puzzling cases. Failure to X-ray, for example, might well be negligence – but even that might not be so, particularly in the light of both public and professional awareness of the major contribution made by diagnostic radiography to the background radiation in developed countries. We can turn again to Lord Denning:[2]

> In some of the earlier cases, the doctor has been criticised for not having taken X-rays with the result that they have sometimes been taken unnecessarily. This case shows that the Courts do not always find that there has been negligence because a patient has not had an X-ray; it depends upon the circumstances of each case.

Only some 1% of radiographs taken of the ankle in casualty departments demonstrate a fracture and, of these, a high proportion would have healed in the absence of identification. The approach to and the solution of such problems is by no means easy.[3]

Langley v Campbell[4] and *Tuffil v East Surrey Area Health Authority*[5] provide instances of successful actions against doctors on the basis of failure to diagnose

---

17 In *Crinon v Barnet Group Hospital Management Committee* (1958) Times, 19 November, the judge said of misdiagnosis: 'Unfortunate as it was that there was a wrong diagnosis, it was one of those misadventures, one of those chances, that life holds for people.' Courts – and patients – might be less inclned to take such a view today.

18 *Chin Keow v Government of Malaysia* [1967] 1 WLR 813 (failure to enquire as to the possibility of penicillin allergy); *Coles v Reading and District Hospital Management Committee* (1963) 107 SJ 115 (failure to immunise).

19 *Giurelli v Girgis* (1980) 24 SASR 264, discussed by Jones *Medical Negligence* (1991) p 117.

20 *Barnett v Chelsea and Kensington Hospital Management Committee* [1969] 1 QB 428, [1968] 1 All ER 1068; *Cavan v Wilcox* (1973) 44 DLR (3d) 42.

1 *Gardiner v Mounfield and Lincolnshire Area Health Authority* [1990] 1 Med LR 205.

2 In *Braisher v Harefield and Northwood Hospital Group Management Committee* (13 July 1966, unreported), CA. See H Jellie [1966] 2 Lancet 235.

3 B Jennett 'Some Medico-legal Aspects of the Management of Acute Head Injury' [1976] 1 BMJ 1383.

4 (1975) Times, 6 November.

5 (1978) The Times, 15 March, p 4.

correctly the nature of the patient's complaint. In *Langley*, the patient had returned from East Africa shortly before the development of symptoms. The general practitioner failed to diagnose malaria and negligence was found, the judge accepting the evidence of a relative who said that the family had suggested such a diagnosis to the doctor. In *Tuffil*, the patient had spent many years in a tropical climate; the doctor failed to diagnose amoebic dysentery which proved fatal. This failure to diagnose was held to be negligence on the doctor's part.

An example of an unsuccessful claim of this sort is provided by *Whiteford v Hunter*.[6] The defendant in this case had diagnosed carcinoma of the bladder, a diagnosis which was subsequently found to be incorrect. An important question was whether the defendant should have used a cystoscope: he did not have one in his possession and it would have been difficult to obtain one. The court found that there was no negligence in the misdiagnosis, holding that the defendant had used methods which were in common use at the time.

In cases where a doctor is doubtful about a diagnosis, good practice may require that the patient be referred to a specialist for further consideration of the case. It may be difficult for a doctor to know when to seek specialist advice – a fact explicitly acknowledged in the case of *Wilsher v Essex Area Health Authority*[7] – but in a case of doubt it is undoubtedly safer for a doctor to refer to a specialist.[8]

Negligence in treatment

The most important distinction to be made here is that between a medical mistake which the law regards as excusable and a mistake which would amount to negligence. In the former case, the court accepts that ordinary human fallibility precludes liability while, in the latter, the conduct of the defendant is considered to have gone beyond the bounds of what is expected of the reasonably skilful or competent doctor.

The issue came before the courts in the case of *Whitehouse v Jordan*.[9] In this case negligence was alleged on the part of an obstetrician who, it was claimed, had pulled too hard in a trial of forceps delivery and had thereby caused the plaintiff's head to become wedged with consequent asphyxia and brain damage. The trial judge held that, although the decision to perform a trial of forceps was a reasonable one, the defendant had in fact pulled too hard and was therefore negligent. This initial finding of negligence was reversed in the Court of Appeal and, in a strongly worded judgment, Lord Denning emphasised that an error of judgment was not negligence.[10] Implicit in Lord Denning's remarks was a strong policy based unwillingness to find negligence against doctors, an unwillingness which is to be seen in a number of the earlier judgments of the same judge.[11] When the matter came on appeal before the

---

6 (1950) 94 SJ 758, HL. Note 'at the time'; such an error would be indefensible today.
7 [1987] QB 730 at 777, [1986] 3 All ER 801 at 833.
8 This would be especially so where the doctor was unable to explain some aspect of the patient's condition: *MacDonald v York County Hospital Corpn* (1973) 41 DLR (3d) 321; (1976) 66 DLR (3d) 530 (S Ct Can).
9 [1981] 1 All ER 267, [1981] 1 WLR 246, HL.
10 [1980] 1 All ER 650 at 658, CA.
11 For further instances, see G Robertson '*Whitehouse v Jordan* – Medical Negligence Retired' [1981] 44 MLR 457.

House of Lords, the views expressed by Lord Denning on the error of judgment question were rejected. An error of judgment could be negligence if it is an error which would not have been made by a reasonably competent professional man acting with ordinary care. As Lord Fraser pointed out:

> The true position is that an error of judgment may, or may not, be negligent; it depends on the nature of the error. If it is one that would not have been made by a reasonably competent professional man professing to have the standard and type of skill that the defendant holds himself out as having, and acting with ordinary care, then it is negligence. If, on the other hand, it is an error that such a man, acting with ordinary care, might have made, then it is not negligence.[12]

In the event, the House of Lords held that there had not, in any case, been sufficient evidence to justify the trial judge's finding of negligence on the part of the defendant.[13]

Gross medical mistakes will almost always result in a finding of negligence. Operating mistakes such as the removal of the wrong limb or the performance of an operation on the wrong patient are usually treated as indefensible and settled out of court; hence the paucity of decisions on such points.[14] Use of the wrong drug or, often with more serious consequences, the wrong gas during the course of an anaesthetic will frequently lead to the imposition of liability, and in some of these situations the res ipsa loquitur principle (see below) may be applied.[15]

Many cases deal with items of operating equipment being left inside patients after surgery. In these, generally known as the 'swab cases', the allocation of liability is made according to the principle laid down in the locus classicus of the law on this point, the decision in *Mahon v Osborne*.[16] In this case, as in subsequent decisions, the courts have shown themselves unlikely to dictate to doctors in a hard and fast way the exact procedure that should be used towards the end of an operation in order to ensure no foreign bodies are left in the patient. At the same time, however, it is clear that the law requires that there should be some sort of set procedures adopted in order to minimise the possibility of this occurring. Overall responsibility to see that swabs and other items are not left in the patient rests on the surgeon; he is not entitled to delegate the matter altogether to a nurse.

This point was emphasised in *Mahon* by Goddard LJ who said:

> As it is the task of the surgeon to put swabs in, so it is his task to take them out and if the evidence is that he has not used a reasonable standard of care he cannot absolve himself, if a mistake has been made, by saying, 'I relied on the nurse'.[17]

12 [1981] 1 All ER 267 at 281; (1980) 1 BMLR 14 at 30.
13 A misjudgment will also be negligent if it is in respect of something 'lying within the area where only a sound judgment measures up to the standard of reasonable competence expected': *Hendy v Milton Keynes Health Authority (No 2)* [1992] 3 Med LR 119 per Jowitt J at 127.
14 An example is *Ibrahim (a minor) v Muhammad* (21 May 1984, unreported), QBD in which a penis was partially amputated during circumcision; only the quantum of damages was in dispute.
15 *Strangeways-Lesmere v Clayton* [1936] 2 KB 11, [1936] 1 All ER 484; *Collins v Hertfordshire County Council* [1947] KB 598, [1947] 1 All ER 633; *Gray v Mid Herts Hospital Management Committee* (1974) 118 SJ 501.
16 [1939] 2 KB 14, [1939] 1 All ER 535, CA.
17 [1939] 2 KB 14 at 47, [1939] 1 All ER 535 at 559. Scott LJ, however, qualified this by pointing out that it might be necessary to dispense with normal precautions in an emergency.

In the later case of *Urry v Bierer*,[18] the Court of Appeal confirmed that the patient was entitled to expect the surgeon to do all that was reasonably necessary to ensure that all packs were removed and that this duty required more than mere reliance on the nurse's count.

The problem of the novice   The degree of expertise possessed by a medical practitioner obviously depends to a considerable extent on his experience and the argument has been put forward that the standard of competence of a newly qualified doctor will be less than that expected of an experienced practitioner. Although this may be the day-to-day expectation, it is not that of the law. The strict application of the *Bolam* principle[19] would lead the courts to expect the doctor to show that degree of skill which would be shown by the reasonably competent professional man. This is an objective standard and it is therefore irrelevant whether the doctor has qualified the day before or ten years before the alleged incident of negligence – it should make no difference to the way in which his conduct is assessed.

The issue was addressed in the case of *Wilsher v Essex Area Health Authority*.[20] The plaintiff had been born prematurely and had been admitted to a specialised neonatal intensive care unit. Extra oxygen was administered by junior hospital doctors who made an error in monitoring the arterial oxygen tension. It was claimed that this could have caused the virtually blinding condition of retrolental fibroplasia which occurred. It was argued by the defendants that the standard of care expected of the junior doctor was not the same as that of his experienced counterpart. Extensive use, it was said, had to be made of recently qualified medical and nursing staff and it was unavoidable that such staff should 'learn on the job'; it would be impossible for public medicine to operate properly without such arrangements and to do otherwise would, ultimately, not be in the best interests of patients. The judgments in the Court of Appeal are not free of ambiguity. The majority of the judges maintained that the public were entitled to expect a reasonable standard of competence in their medical attendants. The decision of Mustill LJ, however, makes it clear that he, at least, was prepared to define the standard of care according to the requirements of the post. An inexperienced doctor occupying a post in a unit which offered specialised services would, accordingly, need that degree of expertise expected of a reasonably competent person occupying that post; the defendant's actual hospital rank – house officer, registrar etc – would not, therefore, be relevant in the determination.

Glidewell LJ also stressed the importance of applying an objective standard which would not take account of an individual doctor's inexperience. The apparent harshness of this is, nevertheless, mitigated by his suggestion that the standard of care is very likely to be met if the novice seeks advice or consults with his more

---

18 (1955) Times, 15 July, CA. For discussion of further swab (and forceps) cases see M A Jones *Medical Negligence* (1991) p140.

19 *Bolam v Friern Hospital Management Committee* [1957] 2 All ER 118, [1957] 1 WLR 582, QBD.

20 [1987] QB 730, [1986] 3 All ER 801, CA. For discussion of this case, see I Kennedy and A Grubb *Medical Law: Text with Materials* (2nd edn, 1994) p 445. A lower standard of care for novices was proposed in the Australian case of *Cook v Cook* (1986) 162 CLR 376, in which it was held that an inexperienced driver might not be judged on the same standard as others. In this case, however, there were special features in the relationship between the parties.

experienced colleagues when appropriate. Even so, this apparently simple solution does not answer the question which many juniors may ask – how am I to be so experienced as to know when I should be uncertain? And, if I cannot tell this, am I to ask my seniors before I make *any* important decision? And this question effectively forces us back to accepting a standard of care test which is based on the doctor of similar experience irrespective of the post in which he operates. Conversely, however, an experienced doctor occupying a junior post would be judged according to his actual knowledge rather than by the lower standard of the reasonably competent occupant of that post – the rationale being that, by reason of his superior expertise, he would be more able to foresee the damage likely to arise from any negligent acts or omissions.[1] It is important to bear in mind that *Wilsher* was very much concerned with specialist units and there is no certainty that the judgments are applicable, say, to the general practitioner in so far as delegation of responsibility, hierarchical organisation and the like are particular features of hospital practice. Hospital authorities cannot, of course, rely too much upon junior employees; the principles of vicarious liability will, by themselves, prevent this. As Lord Denning said in *Jones v Manchester Corpn*:

> It would be in the highest degree unjust that the hospital board, by getting inexperienced doctors to perform their duties for them, without adequate supervision, should be able to throw all the responsibility on to those doctors as if they were fully experienced practitioners.[2]

Delegation of responsibility to another may, however, amount to negligence in certain circumstances. A consultant could be negligent were he to delegate responsibility to a junior in the knowledge that the junior was incapable of performing his duties properly.

A junior to whom responsibility has been delegated must carry out his duties as instructed by his superior in order to avoid liability. If he chooses to depart from specific instructions, he will be placing himself in a risky position in the event of anything going wrong.[3] At the same time, there may be circumstances in which he is entitled to depart from instructions; obedience to manifestly wrong instructions might, itself, be construed as negligence in some cases.

Protecting the patient from himself
In certain circumstances, it is part of the duty of care of doctors and nurses to predict that patients may damage themselves as a result of their medical condition. The extent of the duty to safeguard against such damage is problematical and the decisions have not all gone the same way. In *Selfe v Ilford and District Hospital Management Committee*,[4] the plaintiff had been admitted to hospital after a drug overdose. Although he had known suicidal tendencies, he was not kept under

---

1 See *Wimpey Construction UK Ltd v Poole* [1984] 2 Lloyd's Rep 499.
2 [1952] 2 QB 852 at 871, [1952] 2 All ER 125 at 133, CA.
3 *Junor v Inverness Hospital Board of Management and McNicol* (1959) Times, 26 March, HL.
4 (1970) 114 SJ 935.

constant observation and climbed on to the hospital roof while the two nurses on duty were out of the ward; he fell and was injured. Damages of £19,000 were awarded against the hospital.

By contrast, the plaintiff in *Thorne v Northern Group Hospital Management Committee*[5] failed to win an award of damages for the death of his wife who had left a hospital in suicidal mood. In this case the patient had slipped out of the hospital when the nurses' backs were turned, returned home and gassed herself. The court took the view that, although the degree of supervision which a hospital should exercise in relation to patients with known suicidal tendencies is higher than that to be exercised over other patients, they could not be kept under constant supervision by hospital staff.

In *Hyde v Tameside Area Health Authority*[6] the Court of Appeal overturned a High Court award of substantial damages to a plaintiff who, believing he had cancer, made a suicide attempt in hospital. Not only did the court take the view that there had been no breach of duty on the part of the defendants, but Lord Denning stressed in his judgment that there were strong policy grounds why damages should not be awarded in respect of attempted suicide. Nowadays, that would probably be a minority view.

In *Kirkham v Chief Constable of Greater Manchester*[7] an appeal to the ex turpi causa principle – which may exclude liability where the plaintiff's act is in some way immoral – was rejected. It was held that the award of damages in respect of a suicidal death caused no affront to the public conscience – at least when the mind of the suicide was in some way unbalanced.

Res ipsa loquitur

Because it may be difficult in many personal injury actions to establish negligence on the part of the defendant, plaintiffs occasionally have recourse to the doctrine of res ipsa loquitur. This doctrine does not shift the onus of proof to the defendant as is sometimes suggested; what it does achieve is to give rise to an inference of negligence on the defendant's part.[8] If the defendant cannot then rebut this inference of negligence, the plaintiff will have established his case. It follows from this that it is considerably easier for the plaintiff to succeed in his claim when res ipsa loquitur applies.

The doctrine is most useful in cases where damage has occurred in an incident involving machinery or in the context of damage suffered while the plaintiff was involved in some sort of complex process. It applies only where the plaintiff is unable to identify the precise nature of the negligence which caused his injury and where no explanation of the way in which the injury came to be inflicted has been offered by the defendant. The injury itself must be of such a kind as 'does not

5 (1964) 108 SJ 484. A similar decision was taken in the Scottish case *Rolland v Lothian Health Board* (1981) unreported, Outer House, per Lord Ross.
6 [1981] CLY 1854, 2 PN 26, CA.
7 [1989] 3 All ER 882; affd [1990] 2 QB 283.
8 There has been some debate as to the precise effect of res ipsa loquitur, but the current weight of opinion favours the view outlined here: see *Ng Chun Pui v Lee Chuen Tat* [1988] RTR 298, PC. For discussion, see J Fleming *The Law of Torts* (8th edn, 1992) p 322; D Giesen *International Medical Malpractice Law* (1988) p 515.

normally happen' in the circumstances unless there is negligence. Thus, in a case of neurological damage following difficult aortography,[9] the plea of res ipsa loquitur was rejected on the grounds that the injury sustained was of a kind recognised as an inherent risk of the procedure.

The doctrine's application in medical cases may still be particularly apt because of the difficulty that the ordinary plaintiff sometimes experiences in unravelling the cause of an injury sustained during technical procedures of which he has little understanding; indeed, he may well have been unconscious at the relevant time. It may also be seen as a potential corrective to the tendency of the medical profession to 'close ranks' when one of their number is accused of negligence. In general, however, there is a marked reluctance on the part of the courts to apply the res ipsa loquitur principle, and this is certainly evident in medical negligence cases. As Megaw LJ said:

> [if one were to accept the view that negligence was inevitably proved if something went wrong and it was unexplained], few dentists, doctors and surgeons, however competent, conscientious and careful they might be, would avoid the totally unjustified and unfair stigma of professional negligence probably several times in the course of their careers.[10]

An unsuccessful attempt to raise the doctrine of res ipsa loquitur was made in *Ludlow v Swindon Health Authority*[11] in which it was stressed that the plaintiff had to establish facts which, if unexplained, would give rise to an inference of negligence. In this case the plaintiff claimed to have regained consciousness during a Caesarean section operation and to have experienced intense pain. She failed, however, to establish that the pain arose at a stage during which halothane should have been administered; there was, accordingly, no inference of negligence in the administration of the anaesthetic. Nevertheless, there are cases where the injuries sustained by the patient are of such a nature that there is an inescapable inference of negligence. The Canadian case of *MacDonald v York County Hospital Corpn*[12] provides an example. In this case, the plaintiff was admitted to hospital for treatment of a fractured ankle and left with an amputated leg. All the requirements of res ipsa loquitur were present: a leg is not usually lost in such circumstances unless there is negligence; the plaintiff was not able to explain what had happened, nor was the defendant; and the plaintiff had identified the doctor whose negligence must have been responsible for the injury.

Similarly, in *Cassidy v Ministry of Health*, the doctrine was applied in an English case in which the plaintiff went into hospital for an operation to remedy Dupuytren's contracture of two fingers and came out with four stiff fingers. Denning LJ (as he then was) expressed the view that the plaintiff was quite entitled to say:

---

9 *O'Malley-Williams v Board of Governors of the National Hospital for Nervous Diseases* (1975) unreported, cited in 1 BMJ 635.
10 *Fletcher v Bench* (1973) unreported, cited in 4 BMJ 117, CA.
11 [1989] 1 Med LR 104.
12 (1972) 28 DLR (3d) 521.

I went into hospital to be cured of two stiff fingers. I have come out with four stiff fingers and my hand is useless. That should not have happened if due care had been used. Explain it if you can.[13]

Although res ipsa loquitur will not be applied automatically, there are several 'swab cases' – as discussed above – in which it has been successfully invoked. In *Mahon v Osborne*,[14] for example, the court held that the patient could know nothing about swab procedures in the operating theatre and it was therefore for the surgeon to show that he exercised due care to ensure that the swabs were not left there.

Causation

As if the problems of fault were not enough, it will do the plaintiff no good to establish negligence on the part of a defendant doctor unless he is able to prove that the damage he has suffered was caused by that negligence. This may be particularly difficult in the context of medicine where there may be a variety of possible independent explanations for the occurrence of a condition. Thus, if a person brings an action for 'nervous shock', it may well be arguable that the symptoms complained of are those of a psychiatric state which existed before the claimed precipitating event. Some assistance in this respect was provided to the plaintiff through the Scottish case of *McGhee v National Coal Board*[15] in which it was held that liability will be imposed if it can be established that the negligence of the defender materially increased the risk of the plaintiff being damaged in the way in question.[16]

This principle was endorsed in *Clark v MacLennan*[17] in which it was held that, where there was a precaution which could have been taken to avoid the precise injury which occurred, the onus was then upon the defendant to establish that his failure to take this precaution did not cause the plaintiff's injury. This 'recognised risk avoidance' concept brings us very close to that of res ipsa loquitur which, as we have seen, the courts are reluctant to apply. This antipathy was demonstrated in the very comparable case of *Ashcroft v Mersey Health Authority*[18] which was heard at much the same time as *Clark*. Here, the plaintiff underwent a relatively straightforward and commonplace operation to remove granulation tissue – the result of chronic infection – from the ear; she sustained a severe paralysis of the facial nerve. Opinion was divided as to whether the surgeon had negligently pulled too hard on the nerve or whether the injury was an unfortunate accident. In the result, Kilner Brown J was, with obvious reluctance, unable to shift the burden of proof and found that, on a

---

13 [1951] 2 KB 343 at 365, [1951] 1 All ER 574 at 588, CA. Other medical cases in which res ipsa loquitur has applied include: *Saunders v Leeds Western Health Authority* (1984) 129 SJ 225, [1993] 4 Med LR 355. *Cavan v Wilcox* (1973) 44 DLR (3d) 42 and *Holmes v Board of Hospital Trustees of the City of London* (1977) 81 DLR (3d) 67.
14 [1939] 2 KB 14, [1939] 1 All ER 535, CA.
15 [1972] 3 All ER 1008, [1973] 1 WLR 1, HL.
16 [1972] 3 All ER 1008 at 1011, [1973] 1 WLR 1 at 4, per Lord Reid.
17 [1983] 1 All ER 416.
18 [1983] 2 All ER 245.

balance of probabilities, there was no negligence. The correctness of this view was later confirmed in *Wilsher*[19] where the House of Lords went so far as to reverse the opinion of the Court of Appeal and to order a retrial on the grounds that the coincidence of a breach of duty and injury could not, of itself, give rise to a presumption that the injury was so caused:

> Whether we like it or not, the law . . . requires proof of fault causing damage as the basis of liability in tort.[20]

The difficulty for the plaintiff in *Wilsher* lay in the fact there were five possible causes for the condition with which he was afflicted. One of these was medical negligence but it could not be established that this *possible* cause actually made a material contribution to the injury. It might have done so, but this fact still required to be proved by the plaintiff. The House of Lords discarded the notion that *McGhee v National Coal Board* [1] constituted an authority for transferring the onus of proof to the defendant. *McGhee* was to be distinguished from *Wilsher* in that there were several agents which could have caused the injury in the latter but only one in the former.[2] This provided an exceptional inference as to cause and, as a result, *McGhee* positively affirmed that the onus of proving causation lies on the pursuer or plaintiff.

A similar point as to proof of causation was made in the lengthy and complicated litigation over pertussis vaccination. In *Loveday*,[3] the court held that establishing a mere chance that the vaccine might cause brain damage in children did not discharge the obligation on the plaintiff. It is to be noted, parenthetically, that the decision in *Loveday* was not the last word on pertussis vaccine; in *Best v Wellcome Foundation Ltd*, the Supreme Court in Ireland awarded £2.75m to a young man who had suffered brain damage after its administration.[4] The decision is likely to encourage further litigation elsewhere – although the ground for the award was that the particular batch of vaccine used was substandard and should not have been released on the market. Future litigants will still have to prove that, on the balance of probabilities, their injuries were caused by the vaccine per se.

In a rather similar causation problem, both the Court of Session and the House of Lords have declared that a judge was not entitled to propound his own theory of a causative link between an overdose of penicillin and deafness; the weight of the evidence in *Kay* was that the causative factor was the meningitis for which the penicillin had been prescribed.[5]

---

19 *Wilsher v Essex Area Health Authority* [1988] AC 1074, [1988] 1 All ER 871, HL.
20 [1988] AC 1074 at 1092, [1988] 1 All ER 871 at 883, per Lord Bridge.
 1 [1972] 3 All ER 1008, [1973] 1 WLR 1.
 2 See the dissenting opinion of Browne-Wilkinson V-C in *Wilsher v Essex Area Health Authority*, [1987] QB 730 at 779, [1986] 3 All ER 801 at 834, CA. For discussion of the issue, see J Fleming 'Probabilistic Causation in the Tort Law' (1989) 68 Can BR 661.
 3 *Loveday v Renton* [1990] 1 Med LR 117.
 4 Irish Supreme Court, 3 June 1992. Reported by D Brahams 'Court Award for Pertussis Brain Damage' (1993) 341 Lancet 1338; C Dyer 'Man Awarded Damages after Pertussis Vaccination' (1993) 306 BMJ 1365.
 5 *Kay's Tutor v Ayrshire and Arran Health Board* [1987] 2 All ER 417, 1987 SLT 577, HL.

An interesting variation on the causation theme was reintroduced in *Hotson*.[6] Here, the plaintiff was, admittedly, negligently treated following traumatic avulsion of the head of the femur and developed avascular necrosis. However, there was a 75% chance that this lesion would develop even in the event of correct diagnosis and treatment. The trial judge concluded that the matter was simply one of quantification of damages and the Court of Appeal upheld the view that the mistreatment had denied the plaintiff a 25% chance of a good recovery. Damages were awarded and reduced accordingly. The House of Lords, however, declined to measure statistical chances[7] and concluded that it was the original injury which caused the avascular necrosis. Lord MacKay expressed the true situation:

> . . . the probable effect of delay in treatment was determined by the state of facts existing when the plaintiff was first presented at the hospital . . . If insufficient blood vessels were left intact by the fall, he had no prospect of avoiding complete avascular necrosis whereas if sufficient blood vessels were left intact . . . he would not have suffered the avascular necrosis.[8]

or, as put in The Times transcript,[9] what was meant by a chance was that if 100 people had suffered the same injury, 75 would have developed avascular necrosis and 25 would not. Thus, on the balance of probabilities, the plaintiff fell into the larger group – there being no evidence that he was one of the fortunate 25% who could benefit from treatment – and, consequently, his injury could not be attributed to the negligence of the defendants. It would be different if 51% of people sustaining the sort of injury which the plaintiff suffered could be treated with, say, a 20% chance of success. Then, on the balance of probabilities, the plaintiff would have fallen into that group of 51%, and, if a hospital negligently failed to offer him the treatment, he would have personally lost that 20% chance of a successful outcome. Whether that 20 per cent loss is something which should attract compensation in the form of 20% damages is left open by the decision in *Hotson*.

Damages for a loss of chance have been awarded in the United States. In *Falcon v Memorial Hospital*,[10] the Supreme Court of Michigan awarded damages for the wrongful death of a woman who would have had a 37.5% chance of survival had she been treated effectively. The court held that the physician's inaction had elided any chance of survival and that the appropriate measure of damages was equal to the chance of survival multiplied by the total damages available for wrongful death.

6 *Hotson v East Berkshire Area Health Authority* [1987] AC 750, [1987] 2 All ER 909, HL. A similar claim was dismissed in the early Scottish case of *Kenyon v Bell* 1953 SC 125. For discussion, see D T Price 'Causation – The Lords' "Lost Chance" ' (1989) 33 ICLQ 735.

7 Statistical chances and personal chances are quite different matters: T Hill 'A Lost Chance for Compensation in the Tort of Negligence by the House of Lords' (1991) 54 MLR 511. The author regrets the fact that the House of Lords appears to leave open the possibility of future successful actions based on a *personal* loss of chance.

8 [1987] AC 750 at 785, [1987] 2 All ER 909 at 915.

9 (1987) Times, 6 July.

10 462 NW 2d 44 (Mich, 1990). See also the earlier case of *Herskovits v Group Health Co-operative of Puget Sound* 664 P 2d 474 (Wash, 1983) in which the court allowed a claim for damages in respect of a cancer patient's loss of a 14% chance of survival for more than five years.

Injuries caused by medical products

The extensive use of drugs and other medical products in modern medical practice, coupled with the wide variety of available substances and devices, inevitably leads to a high incidence of injuries for which they are responsible. The number of persons affected will be small in some instances due to the speedy detection of the dangers and the rapid withdrawal of the products concerned. In others, the scale of the claims may be astronomic, an example being the series of actions brought against manufacturers of intrauterine devices.[11] For these reasons, the question of compensation becomes an intensely political issue, as it has done in relation to HIV-contaminated blood and certain tranquillisers.

Compensation for injury caused by products is now largely regulated in the United Kingdom by the Consumer Protection Act 1987. This derives from the European directive on product liability,[12] the aim of which was to create strict liability for most injuries which were caused by defective products; this policy had long been advocated by commentators on compensation for personal injury. Under the terms of the Act, strict liability is borne primarily by the manufacturer of a defective product although the suppliers will also be held liable if they cannot identify the manufacturer. Products include the components and raw materials from which a product is made and, in certain circumstances, a doctor may be a supplier of a drug. Despite strong protests from the industry, pharmaceutical products are not exempted from the system of strict liability. A drug will now be regarded as defective if it fails to measure up to that degree of safety which 'persons generally are entitled to expect' (s 3(1)).

In some circumstances, the manufacturer will be able to call on a development risk – or, in American terms, a 'state of the art' – defence. Section 4(1)(e) of the 1987 Act provides that the manufacturer will not be liable if he can show 'that the state of scientific and technical knowledge at the relevant time was not such that a producer of products of the same description as the product in question might be expected to have discovered the defect if it had existed in his products while they were under his control'. The aim of this defence is to relieve manufacturers of liability when the existence of a defect was undiscoverable at the time.[13] Expert evidence will be important in deciding whether a manufacturer has attained this goal; it is probable that the Act will not require the highest possible standards. It is suggested, for example, that a manufacturer would not reasonably be expected to know of and to act on an obscure report in a foreign language.

Is a manufacturer entitled to market a drug which will be beneficial to many but which he knows may cause harm to a minority? The traditional approach to this issue is by way of balancing the prospective benefit and risk. In general, sensitive users will have no claim to compensation if it is in the public interest that the drug should be available; much would then depend upon the presentation of the product and the nature of any warnings given. The Act (s 3(2)(b)) also stipulates that, in assessing

11 G R Thornton 'Intrauterine Devices: Malpractice and Product Liability' (1986) 14 Law Med Hlth Care 4.
12 Council Directive 85/374/EEC.
13 C Newdick 'The Development Risk Defence of the Consumer Protection Act 1987' (1988) 47 CLJ 455. See also C J Stolker 'Objections to the Development Risk Defence' (1990) 9 Med Law 783.

what constitutes defect, consideration must be given to what might reasonably be expected to be done with or in relation to the product. Thus, for example, it might reasonably be expected that children could gain access to drugs intended for adult use only. It is, however, unlikely that, say, suicide could be reasonably anticipated by the manufacturer.

The litigation relating to transmission of HIV infection through contaminated blood products has been taken in breach of a statutory duty under the National Health Service Act 1977 and in negligence;[14] nevertheless, it raises questions as to whether strict liability now applies to human blood and its derivatives. While, say, concentrated Factor VIII would clearly be a pharmacological product, it is less easy to see unmodified blood as such. A reading of the 1987 Act, ss 1(2) and 45(1), however, indicates firmly that blood would be a substance included within its scope – blood being a naturally occurring substance which has not been manufactured but which has been won or abstracted.[15] In terms of the Act, the Blood Transfusion Service would normally be the producer of the 'product' but the hospital, or even the individual doctor, responsible for its transfusion would be the supplier. The application of strict liability to blood transfusion has, inevitably, been considered at greatest length in the United States where the principle has been applied in some courts but where, in general, transfusion has been looked upon rather as the provision of a service than of a product,[16] thereby attracting potential actions in negligence – which would, of course, still be available outside the Act in the United Kingdom.[17] Clark[18] says that the majority of the United States have legislated to the effect that the supply of human blood is a service rather than a sale; the concept of 'sale' perhaps makes the distinction more urgent there than it is in the United Kingdom.

From the point of view of the doctor or the pharmacist, the major concern over strict liability laws lies in the need to ensure that the manufacturer can be adequately identified in order to avoid claims being made against himself as supplier. This might entail elaborate bureaucratic procedures and the fear has been expressed it could lead to further development of the practice of defensive medicine. An interesting American twist is shown in *Oskenholt v Lederle Laboratories*[19] where a doctor, having been successfully sued for prescribing a faulty drug, himself brought an action against the manufacturers for damage to his professional reputation – another example of the worm turning!

Criminal negligence

Medical negligence is predominantly a civil matter, but a spate of prosecutions have served to remind doctors of the fact that the loss of a patient may sometimes lead to

14 D Brahams 'Confidential Documents in HIV/Haemophilia Litigation' (1990) 336 Lancet 805.
15 Most commentators as we have been able to find agree with this analysis in general. See, in particular, A M Clark *Product Liability* (1989) ch 3. C Dyer 'Strict Liability Arrives: Significance for Doctors' (1988) 296 BMJ 635 is less certain, as is M A Jones *Medical Negligence* (1991) p 292, n 4.
16 Eg *Coffee v Cutter Biological* 809 F 2d 191 (1987)
17 The supply of HIV infected blood was the subject of common law-based litigation in the Australian case of *H v Royal Alexandra Hospital for Children* [1990] 1 Med LR 297.
18 A M Clark *Product Liability* (1989) p 62.
19 656 P 2d 293 (Ore, 1982).

criminal prosecution. Such prosecutions used to be rare; their increase points to heightened interest in the external regulation of medicine and to a diminution in the professional immunity which doctors may previously have enjoyed. In some respects, this process is healthy; in others, it is a matter for regret. The principle that doctors, and indeed all professionals, should be accountable for their failures is entirely acceptable; what is more dubious is that the criminal law, and particularly manslaughter prosecutions, should be the instrument chosen to perform that task. We believe that there should be no criminal liability for negligence and that the minimum threshold for the invocation of criminal sanctions should be recklessness. We explore the implications of this below.

Criminal liability for negligence is effectively limited to prosecutions for manslaughter. The level of negligence which the doctor must have manifested is considerably above that at which civil liability may be incurred. Traditionally it has been defined as 'gross' or 'extreme' negligence and sometimes, somewhat tautologically, as 'criminal negligence'; the essential concern is that it surpasses the civil test, as was stressed in *R v Bateman*:

> In order to establish criminal liability, the facts must be such that . . . the negligence of the accused went beyond a mere matter of compensation between subjects and showed such disregard for the life and safety of others as to amount to a crime against the State and conduct deserving punishment.[20]

This, of course, does not answer the question of when conduct goes beyond the compensation level but it is probably impossible to be much more specific. It is clear that what is required is conduct which gives rise to a sense of outrage – or to the conclusion that the accused deserves *punishment* for what he did. Such a conclusion, though, is likely to be articulated in terms of a lack of regard for the patient's welfare or safety – and therein lies the problem. If criminal negligence is defined in terms of a deliberate exposure of the patient to some form of risk, then we are in the realms of recklessness rather than negligence.[1] It is one thing to punish a person for subjective recklessness; it is quite another to punish for objective negligence. In the former case the accused has effectively said: 'I knew of the risk of harm but did not care'; in the latter, he may have been quite unaware of any risk at all – the damage caused may have been the result of incompetence or ignorance, neither of which qualities necessarily deserve punishment.

The conduct involved in recent cases has ranged from an apparent indifference with all the features of recklessness at one extreme, to mere inexpertise at the other. In *Saha and Salim*,[2] two doctors administered an astonishing cocktail of drugs to a remand prisoner who died as a result. They were both convicted and sentenced to a

---

20 [1925] All ER Rep 45 at 48, 19 Cr App Rep 8 at 11, per Lord Hewart LCJ.
  1 A difficulty which the courts have acknowledged in those decisions where gross negligence manslaughter appears to have been replaced by reckless manslaughter: *R v Seymour* (1983) 76 Cr App R 211; *Kong Cheuk Kwan v R* (1985) 82 Cr App Rep 18.
  2 1992, unreported; see D Brahams 'Death of Remand Prisoner' (1992) 340 Lancet 1462.

term of imprisonment. By contrast, the conviction of two young and relatively inexperienced doctors for the manslaughter of a patient to whom they had incorrectly administered cytotoxic drugs was greeted with concern in medical circles and was, in due course, quashed by the Court of Appeal. Somewhere in between lies the case of *R v Adomako*[3] in which an anaesthetist failed to notice the fact that his patient was in distress when this would have been glaringly obvious to any competent practitioner. There was conflicting evidence on the question of whether the accused was out of the theatre at the time; if he had been, and if there had been a failure on his part to make adequate arrangements for the monitoring of the patient, then that would surely have amounted to a degree of recklessness which was strongly deserving of punishment. If, however, he was merely incompetent, it might be more difficult to argue for his conviction of manslaughter – although, undoubtedly, professional sanctions would still be needed. These cases were heard together on appeal[4] when it was held that the proper test in manslaughter cases based on breach of duty was that of gross negligence rather than recklessness.[5] In contrast to that of the two young doctors, Dr Adomako's appeal failed.

As the criminal law now stands, a grossly incompetent doctor is liable to conviction despite the fact that there is no element of subjective wrongdoing on his part. This might well be considered inappropriate.[6] The alternative view is that the law should protect the public and that prosecution represents one way of controlling those who cannot meet minimal professional standards. No one would contend that incompetence, as understood here, merits imprisonment; but a successful prosecution, coupled with token sentencing, at least ensures that the case *must* come to the attention of the General Medical Council.

If concern is felt in the United Kingdom over the prosecution of, often junior, doctors for causing the deaths of patients, it might well be multiplied in New Zealand where, under the Crimes Act 1961, criminal liability may be imposed on a doctor who merely fails to show 'reasonable knowledge, skill and care' in the treatment of his patients. This extraordinarily low threshold of liability was applied in *R v Yogasakaran*[7] and confirmed on appeal to the Privy Council.[8] In this case, an anaesthetist had not checked the label on an ampoule of a drug which he injected into a patient. The ampoule was of the appropriate shape and size and was in the right place on the trolley but, for some reason unconnected with the anaesthetist, contained the wrong drug. Presumably the same result would have been achieved if the anaesthetist had, in fact, read the label but had read it

3 [1991] 2 Med LR 277.
4 *R v Prentice*, *R v Adamako*, *R v Holloway* [1993] 4 All ER 935, sub nom *R v Holloway*, *R v Adomako*, *R v Prentice and Sulman* [1993] 4 Med LR 304. See C Dyer 'Manslaughter Verdict Quashed on Junior Doctors' (1993) 306 BMJ 1432.
5 [1993] 4 Med LR 304 at 310, [1993] 4 All ER 935 at 943, per Lord Taylor following *Andrews v DPP* [1937] AC 576, [1937] 2 All ER 552, HL and *R v Stone and Dobinson* [1977] QB 354, [1977] 2 All ER 341.
6 For expansion of this argument, see A McCall Smith 'Criminal Negligence and the Incompetent Doctor' (1993) 1 Med L Rev 336.
7 [1990] 1 NZLR 399.
8 See D B Collins 'New Zealand's Medical Manslaughter' (1992) Med Law 221.

wrongly. Such a common mistake can hardly be seen as justification for convicting a person of a crime which carries with it a very deal of moral opprobrium – it would surely be better investigated by the Medical Practitioners' Disciplinary Committee.

10 Consent to treatment

The paternalist might argue that there are many examples in medical practice of situations in which treatment is justified in the teeth of the patient's objection. Arguing from such a position – that the patient may be unable to appreciate that a particular treatment is in his best interest – the decision of the doctor to impose it is seen as serving the patient's interest in spite of what may turn out to be short-term objections. This, a paternalist would hold, cannot be wrong. Good health and physical comfort are preferable to ill health and physical discomfort: a patient will thus be happier treated than untreated.

Such arguments can, however, be sustained only in very limited conditions such as when the patient is in an irrational state because of impaired or disturbed consciousness. Restraining a delirious patient is justifiable paternalism, as is the action of clearing the air passages of one who is about to choke to death. The intervention is justified by the conviction that this is what the patient would want, were he fully rational, or that such treatment is needed to restore him to a position in which he can make up his own mind.

The case for imposed treatment can also be couched in social terms. Illness is costly to the community and the individual is not entitled to refuse treatment which may minimise this cost. The community may have to support the family of a person who dies as a result of refusing treatment. Non-voluntary intervention is, thereby, justified. This argument is, however, also weak. Society may, indeed, be saved certain costs if a life is preserved but it can be argued that the damage resulting from coercion convincingly outweighs that which it seeks to avert. A coercive society can be most cost-effective – but this does not mean it is most desirable.

A possible, although uncommon, exception to this rejection of the social cost argument exists when a person is found to be suffering from a highly infectious and dangerous illness; few would then argue that he should be allowed to refuse treatment if such treatment is the sole way to reduce the risk of spreading the disease. Here, the only caveat to the application of coercive treatment is that it should be as non-coercive as is compatible with containment of the threat.

Non-consensual treatment

The legal justification
The common law has long recognised the principle that every person has the right to have his bodily integrity protected against invasion by others. Only in certain narrowly defined circumstances may this integrity be compromised without the individual's consent – as where, for example, a parent or guardian applies justifiable

corporal punishment or where physical intrusion is involved in the carrying out of lawful arrest.

The seriousness with which the law views any invasion of physical integrity is based on the strong moral conviction that everyone has the right of self-determination with regard to his body. Unless there is consent to an act of touching by another, such an act will – subject to the principle de minimis non curat lex – constitute a battery for which damages may be awarded. Consent can make physical invasion lawful but the reality of such consent may be closely scrutinised by the law and is, anyway, subject to certain policy limitations. Consent will not normally render legitimate a serious physical injury. Thus, it was held by Swift J in *R v Donovan*:

> As a general rule to which there are well established exceptions, it is an unlawful act to beat another person with such a degree of violence that the infliction of bodily harm is a probable consequence and, when such an act is proved, consent is immaterial.[1]

In medical treatment, every touching of the patient is potentially a battery on that patient. The classic expression is that of Cardozo J:

> Every human being of adult years and sound mind has a right to determine what shall be done with his own body; and a surgeon who performs an operation without the patient's consent commits an assault.[2]

It is the patient's consent – either implied or expressed – which makes the touching legally innocuous and there is no doubt that surgical interference is covered by this principle.[3] The theory, then, is quite simple – the reality is somewhat different. Much litigation in common law countries has focused on the consent issue over the past decade and, as a result, the doctrine of informed consent, as it has come to be called, has assumed a significant role in the medical negligence debate. As will be seen later in this chapter, it is a doctrine which lies surprisingly uneasily in the medico-legal ambience of the United Kingdom.

Is consent always necessary?

As a general rule, medical treatment, even of a minor nature, should not proceed unless the doctor has first obtained the patient's consent. This consent may be expressed or it may be implied, as it is when the patient presents himself to the doctor for examination and acquiesces in the suggested routine. This principle applies in the overwhelming majority of cases but there are limited circumstances in which a doctor may be entitled to proceed without this consent. Essentially, these can be subsumed under the heading of non-voluntary therapy which has to be distinguished from involuntary treatment. The latter implies treatment against the patient's

---

1 [1934] 2 KB 498 at 507. Endorsed in *R v Brown* [1993] 2 All ER 75, HL.
2 *Schloendorff v Society of New York Hospital* 105 NE 92 (NY, 1914).
3 *A-G's Reference (No 6 of 1980)* [1981] QB 715, [1981] 2 All ER 1057. The Scots equivalent, albeit indirect, lies in *Smart v HM Advocate* 1975 SLT 65.

expressed wishes; the occasions on which this would be ethical are, indeed, very few although a case can be made out when the interests of a third party or of society itself are involved. Non-voluntary treatment is that which is given when the patient is not in a position to have or to express any views as to his or her management. This clearly covers circumstances in which treatment in the absence of consent is more easily justified. They include, first, when the patient is incapable of giving consent by reason of unconsciousness; second, when the patient is a minor; and, finally, when the patient's state of mind is such as to render an apparent consent invalid.

The unconscious patient

It is possible to see non-voluntary treatment as proceeding with consent, although that consent is not expressed. Thus, when an unconscious patient is admitted to hospital, the casualty officer may argue that his consent could be implied or presumed on the grounds that if he were conscious he would probably consent to his life being saved in this way. This may be true but, while the majority of patients could be expected to endorse the decision to treat in such circumstances, it is a rather fictitious way of approaching the problem[4] – although the principle of negotiorum gestio, which is, essentially, that a person expects another to do his best for him, might be applied in this situation in Scotland.

An easier approach is to apply the necessity principle. It is widely recognised in both criminal and civil law that there are certain circumstances in which acting out of necessity legitimates an otherwise wrongful act. The basis of this doctrine is that acting unlawfully is justified if the resulting good effect materially outweighs the consequences of adhering strictly to the law. In the present context, the doctor is justified, and should not have criminal or civil liability imposed upon, him if the value which he seeks to protect is of greater weight than the wrongful act he performs – that is, treating without consent.

Necessity will be a viable defence to any proceedings for non-consensual treatment when an unconscious patient is involved and there is no known objection to treatment. The treatment undertaken, however, must not be more extensive than is required by the exigencies of the situation – we do well to remember what Lord Devlin said, albeit in a rather different context: 'The Good Samaritan is a character unesteemed in English law'.[5] A doctor cannot, therefore, 'take advantage' of unconsciousness to perform procedures which are not essential for the patient's survival. This was established in two well-known Canadian cases where the courts explored the distinction between procedures justified by necessity and those which are merely 'convenient', a distinction which would, in all probability, be followed by the British courts.

In the first of these, *Marshall v Curry*,[6] the plaintiff sought damages for battery against the surgeon who had, in the course of an operation for a hernia, removed a testicle. The surgeon's case was that the removal was essential to a successful

---

4   The use of a legal fiction of this sort was disapproved in *Marshall v Curry* [1933] 3 DLR 260 at 275. P D G Skegg *Law, Ethics and Medicine* (1984) is a most valuable reference; the particular point is discussed at p 99.

5   Lord Devlin *Samples of Law Making* (1962) p 90.

6   [1933] 3 DLR 260.

operation and that, had he not done so, the health and life of the patient would have been imperilled because the testis was, itself, diseased. Taking the view that the doctor had acted 'for the protection of the plaintiff's health and possibly his life', the court held that the removal of the testicle was necessary and that it would have been unreasonable to put the procedure off until a later date. By contrast, in *Murray v McMurchy*,[7] the plaintiff succeeded in an action for battery against a doctor who had sterilised her without her consent. In this case, the doctor had discovered during a Caesarean section that the condition of the plaintiff's uterus would have made it hazardous for her to go through another pregnancy and, although there was no pressing need for the Fallopian tubes to be tied, the doctor went ahead with the procedure. The court took the view that it would not have been unreasonable to postpone the sterilisation until after consent had been obtained in spite of the convenience of doing it on the spot.[8]

The principle that emerges from these two cases is that a doctor is justified by necessity in proceeding without the patient's consent if a condition is discovered in an unconscious patient for which treatment is necessary in the sense that it would be, in the circumstances, unreasonable to postpone the operation to a later date. If, however, it is possible to put off any treatment until the patient is in a position to give consent, the postponement of treatment is to be preferred. The distinction is, nevertheless, often delicately balanced – particularly in the light of the sometimes vague terms of written consent forms. In an unreported Scottish case[9] the patient signed to the effect: 'I hereby give permission for myself to have a general anaesthetic and any operation the surgeon considers necessary.' The operation proposed was the comparatively simple removal of a supposed branchial cyst but, on exploration, the 'cyst' was found to be a carotid body tumour. Removal of such a mass is a far more difficult procedure and the patient, in fact, sustained paralysis of half his body. The Inner House concluded that permission was not limited by seriousness and that the patient had consented to any operation to the end of removing the swelling: 'Consent must be read as covering any operation considered by the surgeon at the time to be in the patient's interest' (per Lord Robertson); none the less, the three judges concerned could all foresee different conclusions if the operation was outwith the procedure contemplated by the patient. It is less certain that such a decision would be reached elsewhere, particularly in the United States where, in respect of such consent forms, it has been considered that: 'the so-called authority is so ambiguous as to be almost completely worthless'.[10] The increasing

7 [1949] 2 DLR 442. *Devi v West Midlands Regional Health Authority* [1981] CA Transcript 491 provides an almost exact British parallel.
8 Such cases seem still not infrequent and, although the formation of such pressure groups is increasingly common, it is significant that a charity – the Hysterectomy Legal Fighting Fund – has recently been established in the United Kingdom. At the time of writing, publicity has been given to a case in which it is alleged a uterus removed for the treatment of endometriosis contained an 11-week fetus: C Dyer 'Woman Sues after Hysterectomy and Abortion' (1993) 307 BMJ 754. See also D Brahams 'Unwanted Hysterectomies' (1993) 342 Lancet 361.
9 *Craig v Glasgow Victoria and Leverndale Hospitals Board of Management*, 1st Division, (22 March 1974, unreported). See J A Cameron *Medical Negligence: An Introduction* (1983).
10 *Rogers v Lumbermens Mutual Cas Co* 119 So 2d 649 (La, 1960).

prevalence of such attitudes has resulted in the publication as recently as 1990 of a model consent form to be used throughout the British National Health Service.[11]

Proxy consent and the consent of minors

It is possible that a member of the family may be at hand when a patient is unconscious. In such a case, it may be wise for the doctor to obtain the agreement of a close relative largely in order to discover any anticipatory choice on the part of the patient or other details which might affect a clinical decision. It is, however, now clear that, in the case of an adult patient, the next of kin has no *legal* right to consent to or refuse consent to treatment.[12] Indeed, the doctor who delays unreasonably while seeking the support of the next of kin is misconceiving the law. None the less, the doctor's position is often not easy and, provided that it involved no adverse effects, the fact that the spouse's or relatives' agreement had been obtained could be of value in that it would diminish the likelihood of the patient feeling aggrieved at the invasion of his or her privacy.[13]

Proxy *consents* are truly valid only when the patient has given express authority to another person to give or withhold consent on his behalf or when the law invests a person with such power. The commonest example of the latter would be that of parent and child. When proxy consent of this sort is available, the person vested with the power must use it reasonably; the unreasonable withholding of consent may justify a third party's ignoring such withholding, although this might well be a hazardous course to adopt in the absence of judicial support.

A common occasion on which parents refuse to give consent to the medical treatment of their children is when they disapprove of such treatment for religious reasons. The capacity of the 'mature minor' to consent to treatment on his or her own behalf is discussed in some detail below; here, we are concerned only with the child who is evidently too young to take important decisions of the quality of accepting a blood transfusion. A doctor taking steps to administer such life-saving treatment to the child against the wishes of its parents could rely upon the common law as above – and the current judicial climate is such that we believe a decision taken in good faith in the best interests of a child would, save in very unusual circumstances, be upheld by the courts[14] – and this is the choice hospital authorities will, in general, adopt. It is also technically possible for the medical advisers to initiate care proceedings when parents refuse to consent to life-saving medical treatment; the appropriate local

---

11 NHS Management Executive *A Guide to Consent for Examination or Treatment* (1990). It is possible to make out an argument, based on *Sidaway* (see p 241 below), that it is wrong in law to require such detailed consent; see C Heneghan 'Consent to Medical Treatment' (1991) 337 Lancet 421. We suggest that it would be unwise to put it to the test.

12 *Re T (Adult: refusal of medical treatment)* [1992] 4 All ER 649 at 653; (1992) 9 BMLR 46 at 50, CA, per Lord Donaldson MR.

13 All the United States have enacted 'Good Samaritan' legislation aimed at protecting the doctor giving emergency roadside treatment; it can be argued that this interference with access to the courts is both unnecessary and unconstitutional – B Sullivan 'Some Thoughts on the Constitutionality of Good Samaritan Statutes' (1982) 8 Amer J Law Med 27. See also Australian legislation: Voluntary Aid in Emergency Act 1973 (Queensland), Ambulance Services Act 1976, s 14A (NSW).

14 By extrapolation from *Re F* [1990] 2 AC 1, sub nom *F v West Berkshire Health Authority* [1989] 2 All ER 545, HL (the *Bolam* principle, see p 200, would, presumably, dictate the outcome).

authority or the court may then be able to consent to the proposed procedure[15] or to apply for a specific issue order.[16] An alternative approach would be invite the High Court to exercise its inherent jurisdiction and to negate the parental decision because the that power had been exercised unreasonably. There is, at present, some confusion as to the priority to be given to these possible tactics. In *Re O*,[17] it was held that the inherent jurisdiction of the High Court was the most appropriate legal framework within which to consider a contested issue relating to emergency treatment for a child. Only a few months later, however, another judge of the Family Division opted for the invocation of a specific issue order.[18] The difference is, however, largely a matter of the interpretation of a statute and its more subtle limitations; it was admitted in *Re R* that the inherent jurisdiction of the court was always available should its statutory jurisdiction be found wanting. It is to be noted that neither court was in any doubt that blood transfusion should be authorised when medical considerations dictated the need.

Although there would be little public sympathy for parents who refuse on religious grounds to consent to blood transfusion for a perilously ill child, it would be a mistake to reject their position out of hand. The refusal of blood in such circumstances may seem to many to be irrational and pointless, but there is no doubt that it is a strongly held minority position. Ignoring it involves overriding religious convictions and this is a major step in a free society. Such action also entails a significant interference with the principle that parents should have freedom to choose the religious and social upbringing of their children. These factors certainly suggest caution but are outweighed by the counter-arguments that there has been a redefinition of the role of the parents in respect of control of their children and that it is no longer possible to regard them as having an almost absolute power: 'Parental rights to control a child', said Lord Fraser, 'exist not for the benefit of the parent but for the child.'[19] The community interest in the welfare of children is demonstrated in a number of ways, some more draconian than others. Society is prepared to remove a child from its parents if it is in moral or physical danger; the child whose life is endangered by parental refusal of consent to medical treatment may be removed from its home on precisely the same grounds as may be the battered child. Any difference in the two cases lies in motives. The parent withholding consent may be doing so for what he sees as good reasons and in the interests of the child; the parent who neglects his child is unlikely to feel the same. In spite of this difference, however, there must be few who will see the parents' good faith as justifying the imperilling of the child's life; death of a child in such circumstances might result in prosecution of the parents for manslaughter[20] – as was said in a well-known American case:

15 Children Act 1989, s 31; Social Work (Scotland) Act 1968, s 44.
16 Children Act 1989, s 8(1).
17 *In Re O (a minor)(medical treatment)* [1993] 2 FLR 149, [1993] 4 Med LR 272.
18 *Re R (a Minor)(Blood Transfusion)* [1993] 2 FCR 544. For discussion of the procedural 'route', see C Gilham 'The Dilema of Parental Choice' (1993) NLJ 1219.
19 In *Gillick v West Norfolk and Wisbech Area Health Authority* [1986] AC 112, [1985] 3 All ER 402, (1985) 2 BMLR 11, HL. Following Lord Denning MR in *Hewer v Bryant* [1970] 1 QB 357 at 369, [1969] 3 All ER 578 at 582: 'Parental rights start with the right of control and end with little more than advice.' See also footnote 5 below.
20 *R v Senior* [1899] 1 QB 283. A recent English conviction is reported by D Brahams in 'Religious Objection versus Parental Duty' (1993) 342 Lancet 1189.

Parents may be free to become martyrs themselves. But it does not follow that they are free in identical circumstances to make martyrs of their children.[1]

The questions of positive consent to and refusal of medical and surgical procedures by relatively mature minors in the absence of parental authority – or, indeed, knowledge – is, however, by far the most controversial issue in this field. The status of the minor between the ages of 16 and 18 is now almost settled and we return to it briefly below; discussion is, here, confined to the child below the age of 16. The common law does not exclude such a child giving consent but the validity of that consent has to be considered in the light of the pivotal case of *Gillick v West Norfolk and Wisbech Area Health Authority*.[2] Although, as is well known, that case was specifically concerned with the provision of contraceptives (and is also discussed under that heading and under confidentiality, pp 94, 179 above), many of the points made in the majority opinions can be taken as relating to the consent of minors to medical treatment as a whole – indeed, the term '*Gillick* competent' is now part of medico-legal lore.[3]

The dominant opinion[4] was that the parental right to determine whether or not their minor child below the age of 16 years will have medical treatment 'terminates if and when the child achieves a significant understanding and intelligence to enable him or her to understand fully what is proposed' but, until the child attains such a capacity to consent, the parental right to make the decision continues save only in exceptional circumstances.[5] Despite the general tenor of his judgment, Lord Scarman affirmed that: 'Parental rights clearly exist and do not wholly disappear until the age of majority.' It can be taken as being now accepted that a doctor treating a child should always attempt to obtain parental authority but that, provided the patient is capable of understanding what is proposed and of expressing his or her wishes, he may, in exceptional circumstances, provide treatment on the basis of the minor's consent alone. The decision to do so must be taken on clinical grounds and, clearly, must depend heavily on the severity and permanence of the proposed therapy.[6] The concurrence of Scots law on this question has scarcely been disputed; it is now confirmed – and, in some ways, extended – in the Age of Legal Capacity (Scotland) Act 1991, s 2(4).

The court in *Gillick* took the view that it would be a question of fact to be decided in each case whether a child seeking advice had sufficient understanding to give a consent valid in law. An illustration of this is provided by a case in which the court agreed that a schoolgirl aged 15 should be allowed to have an abortion against the wishes of her parents. Butler-Sloss J said: 'I am satisfied she wants this abortion; she understands the implications of it.'[7]

1   *Prince v Massachusetts* 321 US 158 (1944).
2   [1986] AC 112, [1985] 3 All ER 402, (1985) 2 BMLR 11, HL.
3   *Re R (a minor)(wardship: medical treatment)* [1992] Fam 11 at 23, (1991) 7 BMLR 147 at 156, CA, per Lord Donaldson.
4   [1986] AC 112 at 189, [1985] 3 All ER 402 at 423, per Lord Scarman.
5   A similar approach by Lord Denning MR in *Hewer v Bryant* [1970] 1 QB 357, [1969] 3 All ER 578 was strongly approved and the common law position in Canada, as expressed in *Johnston v Wellesley Hospital* (1970) 17 DLR (3d) 139, was also quoted.
6   For a critical review of the *Gillick* decision with particular reference to the doctor's situation, see G Williams 'The *Gillick* Saga' (1985) 135 NLJ 1156, 1179.
7   *Re P (a minor)* [1986] 1 FLR 272, (1982) 80 LGR 301.

Thus, the problem of consent to treatment by minors is, to all intents, settled and is well understood. We have not, however, yet touched on refusal of treatment. This is a comparatively novel issue and one which has aroused considerable controversy. We return to it in a discussion of recent cases below.

The mentally incompetent

A proportion of non-consensual treatment which can be provided for involuntary mental patients is proscribed by statute and is discussed further at p 391. All such therapy is, however, specifically limited to treatment of the mental condition. Treatments of unrelated physical conditions are excluded and a therapeutic lacuna remains – how can treatment be provided legitimately to persons who are unable to consent to it?

We have already seen some of the difficulties entailed in the series of sterilisation operations which have come to the notice of the courts (see chapter 4). Nevertheless, it is these very cases which have served to clarify the medical position. In *Re F*,[8] it was clearly stated that a doctor can provide treatment for a mentally handicapped person in the absence of consent so long as that treatment is in the patient's best interests – and a line of decisions have supported that view and, indeed, extended its scope. It is, however, doubtful if this professionally orientated approach acts to the advantage of the mentally handicapped; this is despite the fact that the confusion arises, at least in part, from progressive changes on mental health legislation which have been designed, with the best of intentions, to restore autonomy to the mentally impaired[9] – not the least significant of these being the removal of the courts' parens patriae jurisdiction in the Mental Health Act 1959. Neither does it provide the necessary security for the medical profession. At the present time, the Law Commission has prepared a consultation paper covering the whole spectrum and has added its own recommendations.[10] The great majority of these follow the anticipated lines and include an obligation on the doctor to consult the nearest relative so as to achieve a 'best interests' decision and to obtain his or her consent – as opposed to the current agreement; there is also a call for the appointment of decision-making proxies. The commission does, however, propose the formation of a 'judicial forum' which will decide, inter alia, on the provision of major and sensitive treatments. It is this, perhaps particularly, which demonstrates the dilemma involved in defining medical 'art' in terms of a statute – how is the state to satisfy the concerns and aspirations of all parties without strangling the therapeutic service with bureaucracy?[11] These are, however, early days in the evolution of a new framework and further discussion at this point would probably prove unprofitable.

---

8 *Re F (mental patient: sterilisation)* [1990] 2 AC 1, sub nom *F v West Berkshire Health Authority* [1989] 2 All ER 545.
9 See, for example, C Dyer 'Who Decides for Those Who Can't?' (1991) 302 BMJ 1352.
10 Law Commission *Mentally Incompetent Adults and Decision-making* (Consultation Paper No 128, 1993). The matter is discussed by the Scottish Law Commission in *Mentally Disabled Adults* (Discussion Paper No 94, 1991).
11 For discussion from the medical aspect, see 'Mental Incapacity and Medical Treatment' (1993) 341 Lancet 1123.

The recent cases

The interval between the previous edition of this book and this one has provided a remarkable series of cases which have served to draw together, and indicate judicial attitudes to, non-voluntary treatment involving minors, mature minors and doubtfully incompetent adults.

The first, although not chronologically, which is of importance in the present context is *Re J*.[12] This case concerned a 16-month-old brain damaged child whose condition was such that his medical attendants considered it inappropriate to provide invasive intensive care in the event that he suffered a life-threatening event. The boy's mother sought, and obtained, an order that such treatment should be given if it served to prolong his life. This order was immediately stayed and, later, the Court of Appeal upheld an appeal against the order. The significance of *Re J* is that, in restating[13] in the clearest terms that the medical profession could not be required to undertake treatment against its clinical judgment, it lays a base-line that, while *consent* to treatment is essential, there is no concurrent right to *demand* treatment. In short, there are 'checks and balances of consent and willingness and ability to treat'.

Re R[14] is something of a landmark case as it constitutes the first time that the concept of the mature – or *Gillick* competent – minor has been tested in the United Kingdom courts; it also raises, but scarcely resolves, the relationship between consent to and refusal of treatment. Briefly, the case concerned a 15-year-old girl whose increasingly disturbed behaviour required sedative treatment. However, during her lucid phases – in which she appeared rational and capable of making decisions – she refused her medication and the local authority instituted wardship proceedings, the intention being to seek authority to provide anti-psychotic treatment whether or not she consented. R appealed against an order to that effect which had been obtained.

The Court of Appeal first disposed of the distinction, if any, between parental powers and those of the court in wardship and concluded that the latter were wider; the court could override both consent and refusal of treatment by the ward if that was considered to be in his or her best interests. The court then further distinguished *Gillick* which was concerned with the developing maturity of normal children; the test elaborated in that case could not be applied to a child whose mental state fluctuated widely from day to day. But the aspect of the case having by far the most general significance lay in its definition of parental powers. Essentially, Lord Donaldson MR considered that the parental right which *Gillick* extinguished was to *determine* the treatment of a mature minor – and this was considered to be wider in its implications than a right to consent in so far as it included the right of veto. In explanation, Lord Donaldson introduced the concept of consent providing the key to the therapeutic door and of there being, in the case of the mature minor, two keyholders – the minor and its parents. Consent by either *enabled* treatment to be

---

12 *Re J (a minor)(wardship: medical treatment)* [1992] 2 FLR 165, (1992) 9 BMLR 10.

13 The proposition had been previously stated in *Re J (a minor)(wardship: medical treatment)* [1991] Fam 33 at 41, (1992) 6 BMLR 25 at 30 and in *Re R (a minor)(wardship: medical treatment)* [1992] Fam 11 at 26, (1992) 7 BMLR 147 at 154 both per Lord Donaldson MR. The trial judge in the present case interpreted these remarks as not binding.

14 *Re R (a minor)(wardship: medical treatment)* [1992] Fam 11, (1992) 7 BMLR 147, CA.

given lawfully but did not, in any way, *determine* that the child should be treated. Lord Donaldson was later to regret his keyholder analogy in so far as keys can lock as well as unlock doors. It seems to us to be acceptable so long as it is modified to imply that refusal on the part of the child effectively means that the child has thrown away its key to a locked door; it is then only prudent that there should be a second key available as a fire precaution.

Re R raised a storm of academic protest. This was not, primarily, as to the assessment of mental incompetence which the court considered should be based on the general condition of the patient rather than that at a given moment in time; nor was there great exception to the definition of the court's authority in wardship – which will, in any event, be less commonly invoked since the coming into force of the Children Act 1989. Rather, the criticism was directed at the retention of the parental right to give consent in the face of the child's refusal – an interpretation of the law which Kennedy described as 'driving a coach and horses through *Gillick*'.[15] But is this, in fact, so? Lord Donaldson's distinction between a parental ability to determine a minor's treatment – which Lord Scarman considered to be overtaken by the child's developing maturity[16] – and to consent to treatment is a legitimate one and, as we have seen, a corresponding obligation to apply that treatment was firmly rejected. Moreover, the Master of the Rolls was, arguably, doing no more than interpreting the statute law of England. The Family Law Reform Act 1969, s 8(1) gives the minor aged 16-18 powers of consent to medical and surgical treatment equivalent to those of an adult. Section 8(3), however, goes on to say:

> Nothing in this section shall be construed as making ineffective any consent which would have been effective if this section had not been enacted.

It has been widely assumed that this section does no more than confirm the common law right of competent minors to decide these questions for themselves. We have always doubted this, largely because, if this is the correct interpretation, there was never any need for s 8(1) – a view which was endorsed by the absence of any such statute in Scotland prior to the Age of Legal Capacity (Scotland) Act 1991.[17] The better view, in our opinion, is that a parental right to consent on behalf of a child existed before 1969 and that s 8(3) preserves that right; this seems to have been Lord Donaldson's interpretation[18] – one which formed the basis of his opinion. The academic response to *Re R* demonstrates, above all, the difficulties which arise when attempting to apply general philosophical principles to particular medical cases. The opinion may have further muddied the murky waters of *Gillick* but what was the

---

15 I Kennedy 'Consent to Treatment: The Capable Person' in C Dyer (ed) *Doctors, Patients and the Law* (1992) ch 3. See also A Bainham 'The Judge and the Competent Minor' (1992) 108 LQR 196 – which is concerned more with the Family Law Reform Act 1969, s 8(1) rather than s 8(3).

16 In *Gillick* [1986] AC 112 at 188, [1985] 3 All ER 402 at 423, (1985) 2 BMLR 11 at 37, HL.

17 The Age of Legal Capacity (Scotland) Act 1991, s 2(4) gives statutory power, which is rather wider even than that envisaged in *Gillick*, to the mature minor under the age of 16 to consent to medical treatment. The section is, however, *enabling* in that it provides an exception to the general rule that a person under 16 has no capacity to enter into any legal transaction. For the application of the English case law to Scotland, see L Edwards 'The Right to Consent and the Right to Refuse: More Problems with Minors and Medical Consent' [1993] Juridical Rev 52.

18 [1992] Fam 11 at 24, (1991) 7 BMLR 147 at 156.

alternative? This could only have been to accede to the minor's right to refuse treatment when competent and to treat her when incompetent under the mantle of necessity. This is not only bad medicine; it also smacks of a 'cat and mouse' approach which cannot be ethically sustainable. It might have been better to confine the ratio to such narrow issues and to regard the remainder of Lord Donaldson's speech as obiter; but the Master of the Rolls, albeit with some reservations, consolidated his position in the next case – *Re W*.[19]

Re W takes us one step further down the road of consent in that it concerned a 16-year-old girl who, therefore, came within the provisions of the Family Reform Act 1969, s 8(1) which states:

> The consent of a minor who has attained the age of sixteen years to any . . . medical . . . treatment which, in the absence of consent, would constitute a trespass to the person, shall be as effective as it would be if he were of full age; and where a minor has by virtue of this section given effective consent to any treatment it shall not be necessary to obtain any consent for it from his parent or guardian . . .

W was suffering from anorexia nervosa and was refusing all treatment despite a rapid deterioration in her health. The Court of Appeal supported an order that she be treated in a specialist unit but, in essence, did so on the clinical grounds that the disease is capable of destroying the ability to make an informed choice – the wishes of the minor thus constituted something which, of themselves, required treatment. In the course of the judgments, however, several general issues were either clarified or reinforced. First, it was reiterated that the court had extensive powers in wardship and that these existed irrespective of the provisions of the Family Law Reform Act 1969, s 8(1). Moreover, Lord Donaldson held that the exercise of the court's power to make a specific issue order did not conflict with those sections of the Children Act 1989 which give a mature minor the right to refuse psychiatric or medical treatment in defined circumstances.[20] All the opinions emphasised that this attitude did not conflict with *Gillick* which was concerned with *parental* powers only. Second, the court disposed in clear terms of the relationship of consent to refusal of treatment with particular reference to the 1969 Act. Lord Donaldson said:

> No minor of whatever age has power by refusing consent to treatment to override a consent to treatment by someone who has parental responsibility for the minor and a fortiori a consent by the court.[1]

and we have Balcombe LJ:

> I am quite unable to see how, on any normal reading of the words of the section, it can be construed to confer [an absolute right to refuse medical treatment] . . . That the section did

19 *Re W (a minor)(medical treatment)* [1992] 4 All ER 627, (1992) 9 BMLR 22.
20 This has been clearly restated in *South Glamorgan County Council v B and W* [1993] 1 FLR 574, (1992) 11 BMLR 162.
1   [1992] 4 All ER 627 at 639, (1992) 9 BMLR 22 at 36.

not operate to prevent parental consent remaining effective, as well in the case of a child over 16 as in the case of a child under that age, is apparent from the words of sub-s (3).[2]

This is, of course, a legal decision and it is true, as Balcombe LJ himself said, that, in logic, there can be no difference between an ability to consent to treatment and an ability to refuse treatment. But is there not a clear practical distinction to be made? It is reasonable to suppose, paternalistic though it may sound, that a qualified doctor knows more about the treatment of disease than does a child. Thus, while consent involves acceptance of an experienced view, refusal rejects that experience – and does so from a position of limited understanding. Furthermore, a refusal of medical treatment may close down the options – and this may be regretted later in that the chance to consent has now passed. The implications of refusal may, therefore, be more serious and, on these grounds, refusal of treatment may require greater understanding than does acceptance. A level of comprehension sufficient to justify refusal of treatment certainly includes one to accept treatment but the reverse does not hold; the two conditions cannot be regarded as being on a par.[3]

What is clear from both *Re R* and *Re W* is that, rather like Lord Denning before him, Lord Donaldson was concerned to protect the medical profession from the fire of litigation – his reference to consent providing a flak-jacket for the doctor demonstrates this vividly. It is, therefore, possible to criticise the two decisions as concentrating on this aspect and taking insufficient notice of the developing autonomy of adolescence. None the less, all the speeches in both cases are at pains to emphasise the importance of respecting the minor's wishes – and of giving them increasing value with increasing maturity. What they do is to emphasise that they are not absolute; but their tenor is such as to retain the concept of the mature minor very firmly and to insist that this is breached only in exceptional circumstances. It is very unlikely that future cases will be regressive in this sense.

The Court of Appeal was not yet done for it still had to consider the adult who refuses treatment – this it did in *Re T*.[4] *Re T* appears to have been the first adult Jehovah's Witness case to have come before a British court. The case itself was fairly unexceptional. A pregnant woman was involved in a car accident and, after speaking with her mother, signed a form of refusal of blood transfusion. Following a Caesarian section and the delivery of a stillborn baby, her condition deteriorated and a court order was obtained legalising blood transfusion on the grounds that it was manifestly in her best interests; the declaration was upheld by the Court of Appeal. The fundamental decision was to the effect that an adult patient who suffers from no mental incapacity has an absolute right to consent to medical treatment, to refuse it or to choose an alternative treatment[5] – 'it exists notwithstanding that the reasons for making the choice

---

2 [1992] 4 All ER 627 at 641, (1992) 9 BMLR 22 at 37, 38. I Kennedy 'Consent to Treatment: The Capable Person' in C Dyer (ed) *Doctors, Patients and the Law* (1992) regarded Lord Donaldson's refusal in *Re R* to accept refusal and consent as twin aspects of the single right to self-determination as bordering on the perverse; this was because he had no stated support. The presence of such support in *Re W* serves to fill the lacuna.

3 This line of reasoning was adopted by the court in *Re E (a minor)* (1990) 9 BMLR 1. For a contrary clinico-legal view, see J A Devereux, D P H Jones and D I Dickenson 'Can Children Withhold Consent to Treatment?' (1993) 306 BMJ 1459.

4 *Re T (adult)(refusal of medical treatment)* [1992] 4 All ER 649, (1992) 9 BMLR 46, CA.

5 The only possible qualification mentioned by Lord Donaldson – where the choice might lead to the death of a viable fetus – has been discussed at p 138.

are rational, irrational, unknown or even non-existent'.[6] How, then, did the court arrive at its decision to support the provision of apparently involuntary treatment?

First, of course, it had to transform involuntary treatment into non-voluntary. This it did by finding that T's mental state had deteriorated to such an extent that she could not make a valid choice as between death and transfusion – and if there was doubt as to how the patient was exercising her right of self-determination, that doubt should be resolved in favour of the preservation of life.[7] But an additional factor of great importance to the doctors was added when it was stated that the effects of outside influence on a patient's refusal have to be taken into consideration: in short, the question of whether the patient means what he or she says has to be posed – and whether the decision was reached independently after counselling and persuasion or whether the patient's will was overborne is a matter to be decided by the doctors. At first glance, this looks suspiciously like opening the door to involuntary treatment – that is, until one comes to Staughton LJ who said:

> I cannot find authority that the decision of a doctor as to the existence or refusal of consent is sufficient protection, if the law subsequently decides otherwise. So the medical profession . . . must bear the responsibility unless it is possible to obtain a decision from the courts.[8]

Since this will be possible only rarely in an emergency, *Re T* seems to place a well-nigh intolerable burden on the doctors, not all of whom in the middle of the night will be of consultant status. What, for example, is the young houseman to make of Lord Donaldson:

> . . . what the doctors *cannot* do is to conclude that, if the patient still had the necessary capacity in the changed situation [he being now unable to communicate], he would have reversed his decision . . . What they *can* do is to consider whether at the time the decision was made it was intended by the patient to apply in the changed situation.[9]

One of us, at least, is grateful that he is no longer likely to be faced with an uncompleted suicide attempt in a busy casualty department! Even the law is undecided on the definition of undue influence and, again, neither Lord Donaldson[10] nor Butler-Sloss LJ[11] make it any easier by including parents and religious advisers among those whose relationship might more readily lend themselves to overbearing the patient's will than others. The law, in fact, seems to have comparatively little difficulty in discounting religious belief. T was considered to be, at best, an

---

6 [1992] 4 All ER 649 at 653, (1992) 9 BMLR 46 at 50, per Lord Donaldson MR. For a recent example in a schizophrenic patient, see *Re C (adult: refusal of medical treatment)* [1994] 1 All ER 819, (1993) 15 BMLR 77.

7 For an example of the difficulty given a patient of marginal mental capacity, see A N Wear and D Brahams 'To Treat or Not To Treat: The Legal, Ethical and Therapeutic Implications of Patient Refusal' (1991) 17 J Med Ethics 131.

8 [1992] 4 All ER 649 at 670, (1992) 9 BMLR 46 at 68.

9 (1992) 9 BMLR 46 at 60.

10 (1992) 9 BMLR 46 at 62.

11 (1992) 9 BMLR 46 at 65-66.

uncommitted Jehovah's Witness and we have Ward J in *Re E*[12] saying of a 15-year-old '*Gillick* competent' boy who was refusing blood transfusion:

> I respect this boy's profession of faith, but I cannot discount at least the possibility that he may in later years suffer some diminution in his convictions.

Yet one feels that parents ought to be able to take seriously their duty to look after not only the physical but also the spiritual well-being of their children free from the potential accusation of exercising undue influence. *Re T* is, in our opinion, the least satisfactory of this series of cases and it is to be noted that, in contrast to *Re R* and *Re W*, leave to appeal to the House of Lords was granted.

Other vulnerable groups

It is everywhere agreed that, to be valid, consent should be free, rational and unfettered; thus, prisoners constitute a further group which deserves special consideration.

The status of prisoners has been referred to briefly in chapter 1. It will be seen from this that it could be held that the incarcerated can never give a valid consent to treatment in that an element of coercion is implicit in the prison doctor/patient relationship. This proposition was considered in *Freeman*,[13] the decision in which greatly restricts this line of argument. The case turned in large measure on its own facts but the suggestion that the position of the prison psychiatrist vis-à-vis his patient voided a general consent was rejected; it was further stated that 'it was not open for it to be argued for the plaintiff that "informed consent" was a consideration which could be entertained by the courts'. While we believe that this latter opinion derived from a semantic misinterpretation of the concept which is discussed in detail below, the judgment clearly indicates that, in the absence of overt coercion, the restricted circumstances in which a prisoner's consent to treatment is given will be unlikely to affect the validity of that consent in law. An action for trespass is open to those in detention when consent to treatment has not been given[14] but mere negligence in obtaining that consent (see below) will not brand the trespass as being coercive or oppressive.

Consent to testing for HIV infection

The question of whether tests for HIV infection can be undertaken without the consent of the patient has always been controversial.[15] There may be times when a

---

12 *Re E (A minor)* (1990) 9 BMLR 1 at 8 – Ward J did say he wished to avoid notions of undue influence. Perhaps feelings are not as strong as they once were: 'of all influences religious influence is the most dangerous and powerful' – *Allcard v Skinner* (1887) 36 Ch D 145 at 183, [1886-90] All ER Rep 90 at 99-100, per Lindley LJ, referred to by Butler-Sloss LJ in *Re T (adult)(refusal of medical treatment)* [1992] 4 All ER 649 at 667, (1992) 9 BMLR 46 at 65.

13 *Freeman v Home Office (No 2)* [1984] QB 524, [1984] 1 All ER 1036.

14 *Barbara v Home Office* (1984) 134 NLJ 888.

15 See K M Boyd 'HIV Infection: The Ethics of Anonymised Testing and of Testing Pregnant Women' (1990) 16 J Med Ethics 173. The position in the United States, and elsewhere, where AIDS is a notifiable disease, may well be different and is not considered here; see D H J Hermann 'Liability Related to Diagnosis and Treatment of AIDS' (1987) 15 Law Med Hlth Care 36. For general discussion of blood testing, see A Grubb and D S Pearl *Blood Testing, AIDS and DNA Profiling: Law and Policy* (1990).

doctor would wish to carry out such tests as part of a responsible diagnostic routine but, at the same time, be reluctant to alarm or embarrass his patient by disclosing his intention. Equally, the HIV status of a patient might be an issue after a needle-stick injury or blood contamination of medical personnel; the need to know could be urgent, yet the patient might refuse to consent to testing. The legal problem is the same in each instance: does HIV testing exceed the bounds of any consent which the patient has already given to therapeutic or diagnostic investigation?

The General Medical Council has firmly rejected HIV testing in the absence of specific consent save in the 'most exceptional circumstances'.[16] The council believes that specific consent is required because of the serious social and financial consequences that may follow a positive diagnosis; each patient should have the opportunity to evaluate these consequences as they affect him personally. Non-consensual testing is permissible, in the Council's view, only where it has not been possible to obtain consent and the health of others than the patient is endangered – although the memorandum defines neither 'possible' nor 'other persons'; the Council also agrees that the best interests of a child may dictate testing even in the face of parental objection. Such advice carries great ethical weight but does not help as to the legality of such testing. Here, conflicting advice has been offered to doctors in the United Kingdom. Legal opinion sought by the Council of the British Medical Association was to the effect that, not only was non-consensual testing impermissible but also, to do so, might well constitute an assault;[17] by contrast, the Central Committee for Hospital Medical Services has been advised that the doctor may exercise his clinical judgment unless the patient asks specifically about HIV testing;[18] finally, the Medical Defence Union obtained an opinion which eliminated the possibility of assault once permission for venepuncture had been given but, nevertheless, thought that, save in exceptional circumstances – as, for instance when the expectation of a positive result was very low – specific consent for HIV should always be obtained.[19]

In seeking a way through these divergent opinions, we take the view that a patient who consults a doctor gives tacit consent to the carrying out of those diagnostic tests that the doctor considers necessary – the patient's consent to each and every test to be performed on a blood sample need not be obtained and it is unreal to speak of 'informed consent' in this context. This is not a unique view – as Dyer has reported: 'Some lawyers have suggested that patients with a "perplexing presentation" might be taken to have given an implied consent to any tests designed to find out what was wrong with them'.[20] The essential question is whether the HIV test is of such a nature as to remove it from the scope of those tests to which the patient may be said to

---

16 General Medical Council *HIV Infection and AIDS: The Ethical Considerations* (revised 1993).
17 M Sharrard and I Gatt 'Human Immunodeficiency Virus (HIV) Antibody Testing' (1987) 295 BMJ 911.
18 HMSC *Advice re HIV Testing* (1988) discussed by C Dyer 'Another Judgment on Testing for HIV Without Consent' (1988) 296 BMJ 1791.
19 Medical Defence Union *AIDS: Medico-Legal Advice* (1988). These three opinions are discussed in detail by J Keown 'The Ashes of AIDS and the Phoenix of Informed Consent' (1989) 52 MLR 790.
20 C Dyer 'Testing for HIV: The Medicolegal View' (1987) 295 BMJ 871. D Brahams 'Human Immunodeficiency Virus and the Law' [1987] 2 Lancet 227 shares our view so long as consent to test for HIV infection has not been specifically withheld.

consent implicitly – reportedly, it would not be excluded, say, in Germany.[1] It is true that HIV tests carry major emotional, financial and social significance; moreover, the disease to be diagnosed is currently untreatable – which distinguishes the test from one for, eg, syphilis. The same could, however, be said for a hypothetical test which demonstrated the presence of incurable malignant disease. It would not be necessary for the doctor to obtain specific consent to undertake such a test, yet it could have consequences similar to a test for HIV infection. The similarity is, however, not absolute – the major distinction being that, irrespective of the result, the mere fact that an HIV test has been undertaken carries serious insurance implications and has to be disclosed as a condition of most policies (see chapter 1). This certainly constitutes grounds for putting the HIV test into a separate category but it is doubtful if it is a sufficiently powerful argument to exclude absolutely all testing for which no specific consent was given. None the less, the patient could argue that, had he been informed of the doctor's intention, he would not have consented to giving the sample; in such circumstances, an action for negligence might be available under the general terms of the consent doctrine (see p 236). The critical condition here is that he was informed – insurance and comparable complicating factors do not arise if the patient is ignorant of the facts. Thus, there may be many, perhaps a majority of, cases in which non-disclosure would be good medical practice and, as Keowan has stressed, the legality of non-disclosure is then measured in *Bolam* terms – would the action be supported by a responsible body of medical opinion? (for discussion of the principle, see p 241 below). Judging by the fact that a motion in favour of non-consensual clinical testing was passed by a vote of 183-140 at the 1987 annual representative meeting of the British Medical Association,[2] this support might be available despite the fact that the council of the BMA did not support the resolution. The arguments in favour of this practice, of course, meet stiff opposition in the face of a positive result and we accept that this does raise considerable difficulty. Is it, however, sufficient to overcome the evident advantages of being able to investigate the patient without, at the same time, distressing him or her unnecessarily? One way out of the impasse might be a policy of obtaining retrospective consent and, if this is not forthcoming, of maintaining secrecy. This, of course, is, at least, ethically dubious; much would depend on whether one sees a moral distinction between deception and lying.[3] But there is not a chasm of difference between silence when one strongly suspects a diagnosis and silence when one knows the answer; such a practice, although philosophically suspect, might be seen as benign pragmatism.

All the above discussion relates to consent within the clinical setting and the patient's advantage; there can, in our opinion, be no vacillation if the advantage of testing is to another party – express consent would have to be obtained in such circumstances and action in its absence would have to be defended on the grounds of necessity or public interest. Would the public interest justify coercive routine testing of some or all health carers? There is clearly a tendency in this direction in

1 H L Karcher 'Doctors and HIV: An International Perspective. 1 – Germany' (1991) 302 BMJ 195.
2 British Medical Association 'HIV Antibody Testing: Summary of Guidance' (1987) 295 BMJ 940.
3 See the useful debate J Jackson 'Telling the Truth' (1991) 17 J Med Ethics 5, 'On the Morality of Deception – Does Method Matter?' (1993) 19 J Med Ethics 183 vs D Bakhurst 'On Lying and Deceiving' (1992) 18 J Med Ethics 63.

the United States[4] which has been resisted in the United Kingdom both by the government and by the medical profession. In practice, it would be an ineffective way of solving a problem which, as we have seen, is, to all intents, insignificant. It is more than doubtful if it would be morally defensible to spend millions of pounds of health service money[5] on exorcising such an ephemeral spectre.

The issue of contamination of the health carer has been raised by the Royal Colleges of Surgeons of England and of Edinburgh.[6] The principle of the need to obtain consent to testing before operation, even in an emergency, from a high-risk patient was emphasised but the colleges agreed to support any surgeon who undertook non-consensual testing in the interests of seriously contaminated theatre staff – serious contamination and high-risk being, again, left to the individual surgeon's interpretation. It was said that testing before the patient had recovered from the anaesthetic could count as an assault; we confess to some difficulty in accepting this – it is hard to see where would be the element of assault provided no special invasion were made for the express purpose of obtaining the blood sample. In the current climate, however, it might be hard to justify a failure to wait the few minutes needed for the patient's recovery in order to carry out a relatively lengthy test; the situation, however, seems to be one of more theoretical than practical importance.

Anonymised HIV testing, which may be of great epidemiological importance, is less controversial but still raises ethical issues.[7] Such tests involve either taking blood or saliva from random groups of patients who fall into no particular high-risk group or using blood samples that have been obtained for other purposes. The morality of random testing for a specific condition depends, to a large extent and as discussed above, on what would be done in the event of a positive result. The dilemma can be overcome by total anonymisation but this only substitutes one potential immorality by another – the knowledge obtained cannot now be used for the benefit of the individual; obtaining useful epidemiological evidence at the expense of the deliberate exclusion of any means of helping both those who are found to be infected and their contacts is a process fraught with ethical problems. In general, however, the positive advantages of investigation seem to outweigh such objections provided that those tested are informed that their blood may be subjected to anonymised testing of any sort.

Proceeding without consent – the consequences

Non-consensual medical treatment entitles the patient to sue for damages for the battery which is committed. It is also possible to base a claim on the tort of negligence, the theory being that the doctor has been negligent in failing to obtain the consent of the patient. There are important differences between the two forms

---

4   M Morris 'American Legislation on AIDS' (1991) 303 BMJ 325.
5   K Tolley and J Kennelly 'Cost of Compulsory HIV Testing' (1993) 306 BMJ 1202.
6   A Walker 'Surgeons and HIV' (1991) 302 BMJ 136.
7   See K M Boyd 'HIV Infection: The Ethics of Anonymised Testing and Testing of Pregnant Women' (1990) 16 J Med Ethics 173.

of action which have given rise to much legal debate. The issue is, however, now settled and the law is reasonably clear.

An action for battery arises when the plaintiff has been touched in some way by the defendant and when there has been no consent, express or implied, to such touching. All that the plaintiff need establish in such an action is that the defendant wrongfully touched him. It is unnecessary to establish loss as a result of the touching and, therefore, there is no problem of causation of damage to be overcome. By contrast, in an action based on the tort of negligence, the plaintiff must establish that the defendant wrongfully touched him and that the negligence of the defendant in touching him without consent has led to the injury for which damages are sought. There is thus a problem of factual causation to be tackled and, for this reason, the action for battery is an easier option from the plaintiff's point of view. The measure of damages recoverable will also be different. All direct damages are recoverable in battery; only those damages which are foreseeable may be recovered in an action for negligence. Thus an unforeseen medical complication arising from the procedure in question may be something for which damages are recoverable in battery but not in negligence. Clarification of the circumstances in which each action is available was provided by the Supreme Court of Canada in *Reibl v Hughes*[8] and in the first apposite English case of *Chatterton v Gerson.*[9]

An action for battery is appropriate where there has been no consent at all to the physical contact in question. Thus, an action for battery is the suitable remedy if a patient has refused to submit to a procedure but the doctor has, nevertheless, gone ahead in the face of that refusal. A number of Canadian cases illustrate the typical circumstances. Actions were sustained in *Mulloy v Hop Sang*,[10] where the plaintiff's hand was amputated without his consent; in *Allan v New Mount Sinai Hospital*,[11] where the plaintiff had an anaesthetic injected into his left arm in spite of his objection to this procedure; and, as a final illustration, in *Schweizer v Central Hospital*,[12] in which the surgeon performing an operation on the back of a plaintiff whose consent was related to an operation on his toe was held liable for battery. It will be seen that, in all of these cases, what the doctor actually did was quite unconnected with the procedure to which the patient had consented: there was no consent to an operation of the 'general nature' of that which was actually performed – thus, they lay within the courts' policy of restricting battery actions to acts of unambiguous hostility.

A claim based on negligence is apt when the plaintiff has given his consent to an act of the general nature of that which is performed by the defendant but there is a flaw in this consent and, as a result, there is no consent to certain concomitant features of the act of which he was unaware. The negligence lies in a failure to apprise the patient of such features as a result of which he has sustained damage; the damage is not due to negligent performance but results from a mishap which, in this instance, was a recognised potential hazard of the procedure. The distinction

8 (1980) 114 DLR (3d) 1 at 10, per Laskin CJ.
9 [1981] QB 432, [1981] 1 All ER 257. See also *Hills v Potter* [1983] 3 All ER 716, [1984] 1 WLR 641.
10 [1935] 1 WWR 714.
11 (1980) 109 DLR (3d) 634.
12 (1974) 53 DLR (3d) 494.

between the two forms of action was sharply outlined in *Reibl v Hughes* by Laskin CJC who remarked in his judgment:

> I do not understand how it can be said that the consent was vitiated by the failure of disclosure of risks as to make the surgery or other treatment an unprivileged, unconsented to and intentional invasion of the patient's bodily integrity.   I can appreciate the temptation to say that the genuineness of consent to medical treatment depends on proper disclosure of the risks which it entails, but . . . unless there has been misrepresentation or fraud to secure consent to the treatment, a failure to disclose the attendant risks, however serious, should go to negligence rather than battery.[13]

Similarly, it was emphasised in *Chatterton v Gerson* that an action for trespass to the person is inappropriate once the patient is informed in 'broad terms' of the nature of the procedure and consent is given; an action for negligence is the proper remedy if there is a failure to disclose risks.

The negligence action – causation problems

In essence, the aggrieved patient is claiming: 'You did not inform me of the risk which has eventuated; but for your failure, I would not have consented to the procedure; you have failed in your duty of care and, as a result, I have sustained injury.' The problem in negligence actions based on a lack of consent is, therefore, that of causation – the court must be satisfied that the defendant's failure to obtain the valid consent of the patient was, in fact, the cause of the patient's injury. To satisfy this requirement, the patient must prove he would not have given his consent had he had the information of which he was allegedly deprived.

There are several ways by which the strength of the plaintiff's case can be assessed. The first involves a purely subjective judgment – that is, what would that particular patient have considered to be adequate information? This is clearly open to the abuse of hindsight. It will be only too easy for a plaintiff, once he has suffered damage, to allege that he would not have given his consent when, in reality, he may well have been quite prepared to do so, even with full knowledge of the risks entailed – as a Californian court had it: 'Subjectively he may believe [he would have declined treatment] with the 20/20 vision of hindsight but we doubt that justice will be served by placing the physician in jeopardy of the patient's bitterness and disillusionment.'[14] The subjective standard is weighted overwhelmingly in favour of the plaintiff and only a few jurisdictions have accepted it.[15]

An alternative objective approach is to postulate a standard based on a reasonable patient. Would the reasonable patient have given his consent when confronted with full information of the risks and difficulties of the procedure in question? If the answer is Yes, then it may be inferred that the plaintiff himself would have

---

13 (1980) 114 DLR (3d) 1 at 10-11.

14 *Cobbs v Grant* 104 Cal Rptr 505 (1972).

15 The subjective standard was certainly used by the New Zealand Court of Appeal in *Smith* [1964] NZLR 241 SC; revsd [1965] NZLR 191 (NZCA), fn 15, p 243 below but there was no argument on the point in this very early case; a clear Antipodean preference for the subjective standard is to be found in the New South Wales Court of Appeal decision: *Ellis v Wallsend District Hospital* [1990] 2 Med LR 103.

consented. This, like all objective tests, has the disadvantage of being potentially unfair to the plaintiff. There may be specific circumstances which are unique to the individual and it may well be that he genuinely would not have consented. To apply the objective standard might, then, be equally unsatisfactory: 'if it is Utopian to think one must concentrate on the particular patient, the law should surely be aiming at Utopia.'[16] The reasonable patient test has practical value in that judges are, themselves, patients and can, therefore, assess the evidence at first hand rather than by proxy; at the same time, this introduces the element of personal prejudice and, in *Maynard v West Midlands Regional Health Authority*,[17] the trial judge was considered to have been in error in preferring one body of medical opinion to another.

A third, compromise, possibility exists. The court may opt for an objective approach but qualify it by investing the hypothetical reasonable patient with the relevant special peculiarities of the individual plaintiff. In this way the edge is taken off the objective test while the pitfalls of the purely subjective approach are avoided. This solution is increasingly favoured in the criminal law relating to the plea of provocation.

The courts in Canada vacillated between the alternatives of the objective and subjective approaches.[18] Finally, in *Reibl v Hughes*,[19] the Supreme Court came down in favour of the compromise solution. The effect of this is that the starting point is to determine the extent to which the balance of risks was, medically speaking, in favour of the treatment in question. This allows a decision to be made as to whether a reasonable patient would have consented and, that done, the court can proceed to look at the particular patient's condition. Here the judgment in *Reibl v Hughes* emphasised the importance of taking into account the patient's questions to the doctor, as these will demonstrate his concerns and will better enable the court to assess what a reasonable patient in the plaintiff 's position would have done.

The concept of informed consent

The discussion thus moves irresistibly to the issue of 'informed consent' – one which will always remain a classic example of the importation of a medical philosophy from across the Atlantic. Its progress has, in fact, been remarkably slow. Thus, while the first mention of 'informed consent' in the English courts seems to have been as late as 1981.[20] the seed was sown in America in 1957 in the case of *Salgo*.[1] Here, the court concluded that the doctor had a duty to disclose to the patient 'any facts which

16 K McK Norrie 'Informed Consent and the Duty of Care' 1985 SLT 289. Or achieving 'the ethical optimum of patient autonomy' as put by M Brazier 'Patient Autonomy and Consent to Treatment: The Role of the Law ?' (1987) 7 LS 169.
17 [1985] 1 All ER 635, [1984] 1 WLR 634, HL. A rather similar judicial foray into medical decision-making was rejected on appeal in *Gold v Haringey Health Authority* [1988] QB 481, [1987] 2 All ER 888, CA.
18 See, for example, *Male v Hopmans* (1967) 64 DLR (2d) 105; *Kelly v Hazlett* (1976) 75 DLR (3d) 536.
19 (1980) 114 DLR (3d) 1.
20 *Chatterton v Gerson* [1981] QB 432, [1981] 1 All ER 257.
1 *Salgo v Leland Stanford Junior University Board of Trustees* 317 P 2d 170 (Cal, 1957).

are necessary to form the basis of an intelligent consent by the patient to the proposed treatment'.[2] It is unfortunate that the phrase 'intelligent consent' was replaced in a later passage related to therapeutic privilege (see p 239, below):

> In discussing the element of risk, a certain amount of discretion must be employed consistent with full disclosure of facts necessary to an *informed* consent'[3] (our emphasis).

Informed consent was later made a requirement for all state-funded research work following a series of allegations that potentially dangerous experiments were being conducted without the consent of the experimental subjects.[4] Silverman maintains that there are, thus, two distinct forms of 'informed consent' and, certainly, this must be so as to the assessment of the quality of the information provided. Such a review *must* be prospective in the case of research whereas it can only be retrospective, for example by way of litigation, in respect of day to day patient management.

In either event, informed consent introduces a new element to medical treatment. It is no longer a simple matter of consent to a technical assault; consent must now be based on a knowledge of the nature, consequences and alternatives associated with the proposed therapy. Bray J's definition has gone relatively unchallenged[5] across the United States but it is still no more than a broad expression of principle. It goes no way to explaining either what counts as informed consent or how we tell that the circumstances surrounding a given event satisfy the requirements.[6] In so far as it defines a doctor's duties rather than the patient's reaction, the phrase is a misnomer[7] which, we believe, has been applied in medical writing and, indeed, in official publications with inadequate exploration of its meaning. The concept recalls the remarks of Frankfurter J, albeit in a completely different context:

> A phrase begins life as a literary expression; its felicity leads to its lazy repetition; and repetition soon establishes it as a legal formula indiscriminately used to express different and sometimes contradictory ideas.[8]

Thus, we suggest that, when Dunn LJ said in the fundamental United Kingdom case of *Sidaway*: 'The concept of informed consent forms no part of English law',[9] he may well have been referring to consent based on a subjective patient test – for no one would deny that 'information' must be nowadays be passed from doctor to patient in the United Kingdom. Yet, similar disclaimers have been repeated more

2   Per Bray J.
3   We are indebted to W A Silverman 'The Myth of Informed Consent: In Daily Practice and in Clinical Trials' (1989) 15 J Med Ethics 6 for many of the historical facts.
4   Surgeon General's Memorandum *Clinical Investigations Using Human Subjects* (1966).
5   Eg *Harnish v Children's Hospital Medical Center* 387 Mass 152 (1982) where the phrase 'intelligent decision' was used.
6   G R Gillett 'Informed Consent and Moral Integrity' (1989) 15 J Med Ethics 117.
7   T K Feng 'Failure of Medical Advice: Trespass or Negligence' (1987) 7 LS 149.
8   *Tiller v Atlantic Coast Line Railroad Co* 318 US 54 (1943) at 68.
9   *Sidaway v Board of Governors of the Bethlem Royal Hospital* [1984] QB 493 at 517, [1984] 1 All ER 1018 at 1030, CA.

recently both in England[10] and in Scotland[11] – and have been echoed in Australia[12] – and the legal definition has become no clearer. The phrase 'informed consent' is, however, now part of the lore of medical ethics; we must therefore accept it and consider the basic nature of the information that has to be given in order to validate consent to medical treatment.

What needs to be disclosed?
Looked at from the ethical point of view, the matter is one of self-determination. A person should not be exposed to a risk of damage unless he has agreed to that risk and he cannot properly agree to – or, equally importantly, make a choice between – risks in the absence of factual information. The twin problems to be resolved are, therefore, by what general standard should the information be judged and, within that, to what extent must or should particular details be divulged?

The general standards available are conveniently described as the 'patient standard' and the 'professional standard'. The former has already been described above in the wide context of consent to battery. Precisely the same principles apply to counselling. Thus, the extreme of this school of thought would hold that, given a rational patient, the doctor must reveal all the relevant facts as to what he intends to do. It is not for him to determine what the patient should or should not hear. Obviously, there must be some medical assessment of what is or is not significant but, apart from the exclusion of irrelevant material, the patient should be as fully informed as possible so that he or she can make up their minds in the light of all the relevant circumstances.

This approach most fully satisfies the requirements of self-determination but can be criticised on the grounds that it leaves little scope for the exercise of clinical judgment by the doctor. It is for this reason that even those most dedicated to patient autonomy will allow the doctor the 'therapeutic privilege' to withhold information which would merely serve to distress or confuse patient.

This concession applies only to specific items selected by the doctor for specific reasons. It does not run as far as acceptance of the alternative ethical approach to disclosure of information – that is, one based on the professional standard. Here, counselling and informing are regarded as an integral part of clinical management; the extent and detail of the information supplied is a matter for decision by the doctor who is, therein, subject to the same duty of care as when prescribing or operating. It follows that, whichever standard is adopted, litigation based on inadequate information must be taken in negligence. Any difference lies in the test to be applied. Given a patient standard, the quality of information will be judged from the viewpoint of the

10 'English law does not accept the transatlantic concept of informed consent' per Lord Donaldson in *Re T(adult)(refusal of medical treatment)* [1992] 4 All ER 649 at 663, (1992) 9 BMLR 46 at 61, CA. The use of the word 'transatlantic concept' is, itself, misleading as probably the majority of the United States still hold to the professional standard (see p 240 below).
11 '[T]he law . . . has come down firmly against the view that the doctor's duty to the patient involves at all costs obtaining the informed consent of the patient to specific medical treatments': *Moyes v Lothian Health Board* 1990 SLT 444 at 449, [1990] 1 Med LR 463 at 469, per Lord Caplan.
12 '. . . nothing is to be gained by reiterating . . . the oft-used and somewhat amorphous phrase "informed consent" ': *Rogers v Whitaker* (1992) 109 ALR 625 at 633, [1993] 4 Med LR 79 at 83 (High Court of Australia), per Mason CJ et al.

prudent – or the particular – patient; under the professional standard, it will be that of the prudent doctor.

The choice between a 'patient standard' and a 'professional standard' is a difficult one. There must be respect for the patient's legitimate interest in knowing to what he is subjecting himself but, at the same time, there will clearly be cases where a paternal approach is appropriate. In addition, the practicalities of the situation must be borne in mind. Although it might be ethically desirable for patients to be as fully informed as possible, the time spent in explaining the intricacies of procedures could be considerable, particularly if a doctor is expected to deal with remote risks. Doctors – and, particularly, doctors operating in a national health service – simply do not have the time to spend on unduly lengthy explanations of all the ramifications of treatment and many would regard the practice as unnecessarily disturbing for the patient.[13] It has also been pointed out that adherence to a professional standard provides a coherent body of principles;[14] courts that are subject to this standard are, therefore, at least less likely to be inconsistent in their judgment of disputes.

The cases
Whatever standpoint one takes on this matter, a decision of some court can be found to endorse one's preferred approach. Within the Commonwealth, there are decisions ranging from the endorsement of the deliberate medical lie to the acceptance of the extreme patient-orientated approach which emphasises complete disclosure of risk. The United States, with its 51 independent jurisdictions, provides a useful overall view. Although a majority of the states still apply a professional standard, there is a recognisable national drift towards that of the prudent patient. It is worth recapitulating the reasons given for this in a typical transfer case.[15] These included:

(a) that conditions other than those that are purely medical will influence the patient's decision;

(b) that following the whim of the physician is inconsistent with the patient's right to self-determination; and

(c) that the professional standard smacks of anachronistic paternalism.

In addition, the court specifically ruled out the criticism that the prudent patient test obliges the doctor to list every possible complication of the proposed procedure. While this appears superficially disarming, it does, in fact, serve to emphasise that

13 This, and other aspects, have been researched in Sheffield: D D Kerrigan, R S Thevasagayam, T O Woods et al 'Who's Afraid of Informed Consent?' (1993) 306 BMJ 298 and was found to be unmerited. The study, however, concerned the relatively inocuous repair of inguinal hernia – the authors concede that the results could be different in more serious circumstances. For clinical criticism of informed consent, see J S Tobias and R L Souhami 'Fully Informed Consent Can Be Needlessly Cruel' (1993) BMJ 1199.
14 C Newdick 'The Doctor's Duties of Care Under *Sidaway*' (1985) 36 NILQ 243.
15 *Largey v Rothman* 540 A 2d 504 (NJ, 1988). The prudent patient standard was set in *Canterbury v Spence* 464 F 2d 772 (DC, 1972). For retention of the professional standard, see *Wooley v Henderson* 418 A 2d 1123 (Md, 1980).

the professional is bound to be unsure of his precise position; as Brazier put it – 'the doctor is left to "second-guess" the courts'.[16]

The way ahead in the United Kingdom is, now, reasonably clear. The starting point must be found in the complementary cases of *Hunter v Hanley*[17] in Scotland and *Bolam v Friern Hospital Management Committee*[18] in England, both of which define the essence of medical negligence. Most of the discussion of informed consent has been couched in *Bolam* terms and we will, for the moment, confine ourselves to that case – always with the caveat that we are following the loose thinking which surrounds that concept; for, as the High Court of Australia has pointed out,[19] consent is relevant to actions framed in trespass or battery, not in negligence which is simply a matter of standards of care. For present purposes, the essential part of the *Bolam* dictum runs: 'a doctor is not negligent if he acts in accordance with a practice accepted at the time as proper by a responsible body of medical opinion.'[20] Since it is agreed that actions based on lack of consent to medical treatment should be taken in negligence, it follows that any argument as to what needs to be disclosed in British medical practice hinges upon whether or not the *Bolam* principle applies equally to both diagnosis and treatment and to the giving of information.

That it did so was upheld both in *Chatterton v Gerson*[1] and in *Hills v Potter.*[2] The acid test, however, came in the seminal case of *Sidaway,*[3] where the proposition was accepted in the court of first instance but was received rather less enthusiastically in the Court of Appeal; there, Sir John Donaldson MR did not regard it as self-evident that the standards applied to diagnosis and treatment should be the same as those applied to disclosure. Concern was expressed that the definition of the duty of care was a matter for the law which 'could not stand by if the profession, by an excess of paternalism, denied their patients a real choice'.[4] The Master of the Rolls's reasons for isolating the advisory duty in this way have been questioned[5] and his colleagues were unable to follow him all the way. Browne-Wilkinson LJ, however, also believed that there was a prima facie duty on the doctor to inform the patient – the assumption of the role of adviser carried with it the duty to disclose material and unusual risks.

The House of Lords, while maintaining a professional standard of disclosure, was, similarly, prepared to modify the existing law in certain respects. Thus, Lord Bridge held:

16 M Brazier 'Patient Autonomy and Consent to Treatment: The Role of the Law?' (1987) 7 LS 169.
17 1955 SC 200, 1955 SLT 213.
18 [1957] 2 All ER 118, [1957] 1 WLR 582.
19 In *Rogers v Whitaker* (1992) 109 ALR 625 at 633, [1993] 4 Med LR 79 at 83.
20 Per McNair J [1957] 2 All ER 118 at 122.
 1 [1981] QB 432, [1981] 1 All ER 257.
 2 [1983] 3 All ER 716, [1984] 1 WLR 641.
 3 *Sidaway v Board of Governors of the Bethlem Royal Hospital* [1984] QB 493 at 517, [1984] 1 All ER 1018 at 1030, CA; [1985] AC 871, [1985] 1 All ER 643, HL.
 4 [1984] QB 493 at 513, [1984] 1 All ER 1018 at 1028, CA.
 5 See, for example, K McK Norrie 'Standards of Disclosure' 1984 SLT 237; I Kennedy 'The Patient on the Clapham Omnibus' (1984) 47 MLR 454.

A judge might, in certain circumstances, come to the conclusion that the disclosure of a particular risk was so obviously necessary to an informed choice on the part of the patient that no reasonably prudent medical man would fail to make it . . .[6]

while Lord Templeman considered that:

. . . the court must decide whether the information afforded to the patient was sufficient to alert the patient to the possibility of serious harm of the kind in fact suffered.[7]

Lord Scarman, however, delivered what was, effectively, a dissenting judgment in which he indicated that: 'it was a strange conclusion if our courts should be led to conclude that our law . . . should permit doctors to determine in what circumstances . . . a duty arose to warn.' He found great merit in the American case of *Canterbury v Spence*[8] in which it was held that, while medical evidence on this matter was not excluded, it was the court which determined the extent of, and any breach of, the doctor's duty to inform. Information includes warning. King CJ, for example, specifically instructed that the doctor's duty extends not only to disclose any real risks in the treatment but also to warn of any real risk that the treatment may prove ineffective.[9]

Two specific aspects of the information issue are confirmed as a result of *Sidaway*. The first is that material risks of a procedure must be disclosed, subject only to therapeutic privilege which a doctor might be required to justify. Following *Canterbury*, a risk can be defined as material if a reasonable person in the patient's position, if warned of the risk, would be likely to attach significance to it. Similarly, it is material if the medical practitioner is, or should reasonably be, aware that the particular patient, if warned of the risk, would be likely to attach significance to it.[10] Quite what that means in relation to chance is impossible to assess and, indeed, generalisations may be inappropriate as the test relates to the circumstances of the particular case. Moreover, significance in this field is a function not only of incidence but also of severity; thus, in *Hopp v Lepp*,[11] it was stated that a risk, even if it is a mere possibility, should be regarded as material if its occurrence causes serious consequences. As to incidence, it was agreed in *Sidaway* that a risk of 10% of a stroke resulting – as was established in *Reibl v Hughes*[12] – was one which a doctor could hardly fail to appreciate as necessitating a warning; but non-disclosure was considered proper in Mrs Sidaway's case when the risk of damage to the spinal cord

---

6 [1985] AC 871 at 900, [1985] 1 All ER 643 at 663, HL.
7 [1985] AC 871 at 903, [1985] 1 All ER 643 at 665.
8 464 F 2d 772 (DC, 1972).
9 *F v R* (1983) 33 SASR 189, SC. Alternative treatments should also be canvassed – particularly if there is a choice between medical and surgical procedures: *Haughian v Paine* (1987) 37 DLR (4th) 624, cited in (1987) 137 NLJ 557.
10 Mason CJ et al in *Rogers v Whitaker* (1992) 109 ALR 625 at 634, [1993] 4 Med LR 79 at 83 (High Court of Australia).
11 (1979) 98 DLR (3d) 464. But in the Australian case *Battersby v Tottman and State of South Australia* (1985) 37 SASR 524, the risk of blindness was considered a subject for obligatory disclosure only in a minority opinion – this may, however, have been because there was a strong possibility of suicide.
12 (1980) 114 DLR (3d) 1.

was of the order of 1% or less. We have to admit to some concern that odds shorter than 100-1 might be regarded as immaterial in the eyes of the law.[13] A great deal will, however, hang on the *patient's* requirements as expressed by way of questioning and we return to this below.

Secondly, *Sidaway* confirmed the 'therapeutic' or professional privilege to withhold information that might be psychologically damaging to the patient. This, again, follows the direction in *Bolam* in which the judge said in his charge to the jury:

> You may well think that when a doctor is dealing with a mentally sick man and has a strong belief that his only hope of cure is submission to electroconvulsive therapy, the doctor cannot be criticised if he does not stress the dangers, which he believed to be minimal, which are involved in the treatment . . . [14]

This principle has been widely adopted and was succinctly described in the influential case of *Smith v Auckland Hospital Board*:[15]

> As it seems to me, the paramount consideration is the welfare of the patient and, given good faith on the part of the doctor, I think the exercise of his discretion in the area of advice must depend upon the patient's overall needs. To be taken into account should be the gravity of the condition to be treated, the importance of the benefits to be expected to flow from the treatment or procedure, the need to encourage him to accept it, the relative significance of its inherent risks, the intellectual and emotional capacity of the patient to accept the information without such distortion as to prevent any rational decision at all, and the extent to which the patient may seem to have placed himself in his doctor's hands with the invitation that the latter accept on his behalf the responsibility for intricate or technical decisions.[16]

It is also clear from *Sidaway* that, by way of exception to this rule, there must be particularly good reasons, which the doctor would have to justify, for failing to answer such questions as the patient puts and that there may, indeed, be a strict obligation to do so. Thus, Lord Bridge held, albeit obiter, that:

> When questioned specifically by a patient of apparently sound mind about risks involved in a particular treatment proposed, a doctor's duty must, in my opinion, be to answer both truthfully and as fully as the questioner requires.[17]

The fact that the patient asked questions revealing concern about the risk would make the doctor aware that this patient did, in fact, attach significance to the risk'[18] – and, hence, affect its materiality; it was certainly this fact which served to turn a 1:14,000

---

13 King JC accepted 200:1 as not being material in *F v R* (1983) 33 SASR 189, SC.
14 [1957] 1 WLR 582 at 590, [1957] 2 All ER 118 at 124, per McNair J.
15 [1964] NZLR 241 SC; revsd [1965] NZLR 191 (NZCA).
16 [1964] NZLR 241 at 250, per Woodhouse J.
17 *Sidaway v Board of Governors of the Bethlem Royal Hospital* [1985] AC 871 at 898, [1985] 1 All ER 643 at 661, HL.
18 Mason CJ et al in *Rogers v Whitaker* (1992) 109 ALR 625 at 631, [1993] 4 Med LR 79 at 82 (High Court of Australia).

chance of blindness into a risk which it was found negligent not to disclose in *Rogers v Whittaker.*

This inference was, however, disturbed in England in *Blyth v Bloomsbury Health Authority.*[19] Here, the trial judge's decision in favour of the plaintiff was reversed on appeal. He was found to be in error in holding that there was an obligation, when asked, to pass on *all* the information available to the hospital; the question of what a patient should be told in response to a general enquiry could not be detached from the *Bolam* test any more than when no such enquiry was made (per Kerr LJ). Kerr LJ went on to say:

> I am not convinced [from *Sidaway*] that the *Bolam* test is irrelevant even in relation to the question of what answers are properly to be given to specific enquiries or that Lords Diplock and Bridge intended to hold otherwise.[20]

The argument in *Blyth* centred largely on some rather obscure therapeutic notes written in the hospital and it is difficult to see from this how widely the opinion would be applied.

The House of Lords' approach in *Sidaway* has been subject to academic criticism,[1] largely because of the uncertainties it left behind. A strong impression remains that the House was not entirely at ease with *Bolam* – only Lord Diplock was prepared to carry it to its conclusion. Yet ranks are closed whenever the principle is directly questioned. Thus, in *Gold*,[2] Schiemann J at first instance attempted to distinguish counselling from treatment and was firmly overruled by the Court of Appeal;[3] elsewhere, it has been held that the court can only reject an expert opinion if it was one that no responsible expert in a comparable position could reasonably hold.[4] This attitude is beginning to take on an atmosphere of stubbornness and is becoming almost unique in face of the now universal acceptance of a patient's right to decide on his or her own treatment. The writing was already on the wall in Canada where, in *Reibl*, it was held:[5]

> [The] scope of the duty of disclosure . . . is not a question that is to be concluded on the basis of the expert medical evidence alone . . . What is under consideration here is the patient's right to know what risks are involved in undergoing or forgoing certain surgery or other treatment.

19 (1985) Times, 24 May, QBD; [1993] 4 Med LR 151, (1987) Times, 11 February, CA. *Blyth* reminds us that the principles derived from surgical cases can apply equally to medication – implied consent to taking a drug cannot be assumed: *Crichton v Hastings* (1972) 29 DLR (3d) 692.
20 [1993] 4 Med LR 151 at 157, Neill LJ concurring at 160.
 1 For full discussion see I Kennedy and A Grubb *Medical Law: Text with Materials* (2nd edn, 1994) pp 184 et seq.
 2 *Gold v Haringey Health Authority* [1988] QB 481, [1987] 2 All ER 888, CA.
 3 The integral nature of medical attendance has been emphasised in other contexts – eg in the management of the mentally incompetent – *Re H (Mental patient)(Diagnosis)* [1993] 1 FLR 28, [1993] 4 Med LR 91.
 4 *Bolitho v City and Hackney Health Authority* (1992) 13 BMLR 111 per Dillon LJ at 132.
 5 (1980) 114 DLR (3d) at 13.

and, in 1983, it was said of warning of therapeutic failure in the Supreme Court of South Australia:

> The ultimate question . . . is . . . whether the defendant's conduct . . . conforms to the standard of reasonable care demanded by the law. That is a question for the court and the duty of deciding it cannot be delegated to any profession or group in the community.[6]

The strongest attack on *Bolam* to date has, however, come from the High Court of Australia where its application to counselling has been firmly rejected in *Rogers v Whitaker*. In that case, we have the majority opinion saying:

> There is a fundamental difference between, on the one hand, diagnosis and treatment and, on the other hand, the provision of advice or information to the patient . . . Because the choice to be made calls for a decision by the patient on information known to the medical practitioner but not to the patient, it would be illogical to hold that the amount of information to be provided by the medical practitioner can be determined from the perspective of the practitioner alone or, for that matter, of the medical profession.[7]

and even more trenchantly, Gaudron J:[8]

> [E]ven in the area of diagnosis and treatment, there is, in my view, no legal basis for limiting liability in terms of the rule known as "the *Bolam* test" . . . [It] may be a convenient statement of the approach dictated by the state of the evidence in some cases. As such, it may have some utility as a rule-of-thumb in some jury cases, but it can serve no other useful function'.

Habits die hard, however, in the United Kingdom and the position in Scotland which was awaited with some interest, has been resolved in a way that leaves little room for doubt.[9] Lord Caplan had this to say:[10]

> In my view . . . the appropriate tests to apply in medical negligence cases are to be found in *Hunter v Hanley* and *Bolam* . . . As I see it, the law in both Scotland and England has come down firmly against the view that the doctor's duty to the patient involves at all costs obtaining the informed consent of the patient to specific medical treatments . . . I can read nothing in the majority view in *Sidaway* which suggests that the extent and quality of warning to be given by a doctor to his patient should not in the last resort be governed by medical criteria.

---

6 *F v R* (1983) 33 SASR 189, SC, per King CJ.
7 (1992) 109 ALR 625 at 632. For a full discussion of the case, see D Chalmers and R Schwartz 'Rogers v Whitaker and Informed Consent in Australia: A Fair Dinkum Duty of Disclosure' (1993) 1 Med L Rev 139; R C Pincus 'Has Informed Consent Finally Arrived in Australia?' (1993) 159 Med J Austral 25; and B McSherry 'Failing to Advise and Warn of Inherent Risks in Medical Treatment: When Does Negligence Occur?' (1993) 1 J Law Med 5.
8 (1992) 109 ALR 625 at 635-636, [1993] 4 Med LR 79 at 84.
9 *Moyes v Lothian Health Board* 1990 SLT 444, [1990] 1 Med LR 463. Two further Scottish cases are known to have failed but are very poorly reported: *Comber v Greater Glasgow Health Board* 1992 SLT 22; *Hsuing v Webster* 1992 SLT 1071. They are reported as news items in (1991) Scotsman, 24 April, p 4.
10 1990 SLT 444 at 449, [1990] 1 Med LR 463 at 468.

It is to be noted that there is a subtle difference between *Bolam* and *Hunter*. The former speaks of a '. . . responsible body of medical opinion'. By contrast, Lord President Clyde gave his third criterion defining medical negligence as a practice which would be adopted 'by no professional man of ordinary skill acting with ordinary care'. McNair J suggested in *Bolam* that any difference was just a question of expression;[11] we, however, support the view that *Hunter* erects an even more formidable hurdle for the pursuer in Scotland than confronts the plaintiff in England.

The consent doctrine in the future

The progress of the consent doctrine in the United States has been steadily in the direction of patient autonomy and has shown signs of overreaction leading, in some instances, to the undue encouragement of malpractice litigation.[12] It has undoubtedly resulted in greater sensitivity on the part of the American medical profession to the need to inform patients of the implications of treatment but this positive result has only been achieved at the price of heightened distrust and an increase in the practice of legalistic and defensive medicine.

There is also no doubt that such fears have had their influence on the British courts – Dunn LJ, for example, considered that the acceptance of 'informed consent' would be damaging to the relationship of trust and confidence between doctor and patient and might have an adverse effect on the practice of medicine.[13] Two judges in the House of Lords in Sidaway admitted their reliance on an article by Robertson[14] in which an American opinion was quoted:

> The requirement of informed consent to medical treatment has, for at least the past two decades, been used as a cloth from which courts slowly have begun to fashion a no-fault system for compensating persons who have suffered bad results from medical treatment.[15]

Robertson himself concluded that 'it is judicial policy, rather than the importance of the patient's rights, which will dictate the future development of the doctrine in the United Kingdom'.

We would hope that this cynical analysis is not entirely true although it is certain that the retention of *Bolam* makes it very likely that the consent-based action will be less widely used in British courts than in those of the United States. Within the United Kingdom, the causation issues are so stacked against the plaintiff in Scotland that, apart from extreme malpractice in *Hunter* terms, success is very improbable.[16] In the most comprehensive study of the consent issue in the United Kingdom currently available, McLean predicts that a 'prudent patient' test will never be

---

11 *Bolam v Friern Hospital Management Committee* [1957] 2 All ER 118 at 122.
12 In *Truman v Thomas* 611 P 2d 902 (Cal, 1980) a doctor was, effectively, held liable for failing to convince a reluctant patient of the importance of a screening test for cancer.
13 *Sidaway v Board of Governors of the Bethlem Royal Hospital* [1984] QB 493 at 517, [1984] 1 All ER 1018 at 1030, CA.
14 G Robertson 'Informed Consent to Medical Treatment' (1981) 97 LQR 102.
15 A Meisel 'The Expansion of Liability for Medical Accidents: From Negligence to Strict Liability by Way of Informed Consent' (1977) 56 Neb L Rev 51.
16 See an anonymous article 'Medical Negligence: *Hunter v Hanley* 35 Years On' 1990 SLT 325.

developed here.[17] Successful negligence actions based on flawed consent are virtually non-existent in the United Kingdom and it is idiosyncratic that the only one we have been able to trace comes from Scotland.[18] Even so, the case was unusual in that damages were awarded on the grounds that the pursuer sustained extra stress and anxiety when the complication, knowledge of which would not have deterred him from treatment, actually arose.

The professional standard is here in Britain for the foreseeable future but not all judges are as sympathetic to the medical profession as was Lord Denning and there is evidence of its incremental erosion in favour of the rights of the patient. The opinion of the Master of the Rolls in the appeal stage of *Sidaway* was, for example, scarcely distinguishable from that expressed in the break-away case of *Reibl*. Difficult as it may be, there is a need for clearer guidance as to the meaning of such words as 'material', 'substantial', 'reasonable' and the like. In *Eyre v Measday*,[19] for example, the patient lost her action largely on the grounds that, if you want to know something, the answer to which would be patently obvious to a reasonable patient, you should ask about it. On the face of it, that would seem to be something of a circular argument; it is asking a lot of someone who is so unreasonable as to fail to see the obvious, to be so reasonable as to perceive the need to ask about it.

A start might well be made by dropping the phrase 'informed consent' in favour of 'rational consent' – or, perhaps better, using the word 'understanding', for a competent adult has every right to make a decision which may appear irrational to others. Both are terms which pay due deference to patient autonomy and, at the same time, provide the doctor with a yardstick as to what is expected of him.[20] There is little doubt that a spirit of confrontation between the medical profession and the public is emerging; it is essential that this be halted and abandoned in favour of the concept of a therapeutic alliance.[1] Diana Brahams[2] perhaps expresses the issue best when she says —

it is up to us to persuade doctors to alter their practice so as to divulge more information routinely and bring their standards up to what a prudent patient would like to know – without intervention of law.

There are, indeed, signs that this is happening. The good doctor is becoming increasingly aware of his patients' aspirations and clinicians are involving their patients more in decision making. The prudent patient and the prudent doctor standards are approximating de facto even if not de jure and, if the professional standard of disclosure supports full disclosure, there should be no gap between what *is* revealed and what *should be* revealed to the patient whichever test is applied. At the end of the day, this may prove to be the better route to follow rather than one suggesting an adversarial relationship.

17 S A M McLean *A Patient's Right to Know* (1989) at p 85.
18 *Goorkani v Tayside Health Board* 1991 SLT 94, [1992] 3 Med LR 33.
19 [1986] 1 All ER 488.
20 The use of other ill-defined terms such as 'effective consent' (Human Fertilisation and Embryology Act 1990, Sch 3) do little more than compound the difficulties.
1 H Teff 'Consent in Medical Procedures: Paternalism, Self-determination or Therapeutic Alliance?' (1985) 101 LQR 432.
2 D Brahams '"Informed Consent" – the Thin End of the Wedge' (1985) 135 NLJ 201.

11 Health resources and dilemmas in treatment

No resources are infinite. Even if a basic material is widely available, the costs of harvesting, treating or assembling it put some restraint on its use; moreover, the manpower required for distribution and exploitation of the finished product is always going to be limited. Applying this to medicine, it is clear that it is well-nigh impossible to provide every form of therapy for everyone – some sort of selective distribution is inevitable.

The logistics of medicine get no easier despite – or, possibly, because of – the massive technological advances of the last half century. Costs of all types are rising, while the world faces persistent economic difficulties. The average span of life is increasing – at least in the developed countries – and, as a result, people need treatment for longer. This treatment is not the 'easy-cure' type appropriate to infectious diseases but is rather a matter of sophisticated care for the results of degenerative change. In addition, the public are better informed on medical matters and are better able to assimilate the information they are given. The choice of treatment is increasingly influenced by the patient's demands with proportionate erosion of the doctor's discretion – in effect, while the latter may wish to treat on a productivity basis, the former views therapy in terms of feasibility.

Somehow, a compromise must be achieved between demand and supply and, although there is little law established on the subject, the distribution of scarce resources poses some of the more complex ethical problems of modern medicine and permeates every aspect of its structure. They are not confined to the higher administrative echelons nor to the more esoteric departments of major hospitals. They may, indeed, arise and be answered subconsciously – every time a doctor travels to visit a patient he is distributing his resources in favour of one priority and this is possibly at the expense of others with which he could have dealt during his non-productive driving time.[1]

Such an example relates to the treatment of individuals. But the ethics of health service distribution can also be considered on a global scale; the problems arising on a national level occupy an intermediate position. We propose examining these as three separate issues.

Global distribution of resources

It is beyond question that the world's medical resources are distributed unevenly, both in material and in human terms. The money to buy the expensive paraphernalia

---

1 This aspect is amplified in R Klein 'Dimensions of Rationing: Who Should Do What?' (1993) 307 BMJ 309.

associated with modern hospital medicine is simply not available in the developing countries; at the same time, there are inadequate facilities for the local training of doctors who must, therefore, travel to obtain experience. The result is a vicious circle in which doctors accustomed to the sophisticated methods of the developed nations return to their own countries only to depart again dissatisfied with what they have found. The response of the richer states is often to attempt to fill the vacuum by supplying the highly complex diagnostic and therapeutic apparatus which characterises modern medicine. But does such well-intentioned aid represent either good medical morals or good medical politics? Morals and politics may, indeed, be synonymous because decisions on priorities of allocation can be translated as 'politics', 'management' or 'clinical judgment', depending on whether one is speaking in terms of international, national or individual needs.

Criticism of this type is not new, nor is it confined to those with a special interest in medical jurisprudence. It has long been realised that it is absurd to spend much effort in eradicating disease in the underdeveloped areas only to allow the population to die of starvation because the necessary farming technology was not supplied at the same time. But the nature of medical aid to the developing countries cannot avoid being politically influenced and is certainly a matter beyond the control of the average doctor or lawyer.[2]

The allocation of national resources

We come closer to personal reality when discussing resource allocation on a national scale and, here, a mass of relevant literature has built up in recent years – much of which admits the near impossibility of a wholly just solution.

The primary problem, which is essentially political, is to establish what share of the national resources is to be allocated to health – and it is the open-endedness of claims to health care that leads to particular difficulties. As David Owen said many years ago:

> All the evidence there is, both national and international, suggests that if [the] need [for health care] is not infinite, it is certainly so large relative to the resources which society is able to provide now and in the foreseeable future that we can never hope to meet it completely.[3]

Ideally, resource allocation should provide equal access to health care for those in equal need. Attempts have been made in recent years to achieve this by systematically correlating the revenue given to the regional health authorities with their needs. These needs were originally based by the Resource Allocation Working Party on the standardised mortality rates which were taken as representing the underlying

2 For a philosophical approach, see R Attfield 'The Global Distribution of Health Care Resources' (1990) 16 J Med Ethics 153. Attitudes are, in fact, changing and far more effort is bing put into resources at the level of primary and paramedical care.
3 D Owen *In Sickness and in Health: The Politics of Medicine* (1976) quoted by D Black 'Paying for Health' (1991) 17 J Med Ethics 117.

morbidity. This, in itself, is open to criticism as it reflects the needs at hospital level rather than those of the provision of primary care which is particularly affected by external factors such as the degree of social deprivation. Nevertheless, RAWP, as the process came to be known, appeared to provide an objective, albeit rough, formula which could be readily understood ; inevitably, it was subject to criticism and the major discrepancies were ironed out slowly.[4] A new formula was introduced in 1991 which weights the age adjusted population of each region by the square root of its standardised mortality rate for those under 75 years old;[5] this was based on empirical findings. One effect is, as pointed out by Sheldon, to open the doors to differential interpretation at sub-regional level and to political lobbying by health authorities who can gain from some of the many variables which can, legitimately, be fed into the resultant equation. Moreover, by their nature, empirical data are unlikely to be fully contemporary. Some explicit measure of macroallocation of national resources is clearly needed – it has been suggested that one result of its use is that vote maximising policies become more obvious and are, thus, more difficult to carry out.[6] Even so, it may well be that it is better left at a relatively unsophisticated level and that further research is directed to how the allocations, once made, are actually used.

When allocation is considered at sub-regional level, equity becomes a less significant factor and gives way to the dictates of demand. This inevitably involves a choice and this choice must be, to some extent, arbitrary. The ethical control of resources then depends, first, upon the broad base of representation on the allocation committee and, second, on the willingness of the constituent members not to press their own interests too hard – a process which has been described, and, to an extent, approbated, as shroud waving;[7] the lay influence of community health councils is important at this point.

In any event, a change in circumstances has been dictated by the passage of the National Health Service and Community Care Act 1990. This establishes the district health authorities as purchasers of health services on behalf of the local population. In this role they must act as good housekeepers and not only provide what the people want but also do this in the most cost-effective manner. The choices can never be easy – is it possible to decide the relative importance between, say, strict economy, the avoidance of suffering or the prolongation of life? And how is one to identify the best route to the intended goal? If, for example, morbidity as a whole is taken as the yardstick, the alleviation of bronchitis and asthma has been found to take precedence; if, on the other hand, one considers total hospital in-patient days, mental health may be the single most important consideration. But to say that mental health and

---

4   N Mays 'Measuring Morbidity for Resource Allocation' (1987) 295 BMJ 703; G Bevan and J Charlton 'Making Access to Health Care More Equal: The Role of General Medical Services' (1987) 295 BMJ 764; J Smith 'RAWP Revisited' (1987) 295 BMJ 1015.

5   Department of Health *Funding and Contracts for Health Services, Working Paper 2* (1989). For discussion, see T A Sheldon, G D Smith and G Bevan 'Weighting in the Dark: Resource Allocation in the New NHS' (1993) 306 BMJ 835 – particularly for the mathematical analysis which is beyond the ambit of this book.

6   See, eg, A Maynard and A Ludbrook 'Applying Resource Allocation Formulae to Constituent Parts of the UK' (1980) 1 Lancet 85.

7   J Rawles 'Castigating QALYs' (1989) 15 J Med Ethics 143.

respiratory disease constitute the most serious burdens on the health service is not necessarily to say that they merit the greatest allocation of resources. There is a strong economic incentive to apply some sort of 'productivity test' in distributing the resources of society; the question is – is it ethical to do so? Analysis of the problem raises some stark and disturbing answers. Thus, it has been said that to reject opportunities to allow natural dying is costly in financial terms – in a health care service with finite resources, it is neither harsh nor unethical to accept the consequences of a financial limit.[8] And the same article expresses the grim reality of political power in the suggestion that to spend a lot on the elderly might not be supported by public opinion if it became known that younger lives were being lost because of inadequate finance.

This immediately draws attention to the major difficulty encountered in any such evaluation based on public opinion – which is that the welfare of the unproductive is likely to be regarded as secondary to that of the productive unless the views of voluntary organisations with specific interests are given particular consideration. The mentally handicapped and the elderly are, in fact, in double jeopardy – not only may they be seen as less deserving of resources but they are less likely to be invited to subscribe to the opinion-making process. Geriatric patients, it is said, would not and should not expect priority over younger patients – which is true enough – but they *would* expect equal consideration. Harris's argument,[9] which sees the saving of life as the main medical objective, is at its strongest when we are considering the use of life years as a parameter for the assessment of the disposal of scarce resources. The choice between a 20-year-old and an 80-year-old may be straightforward to the outsider. But, at the moment of decision, each patient values his or her life equally – and the problem, then, is how to measure that equality. A productivity test, for example, demands that treatment should be both beneficial *and* effective, whereas an evaluation on the basis of social good may conclude that benefit alone is sufficient to justify the resultant costs to the community.[10]

It is inevitable that, so long as there is a restriction on resources – and there must be a limit even in Utopia – some principle of maximum societal benefit must be applied; the individual's right to equality must, to some extent, be sacrificed to the general need. The precise determination of a maximum benefit policy is difficult to make but the decision is societal rather than medical and involves a 'cost-benefit' analysis and all that that entails as to the quality of life.[11] The difficulties are formidable because what we are discussing at this level is essentially 'horizontal resource allocation', or priority setting between different types of service, which

8 G S Robertson 'Dealing with the Brain-damaged Old – Dignity Before Sanctity' (1982) 8 J Med Ethics 173.
9 J Harris 'Unprincipled QALYs' (1991) 17 J Med Ethics 185.
10 M A Somerville ' "Shall the Grandparents Die?": Allocation of Medical Resources with an Ageing Population' (1986) 14 Law Med Hlth Care 158.
11 A particularly poignant example is to be found in the salvage of extremely premature infants. The cost of intensive care has been put at £20,000 for each baby weighing less than 1.5kg and some 50% of these may sustain brain damage sufficient to require life-long support. Would the money be better spent on research into the prevention of prematurity? Office of Health Economics *Born Too Soon* (1992). See L Hunt 'Cost "Dilemma" Posed by Premature Babies' (1993) Independent, 20 January, p 6.

depends not so much on professional medical assessment and advice as on public opinion and on evidence as to cost and effectiveness[12] – and the former, at least, is a fickle measuring instrument. Not only can polls be grossly distorted by the way in which questions are put, but also opinion is very subject to political and other extraneous influences; you do not sell newspapers by agreeing that treatment for varicose veins has a low priority – sales are improved by emphasising the injustice in regarding varicose ulceration as less debilitating than the peptic variety. Attempts made thus far to translate societal attitudes into standardised decision-making[13] seem to achieve less than satisfactory results. The essential dilemma stems from the fact that the categories of choice on which a consensus may be sought are indefinable.[14] The new emphasis on explicitness in rationing strategies is an important development and may lead to surprising results. Preliminary research in Norway, for example, indicates that the public's main concern may well be for equality of access to treatment with comparatively little regard for the final health gain; resource allocators, it has been said, should not take it for granted that their own values are shared by the general public.[15]

Given the absence of any obvious set of principles on which to act and given that the function of district health authorities is, on the one hand, constrained by the regional or higher authority[16] and, on the other, is to provide what the public want, it is unsurprising that the distribution of the scarcer resources is uneven and that the principles invoked in decision-making are uncertain – the factors given most weight have been found to range from the availability of other funding (eg the private sphere) for the service to the more obviously laudable potential for health gain in terms of length and quality of life.[17] In his survey of six districts, Ham found that there was a general reluctance to exclude some services entirely from their contracts. But it is from a review of a service which was *not* provided by some authorities – in this case, in vitro fertilisation – that some of the clearest evidence of the factors likely to be considered influential is to be found. These included:

(a) the presence of a prominent lobbyist for the service and the ready availability of the service;

(b) whether or not a competent public health department could be used to interpret the effectiveness of and need for the service;

(c) whether it represented a true health need;

(d) having decided that there was a need, whether the particular service offered the best way of meeting that need;

12 M Cochrane, C Ham, C Heginbotham and R Smith 'Rationing: At the Cutting Edge' (1991) 303 BMJ 1039.
13 P A Lewis and M Charny 'Which of Two Individuals Do You Treat When Only Their Ages Are Different and You Can't Treat Both?' (1989) 15 J Med Ethics 28.
14 See reply to footnote 13: D Lamb 'Priorities in Health Care' (1989) 15 J Med Ethics 33; also B A Stoll 'Choosing Between Cancer Patients' (1990) 16 J Med Ethics 71.
15 E Nord 'The Relevance of Health State after Treatment in Prioritising between Different Patients' (1993) 19 J Med Ethics 37. Norway is, of course, a fiercely egalitarian society but the same response might well be found in any country having an entrenched national health service.
16 See R Klein 'Dimensions of Rationing: Who Should Do What?' (1993) 307 BMJ 309.
17 See the analysis provided by C Ham 'Prority Setting in the NHS:Reports from Six Districts' (1993) 307 BMJ 435.

(e) notwithstanding the effectiveness of the service, whether it should be purchased at the expense of another unrelated service;

(f) whether valid reasons could be given for selective treatment when supply fell short of demand; and

(g) whether it was right to introduce a service which could not be given to everyone.[18]

Despite the obvious difficulties, we see it as self-evident that some form of cost evaluation in health care is essential at the resource purchasing level, if only to ensure impartiality – pressure groups are bad advocates in that they take no account of the deprivation elsewhere which is the concomitant to success in their own particular sphere. District health authorities are at an early stage in developing priority setting and, as Ham put it, the important practical feature is to concentrate on study as to the appropriateness of the use of services and as to the setting in which they are to be used. We agree with those who believe that the ethical problem does not lie in the application of economics to health resource allocation. It should, rather, be accepted that without such control there is likely to be an unethical maldistribution of resources; as Williams put it, anyone who says no account should be paid to costs is, in reality, saying no account should be paid to the sacrifices thereby imposed on others – and there are no *ethical* grounds for ignoring the effect of an action on other people.[19] Surely, everyone would agree with this – but it still leaves open the question of in which group's favour is a marginal change in resource allocation to be tilted.

Finally, it must, of course, be conceded that societies differ and, while some form of resource rationing is, as we have said, inevitable, no single system will be universally acceptable. Britain has been described as an original sin society[20] in which tribulation in the form of ill-health is expected – a statement which, incidentally, we take leave to doubt the truth of ten years after it was made. The United States, on the other hand, are seen as a society striving for perfectibility of man and dominated by consumerism; the demand for and the use of medical resources are bound to differ widely. That being so, it is, perhaps, anomalous that the one experiment in health care rationing that has come into force as a result of statute should have its origins in the United States.[1] The State of Oregon has, as a result of research including extensive public debate, arrived at an adaptable prioritised list of treatments which will and will not be available under Medicaid and business related

18 S Redmayne and R Klein 'Rationing in Practice: The Case of In Vitro Fertilisation' (1993) 306 BMJ 1521. The issue of in vitro fertilisation is also taken up by The Lancet 'Rationing Infertility Services' (1993) 342 Lancet 251.
19 A Williams 'Cost-effectiveness Analysis: Is It Ethical?' (1992) 18 J Med Ethics 7. See also G Mooney 'QALYs: Are They Enough? A Health Economist's Perspective' (1989) 15 J Med Ethics 148.
20 R Klein 'Rationing Health Care' (1984) 289 BMJ 143. For an updated comparative review, see R G Lee and F H Miller 'The Doctor's Changing Role in Allocating U.S. and British Medical Services' (1990) 18 Law Med Hlth Care 69.
 1 M J Garland 'Justice, Politics and Community: Expanding Access and Rationing Health Services in Oregon' (1992) 20 Law Med Hlth Care 67; S Rosenbaum 'Mothers and Children Last: The Oregon Medicaid Experiment' (1992) 18 Amer J Law Med 97; J Dixon and H G Welch 'Priority Setting: Lessons from Oregon' (1991) 337 Lancet 891. New Zealand and the Netherlands are also investigating possible policies.

private insurance arrangements. We doubt, however, if the Oregon experiment has any direct relevance to the United Kingdom. Quite apart from the very disparate populations involved, the Oregon plan is directed at those who cannot, for financial and other reasons, obtain private medical insurance, whereas the NHS is open to all in the United Kingdom as a right. There may well be valuable lessons to be learnt but, at the moment, we will forego further discussion.

The legal situation

Financial restraints clearly place the Secretary of State in some difficulty in discharging his statutory duty to provide, to such extent as he thinks necessary to meet all reasonable requirements of the NHS, health services including, inter alia, hospital accommodation.[2]

In some ways it is surprising that there have not been more actions brought by patients who feel that the Secretary of State has failed in these duties but, on reflection, it is probable that the dearth of cases results from the extreme improbability of a successful outcome. Such as there are tend to be reported sporadically; the classic action is that of *Hincks*.[3] In that case, patients in an orthopaedic hospital complained that they had waited an unreasonable time for treatment because of a shortage of facilities arising, in part, from a decision not to build a new block to the hospital on the grounds of cost; accordingly, they sought a declaration that the Secretary of State and the health authorities were in breach of their duty. In dismissing the application, Wien J said it was not the court's function to direct Parliament what funds to make available to the NHS and how to allocate them. The duty to provide services 'to such extent as he considers necessary' gave the minister a discretion as to the disposition of financial resources. The court could only interfere if the Secretary of State acted so as to frustrate the policy of the Act or as no reasonable minister could have acted; and no such breach had been shown in the particular case. Moreover, even if a breach was proved, the Act did not admit of relief by way of damages.

The case went to appeal[4] where, as might be expected, the judgment turned on the interpretation of 'reasonable requirements'. Lord Denning MR considered this to mean that a failure of duty existed only if the minister's action was thoroughly unreasonable. It was further thought that we should be faced with the economics of a bottomless pit if no limits in respect of long-term planning were to be read into public statutory duties; the further the advances of medical technology, the greater would be the financial burden placed upon the Secretary of State.

---

2 National Health Service Act 1977, s 3.
3 *R v Secretary of State for Social Services, ex p Hincks* (1979) 123 Sol Jo 436. A rather comparable case of 'hospital economics' is described in very human terms by Bishop B Habgood 'The Ethics of Resource Allocation: A Case Study' (1983) 9 J Med Ethics 21.
4 *R v Secretary of State for Social Services, ex p Hincks* (1980) 1 BMLR 93, CA. The case was discussed in J D Finch *Health Services Law* (1981) pp 38-39, in 'Rationing of Resources' (1985) 290 BMJ 374 and by D Brahams 'Enforcing A Duty to Care for Patients in the NHS' [1984] 2 Lancet 1224. See also C Newdick 'Rights to NHS Resources after the 1990 Act' (1993) 1 Med L Rev 53; F H Miller 'Denial of Health Care and Informed Consent in English and American Law' (1992) 18 Amer J Law Med 37.

Since 1980, however, health authorities have been required to balance their individual budgets.[5] Inevitably, major decisions as to the provision of health care have been moved down one hierarchical step, thus bringing the decision-makers into closer contact with those affected. Society, in the form of the Community Health Council, has a statutory place in the process[6] and, as a corollary, is entitled to judicial review of decisions thought to have been taken improperly. Nevertheless, attempts to extend this privilege to individuals seeking improved access to treatment have foundered consistently on the rock of the reasonableness inherent in the adverse decisions taken.

The paradigmatic case is that of *Walker*[7] which concerned a baby whose surgery had been postponed five times because of a shortage of skilled nursing staff. The trial judge, Macpherson J, commented that the application for judicial review took on the guise of a general criticism of the health service rather than that of an actual attack on the decision of the health authority. He deprecated any suggestion that patients should be encouraged to think the court had a role in cases which sought to compel the authority to carry out an operation that was not urgent; the Court of Appeal confirmed his refusal of the application for review. Within two months, the same health authority was involved in a comparable case, the only major difference being that the child was possibly in greater immediate danger.[8] Reiterating that to be so unreasonable as to come within the jurisdiction of the court, the authority would have had to make a decision that no reasonable body could have reached,[9] Stephen Brown LJ said:

> In the absence of any evidence which could begin to show that there was [such a failure] to allocate resources in this instance . . . there can be no arguable case . . . It does seem to me unfortunate that this procedure has been adopted. It is wholly misconceived in my view. The courts of this country cannot arrange the lists in the hospital . . . and should not be asked to intervene.

While expressing great sympathy with the parents, Stephen Brown LJ suggested that it might have been hoped that the publicity would bring pressure to bear on the hospital and there is no doubt that this effect could materialise – particularly in a life-saving situation. Dyer reported a case of a woman suffering from end-stage renal failure who was refused dialysis facilities; on her being granted legal aid to take the authority to court, an extra £250,000 was made available to the local renal units.[10]

---

5 National Health Service Act 1977, s 97A inserted by Health Services Act 1980, s 6.

6 Eg *R v Tunbridge Wells Health Authority, ex p Goodridge* (1988) Times, 21 May; see also *R v North West Thames Regional Health Authority, ex p Daniels* (1993) Times, 22 June (Community Health Council Regulations (SI 1985/304), r 19(1).

7 *Re Walker's Application* (1987) Times, 26 November, (1987) 3 BMLR 32, CA.

8 *R v Central Birmingham Health Authority, ex p Collier* (6 January 1988, unreported, available on Lexis). The case is discussed by D Brahams 'Seeking Increased NHS Resources Through the Courts' (1988) 1 Lancet 133. See also C Newdick 'Rights to NHS Resources after the 1990 Act' (1993) 1 Med L Rev 53; F H Miller 'Denial of Health Care and Informed Consent in English and American Law' (1992) 18 Amer J Law Med 37 for this case and *Re Walker's Application* (see previous footnote).

9 *Associated Provincial Picture Houses Ltd v Wednesbury Corpn* [1948] 1 KB 223 at 229, [1947] 2 All ER 680 at 683, per Lord Greene MR, CA.

10 C Dyer 'Going to Law to Get Treatment' (1987) 295 BMJ 1554.

Whatever one thinks of the morality of the process, it seems to have been a very successful exercise in 'shroud waving' – and it is to be noted that the money was not 'new' but was plucked from the waiting list fund. The circumstances were such, however, as to raise a real possibility of *Wednesbury* unreasonableness; thus, although the door between the individual patient and the courts may be firmly closed, it is not fully locked.[11]

One problem arising since the last edition of this book concerns the effect of the National Health Service and Community Care Act 1990 on the legal rights of patients and doctors in access to health service resources. For present purposes, the significant feature of the Act is to introduce what appear to be commercial concepts into the provision of care under the NHS. Care now reaches the patient through purchasers – that is, the general practitioners who are encouraged to function as fund holders – and suppliers or hospitals which may become self-governing trusts. There can be no doubt that the new regulations revamp the traditional setting of the health service – though whether this is by way of restricting the medical profession's clinical integrity in favour of managerial expertise or by imposing increased financial responsibility on doctors is open to question.[12]

The fact remains that alterations in structure also alter the confrontational ground and the opportunity for, if not the likelihood of, litigation in terms of health care delivery is now increased. In a most comprehensive review, Newdick[13] has pointed to the difficulties in maintaining the precepts of the National Health Service Act 1977 which are introduced by transferring much of the decision making to managers of both practices and hospitals. Newdick points out that no policy reason exists to abolish the rights that patients currently enjoy and he pleads that the *Bolam* principle be shielded from administrative interference. An interesting observation is that much responsibility will now be laid directly on the family health service authorities who will be exposed to claims in negligence and to judicial review. New avenues to litigation against hospitals are also opened up – for example, has a hospital a duty of care to patients on its waiting list and can it, accordingly, be sued for faulty prioritisation arrangements? And as a coda, Miller, in an equally useful contribution, suggests that patients themselves now have an opportunity to 'shop around' and that failure to explain the lack of a resource may result in actions for negligence based on flawed consent (see p 235).[14]

No actions related to the specific provisions of the 1990 Act have been reported[15] and the forecasts of potential confrontation have something of a 'Doomsday' atmosphere about them – many of the scenarios painted are, at least, very unlikely

---

11 An even more spectacular 'success' concerned Laura Davies who received, and rejected, a liver and small intestine transplant; she was then given a second transplant involving seven organs at a cost estimated as £1m (which is said to have been defrayed by a Middle Eastern potentate). For a critical lay view of such disposal of both financial and organic resources, see K Muir 'Can Saving the Life of Little Laura Really Be Worth £1 million?' (1993) The Times, 22 September, p 15.
12 R Klein 'The Politics of Change' (1991) 302 BMJ 1102.
13 C Newdick 'Rights to NHS Resources after the 1990 Act' (1993) 1 Med L Rev 53.
14 F H Miller 'Denial of Health Care and Informed Consent in English and American Law' (1992) 18 Amer J Law Med 37.
15 There was, for example, no action in negligence in *R v North West Thames Regional Health Authority, ex p Daniels* [1993] 4 Med LR 364, a case brough in respect of the closure of a unit which had agreed to treat a child's rare metabolic disease. The Health Authorities were, however, severely criticised for their administrative failures.

to materialise[16] and there seems no reason why professional health economists should not be subject to their own *Bolam*. But, whether or not the direct influence of economists turns out to benefit a national system of health care delivery, there is little doubt that a main effect of the 1990 legislation is to convert the covert rationing which has always occurred into a process which is open to public scrutiny and debate – and this must be a good thing. The extent of public involvement in the Oregon experiment may never be matched in the United Kingdom but increasing attention is likely to be paid to the voice of the consumer.[17]

A recent poll indicated that more than half the British public favoured unlimited funding of the NHS.[18] While this is clearly impossible, it can be argued that, once it is established that there is a reasonable requirement for a particular service, no further qualification exists upon the Secretary of State's duty to provide it and that inadequate resources do not absolve him from this duty.[19] This may well be so but, in so far as one cannot make a pot of tea without tap water unless one takes the water from the coffee urn, it adds little to the solution of the problem. Clearly, however, a further major ethical dilemma centres on the imposed medical limitations on treatment of the individual and it is to that aspect that we now turn.

Treatment of the individual

In discussion of the medical treatment of the individual, we are faced not with the hypothetical patient who may become ill but with one who is actually at risk. Objectivity is no longer the main arbiter and is replaced by need – itself described as an imprecise and elastic concept – and, in the event of enforced discrimination, the assessment of relative needs dictates a value judgment.

How, then, is that judgment to be made? In practice, many decisions are made instinctively and without the need for profound analysis – thus, the single-handed doctor will unhesitatingly choose the patient in greater pain for treatment despite the fact that this will simultaneously delay the treatment of those in lesser pain. There may well be moral arguments against such a policy – it does, for example, act to the detriment of the stoic – but the circumstances are acute and, the urgency being comparable, the doctor has selected a single criterion on which to base his judgment. Moral agonising is, in practice, reserved for the treatment of chronic, life-threatening diseases not only because they offer the opportunity for analysis but because they attract the use of expensive resources and will consume these for a long time – at which point, the dilemma extends not only to the allocation of resources but also to their withdrawal. In practice, the treatment of chronic renal diseases and of brain injury provide good examples on which to base discussion.

It is easy to say that enough dialysis machines should be made available to treat all cases of chronic renal failure but, in existing circumstances, this may merely

16 For a thoroughly pessimistic appraisal, based on English and American experience, see R D Persaud 'What Future for Ethical Medical Practice in the New National Health Service?' (1991) 17 J Med Ethics 10.
17 M Dean 'The Oregon Trail Reaches Britain' (1991) 338 Lancet 1133.
18 T Groves 'Public Disagrees with Professionals over NHS Funding' (1993) 306 BMJ 673.
19 G P Morris 'Enforcing a Duty to Care: The Kidney Patient and the NHS' (1983) 80 LS Gaz 3156.

mean that some other financially dependent resource must be curtailed. Costs can be cut by, say, changing a policy of hospital dialysis to one of home treatment but the fact of financial restraint is not thereby removed – only its degree is altered. But, at the same time, the modern patient undoubtedly regards access to high technology medicine as his individual right and such a view is readily tenable when there is an urgent need. If the doctor is, perforce, to qualify those rights, his reason for so doing must be beyond reproach and therein lies the problem – which we admit to finding virtually insoluble.

It is possible to discuss the allocation of resources in terms of triage. Triage is a curiously derived expression meaning, in the present context, the separation of casualties into priority treatment groups. It is essentially a military concept, the current British policy being to allocate four categories of casualty ranging from those whose slight injuries can be managed by self-care to those who cannot be expected to survive even with extensive treatment and who are, therefore, treated on a humanitarian basis only; the policy is closely associated with that of casualty evacuation. Triage in this sense is not only good emergency surgical practice but is also ethically acceptable because it is directed to a single discernible end – that is, to win the war or the battle – and we accept that this, in itself, is a morally acceptable objective with which the medical branch of the armed services can quite properly associate itself. It may, however, have unusual applications. The story is told that, with the advent during the Second World War of the new and scarce drug penicillin, instructions were given in an allied army that top priority was to be given for its use in the treatment of venereal disease rather than of battle wounds on the grounds that this represented a maximum return by way of military efficiency. The story may well be apocryphal but it serves to illustrate two features. First, given the fact that there is an easily definable and ethically desirable objective, the logical means taken towards that end may still be suspect. Second, it reinforces the view, which we share, that the concept of triage, which is an emergency procedure, cannot be simply transferred to civilian practice.[20] It may be possible to do so in special circumstances – it is, for example, a recognised practice following a major disaster, when the single most pressing objective is to mitigate the effects of that disaster. But the term triage, and its underlying principles, cannot be used as a convenient substitute, or subterfuge, for resource allocation and should be abandoned for that purpose. What, then, does one put in its place?

Alternative models

There have been many attempts to solve the problem[1] but none are satisfactory – all generalisations fail when applied to the particular but we will briefly outline some

20 Not everyone would agree with this view – eg J Cubbon 'The Principle of QALY Maximisation as the Basis for Allocating Health Care Resources' (1991) 17 J Med Ethics 181. See also K M Boyd and B T Potter 'Priorities in the Allocation of Scarce Resources' (1986) 12 J Med Ethics 197.
1 An exhaustive analysis of the alternatives is given by H J J Leenen 'The Selection of Patients in the Event of a Scarcity of Medical Facilities: An Unavoidable Dilemma' (1979) 1 Internat J Med Law 161. For a more recent appraisal, see M J Langford 'Who Should Get the Kidney Machine?' (1992) 18 J Med Ethics 12.

proposals which have been made. It is, perhaps, easiest to progress from those parameters which we consider to be least appropriate at the individual patient level.

We do not believe that cost benefit should be a major influence here. It needs no profound philosophical analysis to make one appreciate instinctively that it is right to deploy a helicopter to rescue a man on a drifting pleasure raft despite the fact that his danger is of his own making, despite the expense and despite the fact that the helicopter is designed to carry ten persons. The immediacy of the situation has placed a very high value on life which it would be quite immoral to ignore. The value cannot, however, be infinite, otherwise, faced with the choice of saving one man on a raft or ten men in a sinking dinghy, the grounds for the 'value choice' would be equal whereas, in practice, no one would doubt the correctness of choosing the larger number – always provided the operational circumstances were similar. Such choices must, however, be very rare in practice. In the chronic situation, as exemplified by dialysis, we are effectively confronted with a one to one choice between two individuals; at this point it is possible to introduce a cost-benefit argument which takes the form of assessing the relative gain to society of saving one or the other. In practice, this would invoke the use of some formula such as 'earning capacity x (65 – age)'. We believe that neither age nor income group should be primary criteria regulating choice per se – it might be that the aged respond less well to treatment than do others but that would be a different consideration. Such an assessment would, in addition, offend 'moral' practices which have almost attained the force of common law and of which 'women and children first' is an obvious example; women would, in general, come out worst if such objective cost-benefit criteria were to be applied. But this is not to say that some concern for quality or expectation of life should not be thrown into the prognostic balance and this possibility is discussed at p 261.

The corollary to this line of thought is that scarce resources should be distributed on the basis of the 'deserts' or basic merits of the recipients. One aspect of this is discussed further in chapter 14 where we note a United States experiment which attempts to distribute a very scarce resource – human kidneys – to those hospitals which have, themselves, provided organs. While such a system has much to commend it, any benefit accrues to the hospital rather than to the individual patient who still has to be 'chosen' by some other method. Others would look at this criterion from the opposite point of view and would exclude those who could positively endanger the treatment programme – a group who are exemplified by those carrying the virus of hepatitis or of the acquired immune deficiency syndrome. Such reasoning is a purely technical matter and is, in a sense, a criticism of the dialysis unit itself as being unable to contain the potential hazard. A rather more moralistic variant on this theme would hold it to be acceptable for a society which was providing the facility to exclude persons who increased the cost of care through their own choice;[2] while this is certainly arguable, it is a concept that is probably more applicable to communities in which the health of only a proportion is being supported by the taxes paid by the remainder – the beneficiaries of a national health service are more likely to see themselves as all in the same leaky boat.

More often, the assessment of 'deserts' is taken to apply to the intrinsic worth of the subject to society – and, again, we may look at this from the negative or positive

2   H T Engelhardt 'Allocating Scarce Medical Resources and the Availability of Organ Transplantation' (1984) 311 New Engl J Med 66.

aspect. First, there could be patients who, by reason of some other disability, could be regarded as being unlikely to benefit from treatment in a societal sense; this group, however, is essentially included among those falling to be assessed under the 'medical benefit' test and is best discussed within that context. The alternative, positive, approach in the event of shortage of facilities for treatment is to select those who offer the greatest contribution to society now and in the future. In our view, allocation tests which attempt to distinguish between, for example, the philanthropic mafia millionaire and the contestant for an international prize in applied mathematics serve no useful purpose in that they are hopelessly subjective. Choices so based are clearly beyond the capacity or function of the individual doctor – and a 'committee decision', which is sometimes advocated, is no more than a sum of individual subjective assessments; we reject the concept.

The one 'deserts-related' issue which is most commonly raised is that of age. It is very widely held that the older a patient is, the less can he or she command equal opportunity in a competition for therapy. The reasons for this acquiescence differ. Some will rely on the argument 'he's had his innings'; others, more rationally, will point to the fact that results of treatment are generally better in the young than in the old. But simply because the results of coronary surgery are commonly more satisfactory in the middle aged patient does not mean that surgery is not worthwhile in the 75-year-old. There is, moreover, a tendency to forget that not every therapy is effective for a full life-span; if we anticipate a likely five-year survival, it matters not whether the patient was aged 20 or 60. We suspect that the reason underlying the common assumption is that those responsible for decision-making are, by definition, below retiring age; it has been said, rightly, that there is often a wide discrepancy between the optimum solution of a problem from the perspective of society as a whole and that of the individual within that society.[3] Lewis and Charny have tried, by means of an opinion poll, to establish the points at which the public would be prepared to accept age-based choices and, thus, to map out decision-making boundaries which will reflect the values of society as a whole. This is a praiseworthy effort which is obviously open to criticism;[4] for ourselves, while appreciating the value of uniformity and accepting the need for the development of guidelines established by way of wide societal involvement, we find it difficult to support a cold actuarial basis for making what is still a human clinical decision.

Clearly, the most widely acceptable criterion of selection would be that determined by medical benefit.[5] But, once again, this is easier to believe than to put into practice. Unless one is dealing with a recoverable condition – and dialysis, which is providing the main theme for discussion, is only palliative – medical benefit is a relative matter and, moreover, prognosis is unpredictable. It is also difficult to avoid the conclusion that the individual's social status may influence the outcome of any therapy.

But, even if the clinician claims absolute responsibility for allocation of his expertise, he must consider the quality of the life he is extending and it is here that

3   P A Lewis and M Charny 'Which of Two Individuals Do You Treat When Only Their Ages Are Different and You Can't Treat Both?' (1989) 15 J Med Ethics 28.
4   See D Lamb 'Priorities in Health Care' (1989) 15 J Med Ethics 33; P Whitaker 'Resource Allocation: A Plea for a Touch of Realism' (1990) 16 J Med Ethics 129.
5   The choice made, inter alia, by Dr Gillon's remarkably prescient daughter – see R Gillon 'Justice and Allocation of Medical Resources' (1985) 291 BMJ 266. It was also the implicit choice of the court in *Re J (a minor)(wardship: medical treatment)* [1992] 2 FLR 165, (1992) 9 BMLR 10.

he may obtain guidance from – or suffer the interference of – the health economist. Perhaps the greatest influence in this field over the last decade has been the introduction of the concept of quality adjusted life years – or QALYs.[6]

Quality adjusted life years

The principle of the QALY is simple enough. A year of healthy life expectancy is scored as 1 and a year of unhealthy life as less than 1 depending upon the degree of reduction in quality; while death is taken as zero, a life considered to be worse than death can be accorded a minus score. The 'value' of treatment in terms of 'life appreciation' can then be assessed numerically. Thus far, in fact, QALYs seem to be doing little more than expressing the intuitive findings of the competent clinician in a mathematical formula. And therein lies the rub – for the 'quality scoring' will still be founded on a 'best interests' assessment made by a third party and the paternalistic element in that assessment has been scarcely modified. It might, for example, be hard for a middle class doctor not to see a middle class life as being of higher quality than one sustained on social security; a young physician may see a short life on the golf course as preferable to a long one tied to the television set – but this may very well not be the patient's evaluation. It is thus apparent that, at this level, a QALY can only be truly evaluated with the patient's co-operation; it can then be used to decide between two possible treatments for the same condition. This what has been described as 'vertical priority setting' where one is on more level ground in so far as one is comparing like with like.[7] Used in this way, QALYs may actually augment the patient's autonomy by explicitly involving him or her in the process of rational consent to therapy (see p 237). Even so, a note of caution may be sounded as it is not difficult to confuse the objectives. The easy phrase 'not clinically indicated' may mean either that the treatment is not considered to be of overall benefit to the patient or it may imply an inappropriate allocation of resources.[8] The distinction is conceptually important: in the latter case, the professional has a legitimate prior interest in decision making while, in the former, the views of the individual patient are of major significance.

There are other more specific objections to QALYs as they are currently developed. Clearly, they operate to the disadvantage of the aged; they measure only the end-point of treatment without considering the *proportional* loss or gain in the quality of life; and there are parameters other than simple health which need to be fed into the equation. Possibly the most important moral criticism is that the QALY sets no value on life per se.[9] Harris considers that we should be saving as many lives, not life years, as possible – a proposition which simplifies the argument by removing it from the sphere of life-saving treatment which should, then, be apportioned only on a first come, first served basis; we also suggest that the customary use of the term

6   A Williams 'The Economic Role of "Health Indicators" ', in G Teeling-Smith (ed) *Measuring the Social Benefits of Medicine* (1983).
7   M Cochrane, C Ham, C Heginbotham and R Smith 'Rationing: At the Cutting Edge' (1991) 303 BMJ 1039.
8   See T Hope, D Sprigings and R Crisp ' "Not Clinically Indicated": Patients' Interests or Resource Alocation?' (1993) 306 BMJ 379.
9   See, in particular, J Harris 'QALYfying the Value of Life' (1987) 13 J Med Ethics 117; J Rawles 'Castigating QALYs' (1989) 15 J Med Ethics 143.

'life-saving', when what is really meant is 'death-postponing', can lead to false reasoning. What this view certainly does, however, is to emphasise that QALYs can never be used to compare the value of 'life-saving' therapies with those which are merely life-enhancing. Indeed, it may well be asked whether we have any right to pronounce on the quality of other people's lives and, hence, whether abstract formulae should ever be used to compare the management of individual persons or different disease states. We should be very careful lest we find that we have unwittingly written into the equation a constant such as that the mentally handicapped, for example, are, by definition, possessed of less QALYs than are those with no inherent deficit.

In view of these many criticisms, it is not surprising that alternatives to the QALY are being actively sought. One such system is the saved young life equivalent, in which saving the life of a young person and restoring him or her to full health is regarded as the unit of measurement – on the grounds that most people would regard that as the maximum benefit that a single individual can obtain.[10] The comparative values of treatments is than assessed in terms of how many expected outcomes of each treatment would be equivalent to one SAVE. Such a system may or may not be easier to understand than are QALYs; its evaluation would certainly require a vast amount of empirical field-work such as is currently being undertaken in Norway. Our specific criticism would be that, even by its title, it actively promotes 'ageism' which is little more than an unfortunate, though inevitable, incidental to the QALY concept; and, in general – and in common with all such formulae – it reduces persons to numbers and tends to dehumanise medical practice.

This criticism hardens when the health economists tie cost to their preferred process of analysis – something which they must do in order to guide those responsible for macroallocation of resources. It may well be salutary for physicians and surgeons to be forced into knowing the cost-effectiveness of any given procedure. What health economists should not do, in our view, is to attempt to dictate the resolution of clinical problems in financial terms – to allow this is, as Rawles has put it, to condone 'the development by health economists of fairer methods of denying patients treatment'.[11]

To some, a feasible answer to the resource allocation dilemma is to increase the resources;[12] others regard this as a dangerous assumption – Klein, for example, suggests that it is only a slight exaggeration to say that the demand for health care is what the medical profession chooses to make it.[13] We believe that the transfer of funds from nuclear weapon production to health care, while being admirable in itself, does no more than move the problem one incremental stage further. The majority would agree that some form of structured distribution of facilities at microallocation level is essential even though equity and efficiency may, at times, lie together uneasily. QALYs as they stand are no more than aids to decision-making and they are but one of a number of models that are currently being looked at.[14] All are there

10 E Nord 'An Alternative to QALYs: The Saved Young Life Equivalent (SAVE)' (1992) 305 BMJ 875.
11 J Rawles and K Rawles 'The QALY Argument: A Physician's and A Philosopher's View (1990) 16 J Med Ethics 93.
12 J Rawles 'Castigating QALYs' (1989) 15 J Med Ethics 143.
13 R Klein 'Dimensions of Rationing: Who Should Do What?' (1993) 307 BMJ 309.
14 For a summing up, see R Robinson 'The Policy Context' (1993) 307 BMJ 994.

to be developed and improved upon; possibly their most useful current feature is that they trigger debate as to how priorities in health care should be set rationally.

We should exclude from this discussion, and treat as a special case, the patient who is using a scarce resource but who is obtaining no benefit. The most clear example of this is one who is brain damaged and is being maintained in intensive care – a situation discussed in detail in chapter 15 below. We believe that, once treatment is clearly of no avail, it is not only permissible but positively correct to discontinue heroic measures. Of the many reasons for taking this view, the one which is presently apposite is that a resource is thereby released for someone who is likely to benefit.

Random selection

In our search for an equitable and efficient method of providing limited treatment, we have left for discussion only the option of random selection of patients – or of lottery, or 'first come, first served', which come to much the same thing in slightly different circumstances.

Such a policy has the advantage of apparent objectivity and, as we have seen, it could be regarded as the morally desirable choice in the context of potentially fatal disease. It is, however, a bad medical option because it takes no account of the gravity of the patient's condition and no account of medical benefit – 'it concentrates on justice and ignores welfare';[15] moreover, the sheer length of waiting lists may prevent the most acceptable cases from the physician's point of view from ever obtaining treatment. As an option, it is also socially suspect in that it treats human beings as 'things' and pays no attention to human values and aspirations. Finally, its acceptance may be a cloak for no more than abrogation of responsibility. Nevertheless, as we have seen from the Norwegian experience, it may be the way of allocating scarce resources that the public prefer.

It is surprising that there is no recent precedental case law on which to judge the attitudes of society in respect of allocation of resources at the micro, or individual, level. The most likely reason for this is that decisions are taken in good faith and are based on principles which would be acceptable to a responsible body of medical opinion – there is, therefore, no action available in negligence. There is, moreover, a remarkable tendency for well-publicised and apposite instances to be solved pragmatically.[16] For any assistance, we suspect we must go back to the classic case of *US v Holmes*.[17] In this instance, a ship's officer ordered a number of passengers to be ejected from a sinking lifeboat; Holmes, who helped effect the instructions, was convicted of manslaughter. A main argument for the prosecution was that the passengers, at least, should have been chosen by lot. It seems fair to assume that his decision would lend support to a policy of randomisation in the event of competition for scarce medical resources; the inferred element of an 'appeal to God' certainly adds a moral weight to the argument. A rather similar English incident is reported in relation to a ferry-boat disaster. Here, a passenger assumed a position of authority and may well have occasioned the sacrifice of one man in order to save the lives of several other passengers; the case never came to court and the coroner thought that

15 See T Hope, D Sprigings and R Crisp ' "Not Clinically Indicated": Patients' Interests or Resource Alocation?' (1993) 306 BMJ 379.
16 See the report by D Brahams 'When is Discontinuation of Dialysis Justified?' (1985) 1 Lancet 176.
17 26 Fed Cas 360 (1841), No 15383.

such killing would not necessarily be criminal. The commentator, however, considered that such authority as exists is to the effect that the killing of one to save the lives of others cannot be justified or even excused.[18] But such precedents are, at best, only loosely applicable to the present discussion.

As to the withdrawal of resources from a patient already using them, both United Kingdom and United States law is discussed in chapters 13 and 15. It is to be noted, however, that nowhere is there any authority for such action on the grounds of competing medical benefit – that is, that a further latecomer to the scene would be likely to do better. Indeed, there are strong indications that the contrary holds. In *Re J*,[19] Balcombe LJ said:

> I would stress the absolute undesirability of the court making an order which may have the effect of compelling a doctor or health authority to make available scarce resources (both human and material) to a particular child, without knowing whether or not there are other patients to whom the resources might more advantageously be devoted . . . [It might] require the health authority to put J on a ventilator in an intensive care unit, and thereby possibly to deny the benefit of those limited resources to a child who was much more likely than J to benefit from them.

The implication is clear – withdrawal of treatment will only be condoned when the patient can receive no further benefit.

A solution of the insoluble?

We have thus reached a position where no single parameter seems entirely satisfactory. Gordon,[20] in a discussion of the doctrine of necessity, speaks of it as offending 'against the feeling that no human being has a right to decide which of his fellows should survive in any situation'; but, while most would agree with this proposition, doctors cannot opt out of such decisions. Some idea of the complexity of the dilemma was given in an interesting study of dialysis decisions.[1] In this, 40 specimen patients' records were sent to 25 renal units with the request that ten patients be rejected on the grounds of inadequate treatment resources. Only 13 patients would have been accepted in all the units, but, at the same time, none was rejected by all; in the event, it was discovered that six of the ten most commonly rejected cases had already been successfully treated by the authors of the paper! Something of a lottery must operate despite the most earnest endeavours of physicians to improve upon the system.

We have not discussed a final possible criterion of selection – that is, the ability to pay for a resource. The omission probably derives from a natural repugnance to

---

18 Our authority is J C Smith and B Hogan *Criminal Law: Cases and Materials* (4th edn, 1990) p 231. The well-known case of *R v Dudley and Stephens* (1884) 14 QBD 273, [1881-5] All ER Rep 61, CCR was essentially a matter of killing and cannibalism for self-preservation and is too far removed to be appropriate to the present discussion.
19 *Re J (a minor)(wardship: medical treatment)* [1992] 2 FLR 165 at 176, (1992) 9 BMLR 10 at 20.
20 G H Gordon *The Criminal Law of Scotland* (2nd edn, 1978) p 422.
1 V Parsons and P Lock 'Triage and the Patient with Renal Failure' (1980) 6 J Med Ethics 173. In fairness, however, it should be remarked that this is a somewhat dated reference; renal units have become more sophisticated in the last 14 years.

such an idea, particularly among those accustomed to a national health service. But, on reflection, we wonder if a modified concept of this type does not have its attractions as a way of alleviating scarcity while still retaining moral respectability. There is no shortage of dialysis machines from the manufacturing point of view; it is the shortage of money to pay for them within the confines of a 'free' medical service which lies at the root of the problem. In these circumstances, it might not be unreasonable to allow patients to contribute to the purchase of 'engineering hardware' according to their means on the principle that a machine which is bought releases another for the use of others who cannot do so. Such a system operates in the United States as regards dialysis where, admittedly, it was introduced for precisely the opposite reasons – that patients with chronic renal disease would be destroyed financially unless public assistance was given; but whatever the reason, it is probable that the overall provision of dialysis resources is better when distributed as a joint private and public enterprise.

Such a policy would, we admit, be difficult to apply with absolute equity. In particular, it could be argued that it would draw off in an unequal manner the personnel required to operate the machines and who have been trained at public expense. To which one could answer that you do not expect a university graduate in law to accept only legal aid cases. One could also point out that a greater number of cases – of dialysis cases, at least – would be treated at home and that, by and large, the efficiency of domiciliary treatment and the financial status of the patient are closely related. In short, in certain circumstances, there may be a logical case for including private medicine within the public sector with possible benefit to the latter.

We appreciate that, at the end of this fairly lengthy discussion, we have come to little in the way of firm conclusions. We have approached the issues from the position of doctor and lawyer and it is, in some ways, comforting to find that philosophers may be in much the same dilemma.[2] Gillon probably sums up the debate correctly when he implies that, provided decisions are made taking into account fundamental moral values and principles of equity, impartiality and fairness, and provided the bases for decision-making are flexible in relation to the times, then the underlying system is just and is likely to yield just results. Alternatively, we can simply be stoical and acknowledge that: 'to live with circumstances that are unfortunate but not unfair is the destiny of men and women who have neither the financial nor the moral resources of gods and goddesses'.[3]

The responsibility of the individual
No discussion of this type would be complete without a passing reference to the responsibility of the individual to avoid the need for medical resources. The argument that prevention is better than cure has been widely popularised. No one would deny the importance of the theory at all levels but, equally, it is difficult to decide when friendly persuasion ceases and restriction of liberty begins. It follows that a good case can be made out for a right to choose to be unhealthy – and this not

---

2   R Gillon 'Justice and Allocation of Medical Resources' (1985) 291 BMJ 266.

3   H T Engelhardt 'Allocating Scarce Medical Resources and the Availability of Organ Transplantation' (1984) 311 New Engl J Med 66.

only on Kantian but also on utilitarian grounds, for every sudden death in late middle age that is prevented is potentially a long-term occupation of a bed in a psychogeriatric ward; it could well be that the quest for dementia that is inherent in many of the currently popular limitations on habit will turn out to be remarkably cost-inefficient.

What does *not* follow is that there is a concomitant right to health resources when the consequences of that choice materialise. It seems that the public have little sympathy for the cavalier approach – in Williams's experience, the least unacceptable reason for discrimination in prioritisation was that the prospective patients had not cared for their own health.[4] In making such value judgments, however, the public are not constrained by principles of professional ethics and the issue is certainly not so easily solved by health care providers. Various views have been put forward in an interesting debate in the *British Medical Journal* on whether or not coronary by-pass surgery should be offered to smokers.[5] The attitude of the surgeons was conditioned by the poor results obtained in smokers and the fact that they spent longer in hospital. Non-treatment could, therefore, be justified on the grounds that treatment of non-smokers deprived others of more efficient and effective surgery. An alternative medical view was that non-treatment of symptomatic patients is often less effective in terms of overall cost to society than is operation, that there are many other 'self-inflicted' conditions which one would not hesitate to treat and that, at least in some cases, smoking is an addictive condition which merits sympathy. A warning was also sounded that, in regarding those who have brought medical ills upon themselves as, somehow, less deserving, the doctor is coming perilously close to prescribing punishment. We would accept the view expressed that the patient should be offered the chance when a positive therapeutic advantage – albeit a less than ideal advantage – may be attainable. The solution to the problem thus comes down to the 'best interests' of the individual; we believe, moreover, that this is the route that would be taken by the courts were such a case to be litigated – but no doubt *Bolam* would be left holding the stakes.

4   A Williams 'Cost-effectiveness Analysis: Is It Ethical?' (1992) 18 J Med Ethics 7. See also fn 19, p 253 above.
5   'Should Smokers Be Offered Coronary Bypass Surgery?' (1993) 306 BMJ 1047 - M J Underwood and J S Bailey 'Coronary Bypass Surgery Should Not Be Offered to Smokers' at 1047; M Shiu 'Refusing to Treat Smokers Is Unethical and a Dangerous Precedent' at 1048; R Higgs 'Human Frailty Should Not be Penalised' at 1049; J Garfield 'Let the Health Authority Take the Responsibility' at 1050.

12 Treatment of the aged

Old age used to present no particular medico-ethical problems – senescence carried with it an increasing susceptibility to infection and the majority of the aged died at home, within the family circle, having strayed not too far from their biblical allocation of three score and ten years.

Today, the physical health of the elderly is improving along with that of other age groups; longevity itself and the expectation of longevity are both increasing. Recent figures from America are probably valid for most well-developed countries. There, 4% of the population were aged over 65 years at the turn of the century; this proportion had grown to 12.7% by 1990 and is expected to reach 21.8% in 2050 – at which time 5% of the total population will be aged 85 or over. The elderly population is also growing older – while one third of those aged more than 65 were aged more than 75 in 1960, the proportion is likely to be 50% in 2001.[1] The proportion of women enlarges with increasing age; British men reaching the age of 50 in the year 2000 are projected to have a 50% chance of reaching 75 while the proportion for women is likely to be 74%.[2] Improved physical status, however, is not necessarily paralleled by improved mental capacity; indeed, a longer life provides more time during which the inevitable wastage of a limited supply of brain cells can occur. The stage is then set for a swelling proportion of the population which is suffering from various degrees of dementia; this may, itself, be of primary degenerative type or be secondary to disease of the cerebral vasculature. Long-stay is likely when such patients are admitted to hospital and the dilemma in respect of resource allocation scarcely needs emphasis[3] – up to 20% of all medical and surgical beds in the United Kingdom may be occupied by people over the age of 75 years, although the wider use of community hospitals may be improving this particular resource problem. Population projections are now sufficiently sophisticated to indicate the problems likely to be met in deciding the means by which to cope with conditions in the future – and those means cannot be determined on the basis of administrative convenience alone but must involve both ethical and legal considerations.

---

1 E S Cohen 'Realism, Law and Aging' (1990) 18 Law Med Hlth Care 183. Different views can, however, be taken of statistics. M Jefferys (ed) *Growing Old in the 20th Century* (1989), introduction, points out that there were 11 persons aged over 85 per 1,000 United Kingdom population in 1981; there will only be 17 in 2001 – which should not be too great a burden on an advanced society.
2 M Dean 'Towards a Healthy Third Age' (1992) 339 Lancet 1403. The 'third age' referred to here is an artificial category of persons aged 50 to 75.
3 See K Andrews 'Demographic Changes and Resources for the Elderly' (1985) 290 BMJ 1023 for an analysis.

Autonomy and paternalism in the treatment of the aged

The conflict between autonomy – or the exercise of choice – and paternalism – or the efforts of others to protect those who they consider to be in need of protection – lies at the heart of the dilemma and is far more complex in the context of geriatric medicine than it is, say, in the relatively simple field of consent to surgical treatment by a competent adult.[4] The elderly person is constrained in his choice of action by many factors, some of which are endogenous – such as the effects of early dementia – but others of which are extraneous – such as poverty. The impetus to paternalistic protection of the aged, no matter how it is ultimately applied, is likely to come from that person's family and, although the factor may be minimised in individual cases, it remains an undeniable general fact that it is easier to live without the burden of caring for one's ageing parents; children become paternalists in seeking institutional care for their parents and there is no way in which subjectivity can be wholly eliminated from such action. It is arguable that children have no obligation to support their parents[5] and, regrettable as it may seem, such an obligation has never existed in English law; moreover, the common law duty which existed previously in Scotland has been removed by statute.[6] The public is probably insufficiently aware of the extent of intrafamilial abuse of the elderly; the degree of ignorance – or, in this case possibly, of indifference – is comparable to that which applied to child abuse 30 years ago. There can be little doubt that abuse is extensive and that it occurs in various forms including verbal, physical and by way of neglect or deprivation; figures of between 5 and 65% of elderly persons being at risk are quoted, the incidence depending on the criteria used by the reporting agencies.[7] In one prospective study in England, 45% of carers admitted to some form of 'elder abuse'.[8] It follows that any attempt to enforce a filial duty of care for the aged would be likely to exacerbate domestic violence or neglect and, thus, provoke further deterioration in the geriatrics' conditions. Much of the care of the elderly must, therefore, devolve on the medical and social services and both of these must be supported by the law.[9]

Institutional treatment

Medical treatment of the aged in the United Kingdom has, as in all advanced societies, moved a long way since the chronic sick, including those who were simply homeless, were almost arbitrarily assigned to hospital wards which have been described as little more than 'human warehouses'.[10] Attention is now concentrated on maintaining the old person's environment as far as is possible. Such a policy must

4 For an overview see E S Cohen 'Autonomy and Paternalism: Two Goals in Conflict' (1985) 13 Law Med Hlth Care 145.

5 N Daniels 'Family Responsibility Initiatives and Justice Between Age Groups' (1985) 13 Law Med Hlth Care 153. This US article specifically applauds the general direction of geriatric health care in the United Kingdom. Also by the same author *Am I My Parents' Keeper?* (1988).

6 Family Law (Scotland) Act 1985, s 1(1). Cf the reciprocal obligation imposed by Roman Dutch law – P Q R Boberg *The Law of Persons and the Family* (1991) p 267.

7 B Pitt 'Abusing Old People' (1992) 305 BMJ 968.

8 A C Homer and C Gilleard 'Abuse of Elderly People by their Carers' (1990) 301 BMJ 1359.

9 This has been collected in A Griffiths, R H Grimes and G Roberts *The Law and Elderly People* (1990).

10 T Howell 'The Birth of British Geriatrics' (1983) 13 Geriat Med 791.

include as a starting point a system of pre-admission home visits by specialists in geriatric medicine; the fact that an inability to appreciate one's disablement is a concomitant of dementia has also dictated positive case-finding.[11] Both these activities may raise problems of etiquette, if not of ethics, between specialists and general practitioners. Moreover, there is a strong possibility that case finding imposes an excessively heavy load on general practitioners – which may account for the relatively slight impact the Edinburgh example has had on a national scale.[12] Antipathy to institutionalising the psycho-geriatric patient simultaneously calls for improvements in home help. Given a good relationship, much of this can be provided by the family – particularly if they are given assistance. This is available by way of rather complex legislation. In essence, a disability living allowance, divided into care and mobility components, is payable to a person who, inter alia, is so physically or mentally disabled as to require the constant attention of another person by day (or prolonged or repeated attention at night) to assist with his or her bodily functions or for his or her protection from danger. Disability living allowance is payable only if the disability arose before the age of 65; it is replaced by attendance allowance if it arose later – and there is no age limit applied to this benefit.[13] Elective and temporary admission to hospital, thus allowing the carers time for relaxation, can be a most useful adjunct. By and large, however, home assistance must be a function of the social services and the local authority is under an obligation to provide such aid in a 'preventive' mode. This includes help with the design of the house and the provision of meals, facilities for recreation and home helps. Boarding accommodation, which is something less than residential care, can also be provided.[14] It may be that such treatment is cost ineffective and is difficult to apply. The economic return depends to an extent on the degree of dependency – the expense of domiciliary care increases with increased dependency and, at some point, it will become inequitable for a disabled person to expect cost-ineffective support at the expense of others who are, thereby, deprived of care;[15] clearly, however, the wishes – or autonomy – of the subject must be fed into the balance. The current proliferation of privately run nursing homes, which derives from government policy that most institutional care should be provided on a private commercial basis, makes it very difficult to generalise as to the comparative prognosis of those cared for at home and those institutionalised. Inevitably, much depends upon the degree and efficiency of supervision of residential and nursing homes and we return to the subject below.

Nevertheless, some old people, who are fit other than in the mind, must be institutionalised to an extent which will depend upon the severity of dementia. The simplest form of such care is by way of sheltered housing – which may be provided

11 M Arcand and J Williamson 'An Evaluation of Home Visiting of Patients by Physicians in Geriatric Medicine' (1982) 283 BMJ 718.
12 S Barley 'An Uncompromising Report on Health Visiting for the Elderly' (1987) 294 BMJ 595.
13 Social Security Contributions and Benefits Act 1992, ss 71, 75 and 64. These benefits are to be distinguished from invalid care allowance which is paid to the carer (s 70). The rights of married daughters to invalid care allowance have been upheld by the European Court of Justice: *Drake v Chief Adjudication Officer* [1986] 3 All ER 65, [1986] ECR 1995.
14 Health and Social Services and Social Security Adjudication Act 1983, Sch 9, Part II; Social Work (Scotland) Act 1968, s 14. A general duty to care for the welfare of the elderly also rests on the local social service authority (Health Services and Public Health Act 1968, s 45).
15 J G Evans 'Institutional Care and Elderly People' (1993) 306 BMJ 806.

by the local authority, housing associations or as a private venture – but the degree of available supervision is generally so low as to eliminate it as a resort for persons who are anything greatly less than fully independent; sheltered housing might, however, be the ideal refuge for the elderly person who is subject to domestic abuse and, thereby, eligible for priority accommodation.[16] Beyond this, it may be possible to arrange for residential care in accommodation which the local authority has a duty to provide by virtue of the National Assistance Act 1948, s 21. Practice, however, falls short of the theoretical ideal. The local authority has no obligation to provide specialist or hospital type medical facilities in such institutions which are already accepting patients whose requirements exceed those for which this method of disposal was designed; so-called 'Part III accommodation' tends to revert to the conditions which are less than ideal.

The result has been a growth of private homes which has been encouraged by government policy that the local authorities should utilise the private sector.[17] Homes are divided into those which provide only accommodation and those which provide personal or nursing care. It is only the latter which require to be registered under the Registered Homes Act 1984[18] and, as a result, subject to statutory supervision; there has been some disquiet as to the standards of care that is offered in those not so controlled – a problem which appears to exist worldwide. None the less, the extension of private nursing homes, with governmental assistance as to charge has, on the whole, given a satisfactory solution to the scarcity of residential accommodation – perhaps the main contentious issue being that, whereas those admitted to such homes through the national health service are receiving free 'treatment', those placed by the local authority are subject to payment according to means.[19] Paradoxically, however, the academic specialist in geriatric medicine may well regard this institutionalising policy as being likely to counter that of care within the community; moreover, the process is one which, as discussed above, may or may not be wasteful of scarce financial resources.[20] Even so, old people in NHS nursing homes are likely to do at least as well as those in geriatric hospital units,[1] and the number and quality of such units is increasing. Again, however, the modus operandi of the geriatric unit is based on rehabilitation and the return of patients to their natural environment. In 1987, only 7% of those assessed for ideal disposal in Edinburgh were, in fact, admitted to residential care[2] and less than 20% of patients admitted to the geriatric medical wards remained in long-term care. The aim is to adapt

16 Housing Act 1985, s 59. Vulnerability can only be defined following wide-ranging inquiry: *R v Lambeth London Borough Council, ex p Carroll* (1988) 20 HLR 142.

17 Community Care (Residential Accommodation) Act 1992 amending National Assistance Act 1948, s 26.

18 However, small homes (with less than four residents) providing such services must now be registered: Registered Homes (Amendment) Act 1991.

19 J Kellett 'Long Term Care in the NHS: A Vanishing Prospect' (1993) 306 BMJ 846.

20 D Challis, R Darton, I Johnson et al 'An Evaluation of an Alternative to Long-stay Hospital Care for Frail Elderly Patients. II. Costs and Effectiveness' (1991) 20 Age Ageing 245.

1 A Bowling, J Formby, K Grant and S Ebrahim 'A Randomised Controlled Trial of Nursing Home and Long-stay Geriatric Ward Care for Elderly People' (1991) 20 Age Ageing 316.

2 J Rafferty, R G Smith and J Williamson 'Medical Assessment of Elderly Persons Prior to a Move to Residential Care: A Review of Seven Years' Experience in Edinburgh' (1987) 16 Age Ageing 10.

pragmatically to the changes in conditions and abilities which are likely to occur in this category of patients.

The overall management of psychogeriatric patients may seem to be less than satisfactory but the condition is not confined to the United Kingdom. Kapp,[3] writing of the United States, has appealed for some long-absent direction of, and rationality in, long-term care policy. He wrote:

> Our principles and the choices – that must deal simultaneously with the forces of autonomy, quality and cost – that carry out these principles, must be developed and made public.

The resolution of, on the one hand, demands for unlimited long-term care and, on the other, our willingness to arrange payment for the associated benefits are matters of universal concern.

The individual patient

So far, we have considered the problems of the aged in general terms only; they become even more acute when applied to the individual patient. Thus, in the conditions of Part III housing, injuries due to falls and other mishaps in an unsupervised situation are likely to arise; deaths which occur later, and which are no more than temporarily associated, are likely to be the subject of inquiry by either the Coroner or the Procurator Fiscal. Many such incidents may be beyond the control of inadequate staffs notwithstanding their dedication; yet the fear of culpability can rebound to the overall detriment of the patient – 'defensive' action by the nurses may result in unnecessary restraint of their charges.[4] Of greater immediate importance are the ethical problems surrounding those old persons who want to retain their independence and who resist removal to an institution. The danger, then, is double-sided – either the 'cussedness' of old age may be designated as mental illness and the aged person be compulsorily restricted or, as has occurred in some of the United States, the senile dement may be determinedly excluded from the social benefits which are available to those who can lay claim to a recognisable mental illness.

In the United Kingdom, the legal resolution of the problem of compulsory disposal of the inadequate aged person rests, primarily, on the National Assistance Act 1948, s 47. This allows the compulsory removal from their homes of persons who are not mentally ill but who are suffering from grave chronic disease or, being aged, infirm or physically incapacitated, are living in insanitary conditions and are unable to devote to themselves, and are not receiving from other persons, proper care and attention. Removal may be effected in the person's own interest or in order to prevent injury to the health of, or serious nuisance to, other persons. The district

3 M B Kapp 'Financing Long-term Care for the Elderly; Am I *Your* Parents' Keeper?' (1985) 13 Law Med Hlth Care 188. Experience in Australia seems to be similar but rather more satisfactory: T Smith 'Old Age in the Sun' (1984) 288 BMJ 1515.
4 A very full discussion is to be found in S H Johnson 'The Fear of Liability and the Use of Restraints in Nursing Homes' (1990) 18 Law Med Hlth Care 263.

community physician, or community medicine specialist, can apply for a magistrate's order giving seven days' notice of removal. The order allows for detention in a 'suitable hospital or other place' for up to three months; emergency removal for a period of three weeks can be achieved on the recommendation of the community physician if this is backed by another practitioner – who is normally the person's general practitioner.[5] The fact that this accelerated procedure is used in the majority of cases is a cause of anxiety as to the operation of the legislation.

It is estimated that the powers under s 47 are invoked annually no more than some 200 times in England and 15 times in Scotland. The reasons for this marked selectivity are both practical and ethical. As to the former, the order does not provide for compulsory treatment and the subject is likely to be removed to a geriatric hospital rather than to a geriatric unit; worse, admission may be to a general hospital where treatment and investigation are not likely to be strongly motivated and will be looked on as contradictions in terms unless the admission is on the grounds of grave chronic disease. The moral issues were elegantly argued by Gray[6] who, first, questioned the justifiability of removing an elderly person from his or her home for the benefit of 'other persons' – as he pointed out, powers of compulsory home cleaning and the like are already available under the Public Health Acts 1936-1961. Second, the arguments balancing paternalism against personal liberty, which have been discussed above, are raised in a particularly acute form. Third, the use of statutory powers may be little more than a cloak for inadequate social services or family care – which, taken together, are to be preferred to institutionalisation. And finally, and perhaps of greatest importance, there is a strong implication that the powers are based on disapproval of deviant rather than of dangerous behaviour.[7]

The contrary view has been put by Greaves,[8] who concludes that reference to the standard philosophical alternatives do not do justice to the moral issues at stake; he sees the answer to the problem lying somewhere between the application of rational principles and personal prejudices. Greaves gives no firm answer as to how this level is to be achieved but accepts that, in certain circumstances, a decision must be taken by proxy on behalf of the old person – and this is best done by a doctor whose personal ethical sensitivity is unlikely to be suppressed by the blanket application of a principle. Gray,[9] in fact, points out that s 47 was seen as essentially a mechanism for protecting the elderly against the whims of officialdom and the Medical Officer of Health was thought to be the best person to do this. While criticising the Draconian powers available under s 47, he does not believe that it should be repealed – but this is largely because other coercive or frankly immoral practices would evolve in order to persuade old people to resign their homes. There is an ingrained way of public thought that, given the same abnormality, old people 'must' be protected while others merely 'ought' to be so persuaded.

5   National Assistance (Amendment) Act 1951, s 1(1).
6   J A M Gray 'Section 47' (1981) 7 J Med Ethics 146.
7   For further criticism, see J D Fear, P Hatton and E B Renvoize 'Section 47 of National Assistance Act: A Time for Change?' (1988) 296 BMJ 860.
8   D A Greaves 'Can Compulsory Removal Ever Be Justified for Adults Who Are Mentally Competent?' (1991) 17 J Med Ethics 189.
9   J A M Gray 'Section 47 – Assault On or Protection Of the Freedom of the Individual?' 17 J Med Ethics 195.

The alternative procedures must also be considered critically. Foremost among these are the statutory provisions within the Mental Health Act 1983 and the Scottish equivalent of 1984. There are, first, the extensive powers available under s 135 (s 117 in Scotland (S)) whereby a justice, acting on information from an approved social worker, can authorise the police to enter and remove to a place of safety a mentally disordered person who is at risk and living alone (this can only be done in Scotland after a mental health officer or a medical commissioner has been refused entry). The subject can then be detained for only 72 hours and, unsurprisingly, the section is used very rarely.[10] Very much more important are the powers relating to compulsory admission to hospital for assessment (s 2 (s 24(S)) or for emergency assessment (s 4 (s 26(S)). These are discussed in greater detail in chapter 18; for the present it is necessary only to note that there would be little or no difficulty in invoking them in cases where s 47 was appropriate – indeed, the Mental Health Act is seen as the preferred route in an emergency.[11] We take the view, however, that committal under the 1983 and 1984 Acts inevitably classifies the elderly and confused as being mentally abnormal – and, to many, such classification represents a stigma. Despite the simultaneous provision of a recognised system of appeal, the use of what is, effectively, a ruse as a matter of administrative convenience seems to us to be more morally reprehensible than is the use of the more straightforward s 47.

The possibility of an application for guardianship remains[12] – the purpose being to empower the guardian, who may be the local authority, to dictate the place of residence of the disordered person. Once again, the practice is seldom adopted due, largely, to the fact that the essential function of a guardian is to maintain the incompetent in the community; to order removal to residential care is something of a contradiction in terms. Moreover, the guardian has no power to order treatment and the guardianship can be challenged by the subject's next of kin.

Thus, no current way of achieving compulsory residential care of the elderly is wholly satisfactory. The unfortunate result is that, in the majority of cases, legal process is avoided and the elderly person is 'talked into' abrogating his – or more commonly her – independent status.

The removal of an elderly person to a home or hospital does not, of course, solve all treatment dilemmas. He or she may, like any other, refuse to accept treatment. Compulsion from the legal point of view is out of the question, although, in practice, relatives and others may resort to pressure of various sorts to ensure compliance. The position of the doctor, though, is clear: treatment against the will of the patient could constitute an assault in criminal law or an actionable civil wrong. Thought should also be given to the moral inappropriateness of compelling treatment in such cases; few doctors would wish to force treatment upon a patient who is mentally competent and who does not want it.

The position of one who is dementing may, however, be different. Almost by definition, such a patient is unlikely to understand fully the nature of his condition

10 Section 136, which refers to persons in public places, is being used increasingly as residential patients are returned to community care as a matter of public policy.
11 E Murphy 'What to do with a Sick Elderly Woman Who Refuses to go to Hospital' (1984) 289 BMJ 1435.
12 Mental Health Act 1983, s 7.

and the treatment available. It might be argued that an analogy with the unconscious patient is applicable and, in that case, a doctor may justify the non-consensual treatment of his patient on the grounds of necessity or, alternatively, through the doctrine of implied consent. A dementing patient, however, is not unconscious. His comprehension may be affected by dementia but, equally, he may still be capable of holding and articulating views.[13] It might be better, then, to consider such treatment as an acceptable instance of paternalistic intervention of the sort under which children who are incapable of full understanding are treated. An implied consent rationale could be advanced, should specifically legal justification be called for.

The incompetent patient who is admitted to hospital under the Mental Health Acts may be treated compulsorily for the mental disorder which forms the basis of his admission. Treatment for other conditions is not permitted by the legislation unless it can be seen as being part of that which is appropriate for the mental disorder. This apparently restrictive attitude is compensated by the common law – the lawfulness of a doctor operating on, or giving other treatment to, an adult person disabled from giving consent would depend not on any approval or sanction of a court, but on the question whether the operation or other treatment was in the best interests of the patient concerned.[14]

Legal protection

Any demented person, and certainly anyone who needs compulsory admission to an institution, is unlikely to be able to manage his or her affairs. The law has, therefore, made special provision to ensure that the interests of incompetent elderly people are protected. In English law, the task of administering the affairs of such people may be performed by the Court of Protection. This court, which is an office of the Supreme Court of Judicature, has powers under the Mental Health Act to act on behalf of those who are incapable as a result of mental disorder, a category which would include those suffering from dementia. Application for the appointment of a receiver may be made by a relative or by some other person with a legitimate interest in the matter, including a creditor. During the period in which the receiver acts for the incapable person, the court exercises overall control and supervision of his activities.[15] In Scotland, where there is no comparable body solely concerned with these matters, the normal method of dealing with the affairs of an incompetent person is to petition the Court of Session for the appointment of a curator bonis, who carries out the same duties as a receiver in England. Neither the receiver nor the curator bonis has powers over the person of the incompetent, which means that neither would be able to authorise medical treatment on the incompetent person's behalf or to take

13 For an exhaustive study, see M J Gunn 'Treatment and Mental Handicap' (1987) 16 Anglo-Amer L Rev 242.
14 *Re F (mental patient: sterilisation)* [1990] 2 AC 1 at 55, sub nom *F v West Berkshire Health Authority* [1989] 2 All ER 545 at 551, per Lord Brandon, HL.
15 For powers of the Court of Protection, see *Re W (EEM)* [1971] Ch 123 at 143 per Ungoed-Thomas J. Statute, when enforced, will make a new provision for the appointment of an authorised representative with the power to negotiate on behalf of a disabled person with the local authority as to the general provision of welfare services (Disabled Persons (Services, Consultation and Representation) Act 1986).

any action with respect to the living conditions of their charge. In Scots law, the Court of Session has recently affirmed the persistence of its common law facility to appoint a tutor dative, who has such a power over the person, in respect of an adult incompetent; in one such instance, a couple successfully applied for tutorship of their mentally handicapped adult son.[16] There seems no reason why the principle should not be applied more extensively to the incompetent elderly – one advantage being that the powers of the tutor dative can be as limited or as broad as the Court of Session decides.

Outwith the context of these rather formal legal institutions, the law also takes some account of the particular situation of the elderly person. Contractual capacity may be denied to one who cannot understand the implications of a contract and contracts which are entered into by persons whose mind is affected by dementia may, of course, be set aside. Similarly, testamentary capacity is restricted to those who can comprehend the nature and extent of their estate and the claims which people may have upon them. In assessing such capacity, however, the law is not so much concerned to place a psychiatric label on a testator as to determine the impact which an apparent specific delusion may have on the contents of the will.[17]

The rules of testamentary capacity were developed with the interests of others in mind. The same focus of attention can be detected in the other areas of the law in which special regard has been paid to the needs of the elderly. Continuance of the property control arrangements which the elderly person himself has made may now extend beyond the onset of incompetence.[18]

The law protecting the elderly dementing person is, thus, well-intentioned but seriously fragmented; as a result, it is unsatisfactory from the view of both the patient and society. It is against this background that the influential group Scottish Action on Dementia has suggested a new approach via 'mental health panels', each of which would have a mental health reporter who would provide a 'one door' service to the public.[19] The concept and remit would be based on the successful children's panel system which oversees juvenile justice in Scotland. The advantages claimed for such a system are that it would establish a legal right to care and protection while maintaining respect for individual dignity; the existing juvenile procedure is there to be followed and it is one which entails full community awareness and involvement. While the notion is foreign to English thought, it may yet come to fruition north of the Border.

Ethical considerations

There remain for consideration the practical and ethical aspects of the treatment of geriatric patients. These are often discussed in the context of euthanasia which we deal with in chapter 15. The two issues can, however, be distinguished in that, while

16 A D Ward 'Revival of Tutors-dative' 1987 SLT 69. For further, general discussion, see A D Ward *The Power to Act* (1990).
17 *Banks v Goodfellow* (1870) LR 5 QB 549.
18 Enduring Powers of Attorney Act 1985. Similar arrangements are now available in Scotland: Law Reform (Miscellaneous Provisions) Act 1990, s 71.
19 R McCreadie 'Dementia and the Law: A Radical Approach' (1989) (supp) SJ 28.

it is true that many old persons may be suffering from terminal physical disease, an equal or greater number may be the victims of no more than intellectual deterioration; the greater part of geriatric medicine relates to the management of incurable, rather than of terminal, disease. If the patient's best interests represent the therapeutic yardstick – as they should – the inner world of the geriatric must be assessed subjectively and not related to the observer's own youthful or middle-aged experience. The demented but otherwise physically capable old person is not in pain and, for all we know, is passing a reasonably contented life. The parallel in controversial treatment issues is to be found in the uncomplicated Down's syndrome infant who, as we have already argued, is as entitled to medical treatment as is his mentally normal counterpart. Glib phrases such as 'pneumonia is the old man's friend' come easily to the lips in this discussion and can be dangerously emollient unless they are qualified; death may certainly be a blessed relief to the patient in severe pain but problems raised in the treatment, say, of intercurrent infection in the contented dement are of the same order as are those faced by the mentally competent – one wonders if the more honest aphorism is not that 'pneumonia in an old man is his associates' best friend'.

We would, therefore, disagree to an extent with those who, effectively, call for a policy which is generally biased towards non-treatment of the elderly demented patient on grounds of the 'quality of cognitive life'.[20] At one time, this was frequently expressed by including in the hospital notes the instruction 'do not resuscitate'; public reaction was such that the procedure was officially abandoned. Similar instructions to withhold resuscitative measures in the event of cardio-respiratory arrest are known as 'No-code orders' in the United States; their validity was considered in the important case of *Dinnerstein*[1] – a woman suffering from pre-senile dementia who had been so classified. The Appeal Court of Massachusetts took the view that doctors were under no obligation to defy their medical judgment in attempts to rescue patients who were dying naturally and that, in making such decisions, recourse to the courts was unnecessary.[2]

This case, relying, as does British policy, on good medical practice, emphasises the importance of considering each patient as an individual problem. Following our analogy with the newborn, there is a case to be made out for selective non-treatment of the aged – but selection must be based on the individual patient's circumstances rather than on unfeeling demographic rationalisation.[3] The issues crystallise in the place of the elderly in the allocation of resources which, as we have seen, is inevitable in an expanding medical technological ambience – and the arguments are finely balanced. The views of Callahan are particularly interesting in this context.[4] In brief, Callahan sees the need for objective planning if the otherwise certain breakdown in resources is to be avoided. The aged, it is said, have some claim to public funds but these are not unlimited – the goal is a balanced, affordable system of care for the

20 G S Robertson 'Ethical Dilemmas of Brain Failure in the Elderly' (1983) 287 BMJ 1775.
1 *Re Dinnerstein* 380 NE 2d 134 (Mass, 1978). See, for a general review, T A Brennan 'Do-not-resuscitate Orders for the Incompetent Patient in the Absence of Family Consent' (1986) 14 Law Med Hlth Care 13.
2 For attempts in the United States to codify the process, see T E Miller ' Do-Not-Resuscitate Orders: Public Policy and Patient Autonomy' (1989) 17 Law Med Hlth Care 245.
3 For a useful, brief discussion, see 'Do Doctors Short-change Old People?' (1993) 342 Lancet 1.
4 D Callahan *Setting Limits* (1987).

elderly which admits of a good balance between length and quality of life. Effectively, we should see ageing as an inevitable part of life and accept that society discharges its principal duty to the elderly by avoiding premature death. Callahan admits that any serious form of setting limits to treatment will be unpleasant but, since the possibilities of spending money in an attempt to turn old age into permanent middle age are infinite, we should impose an age limit upon ourselves. These views, needless to say, have attracted opposition particularly from those who see the welfare of the individual as transcending a policy of general societal benefit.[5] While we would agree that difficult decisions may have to be taken, we prefer the egalitarian philosophy which will avoid positive discrimination against the elderly.[6] Therapeutic decisions are intensely individual matters which cannot be covered by way of restrictive formulae; age may be one factor in the decision to treat but it cannot be the only factor.

Such problems may confront the surgeon with particular force; the application of the productive/non-productive test (see p 324) must always affect his decision whether or not to operate on the elderly. A negative response to advanced malignant disease may be a simple matter but the improvement in operative techniques is such that the results of elective general surgery in the aged, even of an advanced technological nature such as coronary artery replacement, may be both satisfactory and rewarding – the fact that results may be generally better in the young does not mean that the same procedure in the old is necessarily not worthwhile. It has, in addition, been suggested that relatively risky surgery, offering either good health or a quick death, may be particularly attractive to the old who should not be denied the choice.[7] In any event, it is relatively unlikely that considerations of productivity can be applied to an acute surgical emergency occurring in an elderly patient with no other mortal disease. The only acceptable test is then one of feasibility – there can seldom be an ethical alternative to treatment if it can be given but, inevitably, high morbidity and mortality rates must be accepted.[8]

The dilemma of what to do in the event that a geriatric patient refuses treatment appears to be less urgent in the United Kingdom than it is in the United States – a difference which possibly reflects that which separates the financial consequences of prolonged medical care in the two countries. There can be no doubt as to the rights of the competent adult to refuse treatment under both jurisdictions and these rights would certainly include opposition to forced feeding. The difficulty is that the borderline between competence and incompetence is often indistinct in old age.[9]

5   See, for example, R W Hunt 'A Critique of Using Age to Ration Health Care' (1993) 19 J Med Ethics 19.
6   M A Somerville ' "Should the Grandparents Die?": Allocation of Medical Resources with an Aging Population' (1986) 14 Law Med Hlth Care 158.
7   T Hope, D Sprigings and R Crisp ' "Not Clinically Indicated": Patients' Interests or Resource Allocation?' (1993) 306 BMJ 379.
8   J E Robb, I Murray and C MacKay 'Is Elective Surgery in the Elderly Worthwhile?' (1987) 32 Scot Med J 79; A V Pollock and M Evans 'Major Abdominal Operations on Patients Aged 80 and Over: An Audit' (1987) 295 BMJ 1522.
9   In an interesting unpublished paper, C Heginbotham 'Mental Disorder and Decision Making: Respecting Autonomy in Substitute Judgements' (1992) Paper presented to the UK Forum on Health Care Ethics and the Law, London, the author draws attention to the distinction between capacity, which hinges on cognitive and volitional attributes of the individual, and competence. Capacity, being a necessary, though insufficient, condition for competence is, thus, the more important.

Court judgments or decisions on the part of guardians may be sought in dramatic situations such as the removal of life-support but are unlikely to be invoked for apparently trivial matters like oral feeding; it is probable that many old people, no matter what their situation, are fed with a varying degree of force but the action is taken on the assumption that refusal to eat is non-volitional.   The process is degrading both to the staff and to the patient and, moreover, carries considerable hazard.   It is, however, difficult to see the alternative to compassionate and moderate coercion in such cases.   Positive refusal of treatment by the competent old person is a different matter and one which has attracted considerable attention in the courts of the United States.   There, the right to be let alone has been described as 'the most comprehensive of rights and the right most valued by civilised men'[10] and the courts have, in general, upheld such rights – perhaps the most apposite case being that concerning an 85-year-old, yet alert, man who frankly chose suicide by self-starvation in preference to medical care.[11]   The problem of the management of the partially competent geriatric who depends upon artificial feeding can be more difficult; this is well exemplified in the various stages of *Re Claire Conroy*[12] which we discuss in greater detail at p 340.   Here, it need only be noted that, although the appellate courts disagreed on the definition of medical treatment, both had misgivings as to the possible impact that the decision to abandon nasogastric feeding might have on the general treatment of the mentally handicapped.   Indeed, in attempting to resolve the ethical issues in this area, it has been rightly said that: Society should be wary of moving from a recognition of an individual's right to die to a climate of enforcing a duty to die.[13]   Our sympathy would be with Murphy[14] when she says that loss of dignity derives from the way that we care for our sufferers from dementia, not from the illness itself; the condition is a challenge to society's attitudes to the aged and is to be met by the provision of appropriate facilities.   Unfortunately, this is a counsel of perfection which, in the prevailing economic climate, is unlikely to be followed in the foreseeable future.   We have said it before and it remains true today – the aged have few friends and they cast even fewer votes.

10 *Griswold v Connecticut* 381 US 479 (1965).
11 *Re Plaza Health and Rehabilitation Center of Syracuse*, S Ct, Onandaga Cty, NY, 4 Feb 1984.
12 464 A 2d 303 (NJ, 1983), CA; 486 A 2d 1209 (NJ, 1985), SC. For an overview of US cases, see H L Hirsh and M K Cuneo 'Who shall Live, Who shall Die. Who Decides?' (1986) 5 Med Law 111. See also N Rhoden 'How Should We View the Incompetent?' (1989) 17 Law Med Hlth Care 264.
13 M Siegler and A J Wiesbard 'Against the Emerging Stream' (1985) 145 Arch Intern Med 129.
14 E Murphy 'Ethical Dilemmas of Brain Failure in the Elderly' (1984) 288 BMJ 61.

Death

13 The diagnosis of death

Death is defined in *Chambers Twentieth Century Dictionary* as 'the state of being dead; extinction or cessation of life'. *Steadman's Medical Dictionary* adds to this 'in multicellular organisms, death is a gradual process at the cellular level with tissues varying in their ability to withstand deprivation of oxygen'. There is, therefore, a conceptual conflict between layman and doctor, the latter being forced to accept an academic formula such as death being 'a permanent state of tissue anoxia'. Tissue anoxia arises naturally in two ways – either respiration ceases, in which case there is a failure to harvest oxygen, or the heart fails, when oxygen is no longer distributed to the tissues. In either case, the diagnostic problem lies in the definition of permanence.

In practice, it is astonishing how often the moment of 'death' is perfectly clear. One can tell immediately when a loved one or a carefully observed patient 'dies' in cardiorespiratory terms. The patient has 'breathed his last' and his heart stops beating; this is 'somatic' death. But the individual cells of the body are not dead; they will continue to function until their residual oxygen is exhausted. How long this takes depends upon their oxygen consumption which, in turn, is correlated with their specialised activity. Theoretically, therefore, there should be evidence of cellular death before the state of permanence is accepted but, in practice, the doctor can rely on his senses and on his stethoscope because death is to be expected and is accepted on the vast majority of occasions when it visits. Even so, one is left with the disquieting realisation that brain cells will withstand anoxia for a time, albeit for only a few minutes. If we are to accept the concept of 'brain death' as argued below, we should treat the patient in irreversible cardiorespiratory failure as dying rather than dead – for the true agonal period in natural death is that which lies between cardiac and cerebral failure.

But what if death is unheralded and unexpected? It is common knowledge that the apparent permanence of cessation of the respiration or blood flow can, in many instances, be challenged by physical or mechanical intervention. Thus, sudden heart failure due to the common 'coronary attack' may, in suitable cases, be reversed by electrical stimulation (cardioversion) or by cardiac massage coupled, perhaps, with artificial respiration or ventilation. But, while the patient has been 'saved from the dead', the process of cellular death has been initiated by the temporary failure of oxygen distribution. The majority of organs will recover from such an insult but the cells of the brain are outstandingly the most sensitive to oxygen deprivation in the body and, moreover, they are irreplaceable. Thus, a situation may arise whereby the body as a whole is brought back to life but where it is now controlled by a brain which is damaged to an uncertain degree. The decision to restore an interrupted cardiac function is not, therefore, a simple choice between the good – life – and the bad – death. It poses serious and urgent ethical problems which provide

281

a base from which to discuss the more measured, and in some ways more complicated, issues arising from ventilator deaths.

When death strikes unexpectedly on its second front – by way of acute respiratory failure – it may be countered by the use of artificial ventilation. This may be accomplished by a mechanical respirator which simulates the movements of the chest wall or, more commonly in the context of the present discussion, by a ventilator which forces air in and out of the lungs.

Brain function as a measure of death

The mechanisms underlying acute heart failure and respiratory failure need to be distinguished. Given an adequate oxygen supply, the heart will continue to beat independently of higher control – it did, for instance, commonly beat for some 20 minutes following the broken neck of judicial hanging; the cause of acute cardiac failure, therefore, lies within the heart itself. Respiration, on the other hand, is controlled by the respiratory centre – a nervous 'battery' situated in the brain stem. Moreover, now that acute anterior poliomyelitis ('infantile paralysis') has been virtually eradicated, there are very few extra-cerebral causes of acute respiratory failure that cannot be corrected by the ventilator. Acute respiratory failure of the type which is important in the present context is almost invariably the result of central damage – that is, damage to the brain stem. Oxygenation of the tissues, or cellular life, is thus based on a servo-type mechanism: the heart depends for its own tissue oxygen on the lungs which, in turn, are useless without the heart; together they supply oxygen to the brain which, therefore, cannot function in the absence of competent heart and lungs; the lungs are, themselves, dependent upon a functioning brain stem. The only segment of this triad which cannot be substituted is the brain. There are, therefore, strong logical arguments for defining death in terms of brain death rather than in the generally accepted terms of cardio-respiratory failure. Indeed, Pallis holds that all death is, and always has been, brain stem death and that circulatory arrest just happens to be the commonest way to bring such death about[1] – a point to which we have alluded in the introduction to this chapter. Be that as it may, it is clear that we *must* turn to the brain when the natural functional condition of the lungs – or, occasionally, of the heart – is obscured by the intervention of a machine.

The brain itself is not uniformly sensitive to hypoxia. Simplistically, it can be divided into three main areas: the cortex, which is responsible for our human intellectual existence and is the least able to withstand oxygen deficiency; the thalamus, which roughly regulates our animal existence; and the brain stem, which controls our purely vegetative functions including breathing. The brain stem is least affected by hypoxia; if it is so damaged, it can be assumed, as near certainly as is possible, that the rest of the brain is damaged to a similar or greater extent. Conditions producing hypoxia of the brain may be natural – eg heart failure or internal haemorrhage – or unnatural, including violence or drug overdose. The effect in either case will be general in nature and will affect all tissues of the body but to

1   C Pallis 'Return to Elsinore' (1990) 16 J Med Ethics 10.

an extent less than the brain – such a situation arises from 'shock' resulting from lowered blood pressure or from reduced oxygen intake due, say, to a poorly given anaesthetic. Other causative lesions may be localised within the skull and injure the brain in secondary fashion by occupying the confined space and, effectively, squeezing the vessels carrying the blood. Whatever the cause, the hypoxic damage is irreversible; but further damage is prevented once an efficient oxygen supply is restored. In such a situation, therefore, one can speak of *degrees* of brain damage and resultant coma but not of *stages* of coma because the condition is now no longer progressive. Clinical appearances in a person who is brain damaged but treated will vary with the degree of anoxic insult sustained. Four degrees of coma were recognised by the early French writers:[2] *coma vigile* which represents no more than a blurring of consciousness and intellect; *coma type* and *coma carus* which are characterised by increasing loss of relative functions followed by vegetative functions; and, finally, *coma depassé* – something beyond coma in which all functions are lost and the patient can only be maintained by artificial means.

Thus, while all appropriate cases may properly be given intensive care for the purposes of diagnosis and assessment, it would be well-nigh impossible to justify long-term treatment for a patient who was likely to end up with no cortical and minimal thalamic function remaining – and the identification of such a case presents a formidable technical dilemma.

The decorticated patient falls into the category originally defined by Jennett[3] as the persistent vegetative state – in layman's terms, the 'human vegetable'. Such a person – in whom the cerebral defect may be confined to the neocortex – will have periods of wakefulness but is, nevertheless, permanently unconscious; the state has been described as eyes-open unconsciousness.[4] It is clear that a human who has lost cortical function has, simultaneously, lost his human personality but, in so far as he is capable of existing without mechanical support, he is equally certainly not dead – indeed, he is in some ways more 'alive' than was the fully conscious sufferer from poliomyelitis who existed only by virtue of the respirator. There have been serious suggestions that the decorticated patient should be regarded as dead – may not *homo sapiens* be weakened in its own fight for survival if it devotes strength and resources to maintaining *homo* when he is no longer *sapiens*?[5] While these were very advanced views at the time they were expressed, the 'new wave' of thinking in terms of equating permanent loss of personality with no longer being alive is gaining momentum and relatively wide acceptance.[6] Such an attitude may be tenable in a general discussion on euthanasia – and we return to the subject in chapter 15 – but, when related to the fact of death, it can only confuse the issue and enhance the already strong public apprehension of 'premature grave robbery'; a particularly influential article, for example, concludes that, while neocortical death is compatible with our current concepts of death, it should not be introduced as public policy simply because

2 P Mollard and M Goulon 'Le Coma Depassé' (1959) 101 Rev Neurol 3.
3 B Jennett and F Plum 'Persistent Vegetative State after Brain Damage' (1972) 1 Lancet 734.
4 R E Cranford and D R Smith 'Consciousness: The Most Critical Moral (Constitutional) Standard for Human Personhood' (1987) 13 Amer J Law Med 233. The persistent vegetative state can be distinguished from coma or eyes-closed unconsciousness but this can, at times, be difficult to do.
5 Lord Scarman 'Legal Liability in Medicine' (1981) 74 J Roy Soc Med 11.
6 For a comparatively early exposition, see D R Smith 'Legal Recognition of Neocortical Death' (1986) 71 Cornell LR 850.

the general public would not understand the issues and it would be needlessly divisive for society.[7] We feel strongly that similar considerations should dictate one's attitudes to the anencephalic infant who, in some circumstances, may represent a naturally occurring persistent vegetative state and whose status we discuss more fully in chapter 14. Death must remain an absolute; there is no place for conditional phrases such as 'at death's door' or 'as good as dead'. The definition of death has not changed; and, if we are to alter our diagnostic methods, the diagnosis of death must be as sure as it was when we were using the heart and lungs as its sole parameters.[8]

It follows that, if we are to adjudge death by death of the brain, we must be certain that there is permanent physical damage to the whole brain. This principle has been unintentionally confused semantically by the Harvard group who introduced the term 'irreversible coma'.[9] One's first reaction would be to equate such a condition with the persistent vegetative state – or decorticated patient – but it is clear that the committee was describing what other Americans and, later, the British Royal Colleges dubbed 'brain death'.[10] Even this term is capable of misinterpretation – in particular, it can be taken as including 'partial brain death'. The alternative is to speak only in terms of 'brain stem death', a phrase which derives from the logical assumption that somatic life is impossible in the absence of a functioning brain stem.

Conceptual difficulties still remain which are concerned, for the most part, with such differences as there may be between 'brain stem death' and 'whole brain death'.[11] We are very doubtful if the distinction needs to be emphasised. Natural diseases in the form of destructive primary lesions of the brain stem which do not simultaneously affect the rest of the brain are rare and are either partial in type or, more commonly, rapidly fatal; the 'locked in' syndrome is probably the least uncommon and, certainly, the most terrifying but its existence is well appreciated by neurologists.[12] The only unnatural ways in which brain stem death can reasonably be expected in the presence of a normal cerebrum are following accident, judicial hanging or beheading – none of which are germane to the present discussion. For the rest, it is well-nigh impossible to conceive of a generalised, fundamentally hypoxic condition destroying the brain stem while sparing the highly specialised tissue of the cerebral cortex; and, even were this possible, continued attempts to maintain such a body artificially would be hopelessly non-productive and positively unethical. We believe that the common terms used to define the irreversible

7 R J Devettere 'Neocortical Death and Human Death' (1990) 18 Law Med Hlth Care 96. This paper also summarises the views of others in the field.
8 J M Stanley 'More Fiddling with the Definition of Death?' (1987) 13 J Med Ethics 21.
9 H K Beecher (Chairman) 'A Definition of Irreversible Coma', Report of the ad hoc Committee of the Harvard Medical School to examine the definition of brain death (1968) 205 J Amer Med Ass 337.
10 Conference of Medical Royal Colleges and their Faculties in the United Kingdom 'Diagnosis of Brain Death' [1976] 2 BMJ 1187.
11 C Pallis *ABC of Brain Stem Death* (1983).
12 J M S Pearce 'The Locked In Syndrome' (1987) 294 BMJ 198. For general discussion, see C M C Allen 'Conscious but Paralysed: Releasing the Locked-in' (1993) 17 Lancet 130.

cessation of all brain function – 'brain stem death' and 'whole brain death' – can be regarded as synonymous in both practice and theory.[13]

We do, however, accept that many misconceptions are founded on misunderstanding of the British standards for the diagnosis of brain stem death. These include three equally important phases. First, there is the exclusion of coma being due to reversible causes including drug overdose, hypothermia and metabolic disorders while, at the same time, making a positive diagnosis of the disorder which has caused the brain damage and ensuring that this, in turn, is irremediable. Second, there is the carrying out of a number of tests specifically designed to demonstrate destruction of the several components of the brain stem. Third, there is a carefully controlled system whereby a patient's inability to breath spontaneously is proved. These tests should be repeated although the recommendations are, of necessity, somewhat open on this point and depend, mainly, on the nature of the precipitating condition.

These criteria are sometimes criticised on the grounds that the patient is 'being asked to prove he is alive' rather than that the physician is proving death. Positive tests such as an electroencephalogram (EEG) or an angiogram – by which cessation of the blood flow in the brain can be visualised – are therefore sought and one or other is, indeed, mandatory in some countries of the European Community.[14] It is almost incredible that an EEG, which measures the surface electrical activity of the cerebral cortex, should be positive in the presence of properly performed confirmatory tests for brain stem death but there is no reason why such a test should not be added if it would serve to allay any fears among the next of kin as to the certainty of death.

There is little doubt that public misgiving would be lessened if the purposes of defining brain stem death were more fully understood. Certainly, it is a valuable tool in the provision of high quality organs for transplantation (see chapter 14) but this is only part of the story. The major purpose of the procedure is to establish a consensus through which patients who can no longer benefit can be removed from ventilator support. This is essential if the patient is to die with dignity, if the relatives are to be spared wholly unnecessary suffering and if resources, both mechanical and human, are to be properly apportioned. Accepting brain stem death is not a way of 'hurrying death along'; rather, the ventilator allows the pace of investigation, assessment and prognosis to be slackened; when it comes to the point, the diagnosis of brain stem death is, in the great majority of cases, only confirming what is clear from clinical observation – that the patient is dead.

In view of the very widespread international agreement that exists, it came as something of a surprise to find the Danish Council of Ethics rejecting the principle

---

13 This is often the case in practice. Victorian legislation, for example, speaks in terms of irreversible cessation of all function of the brain (Human Tissue Act 1982, s 41) while, at the same time assessing this using tests for death of the brain stem – and this is acceptable: J L Dixon (chairperson) Parliament of Victoria Social Development Committee *Report upon the Inquiry into Options for Dying with Dignity* (1987).

14 Pallis, see fn 11 above, quoted France, Greece and Italy as so requiring. The United Kingdom, Eire, Belgium, Germany and the Netherlands are said to accept medical criteria alone as being diagnostic of brain stem death. Among countries in which there is specific legal recognition of the brain as an indicator of death are at least 33 of the United States, Canada and the States of Australia although this relates only to transplantation procedures in Queensland and Western Australia.

of brain death in 1989.[15] It may well be that the council has no political power but its observations are useful to look at as an example of the confused thinking which sometimes attaches to the issue. Reduced to a summary, the council's view is that death should be defined in terms of what a particular community regards as death – few people, it states, would refer to a warm, pink body as a corpse; the loss of brain function should be regarded as the irreversible onset and that of cardiac function as the termination of the process of death. Clearly, such a formula can apply only when the patient is maintained on a ventilator and, even within that limited parameter, it positively excludes cardiac transplantation as an ethically acceptable procedure. More dangerously, it tends to perpetuate a suspicion that different concepts of death are being used by the profession and the public and that special criteria apply in association with transplantation.[16] Understanding, or its lack, lies at the root of the problem. Evans, who is a major opponent of the brain stem death concept, has suggested that our moral convictions stand independent of rational account or explanation[17] – and has been criticised for, thereby, rendering philosophical inquiry superfluous.[18] Yet, in simply calling for better 'education' of the public, it is easy to overlook or to minimise the importance of religious and cultural traditions. Transplant operations involving brain dead donors are performed only exceptionally in Japan and a major reason for this must lie in the unique attitude to death that is widely held in that country. The Japanese medical profession, itself, may share some responsibility for the failure to recognise brain stem death; even so, one feels that caution should prevail before centuries of cultural tradition are swept aside in the name of modern medical technology.[19]

Perhaps we *are* 'fiddling with definitions' and should, rather, concentrate on what it is or is not ethical to do with a dying or a dead body. Gillett[20] has summarised the situation in that we do not and cannot require to prolong a life that will never again be engaged with the world; that we require that life to be terminated decently; and that we require that human remains should be treated with respect – and there is much to commend this rationalisation. Within such a framework, the problems of removal from the ventilator become technical rather than ethical. It has been advised that the diagnosis of brain stem death should be made by two doctors, one of whom should be the consultant in charge of the case and the other suitably experienced and clinically independent of the first,[1] but there is no United Kingdom law on the point.

15 B A Rix 'Danish Ethics Council Rejects Brain Death as the Criterion of Death' (1990) 16 J Med Ethics 5.
16 For further commentary on the Danish recommendations, see R Gillon 'Death' (1990) 16 J Med Ethics 3 and D Lamb 'Wanting It Both Ways' (1990) 16 J Med Ethics 8.
17 M Evans 'A Plea for the Heart' (1990) 3 Bioethics 227; 'Death in Denmark' (1990) 16 J Med Ethics 191.
18 D Lamb 'Death in Denmark: A Reply' (1991) 17 J Med Ethics 100.
19 For discussion, see J Nudeshima 'Obstacles to Brain Death and Organ Transplantation in Japan' (1991) 338 Lancet 1063; M Takao 'Brain-death and Transplantation in Japan' (1992) 340 Lancet 1164; K Hoshino 'Legal Status of Brain Death in Japan: Why Many Japanese Do Not Accept "Brain Death" as a Definition of Death' (1993) 7 Bioethics 234.
20 G Gillett 'Fiddling and Clarity' (1987) 13 J Med Ethics 23. For a rather similar US view, see D Wickler and A J Weisbard 'Appropriate Confusion over "Brain Death"' (1989) 261 J Amer Med Ass 2246.
 1 Lord Smith (Chairman of Working Party) *The Removal of Cadaveric Organs for Transplantation: A Code of Practice* (1979). There is such legislation, for example, in the Australian States and in South Africa (eg Transplantation and Anatomy Act 1983 (South Australia), s 24). A very useful protocol for the diagnosis of brain stem death is to be found in M D O'Brien 'Criteria for Diagnosing Brain Stem Death' (1990) 301 BMJ 108.

The legal effect of applying brain stem death criteria

The application of brain stem death criteria has obvious implications as to causation in cases of unlawful killing. But any difficulties disperse once it is conceded that brain stem death means somatic death.[2] It then becomes clear that the effect of intensive treatment has been simply to delay the inevitable result of the initial insult to the brain and there is no break in the chain of causation. This was accepted, first, in America in *People v Lyons*[3] where it was found that the victim of a shooting incident was legally dead before being used as a transplant donor. The British position has been summed up in two leading cases which are discussed further in chapter 15. Thus, in Scotland, it was held:

> Once the initial reckless act causing injury has been committed, the natural consequence which the perpetrator must accept is that the victim's future depended on a number of circumstances, including whether any particular treatment was available and, if it was available, whether it was medically reasonable and justifiable to attempt it and to continue it.[4]

The later English decision was fully confirmatory:

> Where a medical practitioner, using generally acceptable methods, came to the conclusion that the patient was for all practical purposes dead and that such vital functions as remained were being maintained solely by mechanical means, and accordingly discontinued treatment, that did not break the chain of causation between the initial injury and the death.[5]

It is therefore clear that the law has no intention of regarding doctors who remove a brain stem dead patient from the ventilator as being, thereby, responsible for his death.

Although it is doubtful if it was needed, there is now case law which confirms the medical view that persons whose brain stems are dead are, themselves, dead. In the unusual case of *Re A*[6] – in which the parents of a child sought to have him retained on a ventilator for medico-legal reasons – the judge made a declaration that A, who had been certified as brain stem dead, was dead for all legal as well as all medical purposes and that a doctor who disconnected the apparatus was not acting unlawfully; the fact of death was emphasised when the judge held that he had no inherent jurisdiction over a dead child who could not be made a ward of court for the same reason.

The major legal problem still outstanding relates to the precise time that death occurs in such circumstances; there are several issues which depend upon that determination, some of which are likely to cause difficulties in the future.

---

2 Conference of Royal Medical Colleges and their Faculties in the United Kingdom 'Diagnosis of Death' (1979) 1 BMJ 332.
3 Sup Ct No 56072, Alameda Co (Cal, 1974).
4 *Finlayson v H M Advocate* 1978 SLT (Notes) 60 at 61, per Lord Emslie LJ-G.
5 *R v Malcherek; R v Steel* [1981] 2 All ER 422 at 428-429, CA, per Lord Lane LCJ.
6 [1992] 3 Med LR 303.

Lawyers may be inclined to dismiss the problem of when death occurs on the assumption that the time of death can be equated to the time the diagnosis is made or to the time the ventilator support is removed. But a moment's reflection makes it clear that the diagnosis of brain stem death, and the consequent ending of treatment, must be retrospective – death has already occurred and the precise time at which it occurred is unknown and unknowable. Moreover, the choice of the time at which the necessary tests are undertaken is as likely to be based on the criterion of convenience as on anything else. It is difficult to see how the doctor can conscientiously certify the 'date and time of death' but it is easy to think of occasions on which he might be called upon to do so urgently.

The prospect of a victim of violence being ventilated and declared alive or dead either 364 or 366 days after the incident, and, thereby, affecting the possibility of a charge of murder in England, is commonly raised but the idea of such treatment is unreal and the problem must be of academic interest only. Time related factors in the payment of or withholding of life or personal accident insurance policies are far nearer to the mark; one example could concern the application of a suicide clause which would be lifted on a given day. Problems as to the payment of estate duty might also arise.

But the most intractable issue would seem to be that related to succession and the possibility of disputed survival. What is to be said as to the deaths of a husband and wife who are injured in the same accident, who are both ventilated and who are both declared brain stem dead? One thing is certain – survivorship cannot be judged on the basis of the technical diagnosis because the order in which death is determined could well be purely arbitrary. To remove ventilator support from both simultaneously and measure the time for the individual heart to stop beating would be confusing and would raise considerable difficulties in those jurisdictions which allow for *alternative* means of diagnosing death (see below); it is essential to hold on to the premise that the patients have been certified as being *already* dead. It would be wholly illogical to vary one's criteria to accommodate a specific situation – alternative methods in diagnosis are acceptable but double standards of death are not.[7] The rules of succession are bound by statute and, accordingly, this is one aspect of brain stem death which could be subject to legislative action. It seems to us that a positive solution to 'ventilated commorientes' is currently impossible; but a negative direction on the lines that evidence as to the time of removal of ventilator support cannot, by itself, be regarded as sufficient to rebut the statutory presumptions might, at least, be equitable and, at the same time, relieve the doctor of one moral problem.

The ethical position of the doctor
Thus, while we have said that the act of terminating treatment once brain stem death is diagnosed is a technical problem which raises no ethical issues, the time at which this is done unfortunately does so. It is facile merely to remark that the doctor's decisions should be uninfluenced by extraneous factors because, in practice, he can

---

7   See P D G Skegg *Law, Ethics, and Medicine* (1984), ch 9; D Lamb 'Wanting It Both Ways' (1990) 16 J Med Ethics 8.

scarcely avoid being aware of them – and influence is inseparable from awareness. The moral problems posed, say, by insistent pressure from relatives concerned for an insurance policy could be insoluble. A further question arises in respect of how long can a corpse be kept in a state of cellular preservation while still maintaining an acceptable ethical standard. For how long, for example, would it be proper to await a suitable heart transplant recipient? A number of press reports have spoken of brain stem dead women being retained on support for several weeks for the sole purpose of bringing a fetus to viability – it seems, in fact, that four healthy babies have been born as a result. Nevertheless, the basis for these deserves scrutiny – the more extreme are inconsistent with the view that the heart cannot be kept beating for more than a few days after brain stem death has occurred[8] and some doubts as to the diagnosis are inevitable. The most recent example from Germany concerned an unmarried 18-year-old who was only 15 weeks pregnant; the hospital ethics committee (see chapter 16) recommended continuation of the pregnancy – a decision which was, in our view surprisingly, widely supported by all other than women's groups. The fetus did not survive. The President of the Federal Chamber of Physicians is reported as commenting: 'Due to scientific advances, medicine will, again and again, have to infringe ethical borders';[9] the alternative view, which we share, sees such actions as incremental nudges which may, ultimately, push this branch of medicine into areas of doubtful morality unless they are held firmly in check.

The case for legislation

For these and many other reasons, the case for a modern statutory definition of death has been widely canvassed and is applied in many jurisdictions.

The main difficulty in framing legislation is to allow for all modes of death – from the elementarily obvious to the complex ventilator case; it would be absurd to demand that criteria designed for the latter be applied to the former. As a result, most statutes, either existing or proposed, have applied some form of dual criteria of proof of death.[10] A typical expression is to be found in the United States Uniform Determination of Death Act 1980 which reads:

> An individual who has sustained either (1) irreversible cessation of circulatory and respiratory functions, or (2) irreversible cessation of all functions of the entire brain, including the brain stem, is dead. A determination of death must be made in accordance with accepted medical standards.

8 See B Jennett, J Gleave and P Wilson 'Brain Death in Three Neurological Units' (1981) 282 BMJ 533.
9 H L Karcher 'German Doctors Struggle to Keep 15 Week Fetus Viable' (1992) 305 BMJ 1047; A Tuffs 'Keeping a Brain-dead Pregnant Woman "Alive"' (1992) 340 Lancet 1029.
10 D W Meyers *Medico-Legal Implications of Death and Dying* (1981) divides State statutes in the USA into three categories: those which provide for brain death as an express alternative to heart-lung oriented death, those which admit the use of brain-based criteria when a cardio-respiratory diagnosis is obviated by artificial maintenance and those which recognise brain death simply as a means of determining or defining death. All States have now adopted brain death either by statute or by court recognition.

And, as an example of Commonwealth legislation, we quote the Human Tissue Act 1982 (Victoria), s 41:

A person has died when there has occurred:

(a) Irreversible cessation of the circulation of the blood in the body of the person, or

(b) Irreversible cessation of all functions of the brain of the person.

There are similar provisions in the Human Tissue Act 1983 (NSW), s 33.

But, in essence, all these measures do is to spell out good medical practice within a legal framework – and many would feel this to be unnecessary. They lay down no specific methods – these being relegated to codes of practice – and this, we believe, is rightly so; we would certainly agree with the great majority of commentators that any statutory definition of death must be limited to an enabling concept. Medical facilities and expertise alter and do so faster than can the law; it is, therefore, essential that the evaluation of diagnostic techniques remains in the hands of the medical profession. In fact, the ethical, philosophical and social problems inherent in the definition of death seem to have been largely solved in recent years;[11] definitive legislation might do little more than reanimate concerns which have long been put to rest and might, as a result, be self-defeating.

11 C Pallis 'Return to Elsinore' (1990) 16 J Med Ethics 10.

14 The donation of organs and transplantation

The juxtaposition of chapters on the diagnosis of death and on transplantation of organs should not be taken to indicate that they are *necessarily* associated. It is again emphasised that the concept of brain stem death is as important to neurosurgeons, who can now allow their hopeless patients to die in peace, and to the relatives, who can now accept the fact of death with good conscience, as it is to the transplant surgeon. Nevertheless, and despite the relatively recent introduction of new techniques to which we refer later, optimum transplantation – and, with it, maximum saving of lives – depends upon the acceptance of brain stem death; furthermore, the two conditions are closely linked in the public mind. This is, therefore, a not inappropriate point at which to discuss the ethics and legality of a procedure which is now firmly established as accepted medical treatment – transplantation is agreed to be the most cost-effective treatment of end-stage renal disease. Nevertheless, the process still provokes some public disquiet.

Technical aspects of transplantation
There are three major biological hurdles to be overcome in successful transplantation therapy – neutralising the 'tissue immunity' reaction, ensuring that the donated organs are healthy and preserving the viability of those organs in the period between their becoming available and their reception.

A tissue immunity reaction results from the recognition by the body of antigenically foreign material which it will then reject with a degree of determination which depends, to a large extent, on *how* different is the donated tissue from that of the recipient. From this point of view, we can distinguish three main forms of the procedure:

(a) Autotransplantation, or the resiting of portions of the same body. This is effectively limited to skin or bone grafting and poses only the difficulties of highly complex surgery. It is of no concern in the present context.

(b) Homotransplantation, or allografting, which involves the transfer of viable tissue from one human being to another.

(c) Heterotransplantation, or xenografting – that is, the successful transplantation of organs from one species to another.

In the previous edition of this book, we referred to xenografting as being, currently, a practical impossibility and we dismissed a well-publicised attempt in 1984 to transplant a baboon's heart into a human neonate[1] as being so doomed to

1   L L Hubbard 'The Baby Fae Case' (1987) 6 Med Law 385.

failure as to have no practical significance in a discussion of organ replacement therapy. It is doubtful if one should be so cavalier today. The increasing sophistication of immunosuppressant drugs and of immunosuppressant techniques is changing the scene to the extent that a man has survived for 70 days following the transplantation of a baboon's liver.[2] Non-human primates are, however, unsatisfactory as reservoirs of functional organs for many reasons and attention has shifted further to the use of animals which have even less antigenic similarities to man such as the pig.[3] Modern molecular biological techniques have already produced 'transgenic' pigs in which at least one of the mechanisms leading to graft rejection appears to have been eliminated[4] and there is little doubt that clinical trials using such organs will be in train by the time any further edition of our book appears. All of which may be good scientific medicine but, like so many such 'advances', it raises both intuitive and philosophical doubts. Undoubtedly, there is a 'gut' distaste for being maintained by a porcine heart. More importantly, one must wonder at the morality of maintaining and, worse, breeding animals for the express purpose of substituting human bodies until the human brain disintegrates. The simple response that this is no different from eating pork in order to avoid starvation seems unsatisfactory. We feel, however, that the subject – which should include an analysis of the philosophy of speciesism – is too wide for a book of this type. No xenografts have been performed in the United Kingdom; it is to be noted that current government policy on the subject is cautious but not exclusive.[5]

Our concern in this chapter, however, is with homotransplantation or organ replacement as it is generally understood. Here, despite the fact that we are dealing with tissues from the same species, an immunity problem persists because, for practical purposes, no two persons other than monovular twins are genetically identical; the body can still recognise, and will reject, tissues of the same species which are 'non-self'.[6] This intra-species immune reaction can be increasingly well suppressed with the use of the cyclosporine group of drugs and monoclonal antibodies. The general principle remains, however, that such suppression will be effective – and will have less adverse side effects – in proportion to the genetic similarity of donor and recipient. Thus, sibling donation will be especially satisfactory and intrafamilial exchanges in general are likely to show less antigenic discrepancies than are those between random strangers. Other variables, however, intrude and complicate the picture. Immunosuppression is non-specific; therefore, while the graft rejection process is being controlled, other desirable immune reactions – such as the body's defence against microbiological invasion – are also affected. Moreover, the greater the *quantity* of foreign material transplanted, the greater will be the need for immunosuppression and, as a corollary, micro-organisms that are, normally, resisted with ease are increasingly able to establish themselves in the vulnerable

---

2   T E Starzl, J Fung, A Tzakis et al 'Baboon-to-human Liver Transplantation' (1993) 341 Lancet 65. Even so, we remain unconvinced that such a result should be classified as a success.
3   See, for example, D White and J Wallwork 'Xenografting: Probability, Possibility, or Pipe Dream?' (1993) 342 Lancet 879.
4   A James 'Transplants with Transgenic Pig Organs?' (1993) 342 Lancet 45.
5   219 HC Official Report (6th series) col 80, 15 February 1993.
6   The alternative – where the transplanted material attacks the host – is a difficulty of bone marrow transplantation. See A M Denman 'Graft versus Host Disease: New Versions of Old Problems?' (1985) 290 BMJ 658.

body; the most specifically significant of these are viruses which are responsible for certain forms of malignant disease of the lymphoid system. Enhanced success of transplantation therapy is not, therefore, simply a matter of discovering more powerful immunosuppressants.

It is axiomatic that an organ intended as a replacement for a diseased tissue must be normal itself. The practical result is that donors should be relatively young and they must either be living or have died from accident or from localised natural disease which has no effect on the donated tissue. This implies a pragmatic limitation on the age of the donor but this is higher than might be expected – 70 in the case of kidneys, 50 for livers and 40 for donors of hearts[7] – and may be extended.

Viability is that essential element which combines most clearly the technical and ethical problems of transplantation surgery. As has been discussed above, the cells of the body will deteriorate when deprived of oxygen; the process of deterioration can be slowed markedly by chilling the organ, the viability, or competence, of which then depends on the 'warm anoxic time' – that is, the interval between cessation of the circulation and chilling of the specimen. In terms of practical transplantation, it becomes increasingly pointless to transplant a kidney after more than one hour's warm anoxia. Even so, the acceptable cold anoxic time is also finite and varies with the tissue involved – not only as regards its metabolic activity but also as to the urgency with which it must assume full function after transplantation; the heart and lungs can be used up to four hours after harvesting, the liver up to 8-12 hours and the kidneys can be maintained in vitro for more than 24 hours.[8] Imposed delays must, therefore, jeopardise the validity of the operation.[9]

It will be evident that organs can be provided for transplantation by the living or by the dead. Living donation offers many technical advantages – tissue compatibility can be measured at leisure, the operation can be elective and the warm anoxic time can approach zero. In theory, potential cadaver donors are widely available but, in practice, their recovery is capricious and both donor and recipient operations must take on the character of emergency surgery. The recognition of brain stem death, however, offers the possibility of a variation on cadaver donation – the 'beating heart donor' – which bridges the gap between the living and the conventionally dead and carries with it many of the advantages of both types of donor. The legal and ethical limitations of all three methods must be considered.

The living donor

The donation of tissues which can be replaced rapidly – such as blood and bone marrow – presents, in practice, few technical or ethical problems other than that of

---

7   W B Ross 'Increasing Organ Donation – A Review' (1989) 34 Scott Med J 451.
8   J Wallwork 'Organs for Transplantation' (1989) 299 BMJ 1291.
9   Cold perfusion of the whole body or of individual organs in situ is now used to reduce these difficulties. The non-heart beating donor may be returning and improving the supply of organs. J P Cachera, D Y Loisance, O Tavolaro et al ' Hypothermic Perfusion of the Whole Cadaver: A Response to the Question of the Multiple-organ Donor' (1986) 18 Transplant Proc 1407; G Kootstra, R Wijnen, J P van Hooff and C J van der Linden 'Twenty Percent More Kidneys through a Non-heart Beating Program' (1991) 23 Transplant Proc 910.

commercialism to which we refer below. We are concerned here only with non-regenerative tissues.

The legal regulation of living donations in the United Kingdom lies in both common and statute law. As to the former, the starting-point must be the principle that no person is to be deemed capable of consenting to his being killed or seriously injured. The living donation of a heart is, thereby, precluded. This, of course, is the extreme case and, beyond it, legality would depend upon the presumed risk-benefit ratio involved in the procedure – and assessment of this is difficult because the technological boundaries of medicine are always expanding. A few years ago, one would have said the same about the liver as about the heart; today, the use of segments of adult liver in paediatric transplantation therapy is so far beyond the experimental stage that a leading American surgeon can say: 'We estimate that maybe 50 per cent of our paediatric liver transplants will be done that way'.[10] None the less, ethical problems – especially as to the relative risks and benefits to donor and recipient – abound and must now be applied to live donation of lung tissue where perhaps the main precautionary principle should be that live donation of this severity should be used only to supplement cadaver donation.[11] The common law legality and morality of live organ donations which will not necessarily cause grave harm to the donor is now very largely settled. It can be accepted that consent to a surgical operation which is, in itself, non-therapeutic will be valid so long as the consequent infliction of injury can be shown to be in the public interest.[12]

The statutory regulation of live donation is to be found in the Human Organ Transplants Act 1989[13] which creates an offence if a live organ transplant between persons who are not genetically related is undertaken without the agreement of the Unrelated Live Transplant Regulatory Authority (s 2)[14] – an organ being defined as tissue that cannot be replicated. Section 2(2) defines a genetic relationship. This can be so wide – it includes, for example, uncles and aunts by half blood – as to raise the suspicion that family loyalties are preferred to genetic niceties.[15]

An indication of the difficulties involved in attempted statutory control of such a dynamic field as medicine is provided by what is known as the 'domino transplant'. In the treatment of cystic fibrosis, for example, it is clinically more satisfactory to

---

10 G McBride 'Living Liver Donor' (1989) 299 BMJ 1417.   See also P A Singer, M Siegler, P F Whitington et al (1989) 'Ethics of Liver Transplantation with Living Donors' (1989) 321 New Engl J Med 620; C E Droelach, P F Whitington, J C Emond et al 'Liver Transplantation in Children from Living Related Donors' (1991) 214 Ann Surg 428.

11 L R Shaw, J D Miller, A S Slutsky et al 'Ethics of Lung Transplantation with Live Donors' (1991) 338 Lancet 678.

12 *R v Coney* (1882) 8 QBD 534. The obiter remarks of Denning LJ in *Bravery v Bravery* [1954] 1 WLR 1169 at 1180 have been endorsed in *A-G's Reference (No 6 of 1980)* [1981] QB 715, [1981] 2 All ER 1057.

13 An Order in Council made under the Northern Ireland Act 1974 extends the conditions to Northern Ireland.

14 See also particularly Human Organ Transplants (Establishment of Relationship) Regulations 1989 (SI 1989/2107) and Human Organ Transplants (Unrelated Persons) Regulations 1989 (SI 1989/2480).

15 But the fictional paternity and maternity criteria laid down in the Human Fertilisation and Embryology Act 1990, ss 27-29 (see p 55) do not apply for the purposes of the section. It is, however, fair to say that not everyone is uncritical of the current restrictions, eg M Evans 'Organ Donation Should not be Restricted to Relatives' (1989) 15 J Med Ethics 17.

use a heart/lung preparation obtained from a cadaver rather than a lung alone; this leaves the live recipient's heart available for donation. This would almost certainly be used in a non-related context and, thus, would theoretically be illegal without the specific agreement of the statutory authority; yet, so far as we are aware, the lawfulness of such an operation has never been challenged – and nor should it be.

Currently, some 12% of kidney transplants derive from living donors in the United Kingdom and the proportion is far higher in the United States.[16] There can, therefore, be no doubt that the removal of a kidney from a live donor for the purpose of saving the life of a seriously ill patient is covered by the 'public interest' provision and is perfectly legal.[17] This presupposes that the donor is an adult capable of giving a free and rational consent to the operation (see chapter 10). Living donation by children or by the mentally incompetent raises a number of thorny issues – and these reappear in slightly different guise in relation to payment for donations.

The minor as a donor

Donation from children is required surprisingly often and, clearly, the advantages of live donation will apply here as well as they will in the adult situation. The legality of such operations on children below the age of 16 has not been decided by British courts and the issue must thus be considered in the light of the general legal principles applied to the medical treatment of minors. As discussed in chapter 10, consent to an operation on a minor below the age of 16 years should normally be obtained from the parents, subject only to the possible common law rights of the child.[18] Valid parental consent, however, refers to treatment for the advantage of the child; troublesome questions arise in relation to procedures which are not calculated to be to his or her benefit – does parental consent in such circumstances constitute an abuse of parental power?

It has been argued that the principle that a minor cannot legally be subjected to any procedure which is not to his advantage is not an absolute one. It is also possible that a court might consider that the donation of an organ is not only in the public interest but is also in the interest of the minor donor, who will, almost certainly, be a sibling of the recipient. In such circumstances, it might be supposed that it is in the interests of the minor that a member of his family should be saved rather than that his relative should die. This line of argument was successfully pursued in the important American decision in *Strunk v Strunk*.[19] In this case, the donor, who,

16 G D Chisholm 'Time to End Softly Softly Approach on Harvesting Organs for Transplantation' (1988) 296 BMJ 1419.

17 It should be noted that live donation is the preferred method in some societies. In Japan, for example, where, as discussed at p 286, the concept of brain stem death is unacceptable, some 70% of donations are of live type. Virtually all transplants in India are 'live' but this is probably an administrative rather than cultural consequence (see below, p 300).

18 P D G Skegg 'English Law relating to Experimentation on Children' (1977) 2 Lancet 754 took the view that the Family Law Reform Act 1969, s 8 has no application to non-therapeutic procedures and that the rules of non-statutory law do not vary with different categories of persons. The wider implications of *Gillick v West Norfolk and Wisbech Area Health Authority* [1986] AC 112, [1985] 3 All ER 402, HL have been discussed in ch 10.

19 445 SW 2d 145 (Ky, 1969). Although this decision has been applied in other cases, it may not always be so – see *Lausier v Pescinski* 226 NW 2d 180 (Wise, 1975), another case involving a mentally handicapped donor.

although adult, had a mental age of six, was chosen to donate a kidney to his brother who was critically ill. The court came to the conclusion it would be in the donor's best interests for his brother's life to be saved after hearing evidence of the close relationship which existed between the two boys. Consequently, the operation was allowed although the donor was not in a position to give consent.

Other jurisdictions have been less ready to allow the taking of organs from minors. In Canada, for instance, the Ontario Human Tissue Gift Act provides an example of statutory prohibition of donation by minors.[20] A policy of limitation was advised by the Australian Law Reform Commission in their report on transplantation. The commission took the view that the donation by minors of non-regenerative tissue should not be forbidden without exception but that the circumstances in which it should be allowed should be circumscribed. The enabling conditions were suggested as being: when the donor and recipient are members of the same immediate family; when there is independent medical evidence that the prospective recipient will die unless the transplant is carried out; where the parents of the donor (or those in loco parentis) agree to the donation; where the donor has sufficient mental capacity and agrees to the donation; and, finally, when an ad hoc committee consisting of a judge and two other persons comes to the conclusion that the donation is desirable and in the interests of the donor. In the event, none of the individual States accepted this proposal and, instead, applied some of the qualifications to the donation of *regenerative* tissue; it is not lawful in Australia to remove non-regenerative material from the body of a living child for the purpose of transplantation.[1]

While the complete exclusion of minor donors would seem to many to be too extreme, there are powerful reasons why some limits should be placed on the use of children as donors of non-regenerative tissue and very great caution should be exercised in the case of young children in whom there is unlikely to be any significant understanding of what the donation entails. Even if a minor shows a reasonable degree of understanding of the donation and of the risks involved, a sharp distinction is to be made between instances when the recipient is a member of the immediate family and when he is not. It would probably be regarded as ethically acceptable for a minor to be used as a donor in the former case; generosity towards a brother or sister is to be encouraged and may even be regarded as a social duty.[2] The situation is less clear with relatives other than siblings. Should one apply the same rule to a situation where the prospective recipient is a cousin in the first degree? It is possible that the minor donor may be as fond of such a cousin as he is of a brother or sister and the illness of the cousin may be as distressing to him as would be the illness of a sibling. Nevertheless, a policy of limiting approved donation by minors to the immediate family has the attraction of certainty and, in practice, the clinical limitations must be taken into account – donation to an adoptive brother, for example, would be ethically suspect simply because, other than by chance, genetic incompatibility might compromise the success of the operation.

20 B M Dickens *Medico-legal Aspects of Family Law* (1979), p 96.
1   See, for exmple, Human Tissue and Transplant Act 1982, ss 12, 13 (Western Australia). The Human Tissue Act 1983, s 10 (NSW) forbids it by omission.
2   L F Ross 'Moral Grounding for the Participation of Children as Organ Donors' (1993) 21 J Law Med Ethics 251 introduces the interesting concept of the family as an autonomous unit which can aspire to a collective purpose. Intrafamilial donation by a child advances the family's interests, which is a means of promoting the child's own interests.

The law in France[3] illustrates an acceptable compromise statutory position. There, a living minor may only donate to his brother or sister; consent must be given by the donor's legal representative; and the procedure must be authorised by a committee composed of at least three experts two of whom must be doctors, one of whom must have practised for 20 years. If the minor can be consulted, refusal on his part must be respected in all cases. The caution shown by countries subject to both common and civil law jurisdictions is noteworthy and, while statute is either ambivalent or silent on the matter in the United Kingdom, some clarification of the current legal position here has come recently from the Court of Appeal.

The case of *Re W*[4] dealt with consent to treatment by a 16-year-old and was concerned, in the main, with the application of the Family Law Reform Act 1969, s 8(1) (already discussed in greater detail at p 228). The problem of organ transplantation was not in issue but was touched upon by the Master of the Rolls; his views must, we feel, be regarded as obiter but are, nevertheless, persuasive. Lord Donaldson first disposed of the statute on the grounds that the section related to treatment and diagnosis; it could not, therefore, extend to the donation of organs as this did not constitute either condition in respect of the donor. He went on:

> Organ donations are quite different and, as a matter of law, doctors would have to secure the consent of someone with the right to consent on behalf of a donor under the age of 18 or, if they relied on the consent of the minor himself or herself, be satisfied that the minor was 'Gillick competent' in the context of so serious a procedure which would not benefit the minor.[5]

As to the latter, he added, somewhat equivocally: 'This would be a highly improbable conclusion.' The whole passage is, in fact, a trifle confusing as, logically, '*Gillick* competence' applies only to the under 16-year-old whereas s 8(1) of the Act relates to the 16 to 18-year-old. The issue is, however, clarified in a later statement:

> It is inconceivable that [the doctor] should proceed in reliance solely upon the consent of an under-age patient, however 'Gillick competent', in the absence of supporting parental consent and equally inconceivable that he should proceed in the absence of the patient's consent. In any event he will need to seek the opinions of other doctors and may be well advised to apply to the court for guidance . . .[5]

Thus, it would seem that no person in England below the age of 18 can give reliable consent to donation of non-regenerative tissue in the absence of support from parents or the court. A potential right at common law to do so exists and was accepted by the Master of the Rolls in his summary of *Re W*;[6] even so, this right may be of little more than theoretical significance and it would be a brave surgeon who ignored Lord Donaldson's advice. It is, of course, certain that the minor's right to refuse is preserved.

3   Law of 22 December 1976.
4   *Re W (a minor)(medical treatment)* [1992] 4 All ER 627, (1992) 9 BMLR 22.
5   [1992] 4 All ER 627 at 635, (1992) 9 BMLR 22 at 31.
6   *Re W (a minor)(medical treatment)* [1992] 4 All ER 627 at 639, (1992) 9 BMLR 22 at 35.

It appears, in fact, that transplant surgeons in general have pre-empted the Master of the Rolls. Our inquiries indicate that no currently practising British transplant surgeon would accept a live child as an organ donor; only one such instance, involving an identical twin aged 17 years, has arisen in the United Kingdom in the last decade. Only five living minor donors have been used in the Eurotransplant catchment area and none has been recorded in France despite the enabling legislation; similarly, none is recorded by Scadiatransplant.[7] Discussion of the matter, thus, lies on the academic rather than the practical level.

Nothing, however, is static in modern medicine. There have been reports that couples are now having children for the express purpose of providing genetically compatible sibling donors of, at present, regenerative tissue.[8] Whatever one feels about such a practice, the pragmatic answer is that it cannot be prevented. Medico-legally, any such child, when born, would be protected by the rules governing donation by living minors. But speaking ethically, it cannot be denied that the process does little credit to the doctrine of free consent – there is a strong impression that human life is being used as a means.

Patients in the persistent vegetative state

In ordinary circumstances, we would not feel it necessary to distinguish consideration of any single form of cerebral incompetence from our attitudes to the unconscious patient in general. However, such is the current pressure to accept cognitive death as equivalent to somatic death that we feel a word on the persistent vegetative state is needed. It is, perhaps, necessary only to recapitulate our view that, tragic as their state may be, persons in the persistent vegetative state are existing by means of their own cardiovascular system and are not dead – and none of the standard defences of lawful killing could be applied to them. To confuse the concept of brain stem death and to associate the persistent vegetative state with transplantation could only fan any embers of public distrust for 'premature grave robbing' which still remain. There is, of course, no reason why persistent vegetative patients should not be used as organ donors within the existing framework of the law when they die (see p 308 for further discussion); but there can be no question of killing them – or limiting their existence – for the express purpose.[9] Predictably, this view is shared by the British Medical Association.[10]

The donor as vendor

The most urgent issue in living donation is now that of the commercialisation of transplant surgery which is, again, essentially a matter of consent; on this score, it

7   J K Mason 'Legal Aspects of Organ Transplantation' in C Dyer (ed) *Doctors, Patients and the Law* (1992).
8   G McBride 'Keeping Bone Marrow Donation in the Family' (1990) 300 BMJ 1224. The case is discussed by J Rachels 'When Philosophers Shoot from the Hip' (1991) 5 Bioethics 67.
9   Discussed by J Downie 'The Biology of the Persistent Vegetative State: Legal, Ethical, and Philosophical Implications for Transplantation' (1990) 22 Transplant Proc 995.
10 British Medical Association 'Guidelines Relating to the Persistent Vegetative State' reproduced in (1993) Bull Med Ethics, no 89, 8, para 9.

is to be distinguished from payment for cadaver organs – the latter being better considered as an aspect of the availability of organs.

Inevitably, our view on donation for recompense must be coloured by our experience of a national health service. Within that framework, it is difficult to see the sale of organs as other than a way for the rich to obtain priority essential care, the inequity being compounded by the corollary that the poor, who would form the pool of such donors, would be positively disadvantaged in the role of supplier. But it is only fair to remark that those working in a health care system governed by a market economy could see the situation as one in which an anxious buyer meets a willing seller. It is not easy to occupy an objective middle ground.

The problem may have existed in England before 1989 but it was then that it presented acutely. It transpired that impoverished Turkish donors were being recruited and paid to donate their kidneys to genetically and ethnically unrelated recipients; there were wide-ranging repercussions at both legislative and professional levels and these, of themselves, provoke further ethical debate.

The response of the legislature was to rush through the Human Organ Transplants Act 1989 which prohibits the exchange of money, other than legitimate expenses, for the purpose of organ donation by the living (s 1(1)); it is also an offence to advertise for the purpose (s 1(2)). Clearly, however, the legislative intention is to distinguish altruism from commercialism and to approve the former while condemning the latter. The distinction is dictated by the consent doctrine in that it is assumed that a free, uncoerced consent is impossible in the face of financial inducement. To which one might add the widely held moral objection to *any* commercialisation of the human body.

The great majority, and we would include ourselves therein, would accept these restrictions on the individual's power over his or her own body. And yet, cannot this be seen as unacceptable paternalism? Is it impossible that a commercial donor could make his decision in a reasoned manner and on his own altruistic grounds?[11] And who, in quest of unfettered consent, is to distinguish between external financial pressure and moral pressure exerted within the family? It is at least arguable that, in closing the door on the use of an inessential part of one's body for gain, Parliament is striking at the individual publican's autonomy in favour of the corporate pharisee's inner virtue.[12]

The professional reaction was no less positive. The name of one of the doctors concerned was erased from the medical register while the professional freedom of two others was severely curtailed.[13] The General Medical Council has now issued definitive guidelines which include:

> In no circumstances may doctors participate in or encourage in any way the trade in human organs from live donors. They must not advertise for donors nor make financial or medical arrangements for people who wish to sell or buy organs . . . Doctors must also

---

11 It is reported that one of the donors intended to devote the proceeds to the medical treatment of his daughter. See a sympathetic contribution by J Harvey 'Paying Organ Donors' (1990) 16 J Med Ethics 117.

12 For expression of such doubts, see M Evans 'Organ Donation Should not be Restricted to Relatives' (1989) 15 J Med Ethics 17.

13 C Dyer 'GMC's Decision on "Kidneys for Sale" ' (1990) 300 BMJ 961.

satisfy themselves that consent to a donation has been given without undue influence of any kind, including the offer of financial or material benefit.[14]

It has been said that to allow payment would be to open up a traffic in organs. Yet it is difficult to see why this could not be obviated by legalising paid donations only by way of the Unrelated Live Transplant Regulatory Authority. There is some empirical evidence that public opposition to payment is not as strong as might be supposed – between 40 and 50% may find the practice permissible[15] and it has been noted that:

> As long as there are adequate safeguards, any ethical or legal fastidiousness demanding that donation be only gratuitous could condemn the sick.[16]

In any event, a traffic in organs cannot now be confined within one jurisdiction. It is reported[17] that a network for the commercial provision of organs is already in existence; clearly any restrictions on the practice must be international if they are to be effective and the European Parliament has now asked the Council of Ministers to ban the sale of organs throughout the European Community.[18] A British Minister has said that: 'the concept of kidneys for sale is entirely unacceptable in a civilised society',[19] and many would undoubtedly agree – but, at the same time, it is difficult to identify the precise moral basis for so doing.

Moreover, the fact that this is a specifically Western view merits repetition. It is at least arguable that, in a country such as India, where there is no cadaver transplant programme and where long-term dialysis is impracticable, paid organ donation may be not only ethical but also desirable. As has been said, the ethical distinction between allowing one poor and needy citizen to run the risk of brain damage in the boxing ring and denying another the right to sell a kidney may prove hard to define.[20]

Cadaver donations

The deceased has very limited rights as to the disposal of his body in common law and the wishes of the next of kin would normally be supported rather than those of the dead person in the event of conflict. Statute law is, however, replacing common law and the use of cadaver organs and tissues is now regulated in Great Britain by the Human Tissue Act 1961. This provides, in s 1(1), that removal of an organ is

---

14 General Medical Council 'Guidance for Doctors on Transplantation of Organs from Live Donors' (1992) News Review, December, Supplement.
15 A Guttmann and R D Guttmann 'Attitudes of Health Care Professionals and the Public towards the Sale of Kidneys for Transplantation' (1993) 19 J Med Ethics 148.
16 I Davies 'Live Donation of Human Body Parts: A Case for Negotiability?' (1991) 59 Med-leg J 100.
17 A Dorozynski 'European Kidney Market' (1989) 299 BMJ 1182; H D C R Abbing 'Transplantation of Organs: A European Perspective' (1993) 21 J Law Med Ethics 54.
18 A Dorozynski 'Europe Condemns Sale of Organs' (1993) 307 BMJ 756.
19 See J Warden 'Kidneys not for Sale' (1989) 298 BMJ 1670.
20 J Bignall 'Kidneys: Buy or Die' (1993) 342 Lancet 45.

authorised if there has been a specific request to this effect by the deceased; the removal may be for therapeutic, educational or research purposes. In the absence of such a request, s 1(2) provides for the authorisation of organ removal if the person 'lawfully in possession of the body' has, after making such 'reasonable enquiry as may be practicable', no reason to believe that the deceased had expressed any objection to organ removal or that the surviving spouse or 'any surviving relative' of the deceased objects to the body being so dealt with.

The somewhat loose wording of the Act has caused occasional difficulty in its implementation. This was particularly so as to the definition of the person in lawful possession. For some time it was considered that the term implied one with a right to possession, that is, the next of kin. The alternative view is that it refers to the person who has physical possession of the body who is, in practical terms, the hospital administrative officer. This latter interpretation is supported by the wording of other sections of the Act and is now widely accepted by the administration, the legal profession and the British Medical Association but the point has not been tested in the courts. The more recent legislation which has been passed throughout Australia puts the question beyond doubt by vesting the powers in a designated officer within the hospital. Clarity on the point is important in that, were the next of kin to be in lawful possession, they could overrule any specific request made by the deceased. Even allowing for the fact that the relatives have no locus standi to object to the removal of organs under s 1(1) – which is clearly paramount – the doctor is in a difficult position in the event of their objections being voiced. On the one hand, he has legal justification to proceed and he may, rightly, be thinking of the potential recipients. On the other, it would be extremely hard to justify in ethical terms a decision to add further suffering to the bereaved. It is fortunate that such conflicts are very rare in practice but we return to the point when considering the shortfall in organs available for treatment. It should be noted, in passing, that the coroner or procurator fiscal may veto any authorisation if the death comes within their jurisdiction (s 1(5) and (9)).

The concept of 'such reasonable enquiry as may be practicable' is also vague, reasonableness being a matter of highly subjective judgment. The partial solution is to consider what is *un*reasonable – and it would clearly be unreasonable to prolong one's enquiries until the intended donor organ was non-viable. Such a pragmatic approach is, however, less tenable in the context of the beating-heart donor which is discussed below. Finally, the wording 'any surviving relative' is confusingly open-ended and must again be interpreted in a practical sense – the phrase must be taken to mean 'any relative who can reasonably be contacted within the limited time available' which, effectively, limits one to the immediate next of kin. This difficulty has also been noted in Australia where 'next of kin' are specified in order of 'seniority'; responsibility for consent is then vested in the most senior next of kin who can be contacted.[1]

The Human Tissue Act 1961 is unpopular on theoretical and practical grounds within both the legal and medical professions and it is, therefore, interesting to note that at least one academic commentator has questioned whether there is any offence

1   Eg Human Tissue Act 1983, s 4 (NSW).

committed in its non-observance;[2] the same authority suggests that an apparently unauthorised action to save the life of a recipient might be justified on the basis of necessity. From the civil aspect, there seems no reason in principle why an action in tort for nervous shock should not be available to relatives who believe that the conditions of reasonable enquiry have not been met; the majority opinion is that, while such actions have succeeded in the United States, they would be unlikely to do so in the United Kingdom.[3]

Beating-heart donors

It is apparent that the major technical criticisms levelled at the Human Tissue Act 1961 relate to the prolongation of the warm anoxic time entailed in strict adherence to its terms. But such objections are valid only when death is measured by the irrevocable failure of the cardiovascular system. In practice, the overwhelming proportion of cadaver donated material will come from patients who have been maintained on ventilator support and in whom it will be appropriate to reach a diagnosis of death by means of brain stem criteria. There is no logical reason why ventilation should not be continued after death and the heart beat be maintained during an operation for organ donation. The ideal situation of the living donor is thus achieved in a cadaver.

The technical advantages of a beating-heart donation are not in dispute and the process is essential to the success of some transplantations. It may become a legal demand; successful actions for negligence have been raised in the United States in that conventional cadaver donation did not supply the best available treatment. Why, then, is there such antipathy to the procedure?

Much must stem from an inherent revulsion at performing what is a lethal operation amid the conditions pertaining to a living patient but this is irrational once the concept of brain stem death has been accepted – any emotional bias should be directed towards the recipients. Perhaps the major problem lies in the fact that there are still those who, in all good conscience, cannot accept the technical criteria advocated for the diagnosis of brain stem death – and these include some eminent doctors.[4] Some surgeons, while accepting a ventilated donor, will not operate until the patient is disconnected from the machine and shows a flat electrocardiogram. While fully accepting that every doctor is entitled to his own clinical judgment, we do suggest that the subject would be, so to speak, defused were it to be made compulsory for a death certificate to be issued, and the notification handed to the next of kin, before any donation could be effected. This would serve, first, to ease matters for the professionals involved – it is not entirely satisfactory for the surgeon undertaking a beating-heart donation to have to 'satisfy himself by personal examination of the body that life is extinct' (Human Tissue Act 1961, s 1(4)) from

---

2   P D G Skegg 'Liability for the Unauthorized Removal of Cadaveric Transplant Material' (1974) 14 Med Sci Law 53.
3   I M Kennedy 'Further Thoughts on Liability for Non-observance of the Provisions of the Human Tissue Act 1961' (1976) 16 Med Sci Law 49. While we appreciate the pitfalls on the way, we feel that the necessary conditions of proximity would be satisfied if a close relative was confronted with what he or she regarded as a mutilated corpse.
4   N Hodgkinson 'When Does a Beating Heart Die?' (1986) The Sunday Times, 7 December, p 1.

a mere perusal of the hospital notes; secondly, we feel the process would set the minds of the relatives at rest. An alternative is to dissociate the problems of the definition of death from those of transplantation and to legislate purely for the latter contingency. Thus, the Human Tissue and Transplant Act 1982, s 24(2) of Western Australia makes no mention of death but ordains that two medical practitioners with specific qualifications must certify that irreversible cessation of all functions of the brain has occurred before organs can be removed from the body of a person whose respiration and circulation are being maintained artificially.

In any event, relatives must be confused and distraught unless given sympathetic counselling and, in practice, this should always be possible in modern circumstances when, as a result of ventilator support, relatives will have been aware of the impending death for some time and will, no doubt, have been attending at the hospital – transplant co-ordinators are now widely established and can assist in the task to great advantage. Every assistance should be given. Thus, while we accept the view that an electroencephalogram is not necessary to establish the fact of death, we also believe that the relatives should have the right to such evidence should they ask for it. It is only by such adaptations of the principle of informed consent that beating-heart donation will become widely accepted and that, as a consequence, the best therapy will be available to those in dire need.

As noted above, however, in some countries, notably Japan,[5] there is an inherent antipathy to the concept of brain death which is shared to a major extent by the medical profession. A Japanese doctor has, in fact, been charged with murder for performing a cardiac transplant and, although the case was dropped, it did nothing to encourage the evolution of a programme.[6] It is in such circumstances that a return to non-beating heart donation, aided by developments in hypothermic preservation, may be expected.

The availability of suitable organs

It has been calculated that there are enough suitable cadaver kidneys available in America to satisfy the demand but that the requirements are still not met because only one in eight potentially useful organs are obtained in practice.[7] An unsatisfactory situation also persists in the United Kingdom. Over 3,700 patients were awaiting kidney transplants in 1988;[8] the number had risen to 4,340 by the end of 1992 and shows no sign of slackening. It has been reported that nearly half the potential donors fail to become actual donors[9] and it is this deficit which needs to be corrected. The problem has been addressed by a Government Working Party[10] but, as yet, no satisfactory solution has emerged.

5 J Nudeshima 'Obstacles to Brain Death and Organ Transplantation in Japan' (1991) 338 Lancet 1063.
6 M Yamauchi 'Transplantation in Japan' (1990) 301 BMJ 507.
7 For an overview of US attitudes, see H S Schwartz 'Bioethical and Legal Considerations in Increasing the Supply of Transplantable Organs: From UAGA to "Baby Fae"' (1985) 10 Amer J Law Med 397.
8 S M Gore, C J Hinds and A J Rutherford 'Organ Donation from Intensive Care Units in England' (1989) BMJ 1193.
9 Wallwork, fn 8, p 293 above.
10 R Hoffenberg (Chairman) *Report of the Working Party on the Supply of Donor Organs for Transplantation* (1987).

There are essentially two avenues to explore – to reform the law or to change professional and public attitudes. As to the former, it is clear that a main source of cadaver organs under the Human Tissue Act 1961 results from a system of 'contracting in' to the transplant service, something which dictates a conscious effort that many healthy persons – and particularly young persons – find difficult to make. It is widely suggested that the Act could profitably be altered to hold a 'contracting out' position – that is, one in which consent to donation is presumed unless it is specifically withheld. Such a system operates in several European countries – most successfully in Belgium and Austria. Although a good case for the proposition can be made out – especially if it is combined with a right of veto vested in the next of kin, as is the case in Italy and Spain – it carries with it a hint of coercion; we cannot foresee a British government risking such a major policy change, particularly in the light of a recent statement:

> We must accept that nobody has a right to anybody else's organs. If something untoward happens, our organs may be of value to someone else but that should be the result of an altruistic decision about how we want our bodies to be used when we die. It should not be as a result of a right of the recipient . . . It is the responsibility of the living whose organs may be of use to someone else; it is not anyone else's job to claim the organs.[11]

Moreover, objections from the next of kin would probably remain at much the same level as is presently found when the deceased has left no instructions and many doctors would find the resulting pressure on relatives to be distasteful. At the same time, this fear may be being exaggerated to the detriment of the programme. It is quite clear that signing the donor card is a written expression in life of a request that one's body should be used for therapeutic purposes[12] yet the great majority of transplant surgeons will be reluctant to press the matter if the relatives express an objection. While this may be very good and sympathetic medicine, it is, paradoxically, doubtful medical ethics – effectively, the last autonomous wish of the individual is being thwarted simply because he or she is in no position to object. Whether or not a firmer attitude would result in significantly more donations is uncertain, but it is scarcely fair to blame the law for any shortcomings if the law is being disregarded; it has been said, in a slightly different context, that the kidney donor card is not dead but may require intensive care to restore it to more robust health.[13]

Such professional antipathy to or apathy in seeking the co-operation of relatives may be an important factor; this has led to a movement in favour of 'required request' for organ donation – a format which imposes a legal obligation on doctors to seek permission from the relatives for the removal of tissues from suitable dead persons. This is now the subject of federal law in the United States;[14] a Transplant Notification Bill having the same objectives was introduced in the House of Commons in 1988 but made no progress. There is, in fact, considerable debate in the United Kingdom

---

11 188 HC Official Report (6th series) col 1142, 28 March 1991, per Stephen Dorrell.
12 This was the, admittedly extra-judicial, view of Lord Edmund Davies as long as a quarter of a century ago: 'A Legal Look at Transplants' (1969) 62 Proc Roy Soc Med 633.
13 R M R Taylor 'Opting In or Out of Organ Donation' (1992) 305 BMJ 1380.
14 US Public Law 99-509 9318.

as to the efficacy of this type of legislation.[15] Moreover, 'required request' undoubtedly compromises the clinical autonomy of the medical staff concerned. It has to be appreciated that, in addition to the difficulties associated with grieving relatives, maintaining a brain dead beating-heart donor is effort-intensive, particularly as regards multi-organ donation, and facilities may simply not be available in the acute care unit.[16] Even so, it is significant that failure to ask about donation still constitutes the second most important reason for the loss of useable organs.[17]

A recent addition to the melting pot of professional attitudes and ethical values has been the introduction of 'elective ventilation' as a means of widening the supply of organs. Essentially, the concept involves extending the source of donors from accident and emergency departments so as to include the medical wards. Deeply comatose patients dying from strokes or other cerebral medical conditions are transferred to the intensive care unit and are, there, supported until brain stem death supervenes and organ retrieval can be arranged. The procedure was pioneered in Exeter[18] and involved between three and 41 hours' intensive care for eight donors who would, otherwise, have been missed. A rigid protocol was drawn up and the procedure is being elaborated elsewhere.[19] While appreciating the care that has been put into the drafting of the protocol – and accepting the caution expressed by its authors – we feel that the procedure does raise a number of legal and ethical difficulties. As to the former, we wonder if the authority vested in the hospital and the surviving relatives by the Human Tissue Act 1961, s 1(2) can be assumed before a person is dead. That is, perhaps, a minor point and it could be argued that no *authority* is being claimed by consenting to removal to the intensive care unit. Ethically, however – and despite the precondition of deep coma – we wonder if it is right to alter radically the mode of death, and to prolong the dying process, purely for the benefit of others.[20] Whether intensive care beds should be utilised in this way is, in our view, a purely practical matter to be resolved by the doctors in charge. Even so, one cannot exorcise a feeling that death is being pre-empted; it is certain that this

---

15 G D Chisholm 'Time to End Softly Softly Approach on Harvesting Organs for Transplantation' (1988) 296 BMJ 1419 regards it as 'positive'; R M R Taylor and J H Salaman 'The Obligation to Ask for Organs' (1988) 1 Lancet 985 see it as the only answer to a dialysis 'crisis'; A Bodenham, J C Berridge and G R Park 'Brain Stem Death and Organ Donation' (1989) 299 BMJ 1009 are doubtful.

16 But some writers would see these merely as difficulties to be overcome. For particularly trenchant support of required request, see Taylor and Salaman, fn 15 above.

17 S M Gore, D J Cable and A J Holland 'Organ Donation from Intensive Care Units in England and Wales: Two Year Confidential Audit of Deaths in Intensive Care' (1992) 304 BMJ 349.

18 T G Feest, H N Riad, C H Collins et al 'Protocol for Increasing Organ Donation after Cerebrovascular Deaths in a District General Hospital' (1990) 335 Lancet 1133.

19 Eg M A M Salih, I Harvey, S Frankel et al 'Potential Availability of Cadaver Organs for Transplantation' (1991) 302 BMJ 1053. These authors suggest that, realistically, including potential medical donors aged 50-69 would have provided a harvest of 36 kidneys per million population per year which is coming somewhere near the current need for 48 kidneys per million population per year.

20 This is denied on the grounds that it is a corpse that is being ventilated – A Nicholls and H Riad 'Organ Donation' (1993) 306 BMJ 517. But the patients are not dead when the ventilation is instituted.

form of organ husbandry must be very carefully controlled if a backlash of public reaction is to be avoided.[1]

This is of immense overall importance as it is probable that British policy in the quest for more donated organs will depend upon public education for the foreseeable future. One still has to wonder at the basic reasons underlying the refusal of some 30% of relatives to consent to donation[2] – the same public will flock to donate their blood at the sight of a poster advertising an appropriate time and place. Ignorance may be one factor, antipathy on the part of the mass media another and, undoubtedly, the suggestion of ambivalence, as regards both techniques and ethics, among the medical profession plays its part. Attitudes may, however, be changing as the results of the more exotic transplant operations improve. We now believe that the concept of the multiple organ donor should be maximised. It is not easy to enthuse about a treatment whereby one family's joy at the availability of a donor must be balanced against another's tragedy; the public's imagination might well be fired were it generally appreciated that one regrettable death could be compensated by the salvage of four or more lives. This process will undoubtedly be reinforced as increasingly experienced transplant co-ordinators are established as major points of contact with the public.

Payment for tissues

Any discussion on the availability of organs must take into account the possibility of their provision on a commercial basis. We have discussed the ethics of donation for reward by the living and have concluded that this is essentially a matter of valid consent by the donor. But the selling of cadaver organs is, at root, directed to the enticement of the next of kin. Put this way, the proposition can be seen as appealing to the baser human instincts and as something with which the medical profession should have no truck – typically put:

> A shift into any form of commercialism or its currently more fashionable cousin 'rewarded gifting' holds the potential of threatening the entire spiritual structure upon which organ transplantation is based at present.[3]

The possibility is, however, by no means excluded and seems to be gaining momentum in the United States. Manoeuvres to avoid ethical restrictions such as wholesale to kidney banks rather than to individuals have been mooted; standardised cash awards in various forms – such as payment of donors' funeral expenses – have been suggested; and an 'insurance policy' in the form of preferred status is, perhaps surprisingly, the top-ranked option in the United States where over half those responding to a survey approved the introduction of incentives to improve the supply

---

1   G Routh 'Elective Ventilation for Organ Donation – The Case Against' (1992) 8 Care Crit Ill 60. For the opposite view, see C H Collins 'Elective Ventilation for Organ Donation – The Case in Favour' (1992) 8 Care Crit Ill 57.   The British Medical Association takes a very cautious stance – Annual Report 1992.

2   Gore et al, fn 17 above.

3   F T Rapaport 'Progress in Organ Procurement: The Non Heart-beating Cadaver Donor and Other Issues in Transplantation' (1991) 23 Transplant Proc 2699.

of organs.[4] Commenting on this, Peters, who supports payment of a fixed death benefit to donors through an organ procurement organisation, suggests that those in the transplant field have wrongly adhered to certain moral values of their own – values which are not necessarily accepted by those at the giving and receiving end of the process;[5] Sells also points out that antagonism to incentive represents essentially a Western view of ethics as we think they ought to be practised:

> Western societies have prescribed for the rest of the globe without giving much thought, evidently, to the differing ethical and medical circumstances in which our less-affluent colleagues have to operate.[6]

This is not to say that we approve of a traffic in human organs – in fact, we find payment for the organs of the dead far less easy to justify than payment to the living donor. What causes concern, however, is the threat of rampant commercialism governed by market-place economics. Given, however, that the process is strictly controlled – say, through a restructured Unrelated Live Transplant Regulatory Authority – and supposing that it *succeeds* in providing life-saving treatment for those dying on the waiting list, reward for donation of cadaver organs appears in a less scandalous light than it did at first sight.

The fetus or neonate as a transplant donor

Transplantation therapy in the neonatal period is now a standard part of paediatric surgery. Suitable organs, such as the liver, may become available from other newborn infants suffering from fatal conditions; such opportunities are rare but no new issues are then involved because the infant is subject to the conditions of the Human Tissue Act 1961 in just the same way as is the adult or the minor. This, however, is not always so in the case of the fetus who may be involved as an organ donor at maturity or as a cell donor at an early stage of development.

In the former circumstance, the fetus and its organs must be 'viable'. It will be clear from what follows that the legal complications attending fetal transplantation have been greatly modified by the 1990 amendments to the Abortion Act 1967 which, inter alia, permit an abortion on the grounds of fetal abnormality without limit of gestational age (s 1(1)(a)) and absolve the doctor from liability under the Infant Life (Preservation) Act 1929 when terminating a pregnancy within the provisions of the 1967 Act (s 5(1)). Even so, there are moral implications in that a fetal organ donor

---

4 D S Kittur, M M Hogan, V K Thukral et al 'Incentives for Organ Donation?' (1991) 338 Lancet 1441. For support from an unlikely source of payment for cadaveric organs, see G P Smith 'Market and Non-market Mechanisms for Procuring Human and Cadaveric Organs: When the Price is Right' (1993) 1 Med Law Internat 17.

5 T G Peters 'Life or Death: The Issue of Payment for Cadaveric Organ Donation' (1991) 265 J Amer Med Ass 1302. For criticism of his arguments, see E D Pellegrino 'Families' Self-interest and the Cadaver's Organs: What Price Consent?' (1991) 265 J Amer Med Ass 1305. Opposition also comes from R W Evans 'Incentives for Organ Donation' (1992) 339 Lancet 185; 'Organ Procurement Expenditures and the Role of Financial Incentives' (1993) 269 J Amer Med Ass 3113.

6 R A Sells 'Commerce in Human Organs: A Global Review' (1990) 19 Dialysis Transplant 10.

must either be stillborn, which is something of a contradiction in terms, or must be moribund at birth which, effectively, limits the donor to the anencephalic fetus; new ethical ground is, thereby, broken.

The reasons why an anencephalic neonate need not be treated have been considered already in chapter 7, where we have also concluded that it must be allowed a natural death. Two further difficulties arise from this – first, as to the diagnosis of death in such circumstances and, second, as to the unpalatable corollary that the dead neonate or abortus must be reanimated in order to provide undamaged organs. As to the former, the Royal Colleges and their Faculties in the United Kingdom have concluded that: 'organs for transplantation can be removed from anencephalic infants when two doctors who are not members of the transplant team agree that spontaneous respiration has ceased.'[7] On the face of things, this seems to be doing no more than restating a diagnostic test for death which has been, and still is, the norm – moreover, the test is equally applicable to donors, rare in practice, who have been fatally brain damaged during delivery. More importantly, perhaps, it pre-empts suggestions that anencephaly per se should carry a presumption of death[8]- for the surviving anencephalic neonate is in the same position as is the adult in the persistent vegetative state (see chapter 13). It would seem, therefore, to be both unnecessary and impracticable to attempt to introduce a brain death standard. There is, however, a practical difficulty in that fetal tissues – and particularly the heart – are extremely sensitive to 'warm anoxia' – the best results from the small number of cases reported are said to have come from those infants who were placed on life support and the organs used as soon as possible without regard to the existence of brain stem activity.[9] The time required to satisfy the Royal Colleges' criterion of cessation of respiration may, therefore, dictate an unacceptable deterioration in the quality of the donor organs which, in general, must be recovered from a 'beating-heart' donor. But this practice depends, as we have seen, on the acceptance of 'brain stem death' and the transplant surgeon is left with a well-nigh insoluble dilemma – so much so that at least one authoritative commentator has questioned whether it is possible to establish death legally in an anencephalic and, at the same time, preserve the best interests of the recipient of its organs.[10] Attempts to redefine death in the anencephalic as a state of 'brain absence' or to regard such a neonate as 'not being a reasonable creature in being' seem to us to be examples of semantic juggling which should be resisted; the same applies to the more extreme suggestion that the definition of death should be extended so as to include anencephalics as a distinct group[11] – as McCullagh has observed:

---

7 Report of the Working Party of the Conference of Medical Royal Colleges and their Faculties in the United Kingdom on Organ Transplantation in Neonates (1988).

8 D Brahams 'Transplantation, the Fetus and the Law' (1988) 138 NLJ 91.

9 The Medical Task Force on Anencephaly 'The Infant with Anencephaly' (1990) 322 New Engl J Med 669.

10 S McLean 'Facing the Dilemma of a Life and Death Issue' (1991) Scotsman, 26 August, p 9. For a similar US view, see J L Peabody, J R Emery and S Ashwal 'Experience with Anencephalic Infants as Prospective Organ Donors' (1989) 321 New Engl J Med 344.

11 For review, see W F May 'Brain Death: Anencephalics and Aborted Fetuses' (1990) 22 Transplant Proc 885.

Classification as 'dead' will not cause an anencephalic who is breathing to cease doing so . . . One would require also to accept the burial of a spontaneously breathing patient.[12]

The more honest approach is to accept that, at the least, the legality and morality of anencephalic donations are matters for concern and that it is probable that their eventual solution will be founded on strongly utilitarian rather than strict deontological principles.

The implicit result of using the Royal Colleges' criteria is that anencephalic donation must involve some form of 'reanimation ventilation'. This inevitably introduces moral qualms – not the least being that the period of 'deanimation' will be unacceptably short – and, at the end of the day, one has to ask whether the manifest invasion of normal ethical standards is justified by results. It has been estimated that not more than 20 suitable donors will be available each year in the United Kingdom;[13] the surprisingly low yield of organs which would accrue in the United States has been emphasised[14] as has their poor quality and associated distressingly bad therapeutic success rate.[15]

All these factors were considered in what appears to be the only extant judicial consideration of the status of the anencephalic – at least in the English speaking jurisdictions.[16] The circumstances of T's birth were widely publicised. She was born anencephalic and, during her life of nine days, her parents sought to have her declared dead so that her organs could be used to save other lives. The circuit court judge held that she was not brain dead but, nevertheless, gave permission for a single kidney to be removed on the grounds that this was not harming her. This ruling was upheld in the District Court of Appeal but, despite the fact that the baby was now dead, the Supreme Court of Florida then agreed to accept the case as one which 'raised a question of great public importance requiring immediate resolution'. Much of the court's deliberation concerned the common and statute law of Florida but questions of principle were also addressed. Having established that T was legally alive at the relevant time, the parents' request for an additional common law standard of death applicable to anencephalics was considered in the light of current technology. It was held:

Our review of the medical, ethical, and legal literature on anencephaly discloses absolutely no consensus that public necessity or fundamental rights will be better served by granting this request.[17]

and, later:

We acknowledge the possibility that some infants' lives might be saved by using organs from anencephalics who do not meet the traditional definition of 'death' we affirm to-day.

12 P McCullagh *Brain Dead, Brain Absent, Brain Donors* (1993) p 168.
13 See J R Salaman 'Anencephalic Organ Donors' (1989) 298 BMJ 622.
14 See W F May 'Brain Death: Anencephalics and Aborted Fetuses' (1990) 22 Transplant Proc 885, reporting the findings, in particular, of Shewmon.
15 D A Shewmon, A M Capron, W J Peacock and B L Schulman 'The Use of Anencephalic Infants as Organ Sources' (1989) 261 J Amer Med Ass 1773.
16 *Re T A C P* 609 So 2d 588 (Fla, 1992).
17 609 So 2d 588 at 594.

But weighed against this is the utter lack of consensus, and the questions about the overall utility of such organ donations. The scales clearly tip in favor of not extending the common law in this instance.[18]

In the previous edition of this book, we thought that the inevitable ethical price involved in the use of anencephalic donors was one which could be contained within good medical practice – which certainly must involve dissociation of the donors' and the recipients' health care teams.[19] The 'cost/benefit' analysis now inclines us to the view that, in current circumstances, the price is too high. The balance is, however, finely adjusted;[20] there might well be a case for yet further consideration should transplantation techniques improve to the extent that it can be shown clearly that, once obtained, organs from anencephalics offer a genuine prospect of life to those who are otherwise condemned to death.

In such circumstances, the question arises whether a woman can properly choose to carry an affected baby close to term purely to provide transplantable organs. Such a programme appears, at first sight, to be unethical on the grounds that a human being is being used as a means.   Yet, to prevent it could be seen as unreasonable paternalism. A veto not only *might* deprive potential recipients of life but it would also strike a direct blow at a woman's right to control her body. We would not support a total ban on what may be a truly altruistic endeavour – but it must be an aspect of transplantation therapy which would merit very careful scrutiny.

Fetal brain implants

The most recent innovation in this field is the use of fetal neural tissue for the treatment of Parkinsonism[1] in the elderly – and some practitioners have extended this, perhaps prematurely, to the treatment of other degenerative diseases of the ageing brain. Normal adult nerve cells cannot replicate whereas fetal cells are actively growing and multiplying; theoretically, therefore, an implanted fetal cell will grow and provide a source of important cellular metabolites that are often deficient in the aged. It is too early to assess the value of such treatment; it is, indeed, somewhat suspect and The Lancet has called for the United Kingdom to follow the general lead of the United States and to embargo further experimental treatments of this type until those already performed have been evaluated.[2] We are here concerned only with the legal and ethical problems – and see four of these as being of major importance.

In contrast to fetal organs, fetal brain cells must be immature and are ideally harvested at 10-14 weeks' gestation. Thus, the first problem is that, excluding the

18 609 So 2d 588 at 595.
19 M Harrison 'Organ Procurement for Children: The Anencephalic Fetus as Donor' (1986) 2 Lancet 1383. For criticism of the utilitarian view, see A Davies 'The Status of Anencephalic Babies: Should Their Bodies Be Used as Donor Banks?' (1988) 14 J Med Ethics 150.
20 For an international assessment, see L S Rothenberg 'The Anencephalic Neonate and Brain Death: An International Review of Medical, Ethical and Legal Issues' (1990) 22 Transplant Proc 1037.
1 Note that there is a clinical distinction to be made between idiopathic Parkinson's disease and the signs of Parkinsonism which occur in several other conditions: Editorial Comment 'Parkinson's Disease: One Illness or Many Syndromes?' (1992) 339 Lancet 1263.
2 [1988] 1 Lancet 1087. See also C Marwick 'Use of Fetal Tissue in the United States' (1989) 297 BMJ 1357 and associated notations.

rare opportunities derived from natural spontaneous miscarriage – and all commentators accept that there is a clear moral distinction to be made – the process is inextricably linked to abortion. The legal consequence is that fetal brain therapy is largely governed by the Abortion Act 1967; morally speaking, those who are opposed to abortion can accept fetal brain implantation only on the basis that it is desirable to extract some good from an intrinsically bad action if it is possible to do so[3] – and by no means all moralists would agree to such a proposition.[4] Certainly, virtually everyone would agree that a termination of pregnancy and any subsequent transplantation must be dissociated; the prospect of a woman becoming pregnant in order to provide therapeutic material for an aged relative is scarcely acceptable – as Nolan has put it, it involves seeing fetuses as valuable primarily for their medicinal properties rather than for their stunning developmental potential. Second, it is obvious that the individual brain cells must be viable in themselves; can it then be said that the fetus is dead when subjected to surgery? Here, we must rely to an extent on semantic and pragmatic arguments. A 10-14 week-old fetus is not viable – it has no organised heart beat, its lungs cannot conceivably function as oxygenators and, once delivered, it is so clearly not born alive that its existence will go unrecorded save in respect of the abortion regulations; it follows that it is born dead. Moreover, in practice, the technique of abortion will have been so traumatic to the fetus as to preclude any form of life as it is generally accepted. But, be that as it may, it is still very difficult to answer the question 'Is it brain dead?' in the affirmative.

Third, we cannot overlook the revulsion with which most people view any form of tampering with the brain and particularly the idea of 'brain transplants' – as well they might when it is seriously argued that a severed and perfused head might exist more happily than one attached to an aching body.[5] There is, of course, no suggestion that such developments are remotely upon us; nevertheless, the British Medical Association's recommendation that nervous tissue should only be used for transplantation in the form of isolated neurones or tissue fragments[6] should be fully endorsed. Finally, there is some moral repugnance to the use of tissues from the very young to sustain the aged. This is unfair in the present context for the aged are just as entitled to available treatment as is any other population group. But we must ensure that it is true treatment designed to ameliorate specific disease processes. Dr Faustus, in his quest for eternal youth, is scarcely admirable but there are few who have passed middle age who could honestly deny at least a touch of sympathy for his objectives; it is important that we do not seek to force the role of Mephistopheles upon the neurosurgeon.[7]

3 J A Robertson 'The Ethical Acceptability of Fetal Tissue Transplants' (1990) 22 Transplant Proc 1025 argues, persuasively, that the physician using the material has no complicity in obtaining it. The discussion is continued by K Nolan 'The Use of Embryo or Fetus in Transplantation: What There Is to Lose' (1990) 22 Transplant Proc 1029 who concludes that the use of fetal tissues obtained after elective abortion is justified only as a last resort.
4 See R Gillon 'Ethics of Fetal Brain Cell Transplants' (1988) 296 BMJ 1212 for a brief report of expressed attitudes. For extended analysis, see D G Jones 'Fetal Neural Transplantation: Placing the Ethical Debate Within the Context of Society's Use of Human Material' (1991) 5 Bioethics 23.
5 C Fleming 'If We Can Keep a Severed Head Alive . . .' (1988) 297 BMJ 1048
6 Medical Ethics 'Transplantation of Fetal Material' (1988) 296 BMJ 1410.
7 For an excellent review of the agonies of a Research Review Committee, see A S MacDonald 'Foetal Neuroendocrine Tissue Transplantation for Parkinson's Disease: An Institutional Review Board Faces the Ethical Dilemma' (1990) 22 Transplant Proc 1030.

Donation of ovarian tissue

The difficulty of obtaining ova for donation – and still more for research purposes – has been discussed at p 59. It has been disclosed only recently that research on the use of fetal ova to reduce the imbalance – and on the transplantation of fetal ovarian tissue for the treatment of primary infertility – is currently in progress. Research is also ongoing into the use of adult or cadaver tissue for similar purposes. The news provoked a deal of comment – much of which was so critical that it is understood the programme has been halted. It also precipitated the almost emergency publication of a discussion document by the Human Fertilisation and Embryology Authority.[8]

We do not propose to discuss the issues surrounding the donation of adult or cadaver material at this point – many of the questions raised and their answers can be extrapolated from what has already been said. The HFEA document, itself, concentrated largely on the fetus and identified several problems which are comparatively specific to the donation of ovarian – as opposed to any other – fetal tissue. These included, first, the effect of breaking a natural law of biology in that a process of natural selection is by-passed; the survival of abnormal ova might, as a result, be promoted. Second, the effects on any resulting child of discovering his or her somewhat unusual ancestry were considered. And, third, the morality of any process associated with abortion – particularly one aimed at increasing fertility – was questioned.

We have little difficulty with the last consideration, having already accepted that it is right to extract some good from what many would see as a bad practice. This, of course, presupposes that the abortion is neither designed nor timed for the primary purpose of providing donor material. As to the effect on the child, we confess to being unable to understand the pressing need for disclosure of the information. Given reasonable donor selection, it is surely unlikely that a child will question his or her maternity unless encouraged to do so - and we have already criticised the Human Fertilisation and Embryology Act 1990 in this respect (see p 57). The only likely circumstance in which it would be beneficial to the child to be so informed would be when ovum donation was indicated by reason of genetic abnormality in the recipient woman. How and when such information would be given should form part of the pre-operative counselling which would be not only legally required but clinically imperative in the special circumstances. It is the first of these selected considerations which we find to be of greatest significance and difficulty. The risk would seem to be acceptable given both careful clinical and genetic screening of the parents of the fetal donor and adequate embryo selection – in which respect there might be a case for excluding gamete intra-fallopian transfer (GIFT) in such cases. We would, however, be unwilling to chance the hazards of donation from a fetus derived from a natural miscarriage, for such events may well be associated with fetal abnormality; although the stipulation might be offensive to many, we think it advisable that donations should be confined to selected therapeutic terminations.

All of which applies to therapy; there must be even more moral concern if the harvest of ova is intended for research. Here, we are only one stage away from producing embryos for experimental purposes – a process about which we express

8   HFEA Public Consultation Document *Donated Ovarian Tissue in Embryo Research and Assisted Conception* (1994).

our misgivings below (see p 380). The whole scenario, however, raises new and complex problems which, we feel, merit consideration in greater depth than can be provided in what is, effectively, no more than a note inserted at the proof stage of this edition.

15 Euthanasia

The considered and deliberate termination of life has already been reviewed in the special context of neonaticide. Here it is proposed to discuss the subject only in relation to the incurably or terminally ill adult patient. Conditions at each end of life differ significantly from both the legal and ethical viewpoints. Unlike the infant, the adult patient may well be able to express his wishes as to the quality of his own life. In default of this, those responsible for the patient's management have a background of previous abilities and aspirations from which to measure the likely shortfall; clinical decisions can be based on history rather than on clairvoyance. On the other hand, the aged present a bewildering array of mental and physical variations which virtually preclude generalisations as to management – and attitudes to the elderly are inevitably coloured by the fact that their potential for meaningful relationships is waning rather than developing.

The prohibition of the taking of human life is based on fundamental and deeply held ethical and religious convictions. In the Judaeo-Christian tradition, the sanctity of life is founded on the notion that life is a gift over which we have stewardship but no final control. This conviction is expressed in many ways, the common feature of which is that there is a value in life which must be taken as a moral absolute. The right of each person to life is something which is intrinsic to his status as a human being and which is a necessary concomitant of human existence.[1]

Those with a religious outlook defend the concept of the sanctity of life on the grounds that life itself is of divine origin and is, therefore, outwith human disposal. Those who deny the existence of a creator can, however, maintain a similarly strict view.[2] It is not difficult to construct a utilitarian argument in favour of such a position which is founded on the proposition that the consequences of allowing the taking of life are, ultimately, destructive of greater societal happiness.

Nevertheless, few of those who recognise its value will deny that life may be taken in at least some circumstances. The principle of self-defence – either in the private context or in the course of a just war – may admit the killing of others. Similarly, those who would normally condemn murder might, none the less, see legal execution as an appropriate part of the process of criminal justice. In medicine, too, stout opponents of euthanasia may accept the legitimacy of abortion – a process which, by any standards, involves the taking of *some* form of life. We admit the right of a person to commit suicide and do this on the grounds that, in general, the right

---

1   Linacre Centre, Report of a Working Party Euthanasia and Clinical Practice, London (1982) p 37. The rather doubtful authority for this popular religious view is pointed out in K Boyd 'Euthanasia: Back to the Future' (1993) Bull Med Ethics, May, No 88, p 25.

2   For a discussion of non-religious grounds for opposition to euthanasia, see P Foot *Virtues and Vices* (1978) p 33 et seq. A short appraisal for the lawyer is to be found in J Wilkinson 'The Ethics of Euthanasia' (1990) 35 JLSS 243.

FIGURE 2   A DIAGRAMMATIC CONCEPT OF EUTHANASIA

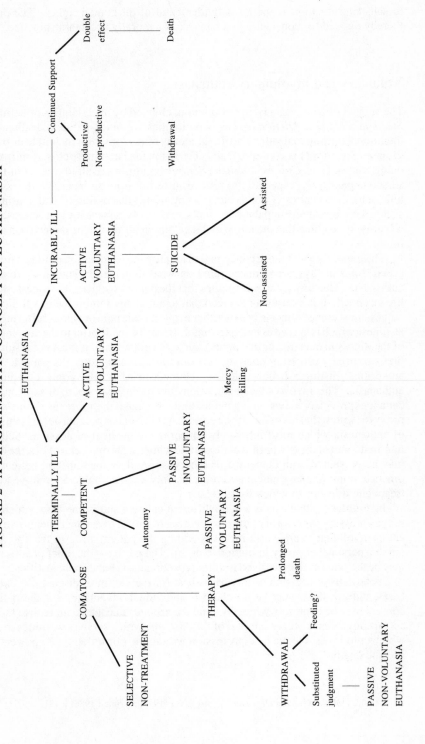

to self-determination is the most fundamental of all human rights. The door is thereby opened for considering euthanasia as a morally acceptable practice.

Voluntary and involuntary euthanasia

The subject of euthanasia is, in our opinion, clouded by uncertainties of definition. *Stedman's Medical Dictionary* has two citations – a quiet, painless death and the intentional putting to death by artificial means of persons with incurable or painful disease. The former is etymologically correct but the latter more closely mirrors the public view. Thus, *Collins' English Dictionary* confines itself to 'the act of killing someone painlessly, especially to relieve suffering from an incurable illness'. To hide behind semantics is obfuscatory. Any useful discussion of euthanasia must accept the – admittedly unpalatable – fact that it involves some form of active killing; it is only by so doing that the moral and legal implications can be reviewed in a clear light.

The major thrust of those concerned to legalise the termination of life on medical grounds has always been concentrated on what is generally known as voluntary euthanasia. This form of words implies that the patient specifically requests that his life be ended. It is everywhere agreed that to attain any semblance of validity, this request must come from one who is either in intolerable pain or who is suffering from an illness which is agreed as being terminal. It may be made prior to the development of the illness in question or during its course. In either case, it must not result from pressure of any sort from relatives or from those looking after the patient. Some authorities[3] distinguish non-voluntary euthanasia as a sub-variety of voluntary euthanasia. This involves the death, ostensibly for his own good, of someone who cannot express any views on the matter and who must, therefore, use some sort of proxy to request that his or her life be ended. As Glover has pointed out, it is this form of euthanasia which most intimately concerns the medical profession. Selective non-treatment of the newborn is one example while, at the other end of life, the doctor may be presented with demented or otherwise senilely incompetent patients. In practice, non-voluntary euthanasia presents only as an arguable alternative to non-treatment, a matter to which we turn later.

Involuntary euthanasia is a quite different concept and is one from which most groups pressing for reform of the law have been careful to distance themselves. An act of involuntary euthanasia involves ending the patient's life in the absence of either a personal or proxy invitation to do so. The motive – the relief of suffering – may be the same as that involved in voluntary euthanasia but its only justification lies in a paternalistic decision as to what is best for the victim of disease. In extreme cases, indeed, there may be no claim to individual advantage – or the patient's consent may be expressly withheld – and the grounds may be no more than those of social convenience. It is examples of this last type which serve as warnings to those who would invest the medical profession with more – or unfettered – powers over life and death.

3　Notably, J Glover *Causing Death and Saving Lives* (1977, reprinted 1986) p 191.

Apart from *R v Adams*[4] which we discuss below at p 329 and *R v Arthur*[5] which we have already considered at p 151, there have been very few truly apposite trials of doctors in the United Kingdom and all have indicated the reluctance of British juries to convict a medical practitioner of serious crime when the charge arises from what they see as his considered medical judgment. In *R v Carr*,[6] a doctor was accused of attempted murder by injecting a massive dose of phenobarbitone into a patient whose lung cancer had been declared inoperable some seven months previously. He was acquitted of the charge but, in the course of the summing-up, Mars-Jones J had this to say:

> However gravely ill a man may be . . . he is entitled in our law to every hour . . . that God has granted him. That hour or hours may be the most precious and most important hours of a man's life. There may be business to transact, gifts to be given, forgivenesses to be made, 101 bits of unfinished business which have to be concluded.

which is as good a comment on misplaced paternalism as is likely to be found. The pattern of acquittal was, however, changed dramatically by the case of *R v Cox*[7] in which a consultant rheumatologist was convicted of attempted murder having, admittedly, injected potassium chloride into an incurably ill patient who died within minutes of the act. The case is discussed in greater detail at p 320.

Active and passive euthanasia

A patient's life may be terminated, or death accelerated, either actively or passively. This distinction – or whether there is, indeed, any true distinction – is one of the most hotly-argued issues in the euthanasia debate and one which can be addressed on either the legal or the moral plane.

Despite the rarity of cases involving the medical profession, there is no ambiguity in the attitude of the law in the United Kingdom towards a positive act of euthanasia. It is summed up in the words of Devlin J:

> If the acts done are intended to kill and do, in fact, kill, it does not matter if a life is cut short by weeks or months, it is just as much murder as if it were cut short by years.[8]

---

4 H Palmer 'Dr Adams' Trial for Murder' [1957] Crim LR 365.
5 The Times, 6 November 1981, pp 1, 12; (1993) 12 BMLR 1.
6 *R v Carr*, The Sunday Times, 30 November 1986, p 1. Another trial concerned with voluntary euthanasia by way of injection of patassium chloride and lignocaine was aborted when the prosecution offered no evidence: *R v Lodwig* (1990) The Times, 16 March, p 3. In Scotland, a doctor who injected an elderly patient with ten times the normal dose of diamorphine was acquitted of culpable homicide - the defence was, however, one of accidental error: *HM Advocate v Watson* (1991) Scotsman, 11 June, p 8, 14 June, p 3.
7 *R v Cox* (1992) 12 BMLR 38.
8 H Palmer 'Dr Adams' Trial for Murder' [1957] Crim L R 365.

and we have Glanville Williams writing: 'The law does not leave the issue in the hands of doctors; it treats euthanasia as murder.[9] While motive is irrelevant, intention is all-important. If a doctor intends to kill, he is as liable to prosecution as is the layman.

There have been recommendations for the introduction of a specific offence of 'mercy-killing'[10] and, although these have not been translated into legislation – and although there is, apparently, no intention so to do[11] – there is an innate reluctance on the part of the courts to convict the genuine 'mercy-killer' of an offence which carries a mandatory sentence of life imprisonment. This is particularly so when relatives have cared for the sick with great devotion and have ultimately decided to release them from misery. In such circumstances, the prosecutor may well exercise his discretion and accept a plea of manslaughter;[12] alternatively, the court may accept a plea of diminished responsibility on the grounds of mental abnormality (see p 412) – psychiatrists are just as ready to diagnose or to infer a reactive depression in the accused.[13]

Until a relatively short time ago, one would have supposed that the public were content with such a practical solution and had little or no wish to see it extended. The euthanasia debate has, however, now been reopened in full force; some of the impetus has undoubtedly come from the Netherlands where many people believe that active euthanasia is widely practised. In point of fact, active euthanasia is still illegal in the Netherlands and the political argument as to its correct status continues.[14] In 1991, it was said that nearly 2% of deaths in the Netherlands resulted from euthanasia; these involved approximately 2300 cases of euthanasia and 400 of assisted suicide each year.[15] The journey towards legislation in Holland has been stormy and, in our opinion, provides a cautionary tale for those intent on a rush down the 'libertarian' slopes. Thus, we have the Royal Dutch Medical Association advocating 'life termination' in 1991 without, apparently, considering whether their proposals conform with Dutch law.[16] From a study undertaken at much the same time, it appeared that medical decisions concerning the end of life were taken in 38% per cent of all deaths – the sole conclusion being that such decisions should get more attention in research, teaching and public debate.[17] Two years later, the Dutch Commission for the Acceptability of Life Terminating Action called for public debate on whether the life of a patient suffering from severe dementia without serious

9 G Williams *Textbook of Criminal Law* (2nd edn, 1983) p 580.
10 See R Leng 'Mercy Killing and the CLRC' (1982) 132 NLJ 76.
11 J Warden 'No New Law Planned on Mercy Killing' (1993) 306 BMJ 1150.
12 For example, *R v Johnson* (1961) 1 Med Sci Law 192. The US experience of similar cases is summarised by L H Glantz 'Withholding and Withdrawing Treatment: The Role of the Criminal Law' (1987/88) 15 Law Med Hlth Care 231.
13 S Dell *Murder into Manslaughter* (1984) p 35 et seq. In *R v Taylor* [1979] CLY 570, a man who battered his autistic child to death was placed on probation for 12 months. Perhaps the most remarkable example comes from the USA where no charges were pressed against a man who held the staff at gun-point while disconnecting his son from the ventilator - see, for example, J D Lantos, S H Miles and C K Cassel 'The Linares Affair' (1989) 17 Law Med Hlth Care 308.
14 M A M de Wachter 'Euthanasia in the Netherlands' (1990) 300 BMJ 1093.
15 H Hellema 'Euthanasia - 2% of Dutch Deaths' (1991) 303 BMJ 877.
16 H Hellema '"Life Termination" in The Netherlands' (1991) 302 BMJ 984.
17 P J van der Maas, J J M van Delden, L Pijnenborg and C W N Looman 'Euthanasia and Other Medical Decisions Concerning the End of Life' (1991) 338 Lancet 669.

physical symptoms might be terminated with or without having executed an advance directive on the point[18] and, in the same year, the concept of life-terminating acts without the specific request of the patient was clearly being accepted as a normal part of medical practice.[19] While such data may suggest a 'slippery slope', the true underlying problem seems to have been that of uncertainty[20] and it was not until 1993 that legislation passed the Second Chamber. The legal position now is that euthanasia, with or without the explicit request of the patient,[1] remains a criminal act and doctors engaging in life-terminating acts will be punishable by penal law unless they conform to relatively strict guidelines.[2] These have not yet been formulated but there is little reason to suppose that they will differ significantly from those which have been followed for some 20 years and which include: that all other treatment options must have been exhausted or refused by the patient; that the patient has made specific requests and that his or her decision is well-informed, free and enduring; that the patient's mental or physical suffering is very severe and without prospect of relief; and that the doctor has taken others into consultation. In the past, even if a prosecution has been brought, the courts have accepted a defence of force majeure – or necessity – when the guidelines have been followed. Thus, despite nearly a quarter of a century's political manoeuvring, the precise legal situation is still unclear. It is said that, following the final acceptance of the 1993 Act by the Senate, doctors are now 'legally obliged to give evidence of a criminal act they have committed' in the face of 'an active prosecution policy' on the part of the justice ministry.[3] Moreover, the extent to which euthanasia is used remains uncertain, largely because many doctors do not refer their cases to the police as is officially required.[4] It is to be noted that both the states of Washington and California have rejected legalised euthanasia[5] – and, at least in the case of the former, this was for fear that the safeguards were inadequate. Such concerns do not appear ill-founded when one reads that a Dutch psychiatrist has been found to be medically justified in assisting the suicide of a physically healthy woman who was depressed[6]- precisely the situation foreseen by those who oppose legalising the termination of life. The

18 H Hellema 'Dutch Doctors Support Life Termination in Dementia' (1993) 306 BMJ 1364.

19 L Pijnenborg, P J van der Maas, J J M van Delden and C W N Looman 'Life-terminating Acts without Explicit Request of Patient' (1993) 341 Lancet 1196. In subsequent correspondence B Pollard suggested that 'the only legal category for LAWER in the Netherlands, as elsewhere, was murder'.

20 See H Rigter, E Borst-Eilers and H J J Leenen 'Euthanasia Across the North Sea' (1988) 297 BMJ 1593; H Rigter 'Euthanasia in the Netherlands: Distinguishing Fact from Fiction' (1989) Hastings Center Report, Spec Supp. Jan/Feb, p 31. The same issue contains a trenchant criticism of the Dutch ethos: R Fenigsen 'A Case Against Dutch Euthanasia' at p 22.

 1 The Dutch have, previously, made a firm distinction between euthanasia, which involves positive action following a well-considered request from the patient for the doctor to end his or her life on account of unbearable and hopeless suffering, and termination of life without request because of, say, mental incompetence. The removal of the distinction has been criticised: H Hellema 'Dutch Confused over Euthanasia' (1993) 306 BMJ 415.

 2 M Spanjer 'Netherlands: Euthanasia Legislation' (1993) 341 Lancet 426.

 3 T Sheldon 'Euthanasia Law Does Not End Debate in the Netherlands' (1993) 307 BMJ 1511.

 4 E Borst-Eilers 'Euthanasia in the Netherlands' Paper presented at the 2nd International Conference on Health Law and Ethics, London, 1989 estimated that between 6,000 and 8,000 terminations are carried out annually but only some 200 are reported.

 5 M Morris 'Washington State Rejects Euthanasia' (1991) 303 BMJ 1223; R Rhein 'California Says No to Euthanasia' (1992) 305 BMJ 1175.

 6 'Mercy-killing Doctor Freed' (1993) Scotsman, 22 April, p 8.

Dutch experience could, in fact, be taken as an object lesson rather than as a paradigm.

It has been reported that 75% of a sample of the British public agreed that the law should allow adults to receive help towards an immediate peaceful death if they suffer from an intolerable physical illness.[7] Against this, a Working Party of the British Medical Association concluded, in 1988, that the deliberate taking of a human life should remain a crime and that the doctor who feels compelled by conscience to end a patient's life must take his chance with the scrutiny of the law. This report has been criticised[8] and an unofficial, though prestigious, body of opinion has come out in favour of carefully controlled euthanasia on the Dutch model.[9] Even so, we remain convinced that such a move is likely to undermine the trust which exists in the ideal doctor/patient relationship. This has been well expressed by Capron:[10]

> I never want to have to wonder whether the physician coming into my hospital room is wearing the white coat (or the green scrubs) of a healer, concerned only to relieve my pain and restore me to health, or the black hood of the executioner. Trust between patient and physician is simply too important and too fragile to be subjected to this unnecessary strain.

How, then, does Dr Cox fit into the mould? His patient had expressed a wish to die and was, indeed, already been categorised as 'not for resuscitation' and seldom has there been so clear an expression of the principle of double effect, or of legal necessity, as that enunciated by the trial judge. At the outset, his summing up laid down the basic law:

> If he injected her with potassium chloride with the primary purpose of killing her, of hastening her death, he is guilty of the offence charged.[11]

and qualified this by:

> If a doctor genuinely believes that a certain course is beneficial to his patient, either therapeutically or analgesically, then even though he recognises that that course carries with it a risk to life, he is fully entitled, nonetheless, to pursue it. If in those circumstances the patient dies, nobody could possibly suggest that in that situation the doctor was guilty of murder or attempted murder.[12]

So, what distinguished Dr Cox from Dr Adams and Dr Arthur? Some aspects of the judge's charge may have had an effect on the jury. They were, for example, exhorted

7 J Dawson 'Easeful Death' (1986) 293 BMJ 1187.
8 For example, R Higgs 'Not the Last Word on Euthanasia' (1988) 296 BMJ 1348.
9 Institute of Medical Ethics Working Party on the Ethics of Prolonging Life and Assisting Death 'Assisted Death' (1990) 336 Lancet 610.
10 A M Capron 'Legal and Ethical Problems in Decisions for Death' (1986) 14 Law Med Hlth Care 141. See also the view of a hospice practitioner R C Twycross 'Assisted Death: A Reply' (1990) 336 Lancet 796.
11 *R v Cox* (1992) 12 BMLR 38 at 39.
12 At 39.

not to be mesmerised by experts and, above all, to hold fast to common sense when assessing intention. Obviously, we can never know the precise reason for the verdict of guilty; it is, however, reasonably safe to assume that, while public opinion in the United Kingdom will give great latitude to the medical profession in its fight against suffering, it is not yet prepared to accept the use of a substance which has no analgesic effect, has no known therapeutic purpose but which is known to be lethal when injected.

Even so, sympathy for Dr Cox was widespread. His judge was clearly anxious to place responsibility for an ill-considered cremation elsewhere and no immediate custodial sentence was imposed; the vice-president of the Voluntary Euthanasia Society castigated what he saw as a supine jury;[13] the General Medical Council was content to admonish him on the grounds that, although his actions had fallen short of the high standards which the medical profession must uphold, he clearly acted in good faith; and the responsible Regional Health Authority offered continued employment subject to certain restrictions.[14] We believe that the jury decision was certainly right in law but that public dissatisfaction ultimately stems from the law's determination to dissociate reasons from intent when faced with unlawful killing[15] – as in the case of Dr Arthur, Dr Cox was certainly not a murderer as the word is commonly interpreted. None the less, for reasons which appear elsewhere in this chapter, we cannot accept that individual doctors should be given free rein in this field in the absence of specific legislation.[16] Moreover, any such legislation must, itself, be suspect – one's distrust lying in what Levin has called the fallacy of the altered standpoint.[17] It has been said that current attitudes to euthanasia are comparable to the attitudes to abortion in the early 1960s;[18] it is precisely the fear that current attitudes to abortion may predict those to euthanasia in the twenty-first century that tempers our intuitive sympathy for both Dr Cox and his patient.

It is, of course, possible to argue the question from the point of view of the patient's autonomy rather than that of the doctor's standards of practice. In so far as the right of the competent adult to refuse life-saving treatment is now established in the United Kingdom[19] and that the right to control one's body has found expression in the decriminalising of suicide, it is but a short step to holding that to refuse assistance in dying to a person who is incapable of ending his or her own life is an affront to that person's rights of autonomy. Just such an issue has been aired in Canada where the Supreme Court, by a majority of 5:4 held that, while this was so,

---

13 C Dyer 'Rheumatologist Convicted of Attempted Murder' (1992) 305 BMJ 731.

14 C Dyer 'GMC Tempers Justice with Mercy in Cox Case' (1992) 305 BMJ 1311.

15 This view is central to the persuasive argument in K Boyd 'Euthanasia: Back to the Future' (1993) Bull Med Ethics, May, No 88.

16 For an interpretation of the relationship between the law and the medical profession see Hoffmann LJ in *Airedale National Health Service Trust v Bland* [1993] 1 All ER 821 at 858, (1993) 12 BMLR 64 at 103, CA: 'The court [has been invited] to decide whether, on medical facts which are not in dispute, [the action] would be justified as being in the best interests of the patient. This is a purely legal (or moral) decision which does not require any medical expertise and is therefore appropriately made by the court'. See also pp 341 et seq below.

17 B Levin 'No Justice in a Merciful Release' (1992) The Times, 24 September, p 12.

18 R Smith 'Euthanasia: Time for a Royal Commission' (1992) 305 BMJ 728.

19 *Re T (adult: refusal of medical treatment)* [1992] 4 All ER 649, (1992) 9 BMLR 46. Reconfirmed in *Re C (refusal of medical treatment)* [1994] 1 All ER 819.

the consequent deprivation of rights was not contrary to the principles of fundamental justice which required a fair balance to be struck between the interests of the state and those of the individual;[20] neither were the liberty and security of the person compromised – one reason being that the provisions in the Criminal Code, s 241 prohibiting assisted suicide were there as a *protection* for the terminally ill who were particularly vulnerable as to their life and will to live:

> There is no certainty that abuses can be prevented by anything less than a complete prohibition [of assisted suicide]. Creating an exception for the terminally ill might therefore frustrate the purpose of the legislation of protecting the vulnerable because adequate guidelines to control abuse are difficult or impossible to develop.[1]

The arguments in Ms Rodriguez's case which concerned the setting up of a mechanism she could use to end her life should she become paralysed as a result of her motor neurone disease, were, in the main, based on Canadian constitutional law and, in particular, related to possible conflicts between the Canadian Charter of Rights and Freedoms the Criminal Code; it is not easy, therefore, to transfer them to the United Kingdom stage. However, the issue was very closely contested and some of the dissenting opinions express important general principles. In particular, the 'floodgates' argument was dismissed not because it might not occur but because a person should not be denied a choice which others have open to them simply on the grounds that, as a consequence, others may then abuse such powers as they already have[2] – each individual person must be treated fairly by the law and not made a scapegoat for the failings of society (per McLachlin J). Finally, the opinion of Cory J merits repetition:

> [D]ying is an integral part of living . . . It follows that the right to die with dignity should be as well protected as is any other aspect of the right to life. State prohibitions that would force a dreadful, painful death on a rational but incapacitated terminally ill patient are an affront to human dignity.[3]

Thus, the arguments for and against assisted suicide are finely balanced but all the dissenting opinions in Rodriguez stressed that it was for Parliament, not the courts, to make such fundamental decisions. Lamer CJ provided a schedule of conditions which could well form a basis for any future United Kingdom legislation.

By contrast with the positive action thus far discussed, passive euthanasia involves the shortening of life through an omission to act. For the reasons given above, we now reject the term 'passive euthanasia' and greatly prefer the concept of selective non-treatment; much confusion is, thereby, eliminated. Nevertheless, there are those who say that any distinction between a commission and an omission

---

20 *Rodriguez v A-G of British Columbia* [1993] 3 WWR 553.
1 At para 43.
2 We do not intend, here, to discuss the bizarre case of Dr Kevorkian in America who is said to have invented and promoted a 'suicide machine' – which brought him before a Grand Jury: D S Greenberg 'Dying, Doctors, and Politics' (1991) 338 Lancet 1446.
3 At para 232.

to act when both have the same effect is no more than an illusion – the responsibility and the intention of the actor are the same.[4] But that is not to say that killing and letting die are, therefore, always morally equivalent. While we see the force of the contrary opinion, we believe that there is a morally significant difference between inactivity and action and that this rests on a firmer base than mere intuition. The essence of discrimination lies in the means to obtain the same end, in that the taking of active steps implies an autocratic control over the way in which the event occurs. The doctor who administers a drug intended to end the life of a suffering patient determines the moment and the manner of the patient's death. The action of the drug changes the physical cause of death and this must be a matter of importance. The process is quite different from allowing another agency – eg illness – to cause death. Activity, moreover, directly confronts those views which concede that death is the one hazard of life which is beyond the ambit of legitimate human intervention.

Suffice it to say that, while only a very small number of physicians would work actively to end the life of a patient, selective non-treatment is practised fairly widely. The medical profession as a whole sees a difference, although the reasons for so doing may be tenuous in the extreme – as one reviewer put it: 'Our gut intuition tells us that there is a difference between active and passive euthanasia and we are not going to be browbeaten into changing our minds by mere logic.'[5] Put in rather less practical terms, philosophical argument has its limits in medical ethics: 'We cannot capture our moral judgments by appeal to argument alone . . . in the area of dying, intuitions and conceptions formed by actual experience must be given weight.'[6] Should the proponents of active euthanasia have their way, very good reasons would have to be given why doctors should be expected to carry out the operations;[7] the Hippocratic Oath is already suffering sufficient erosion and a 'conscience clause' allowing for opt-out would be essential.

As something of an *envoi* to this discussion, we can note that the civil law has also declared its hand. *Re C*[8] concerned the management of a hydrocephalic child as regards the balance to be made between short-term therapeutic gain and needless prolongation of life. The judge at first instance directed that leave be given to the hospital authorities to 'treat the ward to die'. The Court of Appeal considered that such phraseology could not be upheld and the judge, of his own accord, amended his order to read: 'to treat the ward in such a way that she may end her life peacefully'; the Court of Appeal found this perfectly satisfactory.

4   H Kuhse 'A Modern Myth. That Letting Die is not the Intentional Causation of Death' (1984) 1 J Appl Philos 21. R Gillon 'Euthanasia, Withholding Life-prolonging Treatment, and Moral Differences between Killing and Letting Die' (1988) 14 J Med Ethics 115.
5   T B Brewin 'Voluntary Euthanasia' (1986) 1 Lancet 1085.
6   G Gillett 'Euthanasia, Letting Die and the Pause' (1988) 14 J Med Ethics 61. This attitude was challenged by M Parker 'Moral Intuition, Good Deaths and Ordinary Medical Practitioners' (1990) 16 J Med Ethics 28.
7   B Pollard 'Killing the Dying – Not the Easy Way Out' (1988) 149 Med J Austral 312.
8   *Re C (a minor) (wardship: medical treatment)* [1990] Fam 26, [1989] 2 All ER 782, CA.

Allowing the patient to die

While selective non-treatment has gained general acceptance as part of good medical practice, it is clear that it will not find moral endorsement in all its forms. A failure on the part of the doctor to provide his patient with treatment thought to be appropriate to the circumstances might well be considered to be a morally culpable omission. Non-treatment of an infection in a young and otherwise healthy person would undoubtedly constitute such a failure whereas treatment for a bed-ridden elderly patient whose prospects were only those of deteriorating health might, equally, be considered inappropriate.

The issue thus focuses on the distinction between what have become known as ordinary and extraordinary treatments. There is a general consensus, now established in both legal and medical opinion, that the doctor need not resort to heroic methods to prolong the life – or, perhaps better, to prolong the dying – of his patient; considerations of cost and of the distribution of other resources are important here although they must be secondary to the well-being and the dignity of the patient.[9] These principles are embodied in the classic expression of the ordinary/extraordinary treatment test which is to be found in the directive issued by Pope Pius XII in 1957:[10]

> Man has a right and a duty in case of severe illness to take the necessary steps to preserve life and health. That duty . . . devolves from charity as ordained by the Creator, from social justice and even from strict law. But he is obliged at all times to employ only ordinary means . . . that is to say those means which do not impose an extraordinary burden on himself or others.

This statement represents the core of Roman Catholic teaching on the matter and it has been widely accepted through the 35 years of medical progress which have passed since its promulgation. Clearly, however, the difficulty about such a test is to distinguish ordinary treatments from extraordinary and the Pope, himself, qualified 'ordinary' as 'according to personal circumstances, the law, the times and the culture'. Thus, the ordinary/extraordinary test should not and cannot be applied as a general, all embracing rule. Some have, accordingly, suggested that the comparison should be between proportionate and disproportionate therapy; we would take this concept one stage further in preferring the contrast of productive and non-productive means – the test being whether or not a particular treatment is doing the condition any good. This firmly concentrates decision making within the context of the individual patient and his unique condition; such an interpretation is endorsed both by the Anglican Church[11] and by the Roman Catholic Sacred Congregation.[12] Factors such as the physical and psychological pain involved in the treatment, its

9 Two speeches in *Airedale National Health Service Trust v Bland* [1993] 1 All ER 821 at 879, 893, (1993) 12 BMLR 64 at 125, 140, HL indicate that resources can, in certain circumstances, be a legitimate concern of the clinician.

10 (1957) 49 Acta Apostolicae Sedis 1027.

11 Most Rev D Coggan 'On Dying and Dying Well' (1977) 70 Proc R Soc Med 75.

12 *Declaration on Euthanasia* (1980). For further criticism of the ordinary/extraordinary treatment test see N L Cantor *Legal Frontiers of Death and Dying* (1987) p 35.

claim on scarce resources and the general prospects for the patient and his family may all be taken into account in deciding whether or not a treatment is productive.

Non-productivity has recently found expression in the concept of medical futility as a treatment standard. In the litigious battlefield of the United States, however, it seems not to have simplified the issue and is regarded by some as little more than a justification for physicians to impose their values on other involved parties.[13] In other words, what at one time seemed a matter of simple clinical appraisal, now provokes its own conflict with the equally – if not more – important principle of autonomy. Thus, it is possible to define futility as treatment which need not be provided because it is either implausible or non-beneficial. Its application can, however, be held to void patient preferences altogether and may, in fact, dispose of a duty to inform a patient, or the patient's surrogates, of alternative therapeutic programmes. The issue crystallises when the patient demands access to what is regarded as medically futile treatment – a problem which has been solved, at least legally speaking, in the United Kingdom where it has been held that doctors cannot be compelled to treat patients contrary to their clinical judgment.[14] To which opponents would say that it is even less acceptable that physicians should, effectively, allocate resources without the sustaining power of society's judgment. The scope for ethical and legal disagreement is wide and, in the long term, social consensus must be sought on ways to resolve the conflicts engendered by the notion of futility[15] – which we are convinced must come to be accepted in some way. In the meantime, imperfect as the concept may be currently, its practical value should not be discarded for fear of offending what Miles has described as an elitist view of 'autonomy'.

Whose body is it?

The individual's right of self-determination is now virtually established as the determining factor in any situation of conflict – whether it is a problem of abortion, consent to treatment or euthanasia. Yet the question can still be properly asked – are there circumstances in which the wishes of the individual should be looked upon as being qualified by other considerations?

The theologian might well answer Yes; the Roman Catholic church, for example, recognises no right to suicide and declining treatment might be regarded as suicide in certain circumstances. Others might hold that to diminish the seriousness and awe with which we view life is but a step towards the rejection of values which are of crucial importance. We would do well to reflect on the moral steps which are being

---

13 An issue of (1992) 20 Law Med Hlth Care is partly devoted to the subject. We have noted particularly R Cranford and L Gostin 'Futility: A Concept in Search of a Definition' 307; S H Miles 'Medical Futility' 310; A Alpers and B Lo 'Futility: Not Just a Medical Issue' 327; E R Grant 'Medical Futility: Legal and Ethical Aspects' 330.

14 *Re J (a minor)(medical treatment)* (1992) 9 BMLR 10, [1992] 2 FLR 165.

15 For a UK approach, see K R Mitchell, I H Kerridge and T J Lovat 'Medical Futility, Treatment Withdrawal and the Persistent Vegetative State' (1993) 19 J Med Ethics 71. Guidelines are now being drawn up in New South Wales to cover cases in which life support treatment is deemed futile. Life supporting therapy is widely defined and includes chemotherapy, radiotherapy and renal dialysis: NSW Department of Health *Dying with Dignity* (1993) discussed by D John (1993) 306 BMJ 1363.

taken when we pay homage to the cult of self-determination. None the less, the principle of self-ownership is now firmly established and is reflected legally in the offence of battery; any residual limitations of the right to accept or decline treatment are disappearing rapidly[16] – the concept of informed refusal is achieving the same legal standing as that of informed consent in the USA;[17] it is also emerging in Canada.[18] The common law basis for these decisions lies in the assumption that the rights of the competent individual to self-determination will normally outweigh the interests of the state in the preservation of life.

Pioneering statutory action in this field is to be found in the Medical Treatment Act 1988 of Victoria. The Act has two main thrusts. First, it enables a patient to refuse treatment, on either a general or a specific basis, by way of certification; the certificate may be completed only by persons over the age of 18 who were under no inducement or compulsion at the time and who were fully informed as to the consequences of refusal (s 5). Second, it introduces the offence of medical trespass which is committed by a medical practitioner who knowingly treats contrary to the prohibitions of a certificate (s 6); thus, the practitioner cannot plead his own ethos and there is no 'conscience clause'. Simultaneously, however, the Act exonerates the doctor who fails to treat in accordance with a certificate of refusal from professional, criminal and civil liability (s 9).[19]

The Victorian legislation is far-reaching. In particular, no distinction is made between terminal and other illness. Moreover, the right to refuse treatment is unqualified; it is subject neither to the interests of the state nor to those of third parties – non-consensual Caesarean section on behalf of the fetus, for example, now has no place in Victorian medical practice. The Act specifically excludes palliative treatment – or the provision of reasonable medical procedures for the relief of pain, suffering and discomfort (s 3) – from that which can be refused but, at the same time, preserves the patient's rights at common law in this respect. On the face of things, therefore, the Medical Treatment Act 1988 is a particularly firm expression of the doctrine of patient autonomy; it also seems to place a remarkable limitation on the physician's discretion to treat his patient according to his own professional and moral standards.

The moral basis for the treatment of the unconscious or incompetent patient – and particularly of one whose therapy is, at least, unlikely to be productive – is more difficult to assess. So far as we know, there are no legal precedents outside the neonatal field and the wardship jurisdiction to look to in the United Kingdom, where

---

16 In the US, *Fosmire v Nicoleau* 551 NE 2d 77 (NY, 1990). See also the case of Winter – F Charatan ' "Wrongful life" Man Dies' (1990) 300 BMJ 1095 and D Brahams 'Unwanted Life-sustaining Treatment' (1990) 335 Lancet 1209. For the legal position in England, see *Re T (adult: refusal of medical treatment)* [1992] 4 All ER 649, (1992) 9 BMLR 46 and *Airedale National Health Service Trust v Bland* [1993] 1 All ER 821, (1993) 12 BMLR 64, HL.

17 *Re Kathleen Farrell* 529 A 2d 404 (NJ, 1987); *State v McAfee* 385 SE 2d 651 (Ga, 1989) where the right to be helped through the resulting pain was also upheld; *McKay v Bergstedt* 810 P 2d 617 (Nev, 1990).

18 *Malette v Shulman* (1990) 67 DLR (4th) 321 per Robins J A at 328; *Nancy B v Hôtel-Dieu de Québec* (1992) 86 DLR (4th) 385, (1992) 15 BMLR 95.

19 The power to appoint an agent in the event of supervening incompetence is granted in the Medical Treatment (Enduring Power of Attorney) Act 1990. For description of the 1988 Act, see D Lanham 'The Right to Choose to Die with Dignity' (1990) 14 Crim LJ 401.

major reliance is placed on good medical judgment. The more frequent recourse to the law courts in the United States has, however, served to demonstrate certain principles and, at the same time, the difficulties which may be encountered.

The Massachusetts courts, particularly, have wrestled with the problem which they have attempted to solve by applying a 'substituted judgment' test – donning the mental mantle of the patient. In doing so, they raised in a vivid manner the potential for conflict with the medical profession – 'such questions of life and death ... require the process of detached but passionate investigation and decision ... on which the judicial branch of government was created'.[20] Later, however, they made it clear that judicial inquiry was not regarded as a prerequisite to decisions to withdraw treatment and this attitude has now been adopted in several other States.[1]

Certain features of the individual circumstances receive particular attention in the United States. In the first place, great emphasis is placed on intentions which have been expressed in life, not only through the advanced directive (sometimes called the 'living will') – and, now, the concept of the enduring power of attorney – but also by words or attitudes. This is exemplified in the *Eichner/Storar* decisions.[2] In the first of these, the guardian's right to refuse treatment on behalf of an incompetent was upheld on the grounds that the latter had expressed his preferences, albeit only in conversation, when he was healthy. Mr Storar, on the other hand, had never been competent and the appellate court refused his mother's request to abandon blood transfusion therapy for his cancerous condition; it was thought that no one, not even a parent or a sibling, should decide that an incompetent should bleed to death. The authority of an advanced oral directive is, however, not absolute and may be subject to evidence of its being 'clear and convincing'. In the unusual and important case of *Cruzan*,[3] the Supreme Court, ruling for the first time on a case concerning the right to refuse treatment, held that the State was entitled to question the reliability of prestated instructions where its statutory policy strongly favoured the preservation of life. Second, some importance is put on the imminence of death; in general, persons who are likely to survive for more than a year with treatment are maintained on therapy.[4] Third, special attention is given to the persistent vegetative state as regards which it has been held: 'Life expectancy analyses assume that there are still some benefits to be derived from the continued existence of an incompetent patient. That assumption ... is not appropriate in the case of persistent vegetative patients';[5] the prognosis of a year's survival is, then, taken out of the decision-making balance. In many such cases, 'treatment' is no more than a matter of feeding and we return to this problem later in the chapter. For the present, we note that a

---

20 *Superintendent of Belchertown State School v Saikewicz* 370 NE 2d 64 (Mass, 1977).
 1 Eg *Re L H R* 321 SE 2d 716 (Ga, 1984); *John F Kennedy Memorial Hospital Inc v Bludworth* 452 So 2d 921 (Fla, 1984); *Conservatorship of Drabick* 200 Cal App 3d 185 (1988).
 2 *Re Storar* 420 NE 2d 64 (NY, 1981) (consolidating *Eichner v Dillon*).
 3 *Cruzan v Director, Missouri Department of Health* 110 S Ct 2841 (1990). An analysis of the legal effects of *Cruzan* is given in A Meisel 'A Retrospect on *Cruzan*' (1992) 20 Law Med Hlth Care 340. The author cites some 75 'right to die' cases heard in the US courts since 1976. See also F Rouse 'Advance Directives: Where Are We Heading after *Cruzan*?' (1990) 18 Law Med Hlth Care 353.
 4 *Re Claire C Conroy* 464 A 2d 303 (NJ, 1983); on appeal 486 A 2d 1209 (NJ, 1985).
 5 *Re Hilda M Peter* 529 A 2d 419 (NJ, 1987). Withdrawal of treatment from PVS children is also legally acceptable – N K Rhoden 'Treatment Dilemmas for Imperiled Newborns' (1985) 58 S Cal L Rev 1283.

major part of the dilemma of the unconscious patient in the United States relates to the cost of their maintenance; the pressures to regard the persistent vegetative patients as legally dead – or to substitute neocortical death for brain death – are, consequently, very considerable.[6]

Suicide and attempted suicide

No discussion of the right to self-determination would be complete without a reference to suicide. Suicide and attempted suicide are no longer criminal offences.[7] Whether or not this implies a legal right to end one's life is debatable; for present purposes, it can be taken that, at common law, the refusal of life-sustaining treatment is not a matter of attempted suicide.[8] The major interest, here, lies in the relationship of outside agencies to the would-be suicide and, in our particular context, to the standing of the doctor. As to the general outsider, it is now clear that, while counselling or assisting a suicide remains an offence, this can only be illegal if conducted on a basis of immediacy and intent – the impersonal distribution of advice or information is unlikely to attract legal sanction[9] – indeed, books and pamphlets giving detailed instructions on 'self-deliverance' are widely available in both England and Scotland.

Even so, it is the doctor who is most likely to be involved in a personal situation. As has been discussed already with particular reference to the Canadian case of *Rodriguez* (see page 322), he cannot, at present, assist actively in the suicidal process. But can he provide the means for suicide yet leave to the patient the decision to use those means? Can he, in popular terminology, 'leave the pills'? We suggest that, in the legal context, much depends on the method used. It might, for example, be perfectly clear to a patient that he would die were he to use a conveniently located switch to disconnect an electrically operated life-sustaining apparatus; the fatal dose of a drug would be far less obvious and its 'successful' use might depend upon advice from the medical attendant – and, in law, counselling, procuring, aiding and abetting are taken as a whole. The doctor so acting might, therefore, be guilty under the Suicide Act 1961, s 2(1) but the issue would turn on the facts of the individual case and would be closely argued; we are unaware of any such trials in the United Kingdom and doubt very much if a prosecution would succeed. He stands, however, on far less secure *ethical* ground. On the one hand he could be regarded as a moral coward who is unable to carry his convictions to their logical conclusion; on the other, it could be argued that he is providing the means yet firmly placing the responsibility for the decision in autonomous hands – which may be right, but Pontius Pilate still remains a doubtful moral authority.

---

6 R D Mackay 'Terminating Life-sustaining Treatment – Recent US Developments' (1988) 14 J Med Ethics 135. This is not to deny that resources may also be finite within a national health service.
7 Suicide Act 1961.
8 For a discussion of the relationship between suicide and the refusal of treatment, see J Fletcher 'The Courts and Euthanasia' (1987/88) 15 Law Med Hlth Care 223; D Lanham 'The Right to Choose to Die with Dignity' (1990) 14 Crim LJ 401, considers the subject in detail.
9 *A-G v Able* [1984] QB 795, [1984] 1 All ER 277.

The terminally ill patient

In condemning active euthanasia on the grounds which we have identified, we do not suggest that there are not circumstances in which the correct treatment of the patient involves some risk to life – and this is particularly true of the terminally ill. Such persons are beyond curative therapy by definition and treatment becomes a matter of the relief of suffering. The terminally ill patient thus most clearly sets the scene for the application of the philosophical concept of 'double effect'.

The principle of double effect, in simple form, is that an action which has a good objective may be performed despite the fact that the objective can only be achieved at the expense of a coincident harmful effect. This analysis has, however, to be qualified – the action itself must be either good or morally indifferent, the good effect must not be produced by means of the ill-effect and there must be a proportionate reason for allowing the expected ill to occur. It is implicit in this doctrine that the good effect must outweigh the bad and this may involve a value judgment. Thus, it might well be ethically right to administer pain-killing drugs in such dosage as simultaneously shortens the life of a terminally ill patient; it would not be justifiable to give the same dose to a young man with identical pain who stood a reasonable chance of recovery. Lord Edmund Davies[10] put the counter-argument that death is the worst of all evils and, by implication, that it cannot, therefore, be a good objective. Such a view would, however, have little support among moral and religious spokesmen – the Archbishop of Canterbury firmly approved the principle[11] as did Pope Pius XII, with certain limitations, as long ago as 1957;[12] the Sacred Congregation for the Doctrine of the Faith has recently confirmed this view.[13] The legal position now seems reasonably clear.

The seminal case in the United Kingdom is that of *R v Adams*.[14] Dr Adams was thought to have treated a patient, who was incurably but not terminally ill, with increasing doses of opiates. He was tried for murder on her death and was acquitted. In the course of his summing up, Devlin J said:

> The doctor is entitled to relieve pain and suffering even if the measures he takes may incidentally shorten life.

which is a clear direction. Twenty years after the *Adams* verdict, Lord Edmund Davies commented: 'Killing both pain and patient may be good morals but it is far from certain that it is good law.'[15] Williams,[16] by contrast, found the proposition easily justified by necessity. In our view, any conflict has now been resolved. Devlin J's classic direction was followed in *R v Cox*[17] and the latter case was cited with approval by the House of Lords in *Bland*.[18] Treatment of pain undertaken in good faith is lawful; whether it is justified under the essentially moral doctrine of double effect

10 'On Dying and Dying Well' (1977) 70 Proc R Soc Med 73.
11 Fn 11, p 324 above.
12 (1957) 49 Acta Apostolicae Sedis 1027.
13 Fn 12, p 324 above.
14 Fn 8, p 317 above.
15 Commenting on Coggan, fn 11, p 324 above.
16 G Williams *Textbook of Criminal Law* (2nd edn, 1983) p 581.
17 (1992) 12 BMLR 38.
18 *Airedale National Health Service Trust v Bland* [1993] 1 All ER 821, (1993) 12 BMLR 64, HL.

or under the very similar legal principle of necessity is immaterial. We can also look to the important case of *Re C*[19] in which the clinical option to relieve suffering rather than prolong life in the face of accepted terminal illness was reconsidered. This case only came to judicial notice because the patient was a ward of court; we believe, however, that it would be followed as a general principle – there would, in fact, be very few occasions outside wardship in which the courts would expect to be involved. The interesting inclusion of the whole caring team in the decision making process[20] might be thought to be confined to paediatric practice but there is no reason why such a routine should not be extended to hospitals for adults; to do so would not only ensure 'open' decision making, but would also serve to emphasise that the effects of any treatment decisions fall not upon the doctor but on the nursing staff who will care for the dying person.

The incurable patient

The relative simplicity of the euthanasia debate has, thus far, depended upon the use of the adjective 'terminal' which defines a patient status which can only deteriorate. The problems for the doctor become more complex when discussion is extended to the incurably ill whose condition may certainly get worse but which is also likely to remain static for often long times. Many variations on such a state can be envisaged and different therapeutic solutions adduced. There are, however, two overriding considerations likely to influence one's thinking – first, whether the patient is sentient or non-sentient and, second, whether or not the distinction between incurable illness and death depends upon artificial means.

The incapacitated patient

Thus, at one extreme, we have the fully conscious, incapacitated patient able to breathe naturally who is exemplified by the paraplegic or tetraplegic whose condition results from an accident. The clinical and moral solutions here are based on the same principles as relate to the terminally ill but conscious patient – any differences are those of emphasis. In particular, great weight must be given to patient autonomy. Much of the discussion in this area is led by lay people and concentrates on the right to die. Most doctors who have been concerned with disabled persons receiving care and love have, by contrast, been impressed by their tenacity to life and their ability to adapt. This was demonstrated vividly in a study of tetraplegia – a condition which must be as near to wholly intolerable as can be imagined; 18 out of 21 sufferers said that they wished to be resuscitated in the event of their degenerating into coma.[1]

There can be no doubt that it is often undesirable effectively to prolong the process of dying.[2] Nevertheless, it is possible that our attitudes are being moulded

19 *Re C (a minor) (wardship: medical treatment)* [1990] Fam 26, [1989] 2 All ER 782, CA.
20 [1990] Fam 26 at 34, 37, [1989] 2 All ER 782 at 786, 788, per Lord Donaldson MR.
 1 B P Gardner et al 'Ventilation or Dignified Death for Patients with High Tetraplegia' (1985) 291 BMJ 1620. See also M Siegler and A J Weisbard 'Against the Emerging Stream' (1985) 145 Arch Intern Med 129.
 2 A particularly effective series of commentaries is to be found related to E L Schucking 'Death at a New York Hospital' (1985) 13 Law Med Hlth Care 261. See also the papers associated with R F Weir 'Betty's Case: An Introduction' (1989) 17 Law Med Hlth Care 211.

overly in favour of death as an option and there is something to be said for adopting a relatively formal approach to the use of 'Do-not-resuscitate' orders to be effected in the event of cardiopulmonary collapse or coma from other causes. The Royal College of Physicians has drawn up guidelines which indicate that it is inappropriate to attempt to resuscitate patients whose lives are drawing naturally to a close because of irreversible disease,[3] but this leaves open the definition of 'drawing to a close'. Exclusion from resuscitation in British hospitals is said to be more likely in patients with a current diagnosis of malignancy, dementia or pneumonia or with a past or present history of stroke.[4] But at what stage of the disease is the patient with cancer to be regarded as not to be salvaged? How far is any decision dependent on the consent of the patient? What constitutes a high chance of revival for a comfortable and contented existence? – which has been regarded as a criterion for active intervention.[5] To what extent is dementia a contraindication for the benefit of the carers?

The British Medical Association and the Royal College of Nursing have issued a more up-to-date statement which is aimed to promote more discussion –and, it is hoped, uniformity – on the subject in the United Kingdom.[6] In essence, this recommends the following: that a do-not-resuscitate (DNR) decision can be considered when cardiopulmonary resuscitation (CPR) is unlikely to be successful, is contrary to the patient's sustained wishes or is likely to be followed by a quality of life which would be unacceptable to the patient; that in the absence of a decision or of the patient's wishes, resuscitation should be initiated in the event of arrest; that while the overall responsibility for the decision rests with the consultant, the views of the health care staff and the patient's relatives should be canvassed; that discussion of CPR facilities with all patients is not obligatory but sensitive exploration of the wishes of those at risk should be undertaken – and recorded in the hospital notes; that all members of the health care team should be made aware of a DNR order which should, itself, be reviewed regularly; that if the DNR order results from the unlikelihood of any benefit, the clinical decision should be discussed with the patient and others close to him or her; if it derives from quality of life considerations, the views of the patient should be ascertained and, if this is impossible, those of close relatives should be used to assess the patient's best interests. These are clearly little more than points for discussion; they will almost certainly attract criticism – mainly, we suspect, for being too physician orientated. Even so, we doubt if there is any need for legislation on United States lines, given the traditional doctor-patient relationship in the United Kingdom; the possibility was considered by the Parliamentary Select Committee which has reported recently.[7]

3 Working Party of the Royal College of Physicians of London 'Resuscitation from Cardiopulmonary Arrest. Training and Organisation' (1987) 21 J R Coll Physic Lond 175.
4 R M Keating 'Exclusion from Resuscitation' (1989) 82 J R Soc Med 402. For US experience, see S E Bedell et al 'Do-not-resuscitate Orders for Critically Ill Patients in the Hospital' (1986) 256 J Amer Med Ass 233; T E Miller 'Do-not-resuscitate Orders: Public Policy and Patient Autonomy' (1989) 17 Law Med Hlth Care 245.
5 P J F Baskett 'The Ethics of Resuscitation' (1986) 293 BMJ 189.
6 'Cardiopulmonary Resuscitation – A Statement from the BMA and RCN' reported in (1993) Bull Med Ethics, no 86, March, p 3.
7 The House of Lords Select Committee on Medical Ethics did not, in fact, see any need for legislation (HL Paper 21-1, 1994).

Both the double effect doctrine and the productive/non-productive treatment test are available in the management of the incapacitated patient; their rationale needs to be just that much more firmly based than is so in the case of the terminally ill. In our opinion, it is particularly important to ensure that junior doctors in the prime of life are trained to understand the needs of the elderly disabled. The somewhat chilling observation of Rhoads, albeit from across the Atlantic and made some time ago, bears repetition: 'How large a factor is age in deciding to relax therapeutic efforts seems to depend somewhat on the age of the physicians making the decisions.'[8]

The conscious patient maintained artificially

It is fortunate that the interim state – that of mental competence while life is dependent upon a machine – is now rare due to the virtual disappearance of the more serious forms of acute anterior poliomyelitis (infantile paralysis); the least uncommon examples nowadays are those cases of high spinal tetraplegia which cannot be weaned from mechanical ventilation or, as we have seen, cases of motor neurone disease (amyotrophic lateral sclerosis) and the Guillain-Barré syndrome. On the face of things, the problem of what would be the correct action to be taken in the event of a positive request for the doctor to disconnect the mechanical respirator has been eased since the last edition of this book. There is now abundant international case law indicating that not to do so would constitute non-consensual treatment and, accordingly, battery – but the implications of compliance are disturbing. As we discuss later in this chapter, the ethical difficulties concerning the removal of mechanical respiratory support from those who can no longer benefit originate from the *provision* of that support – the primary decision is more important than those which follow as a consequence of that action. But the doctor has virtually no choice of initiative action in the situation now being considered. He is dealing with a conscious but paralysed patient and he must provide support because he cannot know whether an individual patient is going to respond either physically or emotionally to heroic treatment – and, if the doctor does not know, the patient cannot give or withhold his informed consent to setting the therapeutic train in motion. Can the doctor, then, accede to a later request to remove support?

It has been suggested that switching off a mechanical support is an act of omission and, therefore, both morally and legally acceptable. This is, in our opinion, untenable in practical terms. It would be an omission not to switch *on* the emergency supply in the event of a central power failure; that is easily distinguished from a deliberate, premeditated decision to remove the power – one has to *act* to turn off the television and the same will apply to the respirator. Kennedy[9] has pointed out that a well-wisher disconnecting a conscious patient from his respirator would be guilty of homicide or perhaps of abetting suicide – and, in the United States, Mr Linares was, at least, brought before a grand jury.[10] The difference adduced by Lord Goff in *Bland*[11] was that, whereas the doctor was allowing the patient to die from his pre-existing condition, the interloper was actively intervening to stop the doctor from

8 J E Rhoads 'The Right to Die and the Chance to Live' (1980) 6 J Med Ethics 53.
9 I M Kennedy 'Switching Off Life Support Machines: The Legal Implications' [1977] Crim LR 443
10 See Lantos et al, fn 13, p 318.
11 *Airedale National Health Service Trust v Bland* [1993] 1 All ER 821 at 868, (1993) 12 BMLR 64 at 113-114.

prolonging the patient's life. This presupposes that respiratory support is medical treatment, in which case it can be said that there is no logical distinction between stopping renal dialysis at the request of the patient – which would, perhaps, be obligatory – and stopping treatment by artificial respiration. The practical difference must lie in the immediacy and the certainty of death when the respirator is turned off; the care team is, effectively, being asked to suffocate their patient. Lanham[12] has suggested that refusal to turn off a respirator when so requested might be a unique concession to the doctor's ethos allowed within the Victorian legislation which emphatically supports the autonomy of the patient. It is one thing, he says, to prevent doctors from forcing their treatment on an unwilling patient; it is another matter to require them to take what they may regard as unethical positive action to bring a conscious life to an end. Just such a situation was illustrated in a Canadian case[13] in which the court upheld the right of a Guillain-Barré patient to be removed from respirator support. There was, in fact, no dispute as the physician concerned seems to have been anxious to comply with the patient's request. But what if the doctor's Hippocratic conscience forbade him to do so?

Were such a situation to arise in the United Kingdom, it would be a proper case for referral to the court as in the American tradition. At least two apposite cases have been described there. In *McAfee*, a tetraplegic's request for disconnection was not only agreed but his right to professional assistance during the agonal phase was upheld; in *Farrell*, a similar request, and agreement, derived from paralysis due to motor neurone disease.[14] We doubt whether the British courts would adopt a similar attitude in the precise conditions. We believe they would be more likely to give preference to the parallel line of American opinion which held, for example, in *Farrell*, that, in the event of conflict, the patient had no right to 'compel a health-care provider to violate generally accepted professional standards'. What seems clear is that any legislation on the point ought to include a 'conscience clause' which would limit a doctor's liability in such circumstances to transferring the care of his patient to another who would be prepared to carry out the manoeuvre.

The unconscious patient
There remain for consideration those patients who are, again, either capable of a free existence or who depend for survival upon mechanical aids but who are, by contrast, unconscious by virtue of hypoxic brain damage. There are good theoretical and practical reasons for isolating the unconscious patient as a particular ethical problem area. The theoretical basis is summed up in the phrase: 'Consciousness is the most critical moral, legal, and constitutional standard, not for human life itself, but for human personhood.'[15] The unconscious or comatose patient is incapable of fulfilling his human function in a way which transcends the loss of any other capacity. He cannot speak for himself; he cannot consent and decisions on his behalf must be

---

12 D Lanham 'The Right to Choose to Die with Dignity' (1990) 14 Crim LJ 401.

13 *Nancy B v Hôtel-Dieu de Québec* (1992) 86 DLR (4th) 385, (1992) 15 BMLR 95.

14 *Re Kathleen Farrell* 529 A 2d 404 (NJ, 1987); *State v McAfee* 385 SE 2d 651 (Ga, 1989). For comparable medical assistance, see *Bouvia v The Superior Court of Los Angeles County* 179 Cal App 3d 1127 (1986).

15 R E Cranford and D R Smith 'Consciousness: The Most Critical Moral (Constitutional) Standard for Human Personhood' (1987) 13 Amer J Law Med 233.

taken by others and be justified either on a 'best interests' test or by way of substituted judgment. Moreover, as we have discussed under the diagnosis of death, brain substance which is destroyed is destroyed beyond repair and cannot be replicated; the doctor confronted with such injury knows that whatever degree of humanity has been lost is irrecoverable.

We are concerned, here, only with such irreversible damage. This, as we have indicated in chapter 13, may be of such a degree as will allow the patient an independent existence in any condition ranging from intellectual loss to a persistent vegetative state. At this point it is necessary only to reiterate that the last cases, tragic as they may be, still represent 'persons in being'. The law as to killing is unaffected by the mental state of the victim – dements and aments are still protected in so far as the term 'reasonable being' implies no more than 'human being' – and is the same as has already been discussed in relation to the conscious patient. Lord Scarman,[16] while appreciating —

> that there are great social problems not only in the life support of the human vegetable but also in the survival of barely sentient people who cannot look after themselves.

also added:

> there are implications in the right to terminate another's existence of which it is well to be fearful in the absence of a more prolonged analysis of the problem than that which it has received.

This remark was made some time ago and, since then, the topic has been subject to intense scrutiny – albeit with no firm conclusion. 'Irreversible loss of consciousness' may, indeed, 'one day become the mark of death' but that day is not here yet – certainly not in a legal sense. These patients present an extra therapeutic difficulty as, being unconscious, they are free from pain – or, at least, pain cannot be expressed in a manner which makes it treatable; the doctrine of 'double effect' is, therefore, hard to apply. Moreover, the permanently unconscious have strictly limited interests and, in the circumstances, it seems scarcely appropriate to speak of a therapeutic 'best interests test'. Common sense tells us, however, that there can be few instances in medical practice where the productive/non-productive treatment test is as readily appropriate. It is almost beyond argument that patients with this degree of brain damage should not, for example, be ventilated when their respiration fails.[17]

Such difficulty as remains derives from the definition – and demonstration – of *irreversible* damage. As far as the adult is concerned, the diagnosis is usually clear-cut but there are persistent reports of recovery of some function following several months in the vegetative state.[18] Even then, it is generally improbable that the

---

16 Lord Scarman 'Legal Liability and Medicine' (1981) 74 Proc R Soc Med 11.

17 But nothing is certain. It is reported that a US District Court judge has ruled that a hospital must provide aggressive life-sustaining treatment, including ventilation, to an anencephalic infant as and when the mother requests it: M McCarthy 'Anencephalic Baby's Right to Life?' (1993) 342 Lancet 919.

18 For discussion, see a series of papers: K Andrews 'Recovery of Patients after Four Months or More in the Persistent Vegetative State' (1993) 306 BMJ 1597, 'Patients in the Persistent Vegetative State: Problems in their Long Term Management' (1993) 306 BMJ 1600; R Gillon 'Patients in the Persistent Vegetative State: A Response to Dr Andrews' (1993) 306 BMJ 1602.

resultant state would pass either a 'best interests' or a 'substituted judgment' test; the doubt raised is, however, sufficient to indicate the need for a *Bolam* standard of practice (see p 200). Such guidelines have been promulgated by the British Medical Association[19] and include recommendations that: rehabilitation efforts should not be relaxed for six months after the anoxic insult to the brain; the diagnosis of persistence should not be confirmed within 12 months of the incident; the diagnosis should be corroborated by two other doctors independently; and the wishes of the immediate family as to management should be taken into consideration. As to the last point, we strongly support the comments of Lord Goff in *Bland*[20] to the effect that the attitudes of relatives should not be determinative. As in the case of the handicapped neonate (see p 155), pure objectivity is very hard to attain in such circumstances; one of the useful side-effects of a 12-month waiting period is that any conflicts as to management are, meantime, usually resolved.

Undoubtedly, the most difficult management decisions in the case of patients in the persistent vegetative state relate to the provision of alimentation; we return to this specific aspect at p 339.

The patient in intensive care

This brings us to the ultimate stage of human existence – the comatose patient who is unable to sustain his cardiorespiratory functions without the aid of mechanical ventilation.

Kennedy has argued[1] that the ethical dilemmas associated with ventilation apply not so much to the removal of support as to the admission of patients to intensive treatment. The vast majority – perhaps all – of living patients with severe brain damage must be offered such care when they present at hospital. Automatic recourse is for the purpose of facilitating diagnosis and assessment. If a diagnosis of irretrievable functional brain loss is made, there is no legal or ethical objection to regarding the ventilator as no more than part of the diagnostic machinery and dispensing with it once it has served its purpose. But a decision to treat, which, in this case, is within the doctor's clinical choice, is a different matter carrying with it the inescapable consequence that, at some time and for some reason, the treatment must be withdrawn. The critical point for applying the productive/ non-productive ethical test is, thus, at the beginning. With one exception, any later decisions are based on clinical or technical considerations alone.

This exceptional ethical decision relates to the allocation of scarce resources which include machines, beds, doctors and nursing staff, together with the necessary technical back-up. It may be necessary for a resource-based value judgment to be made at some point. Making a choice between patients may be among the doctor's most agonising moments and the weight to be given to economic and policy considerations can only be judged by the individual physician or surgeon on such factors as are outlined in chapter 11.

---

19 British Medical Association *Treatment of Patients in Persistent Vegetative State* (1992).
20 *Airedale National Health Service Trust v Bland* [1993] 1 All ER 821 at 872, (1993) 12 BMLR 64 at 118, HL.
1 I M Kennedy 'Switching Off Life Support Machines: The Legal Implications' [1977] Crim LR 443.

Resources aside, the removal of a patient from ventilation depends, primarily, on a simple alternative – either he is dead or he is not dead. It can be taken that the whole brain is dead once the criteria for brain stem death have been met and we have the authority of the Conference of the Royal Medical Colleges and their Faculties[2] that the individual is dead when the whole brain is dead. In such circumstances, continued treatment is no more than treatment of a corpse – far from being unethical to withhold support, it would be positively immoral to continue other than to serve the purpose of beating heart organ donation or, conceivably, of post-mortem parturition.

However, it may still be proper to discontinue artificial ventilation even if death is not diagnosed. The closely allied considerations of productive/non-productive treatment and of 'death with dignity', untrammelled by tubes and wires, may be regarded by some as being related to the moral sphere and by others as being clinical in nature. Even so, the purely clinical consideration – that the treatment is doing, and will do, no good – will justify removal of support. One of two things may then happen – the patient will either continue to breathe of his own accord or he will die. In the former case, the patient has reverted to the persistent vegetative state, the management of which has already been discussed. Such was the situation and the outcome in the widely publicised and very significant case of Karen Quinlan in which it was established that there was 'no reasonable possibility of her ever emerging from her present comatose condition to a cognitive, sapient state', that 'there would be no criminal homicide in the circumstances' and that death following withdrawal of ventilatory support would 'not be homicide but rather expiration from existing natural causes'.[3] It is true that Ms Quinlan did not die as anticipated. Nevertheless, had she done so, there would have been no moral or legal problem; the outcome would have resulted from a clinical decision taken in good faith and after due deliberation based on a productive/non-productive treatment test. In the current context, there is no need, as there clearly was in the case of the conscious patient, to argue as to whether removal of support is a matter of commission or omission.

Liability for withholding treatment

The Quinlan case settled the problem of criminal liability for ventilation withdrawal in the United States and there have been many later confirmations of this.[4] The position in the United Kingdom was resolved, first through the Scottish case of *Finlayson*[5] and later in the English case of *Malcherek*,[6] both of which have been discussed in relation to causation in chapter 13. Although *Finlayson* was not cited in *Malcherek*, the two decisions have remarkable similarities in that, in excluding criminality, the judges first relied on the concept of good medical practice and, second, declined to define death in both cases. This latter omission might, at first

2   'Diagnosis of Death' [1979] 1 BMJ 332. Legislation to this effect is generalised in the English-speaking world.
3   *Re Quinlan* 355 A 2d 664 (NJ, 1976), per Hughes J.
4   *John F Kennedy Memorial Hospital Inc v Bludworth* 452 So 2d 921 (Fla, 1984); *Re Bertha Colyer* 660 P 2d 738 (Wash, 1983); *Re Nancy Ellen Jobes* 529 A 2d 434 (NJ, 1987).
5   *Finlayson v HM Advocate* 1978 SLT (Notes) 60.
6   [1981] 2 All ER 422, [1981] 1 WLR 690, CA, *R v Steel* being heard simultaneously on appeal.

glance, be interpreted as vacillation on the part of the law; in fact, it reinforces the former principle in leaving the clinical decision firmly in the hands of the clinician.[7]

There is no reason to suppose that these decisions would not be applied in the civil courts and it would now be necessary to prove negligence – with all that entails – before a doctor could be considered culpable of a ventilator death. There are no United Kingdom authorities but a similar policy line has been adopted in the United States.[8]

A need for legislation?

It will be seen that, throughout this discussion, we have tended to the view that there is little need for legislation in respect of the incurably or terminally ill adult patient; the great majority of life or death decisions can be based on good medical practice which is contained by relatively clear legal and moral guidelines. Since the last edition of this book, however, there have been a number of court decisions extending the ambit of non-treatment decisions; at the same time the movement in favour of voluntary euthanasia has gained considerable momentum. Some unease is apparent as to the capacity of the common law to contain what could become moral turmoil and there are a number of advocates of what can be loosely termed 'allowing to die' legislation; we have, ourselves, advocated defining legislation in the case of the neonate in chapter 7. Powerful voices such as those of Lord Browne-Wilkinson and Lord Mustill cannot be ignored. The former asked:

> Should judges seek to develop new law to meet a wholly new situation? Or is this a matter which lies outside the area of legitimate development of the law by judges and requires society, through the democratic expression of its views in Parliament, to reach its decisions on the underlying moral and practical problems and then reflect those decisions in legislation? I have no doubt that it is for Parliament, not the courts, to decide the broader issues which this case raises.[9]

and Lord Mustill expressed his entire agreement.

There are, of course, many hazards in legislating for what are broad moral issues. We have seen from the Netherlands experience that attempts to satisfy all political views result only in confusion for the medical profession. The great majority of 'allowing to die' statutes passed in the United States, particularly in the wake of the *Cruzan* decision, allow for some professional privilege in interpreting instructions and many feel that this represents an actual reduction in patient autonomy. Many years ago, Lappé, discussing the first of these Acts, suggested that, in addition to eroding the patient's rights, legislation may lead to deterioration in standards of care

---

7 Some concern was shown in Scotland when the Solicitor General stated that the prosecuting authorities were not in a position to give an assurance that withdrawing life support would not lead to prosecution: G Duncan 'Doctors Warned about Decision to Withdraw Life Support' (1993) Scotsman, 1 April, p 3. We believe, however, that this was no more than a reminder as to procedure, not as to principle.

8 Eg *Lovato v District Court* 601 P 2d 1072 (Colo, 1979).

9 *Airedale National Health Service Trust v Bland* [1993] 1 All ER 821 at 878, (1993) 12 BMLR 64 at 124, HL.

– by covering poor treatment with the cloak of obedience to a directive – and may lead to the creation of conflict between doctor and patient in so far as both autonomy and paternalism are being simultaneously attacked.[10]

The original California Natural Death Act of 1976 is among those that are, in fact, restrictive. It deals only with 'medical procedures or intervention which utilises mechanical or other artificial means to sustain, restore or supplant a vital function' and can be applied only when 'death is imminent whether or not such procedures are utilised'. US legislation, either enacted or proposed, covers a wide range – from the limited Californian conditions, through the wide acceptance of patient autonomy, subject only to public policy, as in Alabama, to the potential euthanistic permissiveness of Idaho – and none seems entirely satisfactory. Following the attempt at uniformity introduced by the Uniform Rights of the Terminally Ill Act 1985,[11] the Patient Self Determination Act was brought into force in the United States at the end of 1991. The Act is relatively unadventurous and, essentially, lays a duty on hospitals to advise patients of their rights to accept or refuse medical treatment and to execute an advanced directive. The difficulties in drafting in such a complex area are clear from both examples.

To say that legislation will be difficult is not, however, to say that it should not be attempted and we now believe that some form of statutory law regulating 'controlled death' is inevitable, and needed, in the United Kingdom. We have sufficient faith in our legislators to believe that they will stop short of a fundamental alteration of the healing face of medicine. It may be better to start with relatively minor modifications of the law.

In this respect, the very great importance of the advanced directive in the United States is to be contrasted with its lack of standing in British law; the English Enduring Powers of Attorney Act 1985, unlike its American and Australian counterparts,[12] makes no provision for medical control of the incompetent client – nor does the Law Reform (Miscellaneous Provisions) (Scotland) Act 1990, s 71. An advance directive may, however, be useful to the clinician in charge of the case. We believe it should be incumbent upon a lawyer who is aware of its existence to notify the medical attendant of the fact in appropriate circumstances and that it would not be difficult to make this a legal duty by way of statute. There is, in fact, some evidence that lawyers are already accepting the potential validity of the advanced directive – both Lord Keith and Lord Goff clearly expressed their view that an advanced directive spoke as firmly for the incompetent as did consent for the competent.[13] No one would deny the very great difficulties posed by any declaration made some time before it

---

10 M Lappé 'Dying while Living: A Critique of Allowing-to-die Legislation' (1978) 4 J Med Ethics 195.
11 For a full appraisal of this Act, see I Kennedy and A Grubb *Medical Law: Text and Materials* (1989), p p 1137.
12 Eg Durable Power of Attorney Health Care Act 1983 (California) – Kennedy and Grubb, fn 11 above at 1145; Medical Treatment (Enduring Power of Attorney) Act 1990 (Victoria).
13 *Airedale National Health Service Trust v Bland* [1993] 1 All ER 821, (1993) 12 BMLR 64, HL. This appears to have been followed in *Re C (adult: refusal of treatment)* [1994] 1 All ER 819, where it was held to be common ground that a refusal can take the form of a declaration of intention never to consent in the future (Thorpe J at 824).

is put into effect both as to interpretation and activation[14] – changes of mind are part of human nature one can, for example, foresee difficulties for the doctor being required to validate a refusal of treatment as was indicated in *Re T*.[15] But it could be a useful way of edging towards more comprehensive legislation. A specimen 'living will' is reproduced at Appendix G.

Feeding as a part of treatment

We have left to the last what we regard as the most contentious issue in the euthanasia debate – the relationship between the provision of nutritional support and medical treatment. Again, this has been addressed most often in the United States where the uncertainties in the courts have been matched by the inconsistencies in State statutes. Until recently, the problem had been broached publicly in the United Kingdom only in relation to neonatal care when it came to a head with the trial of Dr Arthur (see p 151); although Dr Arthur was acquitted of attempted murder, reaction in the aftermath of the trial was such that we doubt whether instructions are now likely to be given not to feed a neonate who is able to take nourishment by mouth; failure to feed a baby simply because it is likely to be mentally retarded is frankly illegal in the United States, Canada and Australia.[16] Feeding is not, however, a simple concept. As Strong[17] has pointed out, when we speak of providing nourishment, we are referring to a continuum which runs from natural breast feeding through feeding by mouth to seriously invasive procedures which may even entail surgical operation. Once discomfort and danger are introduced, so too is balancing the advantages and disadvantages – or, in practice, applying a productive/non-productive treatment test. The fundamental question is, therefore, at what stage does the natural act of feeding become medical treatment?

There have been a number of apposite court hearings in the United States. The most dramatic of these was the Californian case of Dr Barber and Dr Nejdl, who removed respiratory support and both nasogastric and intravenous feeding lines from a patient in the persistent vegetative state. Their action was taken on the basis of medical expertise and with the consent of the family but, nevertheless, the two doctors were indicted for murder. The charge was dismissed in the lower court but was reinstated on appeal by the prosecution; it was only on appeal from this reinstatement[18] that they were finally discharged, the court not only finding their action justified once treatment was proven to be ineffective but also determining that artificial feeding was part of medical treatment and subject to the same tests as to propriety.

---

14 For recent editorial comment, see T Hope 'Advance Directives about Medical Treatment' (1992) 304 BMJ 398; 'Advance Directives' (1992) 340 Lancet 1321. For a full exposition, see Age Concern Institute of Gerontology *The Living Will* (1988).

15 *Re T (adult: refusal of medical treatment)* [1992] 4 All ER 649, (1992) 9 BMLR 46.

16 See, for example, J E Magnet 'Withholding Treatment from Defective Newborns: Legal Aspects' (1982) 42 Rev du Bar 187; J M Maciejczyk 'Withholding Treatment from Defective Infants: "Infant Doe" Post-mortem' (1983) Notre Dame Law Rev 224; see also the Australian case *Re F*, fn 2, p 154 above.

17 C Strong 'Can Fluids and Electrolytes be "Extraordinary Treatment"?' (1981) 7 J Med Ethics 83.

18 *Barber and Nejdl v Superior Court of Los Angeles County and the People* 147 Cal App 3d 1006 (1983).

Aside from this case taken in the criminal courts, there are a number of decisions in the American civil courts from which to draw the conclusion that treatment and nutrition are steadily being equated in respect of the patient's right to an autonomous choice.[19] The relationship is, however, clearly not absolute and the important case of *Conroy*[20] aptly demonstrates the stresses imposed when the courts are forced into clinical arbitration.

Ms Conroy was an elderly incompetent diabetic, severely malformed and with an intellectual capacity only marginally above that of a person in the persistent vegetative state. Permission to remove her nasogastric tube was sought and granted by the trial court on the grounds that no valid purpose was served by needlessly prolonging a useless life. Although the subject had, meanwhile, died, the finding was appealed and was reversed – the Court of Appeal considering that death following removal of the feeding tube would have been due to dehydration and starvation; this implied active killing and they were not prepared to condone active euthanasia. Great concern was also expressed as to the knock-on effect which might seriously compromise the standards of treatment of the mentally retarded and of the senile demented. Even so, the Supreme Court of New Jersey reversed the appellate decision, holding that —

> artificial feeding by means of a nasogastric tube . . . can be seen as equivalent to artificial breathing by means of a respirator. Both prolong life through mechanical means when the body is no longer able to perform a vital bodily function on its own.[1]

the extrapolation being that the patient has the right to refuse both. While the Supreme Court commended the appointment of a guardian to act as proxy for the incompetent, it still laid down very strict criteria – including investigation by an ombudsman – before such decisions could be taken by the medical staff and the guardian or relatives. It could be that this caution was prompted partially by the fact that Ms Conroy was being treated in a nursing home; later decisions related to hospital patients have not imposed such conditions.

The movement is, thus, towards pure self-determination within a medical ambience. The American courts, as always, place immense importance on prior expression of that determination but have been increasingly prepared to allow surrogate decision making through family or guardian ad litem – and, in doing so, are allowing the application of a 'best interests' test. Purely medical considerations will also apply. Increasing invasiveness carries increasing risk – the complication rate of intravenous hyperalimentation may approach 50%.[2] The solution of the

19 Eg: *Re Severns* 425 A 2d 156 (Del, 1980) (Replacement of nasogastric tube); *Re Mary Hier* 464 NE 2d 959 (Mass, 1984) (Gastrostomy); *Brophy v New England Sinai Hospital* 497 NE 2d 626 (Mass, 1986) (Gastrostomy); *Corbett v D'Alessandro* 487 So 2d 368 (Fla, 1986) (Nasogastric tube); *Re Hilda M Peter* 529 A 2d 419 (NJ, 1987) (Nasogastric tube); Jobes, fn 4, p 336 above (Nasogastric tube). In *Re Requena* 517 A 2d 893 (NJ, 1986), a hospital was ordered to retain a patient who refused to consent to artificial feeding and to honour her decision.
20 *Re Claire C Conroy* 464 A 2d 303 (NJ, 1983); on appeal 486 A 2d 1209 (NJ, 1985).
 1 Per Schreiber J at 1236.
 2 K C Micetich et al 'Are Intravenous Fluids Morally Required for a Dying Patient?' (1983) 143 Arch Intern Med 975. For review, see R S Dresser and EV Boisaubin 'Ethics, Law, and Nutritional Support' (1985) 145 Arch Intern Med 122.

problem is one of balance and has been summarised by Meyers:[3] 'The greater the invasiveness and the more hopeless the prognosis, the less will be the obligation to provide other than misting and manual feeding by mouth.'

And therein lies the important corollary – there is, by implication, a difference drawn between natural and artificial feeding and, so far as we can see, no American court has ever suggested that normal feeding could properly be withheld from someone able to accept it. None the less, even this distinction is over-simplistic. At one extreme, spoon feeding of a reluctant ament can be regarded as invasive and, accordingly, improper treatment; at the other, the instillation of fluid through a tube can be seen as simple care involving no risk – but it can be done only as a *result* of invasion. The difficulties are exemplified in the drafting of the Victorian legislation which includes 'the reasonable provision of food and water' under the heading of palliative treatment – and, therefore, outwith the statutory control of the patient.[4] 'Reasonable', however, is undefined and the position as to the patient's common law rights remains open. An all-embracing solution seems impossible. We can only look to a minimum standard and suggest that, whereas artificial feeding inevitably requires some medical expertise and is, therefore, rightly considered part of selective medical treatment, the provision of food and water by normal means is a matter of skilled nursing care. It may also be seen as the quintessential example of kindness and humanity.

This description is taken from Hoffmann LJ in what became the first United Kingdom case in which the matter was addressed.[5] Anthony Bland was crushed in a football stadium in April 1989 and sustained severe anoxic brain damage; as a result, he relapsed into the persistent vegetative state (see p 283). There was no improvement in his condition by September 1992 and, at that time, the hospital sought a declaration to the effect that they might lawfully discontinue all life-sustaining treatment and medical support measures including ventilation, nutrition and hydration by artificial means; that any subsequent treatment given should be for the sole purpose of enabling him to end his life in dignity and free from pain and suffering; that, if death should then occur, its cause should be attributed to the natural and other causes of his present state; and that none of those concerned should, as a result, be subject to any civil or criminal liability. This declaration – save, for technical reasons, the final clause – was granted in the Family Division essentially on the grounds that it was in AB's best interests to do so; the court considered there was overwhelming evidence that the provision of artificial feeding by means of a nasogastric tube was 'medical treatment' and that its discontinuance was in accord with good medical practice – an absolute view which was to be criticised in the later stages of the case. An appeal was unanimously dismissed in the Court of Appeal. From three exceptionally well-considered opinions, we extract only that of Hoffmann LJ:[6]

---

3   D W Meyers *Medico-legal Implications of Death and Dying*, Cum Supp (1984) p 84. A complete book has been devoted to this single issue: J Lynn (ed) *No Extraordinary Means* (1989).
4   Medical Treatment Act 1988 (Vict), s 3.
5   *Airedale National Health Service Trust v Bland* [1993] 1 All ER 821 at 856, (1993) 12 BMLR 64 at 101, CA.
6   [1993] 1 All ER 821 at 850, (1993) 12 BMLR 64 at 95.

> This is not an area in which any difference can be allowed to exist between what is legal and what is morally right. The decision of the court should be able to carry conviction with the ordinary person as being based not merely on legal precedent but also upon acceptable ethical values.

and, later:[7]

> In my view the choice the law makes must reassure people that the courts do have full respect for life, but that they do not pursue the principle to the point at which it has become almost empty of any real content and when it involves the sacrifice of other important values such as human dignity and freedom of choice. I think that such reassurance can be provided by a decision, properly explained, to allow Anthony Bland to die.

These aspects were very fully explored in the House of Lords, where it was particularly emphasised that, whereas the function of the courts was normally to answer questions of law, they could not, in cases such as these, avoid addressing the ethical, moral and practical issues involved. Here, the fundamental conflict lies in the inevitable distortion of the entrenched principle of the sanctity of life which would result from a decision to terminate treatment of care on which life depended. The majority of the House was able to dispose of this on the grounds that the principle was certainly not absolute; Lord Browne-Wilkinson also asked[8] what was meant by 'life' within that precept. It must surely mean life as it is generally known and we believe that it cannot possibly stretch to include life in the vegetative state. Moreover, since the right to refuse treatment – including life-sustaining treatment – is now firmly part of English law and medical ethics, the principle of the sanctity of life must yield to that of the right to self-determination and, of the many lines of argument considered, it is this which seems to us to bind all five Law Lords most closely together. As Lord Goff put it,[9] the right to self-determination should not be eclipsed by the fact of incompetence – it must always be present. Somewhat surprisingly, the naturally consequential 'substituted judgment' test was firmly rejected in favour of that of 'best interests' but, as we have argued elsewhere,[10] both commonly reach the same end-point and a distinction is needed only rarely. It was emphasised that the issue was not that it was in the patient's best interests to die; rather, the question was whether it was in his best interests to prolong treatment – and, in a case of persistent vegetative state in which the higher brain was known to have liquefied, the answer was clearly No.

This appears to us to embody the most acceptable ethical justification for the withdrawal of treatment in the form of nasogastric feeding. It is also to be noted as being, at base, the *only* justification for dismissing the appeal accepted by Lord Mustill in his highly critical speech. We are less happy with the alternative view of self-determination taken, in particular, by Lord Lowry and Lord Browne-Wilkinson.

---

7 [1993] 1 All ER 821 at 855, (1993) 12 BMLR 64 at 100.
8 [1993] 1 All ER 821 at 878, (1993) 12 BMLR 64 at 125.
9 [1993] 1 All ER 821 at 866, (1993) 12 BMLR 64 at 112.
10 J K Mason 'Master of the Balancers: Non-consensual Treatment under the Mantle of Lord Donaldson' [1993] Juridical Rev 115.

In essence, this started from the premise that non-voluntary treatment was lawful only so long as it was justified by necessity; once necessity could no longer be claimed – by reason of the futility of treatment – further invasion of the patient's body constituted either the crime of battery or the tort of trespass. On this view, any potential medical offence lies not in *withholding* treatment but in *continuing* it to no purpose. This argument has the merits of damping the emotional flames engendered; it does, however, seem to us to be dangerously open-ended in relation to conditions less clear-cut than the persistent vegetative state – a situation which Lord Mustill was clearly anxious to avoid. It is better that a doctor, trained to preserve life, should be required to defend himself against failure to do so rather than for following his natural inclinations. In either event, the assessment of benefit to the patient is a matter of clinical judgment – we return to this below.

It is worth pointing out some of the misgivings which were voiced with varying emphasis in the judgments in *Bland*. Fundamental to the whole discussion was the distinction, if any, to be made between acts and omissions causing death. There was wide agreement that, while there was no moral or logical difference, a distinction was certainly to be made in law. The judges came to a unanimous conclusion, via differing routes, that discontinuance of nasogastric feeding was an omission; such a finding was, of course, essential to accepting that the proposed therapeutic programme was lawful. Second, as we have already discussed, doubt was expressed as to whether the court was the correct forum in which to make such decisions; strong pleas were made that it was for Parliament to decide a policy for practices which were so susceptible to subjective assessment by both doctors and judges.[11] Third, and most importantly in the present context, there was a consensus that, although nasogastric feeding might not, strictly speaking be medical treatment, it formed an inseparable part of general medical care.[12]

We then have to ask what is wrong with regarding the whole issue as a medical matter – having regard to the fact that the Americans find no difficulty in the medicalisation of artificial feeding.[13] Once this premise is accepted, a number of difficulties are simultaneously resolved. The cause of death, for example, remains the disease or injury for which the treatment was being given – the question of novus actus interveniens no longer arises. It also implies that the decision can be made on the basis of clinical judgment alone – something which Lord Keith, at least, was prepared to accept. *Bland* then ceases to be a unique case and can be subsumed within the large number of selective non-treatment decisions which are part of the every-day practice of medicine. A move in this direction was clearly envisaged by Lord Goff when he expressed the hope that, while Sir Stephen Brown P's formula for the routine submission of such decisions to the High Court was currently desirable, a way could be found to relax these requirements so as to limit applications for

---

11 A Select Committee of the House of Lords on 'Medical Ethics' has recently reported on 'euthanasia' – see fn 7, p 331, fn 17, p 161 above.

12 For a forthright criticism of the House of Lords decision, see J M Finnis '*Bland*: Crossing the Rubicon?' (1993) 109 LQR 329.

13 See, for example, B Brody 'Special Ethical Issues in the Management of PVS Patients' (1992) 20 Law Med Hlth Care 104.

declarations to those cases in which there was a special need.[14] The danger, of course, lies in placing too much power in the hands of individual doctors.

While this is a fear which we have already expressed at p 16, it raises one further relevant question – is not *Bland*, in essence, a case concerned with consent to treatment and should it , in fact, be discussed in a chapter headed 'Euthanasia'? We can revert to Hoffmann LJ who said:

> This is not a case about euthanasia because it does not involve any external agency of death. It is about whether, and how, the patient should be allowed to die[15]

a proposition which was given tacit approval by Lord Lowry. We suggest that, once it is accepted, any potential 'slippery slope' towards unlawful killing of the incompetent can be effectively sanded.

Since this chapter was completed, the very comparable case of *Frenchay Healthcare NHS Trust v S*[16] has been decided. This case involved the reinsertion of a gastrosomy tube which had been accidentally dislodged during the treatment of a patient who had been in PVS for over two years; the Court of Appeal decided that it was in S's best interests that the tube was not replaced. *Bland* was closely followed but, although a full report is still not available, the case seems to extend the established principles incrementally – the court was, for example, prepared to cut procedural corners in the face of necessity and there was a suggestion that the evidence as to the totality of the PVS was not as emphatic as was the case in *Bland*; from a reading of the summary report, this did not strike us as being significant. Attention has been drawn to a further distinction between the two cases. Whereas *Bland*'s PVS was due to accident, S's condition may have derived from attempted suicide – a condition which may make a decision to withdraw treatment that much less difficult.[17] On present evidence, *S* seems to us to do little more than demonstrate that appeals to the court are likely to increase in number until a set of guidelines which covers all the subtle variations on the theme of PVS has been established.

Although it is misplaced under the sub-heading 'Feeding', it is appropriate to mention here a parallel case heard in New Zealand.[18] In some ways this was a more difficult case than was that of *Bland* in that the patient, L, was not brain dead; his brain was, rather, disconnected from his body by reason of the Guillain-Barré syndrome which results in degeneration of the peripheral nerve axons leading, in his case, to total paralysis and sensory loss – a condition akin to the 'locked-in' syndrome.[19] His existence depended on artificial ventilation rather than feeding and

---

14 *Airedale National Health Service Trust v Bland* [1993] 1 All ER 821 at 874, (1993) 12 BMLR 64 at 121.

15 [1993] 1 All ER 821 at 856, (1993) 12 BMLR 64 at 101.

16 (1994) Times, 19 January.

17 D Brahams 'Non-renewal of Life Support for PVS' (1994) 343 Lancet 286.

18 *Auckland Area Health Board v A-G* [1993] 1 NZLR 235, [1993] 4 Med LR 239. The Canadian case of *Nancy B v Hôtel-Dieu de Québec* (1992) 86 DLR (4th) 385, (1992) 15 BMLR 95 is distinguished in that Ms B, also suffering from the Guillain-Barré syndrome, was mentally competent and able to request withdrawal of respirator treatment.

19 Fn 12, p 284 above.

the question put to the High Court was in rather starker terms than in the case of *Bland*: would the doctors' action in withdrawing ventilator support make them guilty of homicide?[20]

Thomas J approached this issue through the relatively narrow aspect of whether a doctor is obliged to continue treatment which has no therapeutic or medical benefit notwithstanding that the withdrawal of the treatment may result in the clinical death of the patient. He made the interesting comment that, in a case such as this, all natural life has ceased; it is the *manifestations* of life which are maintained artificially and which are brought to an end by the doctor's intervention. He proceeded on the twin principles of humanity and common sense. On this basis, he concluded that life support provided *only* for the purpose of deferring certain death could not be regarded as a necessary of life; moreover, doctors have a lawful excuse to discontinue treatment when there is no medical justification for continuing that medical assistance. Withdrawal of treatment would not be unlawful if it was carried out within the accepted confines of 'good medical practice' – or adhering to a procedure which provided safeguards against the possibility of individual error. Within this scenario, withdrawal of life support would not be the cause of death *as a matter of law* – and this would coincide with the common sense perception.

Within its narrow parameters, Thomas J's analysis is admirable save, we think, for this final phrase which was introduced largely to spare the blushes of the medical staff. We believe that death certification should be accurate irrespective of emotion. To this end, we suggest that the cause of death following withdrawal of any form of life support depends solely on whether the support was removed before or after brain stem death has occurred. If the body is dead at that time, the cause of death is clearly the original anoxic or other insult sustained by the brain. When, however, a treatment is discontinued solely by reason of its futility, there is nothing to be lost – and much to be gained by way of intellectual honesty – in attributing death, correctly, to 'Lawful withdrawal of life support systems which were necessitated by [the disease]'.

20 Crimes Act 1961, ss. 151(1) and 164, NZ.

Research and Experimentation

16 Biomedical human research and experimentation

At one time, biomedical experimentation using human subjects proceeded almost without comment. The researchers justified their activities as benefiting mankind; the subjects were generally happy to 'oblige' or to be reasonably recompensed; and research was of manageable quantity. Attitudes and conditions have, however, changed. The reaction against paternalistic medicine has gained momentum pari passu with an increasing concern for the rights of the individual; the potential investigations and the instrumental and other means for conducting them have greatly increased; and there has been something of an explosion not only in the production of new therapeutic agents but also in governmental control of their distribution – witness the copious legislation regulating the marketing of medicines. But the greatest single impulse to regulate experiments on human beings sprang from a realisation of the appalling depths which were plumbed in the genocidal era of the Second World War when, undoubtedly, much valuable information was gathered but only at the cost of immense suffering. The awareness of what had happened in the medical laboratories of Nazi Germany and Japan led to a determination that medical research should never again be tainted by such callous disregard for the rights of the individual, and it is this determination which led to the promulgation of international codes on the ethics of research. Such endeavours were not everywhere supported, however, and the end of the Soviet era in Eastern Europe resulted in a frank acknowledgement in a number of countries that medical science in the Soviet Union and its satellite countries had far from met the ethical standards expected in the West.[1] This has been translated into action in Poland, for example, by the introduction of a code of medical ethics which, in a remarkable judgment of the Polish Constitutional Court in 1992 was held to outrank contradictory provisions of the law.[2]

Ethical codes in human biomedical experimentation

The first internationally accepted set of ethical guidelines in this context was known as the Nuremberg code and was a direct result of the war-crimes trials.[3] It is, perhaps, unfortunate that this should be so as it inevitably puts the researcher on the defensive. To minimise this, the tribunal itself adopted the preamble:

---

1 Z Szawarski 'Research Ethics in Eastern Europe' (1992) Bull Inst Med Ethics No 82, 13.
2 The English text of this code is published in (1992) Bull Inst Med Ethics No 82, 13; the decision of the Constitutional Court is discussed by E Zielinska at p 25.
3 References to the various 'Declarations' quoted in this book relate to the text published in A S Duncan, G R Dunstan and R B Welbourn (eds) *Dictionary of Medical Ethics* (2nd edn, 1981).

The great weight of the evidence before us is to the effect that certain types of medical experiments on human beings, when kept within reasonably well defined bounds, conform to the ethics of the medical profession generally . . . All agree, however, that certain basic principles must be observed in order to satisfy moral, ethical and legal concepts.

It was, however, apparent that the medical profession itself should publicly endorse the principles expressed in the ten clauses of the Nuremberg code; this movement culminated in the Declaration of Helsinki – drawn up by the World Medical Association in 1964 and revised several times between 1975 and 1989 – which is reproduced as Appendix F.[4] Many national authorities have attempted to explain or expand upon the basic principles established at Nuremberg and, for the British reader, the most important of these are the comprehensive set of guidelines issued by the Royal College of Physicians of London[5] and the Medical Research Council of 1992.[6] In the European context, the Council of Europe has set out a recommendation which has been adopted by the Council of Ministers.[7]

All such codes have it in common that they appreciate the need for human experimentation while accepting that this can only be accomplished at the expense of some of the subjects' right to self-determination. Moreover, the doctor's ethical position must show some flexibility. The Hippocratic Oath states: 'I will follow that regimen which . . . I consider for the benefit of my patients and abstain from whatever is deleterious and mischievous'; the absolutist could say that this precludes all experimentation on patients yet it is clear that progress in medicine depends upon some form of trial. A balance is needed and must be sought.

What is research?

Research and experimentation are commonly used as interchangeable terms – we, however, believe that there is a distinction to be made. Research implies a predetermined protocol with a clearly defined end-point. Experimentation, by contrast, involves a more speculative, ad hoc, approach to an individual subject. The distinction is significant in that an experiment may be modified to take into account the individual's response; a research programme is more likely to tie the researcher to a particular course of action until such time as its general ineffectiveness is satisfactorily demonstrated.[8]

---

4   Other international codes include the International Ethical Guidelines for Biomedical Research involving Human Subjects published in Z Bankowski and R J Levine *Ethics and Research on Human Subjects: International Guidelines* (1992).

5   Royal College of Physicians of London *Research Involving Patients* (1990). Other useful earlier documents include *Responsibility in Investigations on Human Subjects*, report of the Medical Research Council of 1962-63 (Cmnd 2383).

6   Medical Research Council *Responsibility in Investigations on Human Participants and Material and on Personal Information* (1992). This replaced the statement of the Council of 1962-63.

7   Council of Europe, Committee of Ministers Recommendation No R(90) 3 1990.

8   For discussion, see B M Dickens 'What is a Medical Experiment?' (1975) 113 Can Med Ass J 635; B Gaze and K Dawson 'Distinguishing Medical Practice and Research: the Special Case of IVF' (1989) 3 Bioethics 301.

Research activities can be broadly categorised as clinical research, which is aimed at the improved treatment of a patient or a group of patients and as non-therapeutic – in which the essential object is the furtherance of purely scientific knowledge which may, eventually, have a wider application than patient care. This distinction makes little conceptual difference to the general requirements for ethical research. The mere fact that the research subject, being a patient at the time, may receive benefit does not mean that the programme can be undertaken unregulated by research codes – indeed, the fact that a relatively vulnerable group is involved emphasises the vigour with which controls should be applied. Only the degree of risk to be permitted in proportion to the expected outcome is affected by the nature of the research.

It follows from this classification that research subjects may be of four types: individual patients, a group of patients who are suffering from one particular condition, patients who have no association with the disease or process under review but who are readily available, and, finally, healthy volunteers – a heterogeneous group which is of importance because it may involve other 'captive' populations, including the researchers themselves.

The logical implication of this division of subjects is that researchers should also be categorised. Thus, the individual patient is under the care of a doctor. Any experimentation is, therefore, performed on a care-associated basis and, while there may be difficulties in a hospital setting where 'care' is very much a team concept, the essential doctor/patient relationship is, and should be, maintained. But it cannot be said with reference to any of the other groups that 'the health of my patient is my first consideration' and, consequently, the researchers cannot include the patients' physicians. Even so, when human subjects are involved in medical experimentation, so must doctors be; the danger of non-medical researchers being, not so much callous, as uncomprehending of their subjects' reactions is such that a situation excluding doctors would only be acceptable in the event that the researchers were their own experimental subjects.

The risks involved

All research involves some risk and it is the art of the good investigator to minimise that risk. But there are certain guidelines to be followed which are spelled out in the Declaration of Helsinki (paras 4 and 5) and also in the report of the Royal College of Physicians (paras 5.8 –5.26). A risk/benefit analysis must be undertaken in each case and patients may be involved only when the benefit to them clearly outweighs the inconvenience, discomfort or possible harm which the protocol may impose. The Royal College of Physicians distinguishes between research involving 'less than minimal risk' and that involving 'minimal risk'. The former is the risk of the sort involved in giving a sample of urine or a single venous sample in an adult; the latter arises where there is a reasonable chance of a mild reaction – such as a headache or a feeling of lethargy or where there is a remote chance of serious injury or death. If the level rises above that of minimal risk, then the College takes the view that patients should be involved only if:

(a) the risk is still small in comparison with that already incurred by the patient as a consequence of the disease itself,

(b) the disease is a serious one,

(c) the knowledge gained from the research is likely to be of great practical benefit,

(d) there is no other means of obtaining that knowledge, and

(e) the patient gives a fully informed consent.

The question of whether healthy volunteers may ever be exposed to serious risks in the course of medical research is problematic. The Declaration of Helsinki seems to rule it out in stating in para III.3 that, in non-therapeutic research 'the investigator or the investigating team should discontinue the research if in his/her or their judgment it may, if continued, be harmful to the individual'. This would exclude participation by anyone other than the researchers themselves in hazardous research and would render the use of volunteers unethical in, say, potentially harmful research into the development of vaccines against diseases that may affect the community. Yet there may be those who would accept risks of a very high order for admirable altruistic reasons and it is questionable whether they should be prevented from so doing. There are legal limits to the extent to which consent decriminalises the infliction of harm[9] and it is interesting to speculate whether the consent of a volunteer to a dangerous medical experiment would serve as a defence to a charge of assault or homicide.

The researchers themselves represent the other extreme of risk acceptance. Here, the responsibility rests squarely on the head of department for the safety of his staff but the dedicated work of many physiologists has involved procedures which could not be applied to others; it is doubtful if modern air travel would have been possible in the absence of frankly hazardous work. Great care is essential in the use of the healthy volunteer; it is often difficult not to regard him or her as having equivalent understanding of the procedure as does the experimenter and to proceed on that basis – in fact, the healthy volunteer is more prone to subjective inducements to participate than are others and must be treated accordingly. The problems of volunteers highlight the conditions for informed consent which is discussed further below.

The design of research

All research costs money and causes some inconveniences both to colleagues and subjects. Badly planned research loses all ethical justification if, as a result, the findings are scientifically useless. So much depends upon planning that it is now a requirement for district health authorities to establish and support local research ethics committees whose function it is to approve any experimental project using NHS patients or resources. Such committees wield considerable power in the United States where their function is generally expanded to include therapeutic and

---

9   *A-G's Reference (No 6 of 1980)* [1981] QB 715, [1981] 2 All ER 1057, CA; *Smart v HM Advocate*
     1975 SLT 65.   See also G Williams 'Consent and Public Policy' [1962] Crim LR 74, 154.

prognostic decision making.[10] The situation in the United Kingdom is, however, different. Here, with the occasional exception,[11] committees are established purely to vet research projects and, this, mainly from the point of view of their moral implications as to the use of subjects and of resources. The composition of these committees, along with matters of procedure, are regulated by guidelines issued by the NHS.[12] Each committee should include at least two lay persons, and either the chairman or vice-chairman must be drawn from the lay membership.

The inclusion of 'average citizens' can be seen as no more than a necessary political gesture; on the other hand, lay members may be better placed than professionals to appreciate the effects of different treatments on the day-to-day lives of the patients and their inclusion may, therefore, have definite practical advantages. The overall derivation of committee members is of greater significance. Most committees are institutionalised – some, particularly in the United States, being even of a departmental nature; it is possible that the resulting element of 'self-review' is self-defeating and committees with wider responsibilities would be more appropriate. In the United Kingdom, the setting up by the Nuffield Foundation of a national body – the duties of which will include the monitoring of the activities of ethics committees – goes at least some way towards ensuring consistency of approach in such matters as multicentre trials.

It is not a *legal* requirement that prospective researchers submit their proposals to a local research committee for approval, but there are several reasons why the carrying out of medical research will be effectively impossible without such approval. To begin with, it will not be possible to use NHS patients or resources for an unapproved project. Funding is also likely to be denied unless an ethics committee's *imprimatur* is obtained, and, perhaps of even greater practical importance, the results of unethical research will not be accepted for publication by reputable scientific journals.

The decisions of ethics committees could be subject to judicial review, in the same way as any other administrative decision; a frustrated researcher could therefore pursue a remedy by that route.[13] The aggrieved research subject may also seek redress, in his case most obviously through an action against the researcher.[14] It could be argued that a relationship exists between the committee member and the research subject which is of sufficient proximity to give rise to a duty of care and that

10 For a discussion of procedural aspects of American hospital ethics committees, see 'Ethics Committees' (1992) 20 Law Med Hlth Care: 278 (S M Wolf 'Toward a Theory of Process', 278; J C Fletcher 'Ethics Committees and Due Process' 291; C B Cohen 'Avoiding "Cloudcuckooland" in Ethics Committee Case Review: Matching Models to Issues and Concerns'; B M Dickens 'Ethics Committees, Organ Transplantation and Public Policy' 300). On the implications of the introduction of such committees in the United Kingdom, see A McCall Smith 'Committee Ethics? Clinical Ethics Committees and their Introduction in the United Kingdom' (1990) 17 J Law & Soc 124.
11 'UK's First Hospital Ethics Committee' (1993) Bull Inst Med Ethics No 90, 5, reporting the setting up, within an NHS trust hospital, of an ethics committee with the broad remit of considering any ethical dilemmas arising in the course of hospital activity.
12 National Health Service Management Executive, 'Local Research Ethics Committees' HSG(91) 5 (1991).
13 *R v Ethical Committee of St Mary's Hospital (Manchester), ex p H* [1988] 1 FLR 512.
14 Those injured in the course of pharmaceutical trials may be compensated by the company sponsoring the trial, as recommended by the Association of the British Pharmaceutical Industry in its *Clinical Trial Compensation Guidelines* (1991).

this may, in theory, lead to civil liability in a case where a committee member has failed to exercise due care in the scrutiny of a research proposal. In fact, the courts have tended to avoid imposing liability on those charged with a regulatory role, as has been demonstrated in cases such as *Yeu Kun-yeu v A-G of Hong Kong.*[15] The anxieties of committee members should be allayed, though, by the Department of Health's suggestion that district health authorities give to those members of the local research ethics committees who are not NHS employees an undertaking to the effect that the authority will take full responsibility for those acts which are performed in the context of committee membership. The wording of the indemnity is somewhat limiting, excluding acts performed in bad faith or wilful default and acts of 'gross negligence'. The latter term, in so far as it means anything at all, arguably has no place in such an indemnity.

Controlled trials

Biomedical research almost inevitably involves a controlled trial at some time. The principle is simple – in order to decide whether a new drug or other treatment is better than an existing one, or is preferable to none at all, the new treatment is given to a group of patients or healthy volunteers and not given to as similar a group as can be obtained. The subtleties of experimental design are critical to the success of the project and, as stated above, a badly conceived trial is fundamentally unethical. But even the best designed trial has its built-in moral problem – depending on how one looks at it, on the one hand, a relatively untried treatment which may do harm is being given to one group while, on the other, a treatment which may be of considerable benefit is being withheld from a similar group. In one view, this is ethically unacceptable, as there can be no grounds – other than, possibly, those of limited resources – for withholding a treatment which is believed to be beneficial. The doctor must do his best for patients but the problem is to know what is best and, in particular, to know whether the patient's recovery is being hindered by the restraints of the experimental protocol.[16] The first essential for any controlled trial is, therefore, that it must provide its answer as rapidly as possible and it must be terminable as soon as an adverse effect becomes apparent.   Conflict may arise between statisticians and doctors, with the former possibly insisting on evidence from many more cases – and possibly observed for longer – than the doctor may feel necessary. When, then, should randomised trials stop? At what point does the clinician say that enough is enough and that the evidence of benefit is sufficient to justify the conclusion that a treatment does, indeed, do good? Conversely, at what point does the apparent emergence of an adverse effect dictate that the project be abandoned? The patient involved in such a trial will have been informed that he is possibly being denied a potential benefit or possibly given a placebo – yet his consequent consent will have been based on his trust that there is genuine scientific uncertainty. Once this uncertainty is resolved to the extent of a belief – on, say, a balance of probabilities – that the treatment offers clinical benefit, then it becomes

15 [1988] AC 175, [1987] 2 All ER 705.
16 H Helmchem and B Muller-Oerlinghausen 'The Inherent Paradox of Clinical Trials in Psychiatry' (1975) 1 J Med Ethics 168.

questionable whether it can still be denied to some in a continuing quest for statistical significance.[17] In deciding this question, it is important that the researcher bears in mind the fundamental precept which governs ethical medical research – that one does not use patients as a means to a scientific end but treats them as an end in themselves. Even so, the practical dilemma remains – the clinically orientated researcher stands to see his subsequent report criticised for want of scientific support while the more scientifically minded one sleeps uneasily because he worries that his research has reached an inadequate conclusion. Most good trials include plans for periodic analysis; there is a good case to be made for an independent observer, or the ethical committee itself, being responsible for monitoring the trial from this angle.

Two further features are of major importance in ensuring the objective of a trial – the 'double-blind' technique and randomisation. The former is virtually confined to drug trials. It is almost impossible for a doctor not to have some preference in a choice of treatments; the double-blind trial attempts to eliminate this subjectivity by keeping the assigned therapeutic groups secret from the physicians as well as from the patients. Not only does this dictate that the patient's doctor cannot be the researcher but it also makes it implicit that the ethical justification of the trial is agreed by the 'caring' physicians involved; this leads to considerable difficulty in implementing the second principle – of randomisation – because it involves some form of conscious pre-selection. It has been suggested that no clinical trial can be truly random.[18] Certainly, the subjects, by volunteering, distinguish themselves from those who do not; or it may be necessary to exclude patients on the grounds of the severity of their disease, in which case the trial is limited to establishing the effectiveness of a treatment for the milder forms of the disease.

Randomisation in clinical trials is, in fact, becoming one of the major issues in research; this is particularly so in respect of treatments for cancer. For reasons discussed above, doctors having care – and especially primary care – of patients distrust the process. Most do so for fear that the doctor/patient relationship will be jeopardised; a sizeable minority are, however, concerned with the problems of informed consent.[19] This is discussed in greater detail later but here it can be said that it also has a profound effect on the patient's acceptance of a trialist status. Refusal may be on simple utilitarian grounds but is equally liable to stem from confusion. No randomised therapeutic trial can be ethical unless the professionals genuinely do not know which treatment yields the best results. Given that the doctors are unsure, it may be difficult for the patient to solve what appears to him to be an insoluble problem. The result of the cumulative adverse factors is that accrual rates to important trials are often very low[20] – it is reported that a fundamental research

17 For an analysis, see N Johnson, R J Lilford and W Brazier 'At what Level of Collective Equipoise Does a Clinical Trial Become Ethical?' (1991) 17 J Med Ethics 30. The standards of proof have been compared to the different standards applied in the civil and criminal courts: 'On Stopping a Trial before Its Time' (1993) 342 Lancet 1311.
18 W Rudowski 'World Health Organisation Biomedical Research Guidelines and the Conduct of Clinical Trials' (1980) 6 J Med Ethics 58.
19 K M Taylor et al 'Physicians' Reasons for not Entering Eligible Patients in a Randomised Clinical Trial of Surgery for Breast Cancer' (1984) 310 New Engl J Med 1363. The problem of consent may be particularly acute where the participants in a randomised trial are illiterate or where they do not share the scientific view of the researcher: see M Barry and M Molyneux 'Ethical Dilemmas in Malaria Drug and Vaccine Trials: a Bioethical Perspective' (1992) 18 J Med Ethics 189.
20 M Angell 'Patients' Preferences in Randomized Clinical Trials' (1984) 310 New Engl J Med 1385.

project intended to identify the best treatment for early breast cancer had to be closed after a very low recruitment because the insistence on full informed consent (see below) frightened off both surgeons and patients.[1] Researchers therefore seek devices which will circumvent the confrontation between clinicians and patient and most of these involve some form of pre-selection – or 'pre-randomisation' – prior to discussion of treatment.[2] There are specific ethical and practical objections to such manoeuvres but, in general, it seems doubtfully moral to use what is essentially a ruse in order to obviate an agreed ethical practice which is, in addition, an integral part of the basic principles of the Declaration of Helsinki. The issue is, however, more finely balanced than might be supposed. One perfectly arguable school of thought will hold that this is the penalty we have to accept, 'unless we wish to return to the dark ages when treatment was determined by conceptual rationalism rather than scientific method'.[3] Others would emphasise that care must be taken lest, by attenuating our commitments to present patients in favour of benefits to those of the future, we do not lose overall more than we gain.[4] There is little wonder that the debate persists.

Groups of subjects

There is clearly an advantage, whenever possible, in using healthy volunteers as experimental subjects but, by definition, their use is limited to non-therapeutic research. Somewhat strangely, the Declaration of Helsinki allows for actual patients being used for such purposes. In this context, we believe that the temptation to use a group of persons, who are already under stress and who probably have a sense of obligation to the doctors, simply because of their accessibility, must often bring such research close to unethical practice; non-therapeutic research in patients should be confined to a type which adds no extra burden – for example, through the use of existing blood samples as is discussed below. It has been argued that the use of volunteers is, itself, unjustifiable but we prefer the view that people have a right to exercise altruistic impulses, particularly in a society in which the benefits of free health care are extended to all. None the less, considerable caution is needed, particularly as to the repetitive volunteer who is particularly prone to exploitation even if the researchers are unconscious of this – they may, for example, be quite unaware of marital disharmony caused by frequent absences from home. Motivation of the ever-ready volunteer takes several forms, some good and others bad, and, among these, the problem of recompense looms large. The Declaration of Helsinki is silent on this aspect but it is reasonably certain that, in conditions of present day society, very few volunteers would come forward in the absence of some inducement; large payments would, however, be clearly unethical and a reasonable balance must be set – if for no other reason than to satisfy the needs of randomisation. It might be noted that the Royal College of Physicians Report *Research Involving Patients*

1 M Baum, K Zilkha and J Houghton 'Ethics of Clinical Research: lessons for the Future' (1989) 299 BMJ 251.
2 S S Ellenberg 'Randomization Design in Comparative Clinical Trials' (1984) 310 New Engl J Med 1404. See, in particular, M A Zelen 'A New Design for Randomized Clinical Trials' (1979) 300 New Engl J Med 1242 and, more recently, Editorial Comment 'Zelen Protocols' (1992) 339 Lancet 1574.
3 Baum et al, footnote 1 above.
4 Angell, footnote 20, above.

describes payments to patients as 'generally undesirable' but occasionally acceptable in the case of long and tedious studies.[5] Even in such cases, 'payments should not be for undergoing risk, and payments should not be such as to persuade patients to volunteer against their better judgement'.

The topic of inducement does, however, introduce the problems of the use of special populations because of their easy access, malleability, etc. Students, and particularly medical students, provide an example about whom there is little difficulty: they are intelligent and comprehending, they may well have an active interest in the trial and all educational establishments have very stringently controlling 'ethical committees' to protect against, for example, repetitive use. Much the same could be said for the armed forces, who may be particularly vulnerable to improper research in war or when war threatens – even in 1990 non-consensual trials were allowed on American troops engaged in the Gulf War.[6] The use of prisoners, however, exposes many ethical issues that are based, essentially, on the argument that some advantage, even if only imagined, must accrue to the prisoner participating in a trial; that advantage may be so great as to induce the prisoner to volunteer for research which involves greater discomfort or risk than would be accepted by a free man and, in particular, it may compromise his inalienable right to withdraw from the trial. The arguments are not, however, entirely one way – it is possible to be paternalistic in an attempt to preserve people's autonomy. Thus, prisoners could well resent protective attitudes on the grounds that it is their right to dispose of their bodies and to take such risks as they please that is being compromised. This could be the subject of lengthy debate but we would suggest that the conditions in today's prisons are such that any process which provides some relief deserves, at least, a sympathetic evaluation and, second, that many prisoners might be benefited therapeutically through helping society. But it is also felt that experiments on prisoners should be particularly rigidly controlled by ethical committees, which should always contain lay members with experience in criminology. Nowhere is it more important to observe the maxim: 'the aims do not justify the method – the method must be judged in its own right'.

When comparing treatments, however, the use of patients is axiomatic. This is what the Declaration of Helsinki calls medical research combined with professional care and for which it lays down clear principles. The therapeutic controlled trial must invoke the Geneva principle: 'the health of the patient will be my first consideration.' Rudowski[7] has stated:

A patient is assigned to undergo clinical study when, on the basis of our best judgment, an equal possibility exists that each of the compared methods of treatment will be of advantage to the patient.

This is a minimum standard – a clinical trial is rarely undertaken unless there is good reason to suppose that one therapy will show an advantage over others and

5 Royal College of Physicians *Research Involving Patients* (1990).
6 G J Annas and M A Grodin 'Treating the Troops: Commentary' (1991) 21 Hastings Center Rep (2) 24.
7 W Rudowski 'World Health Organisation Biomedical Research Guidelines and the Conduct of Clinical Trials' (1980) 6 J Med Ethics 58.

particularly over those currently accepted as the best available. The advantage need not be direct; it could, for example, be collateral in that the results of the method were not better but were achieved with less disfigurement or with fewer side effects. Anticipation of advantage can, in general, only be based on laboratory or animal experimentation and, while the view is occasionally expressed that the latter is less moral than is human biomedical research, it represents the first basic principle of the Declaration of Helsinki. The corollary, as we have already emphasised, is that an experimental method must be immediately withdrawn if it is found to be positively deleterious and the patients involved must be transferred, whenever possible, to an alternative regime. The difficulties of such clinical research include, first, the fact that each patient is a unique set of many variables. While a statistical result may be achieved, it would be a remarkably well designed trial which simultaneously solved the problems of the individual exceptions – for example, the patients' preferences may distort a trial unless they are allowed for.[8] Second, the results of the experimental therapies may take a considerable time to filter through and, by then, there may be no turning back. A typical example is provided by the study of the use of folic acid supplements in order to reduce the incidence of neural tube defects in infants. Two pilot studies were undertaken; both showed an apparent marked reduction in recurrence rates in affected families but neither stood up to statistical analysis. The problem then arose as to whether the study should be continued and, if so, was the clinical impression sufficient to render the use of placebos unethical? It was decided that the matter was so important that a major randomised trial was indicated, the intent being to study at least 2,000 pregnancies. In the event, after more than seven years, sufficient information had been gained from 1,195 informative pregnancies. Thus, the trial could now be ended, it being clear that folic acid supplements had no adverse effects but had a significant protective effect as regards fetal neural tube defect.[9]

The use of placebos
A placebo is an inert substance without pharmacological action. The use of placebos is occasionally remarkably successful in straightforward therapeutics but, there, the practice is even more difficult to justify morally than it is in the experimental situation where the use of placebos is sometimes essential. The mere taking of medicine may lead to subjective improvement; this is the 'placebo effect' which must be considered whenever a new drug or procedure is on trial. On the other hand, the trial drug may do more harm than inactivity; but, for psychological reasons, inactivity must involve apparently comparable activity if two regimens are to be properly compared. In either case, the controlled giving of a placebo necessarily involves the deception of patients and this raises some complex issues.

The extreme position is that placebos offend against the fundamental rightness of fidelity.[10] If, as is often the case, there is patient resistance to the use of such

8   C R Brewin and C Bradley 'Patient Preferences and Randomised Clinical Trials' (1989) 299 BMJ 313.
9   MRC Vitamin Study Research Group 'Prevention of Neural Tube Defects: Results of the Medical Research Council Vitamin Study' (1991) 338 Lancet 131.
10 B Simmons 'Problems in Deceptive Medical Procedures: An Ethical and Legal Analysis of the Administration of Placebos' (1978) 4 J Med Ethics 172.

controls, this should not be regarded as an excuse for further deception but rather as an indication that such experiments are unacceptable to society. To which one could reply that a poor experiment is a worse affront to society and that the simple expedient is to leave out those who object. Little is lost – other than, perhaps, absolute numbers – and, as previously discussed, experimental volunteers are, by nature, already a selected group.

More practical objections are based on the effect of the research on patient care; the circumstances in which it is ethical to deprive a patient of treatment must be strictly regulated. It would, for example, be improper to use placebo controls when pain was a feature of the condition under treatment, despite the fact that some patients might derive benefit; many pain killers are available and can be used as reference substances. The basic circumstances in which placebo trials are ethical and, perhaps, necessary are: first, when there is no alternative to the experimental treatment available – it might, for example, be right to include placebo controls in the evaluation of a drug intended for the treatment of the acquired immune deficiency syndrome for which there is no known cure; second, the use of a placebo could be justified when the effect of adding a new treatment to an established one is under study. In the majority of instances, however, the purpose of using placebos is to analyse the effect of a treatment on subjective symptoms rather than on organic disease.

Informed consent

It is apparent that the theoretical baseline for an ethical research programme or therapeutic experiment is drawn on free, autonomous participation by the subject and this, in turn, depends upon 'informed consent', the nature of which has been discussed in chapter 10.

The principles in relation to research are similar to those governing therapy; most philosophers would say that the patient's rights are, if anything, greater in the former situation than they are in the sphere of pure patient management. The standard of information provided must certainly be that of the 'reasonable subject' – if not that of the actual subject – rather than that of the 'reasonable doctor'.[11] Even so, there are many and variable difficulties which make it almost impossible to lay down hard and fast rules – these include the essential need for some measure of ignorance in the trial, the seriousness of the condition being treated, the psychology of individual patients and so on. The complexity is such that in Sweden, for example, while the law lays down that the doctrine of informed consent has to be satisfied, no attempt is made to define the extent of the information given.[12] It is now reported that the requirements for informed consent have rendered controlled trials next to impossible in Germany. Confrontation between the back-room and the coal-face is almost inevitable – The Lancet has expressed it:

> The central dogma [of professional medical ethicists] seems to be that whatever is done for the sake of medical science is alien to the treatment of the individual, and should

11 Detailed requirements are set out didactically by A Herxheimer 'The Rights of the Patient in Clinical Research' (1988) 2 Lancet 1128.
12 G Giertz 'Ethics and Randomised Clinical Trials' (1980) 6 J Med Ethics 55.

therefore be labelled an 'experiment', necessitating informed consent by the patient and adjudication by an ethics committee.[13]

Such general problems are amplified in the practical ambience. It is widely agreed that the patient's consent must be based on four main lines of explanation; the purpose of the experiment, the benefits to the patient and society, the risks involved and the alternatives open to the subject. Who is to impart the information – the patient's physician or the researcher? Should the patient have the benefit of a 'friend' to interpret for him? Should there be confirmation of the consent procedure? It has been fairly widely mooted that, in fact, informed consent is a double-edged weapon – token consent may take the place of the genuine and relieve the researcher of responsibility. Might it not be better to burden the investigator with full responsibility rather than provide such a shield?[14] Many of the states of the United States have enacted 'informed consent statutes', some of which lay down specific disclosure requirements for particular procedures and it was stated in a Canadian case:[15] 'There can be no exceptions to the ordinary requirements of disclosure in the case of research as there may well be in ordinary medical practice.'

These difficulties are highlighted in 'care associated' research when, effectively, the doctrine of informed consent implies that the patient has to choose for himself or herself whether to accept an experimental treatment or to be randomised in a comparative therapeutic trial. The philosophical basis of patient autonomy is perfectly clear but is the ideal end attainable in practice? Ought a patient to be told of a 'last chance' effort? Is the medically naive patient capable of giving consent as required? Can he be expected to understand the risks when the medical profession itself is so divided? Such issues are crystallised in the treatment of cancer, in which respect American legislation as to disclosure is particularly severe[16] – in California, for example, physicians are provided with a summary of medically viable alternative treatments for cancer of the breast which can be used to comply with the relevant statute. Whether such devices are valuable to the patient is doubtful and, while they undoubtedly give protection to the doctors, we can still ask how and why we have reached a situation where that should have to be a major concern.

This is, perhaps, the nub of the problem. We have already noted that a major cancer trial has been abandoned on, mainly, consent-based grounds – and this conclusion was, to an extent, foreseen. In this respect, the working party[17] regarded it as intolerable that the burden of accountability should be placed entirely on the doctors concerned. As things stand, the physician wishing to do his best for the individual patient and, at the same time, for the community at large, is often left in limbo.[18]

13 The Lancet 'Medical Ethics: Should Medicine Turn the Other Cheek?' (1990) 336 Lancet 846.
14 See fn 16, p 354 above.
15 *Halushka v University of Saskatchewan* (1965) 53 DLR (2d) 436.
16 S Taub 'Cancer and the Law of Informed Consent' (1982) 10 Law Med Hlth Care 61.
17 Cancer Research Campaign Working Party in Breast Conservation 'Informed Consent; Ethical, Legal and Medical Implications for Doctors and Patients who Participate in Randomised Clinical Trials' (1983) 286 BMJ 1117.
18 Well described by H A F Dudley 'Informed Consent to Surgical Trials' (1984) 289 BMJ 937.

A remarkable example of how this uncertainty may operate in practice came before a coroner's court inquiring into the death of a female patient – a death due, interestingly enough, to a failure to inform a temporary house officer of the research in progress.[19] It came to light that 15 units were involved in a trial treatment of colonic cancer which involved infusing selected but randomised patients with a potent cytotoxic drug post-operatively; all units had submitted the trial protocol to their ethical committees and 11 had decided that 'informed consent' need not be obtained. The Lancet, while, admittedly, concluding that special consent should have been obtained on the grounds of both variance from standard procedures and the degree of risk involved, summed up the dilemma in a series of questions: when, if ever, can informed consent be dispensed with? if a trial is concerned with the treatment of cancer, how can consent be obtained without adding to the patient's distress? at what stage in the trial should consent be obtained? and, finally, have local ethical committees the authority to override national and international guidelines on the ethics of research? To which we would add – how can you possibly expect a patient to understand such a complex subject? – and The Lancet answers that the patient should not be included in the trial if he or she is not capable of understanding the basic plan of management.

A real problem here is that doubts as to patients' ability to understand complex medical information can very easily result in the striking of an unacceptably paternalistic attitude – sometimes with shocking consequences. Such a situation arose in New Zealand in the course of the Auckland cervical cancer campaign.[20] Here, a senior doctor, believing that cancer in situ would not spread, was strongly of the view that some women with abnormal cervical smear tests were best left untreated. These patients were denied treatment over a period of 15 to 20 years without being told that they were, in effect, involved in a therapeutic experiment. The doctor in charge of the experimental research believed honestly and firmly in his hypothesis, but his failure to obtain consent was severely criticised both by medical colleagues and by the judicial inquiry which was established to investigate the matter; the impact on medicine in New Zealand and, hopefully, elsewhere, has been profound.[1]

The issue of consent still gives rise to disputes. The involvement of a patient in a British randomised breast cancer study without her informed consent led to allegations by the patient in 1988 that she had been 'abused' by the doctors concerned. The Bulletin of the Institute of Medical Ethics took a similar view.[2] By contrast, a leading surgeon, a chairman of an ethical committee and the Assistant

---

19 Coroner's Court, Birmingham, 19 September 1981. Discussed in leading article 'Secret Randomised Clinical Trials' (1982) 2 Lancet 78. See also D Brahams 'Death of Patient who was Unwitting Subject of Randomised Controlled Trial of Cancer Treatment' (1982) 1 Lancet 1028 and 'Clinical Trials and the Consent of the Patient' (1982) 226 Practitioner 1829.

20 Judge S Cartwright *The Report of the Cervical Cancer Enquiry* (1988). Discussed by A V Campbell 'An "Unfortunate Experiment" ' (1989) 3 Bioethics 59.

1 C Paul 'The New Zealand Cancer Study: Could it Happen Again?' (1988) 297 BMJ 533; P McNeill 'The Implications for Australia of the New Zealand Report of the Cervical Cancer Inquiry: No Cause for Complacency' (1989) 150 Med J Austral 264; G Gillett 'NZ Medicine after Cartwright' (1990) 300 BMJ 893.

2 Editorial Comment 'Research Without Consent Continues in the UK' (1988) Bull Inst Med Ethics No 40, 13.

Director of the Cancer Research Campaign argued strongly that it is legitimate to dispense with the informed consent requirements when placing the patient within a trial constitutes good medical treatment.[3] It was suggested that to give a patient full information on such a study might add to her distress and that there are circumstances where the principle of non-maleficence should override that of autonomy. Such views, although motivated by concern for patient welfare are, however, open to the charge that they underestimate the extent to which patients actually want to be informed of what is happening to them; full communication between the patient and researcher is still probably the safer policy.[4]

Research and the incompetent

Particularly difficult ethical and legal problems arise in relation to those patients who cannot give a valid consent to participation in clinical research by virtue of their mental condition. Such patients must be excluded automatically if informed consent is an absolute prerequisite for involvement in research and, yet, this would have the effect of halting valuable lines of inquiry into serious and debilitating diseases. One way round this difficulty is to accept that there are special groups of patients who cannot consent but whose involvement is vital if research into a condition from which they suffer is to make progress. Such patients may be used in research provided that certain safeguards are erected; these would be designed so as to ensure that they were not subjected to appreciable risk or inconvenience and would include the agreement of relatives and/or that of some independent, supervisory party. Although the 'consent' of relatives is of no legal effect in these circumstances, it is an important check in that they may be assumed to have the interests of members of their family at heart. The required approval of an independent authority would cover those instances in which it was suspected that uncaring relatives had been thoughtless.

The Working Party on Research on the Mentally Incapacitated, set up by the Medical Research Council, has accepted that non-therapeutic research on the mentally incapacitated is ethically acceptable, subject to the qualification on risk mentioned above and subject to there being no sign that the subject objects to involvement.[5] Yet, even if we accept the morality of this view, the legal position in such cases is considerably more dubious. As the law stands in both England and Scotland, there can be no legal justification – other than, possibly, that of necessity – for any non-therapeutic invasion of the bodily integrity of an incapacitated person. Research of this type is, therefore, probably unlawful at the present time. Judicial or, better, Parliamentary authority will be needed if it is to become unarguably legal.

The unethical researcher

All that has gone before has assumed that the researcher is acting in good faith with the interests of the profession and of the public at heart. Recently, however, there

3 M Baum, K Zilkha and J Houghton 'Ethics of Clinical Research: Lessons for the Future' (1989) 299 BMJ 251.
4 T M Marteau 'Ethics of Clinical Research' (1989) 299 BMJ 513
5 Medical Research Council *The Ethical Conduct of Research on the Mentally Incapacitated* (1991).

has been a flurry of concern not so much as to research of poor quality – which is distinguished relatively easily – as to frankly fraudulent studies.[6]

Modern doctors are under some pressure in this area. The competitive spirit in high-profile research may lead to unfortunate effects.[7] Elsewhere, the temptation to falsify results or to suppress the truth may be too much for some scientists, particularly when there is a prospect of high earnings from patents. Even in the more mundane reaches of medicine, the senior who publishes frequently is likely to attract more funding than his colleague who does not and the advantage of 'being first' encourages premature reporting. More importantly, advancement in hierarchical medicine now depends heavily on the number of publications to the junior's credit. The fact that this results in ever-escalating multi-authorship is of intra-professional concern only; of far greater public interest is the imposed temptation to look upon an individual patient as a potential notch in one's curriculum vitae. Such influences lead to 'sloppy science' which is, perhaps, understandable. There is, however, no excuse available for the deliberate falsification of results – which are less easy to identify and of which there have been a number of examples.[8] The danger in these cases is that the public, often prompted by the news media, may be led to believe in therapeutic claims which are unsupported by the available data or that, as a result, they may be subjected to valueless or dangerous treatment schedules. The issue is also, understandably, of great interest to pharmaceutical companies, who may be wrongly deprived of profits if a drug is withdrawn from the market on the basis of fraudulent results.[9] This happened in the case of Debendox, which was withdrawn after claims by the Australian gynaecologist, William McBride, that the drug could cause deformities in a small proportion of the children of those women to whom it was administered. An enquiry by the New South Wales Medical Tribunal subsequently concluded that McBride claimed statistically significant results where none, in fact, existed.[10] McBride is reported as saying that he had changed his data in 'the long term interests of humanity',[11] an attempted justification which could appeal to a remarkably wide rage of miscreants. The fraudulent researcher, of course, faces a variety of sanctions. He may be criminally liable for fraudulently obtaining research funds,

6 J Smith 'Preventing Fraud' (1991) 302 BMJ 362 discussing, inter alia, S Lock 'Misconduct in Medical Research: Does it Exist in Britain?' (1988) 297 BMJ 1531. Between 1987 and 1993, ten cases of scientific fraud were processed through the disciplinary committee of the GMC; S Kingman 'GMC Will Fund Misconduct Hearings on Scientific Fraud' (1993) 307 BMJ 1164. The penalties for scientific fraud are severe, and include that of being struck off the register for misconduct: 'Sex, Scandal and Fraud' (1992) 305 BMJ 272.

7 The saga relating to the discovery of the HI virus makes salutory reading – perhaps mainly in favour of a single professional body being responsible for the investigation of such cases. Cf S Connor 'Gallo Guilty of AIDs Misconduct' (1993) 306 BMJ 161 and R Rheim 'US Drops Charges against Robert Gallo' (1993) BMJ 1377.

8 See Smith, fn 6 above.

9 The effect of publication of results – genuine as well as fraudulent – on the stock market has also to be considered. Researchers who also trade in the relevant pharmaceutical shares may find themselves in breach of the Company Securities (Insider Dealing) Act 1985. See D S Freestone and H Mitchell 'Inappropriate Publication of Trial Results and Potential for Allegations of Illegal Share Dealing' (1993) 306 BMJ 1112.

10 M Ragg 'Australia: McBride Guilty of Scientific Fraud' (1993) 341 Lancet 550.

11 N Swan 'Australian Doctor Admits Fraud' (1991) 302 BMJ 1421.

and he could, also, face civil action for any loss incurred by drug manufacturers. In addition, there are powerful professional disciplinary procedures that can effectively end a scientific career.

A closely allied problem is that of experimental treatment. This is an even more contentious subject. Medicine is not always scientific; many advances are made fortuitously or as a result of no more than intuition. The difficulty then becomes that of distinguishing courageous innovation from unethical experimentation – and, human nature being what it is, the answer often depends on the outcome. A vivid example of how differing attitudes and understanding can cloud the issues arose in 1987 when parliamentary questions were asked concerning anaesthesia for children undergoing open heart surgery – emotive words such as 'barbaric' were used. The medical profession was, however, able to point out that the research was humane and that the results had shown the way to improvement in the post-operative status of such infants;[12] the criticisms were withdrawn unreservedly.[13]

We have already noted (at p 291) a less satisfactory defence of an experimental treatment in which a baboon's heart was transplanted into a neonate with congenital heart disease. The parents were unmarried minors and doubts have been expressed as to whether they could give 'informed consent' in the true sense. A consultant summed up the procedure:

> I think this xenograft is premature because I am not aware of any finding in the clinical literature that suggests anything but the prevailing rule – the human body will reject a transplanted animal organ. Baby Fae will reject her baboon heart within the next week or two, and cyclosporine will not prevent it.[14]

Most would agree with this assessment – Baby Fae actually survived for two and a half weeks – but the procedure had been approved by the university's institutional research board and there was some further professional support for the operation. Nevertheless, despite the more recent advances to which we have referred, it does appear to be an example of premature experimental treatment.

At what would seem to be the extreme of dubious practice lies the instance of treating AIDS by an unproven biological method and exaggerating its success in what was described by one consultant as 'the most scientifically unfounded presentation [he had] ever heard'.[15] It is only fair to note, however, that equal criticism was later levelled at the medical profession for failing to bring the matter to the attention of the General Medical Council – doctors have an undoubted distaste for 'shopping' their colleagues but such cases do underline the often expressed concern at the inadequacy of the GMC's powers of investigation.[16]

We are left with the complex problem of whether or not information gained from frankly immoral research should be used for the general good – the classic, and

---

12 J O Forfar and AGM Campbell 'Medicine and the Media' (1987) 295 BMJ 659.
13 B Braine 'MP Apologises' (1988) 297 BMJ 865.
14 Details taken from H S Schwartz 'Bioethical and Legal Considerations in Increasing the Supply of Transplantable Organs: From UAGA to "Baby Fae"' (1985) 10 Amer J Law Med 397.
15 R Smith 'Doctors, Unethical Treatments, and Turning a Blind Eye' (1989) 298 BMJ 1125.
16 The GMC is, itself, concerned at the 'blind eye' mentality. See *Professional Conduct and Discipline: Fitness to Practise* (1993) para 63.

ultimate, examples being data obtained in the concentration camps of the Second World War.[17] The arguments are finely balanced. In the end, we subscribe to the view that the fact that children do not, for instance, now die from certain forms of hypothermia is best regarded as a monument to those who suffered and died to make it possible; if the material is used, they will, at least, not have done so in vain.

Compensation for personal injury in research

The research volunteer who is injured in the course of a medical experiment may resort to a claim for compensation under the law of tort. Such a route, of course, may prove to be difficult: researchers may have taken every precaution to avoid injury and there may therefore be no evidence of negligence. An action based on lack of consent would be unlikely to succeed in the absence of deliberate deception; *Bolam*[18] as modified in *Sidaway*[19] would be as likely to be followed in experimentation as in treatment and a failure of disclosure would probably have to be of a serious nature for it to be regarded as negligence. Although the odds against a plaintiff in such actions are not as long as they were before *Sidaway*, the research subject is in a somewhat unfair situation. Quite apart from the problems of expense or uncertainty, he is entitled to believe he will be looked after in the event of something going wrong – and charity is unpredictable and often ungenerous as a remedy. There is clearly a need for some defined method of compensation as of right, the Pearson Commission (see p 195) favouring strict liability.[20] This is also unsatisfactory from the point of view of the aggrieved subject as it also involves recourse to the courts where the burden of proving causation would fall upon the plaintiff or pursuer. The alternative of a no-fault principle of compensation similar to those schemes discussed in chapter 9 is attractive and, moreover, there would be little or no difficulty in defining an accident within the narrow confines of medical research; but such schemes require funding and administration.

In the United Kingdom, those involved in the funding and regulation of medical research have acknowledged the necessity of compensation outside the framework of tort law and, in theory at least, the injured research subject should be dealt with sympathetically. Some health authorities recommend that ex gratia payments be made under the NHS indemnity scheme and that, where an NHS trust or a health authority has not accepted responsibility for the research investigation, an approach should be made to the sponsoring pharmaceutical company. The Association of the British Pharmaceutical Industry recommends to its members that compensation be paid 'when, on the balance of probabilities, the injury was attributable to the administration of a medicinal product under trial or any clinical intervention or procedure provided for by the protocol that would not have occurred but for the

17 A particularly poignant series of interviews with survivors was published in M Gwyther and S McConville 'Can Good Come from Evil?' (1989) *The Observer Magazine*, 19 November, p 18.
18 *Bolam v Friern Hospital Management Committee* [1957] 2 All ER 118, [1957] 1 WLR 582 in which failure to disclose a minimal risk was not considered negligent.
19 *Sidaway v Board of Governors of Bethlem Royal Hospital and the Maudsley Hospital* [1984] QB 493, [1984] 1 All ER 1018, CA; affd [1985] AC 871, [1985] 1 All ER 643, HL.
20 Report of Royal Commission on Civil Liability and Compensation for Personal Injury (Cmnd 7054, 1978) at para 1341.

inclusion of the patient in the trial'.[1] Compensation is not payable under these guidelines where there has been a significant departure from the agreed protocol, or where there has been a wrongful act on the part of a third party, including a doctor's failure to deal adequately with an adverse reaction. These limitations, together with the non-legally binding nature of the guidelines, mean that the research subject is by no means guaranteed compensation should anything go wrong.

Random sample testing

One aspect of research which has received little consideration concerns the use of samples which have been removed for defined, usually therapeutic, reasons. The use of such samples for other investigations subjects the patient to no further discomfort and, while a patient could undoubtedly make directions as to the disposal of any biological specimen he has provided, this would be by virtue of no more than an inchoate right.[2] It would be reasonable to assume from silence that the patient was indifferent in the matter, yet there is an element of invasion of the patient's privacy in 'finding out things' about him without his consent – no matter how much it might be felt that the geographic distribution of genes or any cultural alterations in body chemistry, for example, might provide useful research projects. But a balance has, again, to be struck since most patients, even if asked, would be uninterested in consent.

The justification of such projects rests on the consequences of a positive finding. At one extreme is the problem of AIDS which we discuss as a separate issue at p 231. At the other, a search for a particular blood group gene in a specific population could make no possible difference to the subjects and would, accordingly, be permissible. But one would have to think carefully before embarking on, for example, a survey of abnormal genetic markers with its consequent possible influences on marriage and having a family.

Other surveys could be of no immediate consequence to the patient but could be of significance were the results to be published. An example would be the routine estimation of blood alcohol as a community study. In the event of the samples deriving from accidents, the results could be of particular interest to the police or insurance companies and would be normally available only by consent of the subjects. Serious consequences might arise if the result of a research project were entered in the notes and these were later subject to disclosure;[3] no research of potentially damaging type would be ethical if there was a chance that the subject and the result could later be associated. Practical problems in this field have, in fact, arisen in the United States in relation to drug screening surveys; preservation of the

---

1   The Association of the British Pharmaceutical Industry *Clinical Trial Compensation Guidelines* (1991).
2   B M Dickens 'The Control of Living Body Materials' (1977) 27 Univ Toronto LJ 142.
3   The evidence might be used in the United Kingdom (*R v Sang* [1980] AC 402, [1979] 2 All ER 1222, HL applied in Australia in *R v Apicella* (1985) 82 Cr App Rep 295, [1986] Crim LR 238, CA) or in Canada (*Wray v R* (1973) 10 CCC (2d) 215) but not in the United States in that it violates the constitutional right to resist self-incrimination.

patient's anonymity must be a determining condition under which specimens are used without express consent for purposes other than those originally stated.

The ultimate disposal of surplus human material is slightly distanced from research but is a problem that is seldom addressed. Given that a surgical specimen has been removed and examined for the benefit of the patient, does it remain the property of that patient or has he effectively abandoned his right to control over that part of his own body? There is no apposite statute law in the United Kingdom – the Human Tissue Act 1961 refers only to the use of body tissues after the subject's death. On the face of it, excised tissue becomes res nullius, although there may well be limits to this – a patient has a perfect right to object to parts of his body being exposed, say, in a museum jar. On the other hand, while he may express a preference, he certainly cannot dictate what is to be done with his specimen. It seems that the most he could insist was that it was returned to him and, in the absence of such a request, he could be assumed to have abandoned his material.[4] There are no property rights in a dead human body[5] and it has sometimes been suggested that there are none in dead human tissue.[6] The matter has not been considered directly in the United Kingdom but its importance is emphasised by the increasing commercial value of human material which follows as biotechnology advances and perpetuated human cell lines become a reality. Some indications in this respect are now available from the decision of the Supreme Court of California in *Moore v Regents of the University of California*.[7] In that case, the subject's spleen was removed as part of the treatment for hairy cell leukaemia; specimens of blood and bone-marrow were also taken on several out-patient visits. Unknown to Moore, a cell line was developed which had a potential market value to be measured in millions of dollars; having discovered this, he sued all those involved in a series of causes of action.

The Supreme Court of California overturned the decision of the Appeal Court and, most importantly, struck out a claim for conversion on the grounds that there were no 'or, at least, very limited' property rights in cells removed from the body. On the other hand, the court held that disposal of the tissue was governed by the doctrine of informed consent and that this, in turn, depended upon a fiduciary duty to disclose all the relevant information to the patient.

It is uncertain how a matter of this nature would be settled under English law. There would not, now, be much disagreement on the fundamental issue of whether it is possible to have property rights in bodily material – urine can be stolen[8] and human hair can be bought and sold. If such rights exist, they must be susceptible to transfer and, specifically, may be transferred to researchers. As Dworkin and Kennedy have argued convincingly, however, the unauthorised use of body tissue

---

4   A very different view is taken by those who are concerned with corporeal resurrection – such as the Natural Death Society – who argue that excised tissue should be available for burial with the cadaver.

5   *R v Sharpe* (1857) 169 ER 959.

6   A matter for regret in an early article by P D G Skegg 'Human Corpses, Medical Specimens and the Law of Property' (1975) 4 Anglo-Amer L Rev 412.

7   793 P 2d 479 (Cal, 1990); discussed by E Scowen 'The Human Body – Whose Property and Whose Profit?' (1990) 1 Dispatches 1. A most sophisticated appraisal is now available in G Dworkin and I Kennedy 'Human Tissue: Rights in the Body and its Parts' (1993) 1 Med L Rev 291.

8   A T H Smith 'Stealing the Body and its Parts' [1976] Crim LR 622.

must constitute a civil wrong. Such a situation must arise only very rarely because, on the vast majority of occasions, the patient will have implicitly abandoned any tissue removed in the course of treatment; an action for conversion could, however, be available if the tissues were used when the patient had explicitly retained ownership – say, on religious or other grounds.[9] Alternatively, an equitable remedy might be available if deception was involved and the fact that his tissues were to be put to commercial use was fraudulently concealed from the patient; we would agree with Scowen's implication that a British court would conclude that the patient should be entitled to a share of the profits arising from an enterprise to which his contribution was an essential prerequisite – although that share might well be proportionate to the expertise and resources contributed by the technologists. Finally, it is still possible that a consent-based action in negligence might be available; it is hard to believe that the court would not see the prospect of a monetary fortune as being something so obviously necessary to an informed decision by the patient that no reasonably prudent professional man would fail to mention it.[10]

The issue of patenting materials based on or incorporating human tissue is very controversial. Patents on animal life forms have been allowed in the United States – although not without considerable opposition from those who see this as an unacceptable reduction of animal life to human control. Here, we see morality doing battle with commercial instincts – with the latter proving rather persuasive. The chances are that the patenting of products derived from human tissue will eventually be seen as permissible provided that human tissue *itself* is not treated as a form of intellectual property.[11]

9 J Finch *Speller's Law Relating to Hospitals* (7th edn, 1994) p 676.
10 See Lord Bridge in *Sidaway v Board of Governors of the Bethlem Royal Hospital and the Maudsley Royal Hospital* [1985] 1 All ER 643 at 663, HL.
11 G Dworkin and I Kennedy 'Human Tissue: Rights in the Body and its Parts' (1993) 1 Med L Rev 291 at 317.

17 Research on children and fetal experimentation

A child is by no means a miniature version of an adult. Children respond differently to drugs, as they do to a number of other treatments, and it is impossible to say that the effect of a particular therapy on an adult will be mirrored when applied to a child. Medical research on children is, therefore, necessary before a treatment can be approved for paediatric use. As in adults, such research may entail not only therapeutic research on sick children but also essential non-therapeutic research on normal control groups; it is this non-therapeutic research which poses the ethical and legal problems.

Such research involves a variety of procedures, ranging from the completely benign – such as weight and height studies – to those which are frankly invasive. As an example of the latter, the Institute of Medical Ethics cites a French project which involved lumbar punctures on newborn infants for non-therapeutic reasons.[1] Such investigations would not be approved by research ethics committees today but procedures that are far less hazardous and uncomfortable still raise questions as to the general acceptability of research in this particular group of subjects.

Non-therapeutic research on children

The essential difficulty with non-therapeutic research on children lies, again, in the question of consent. An adult may be able to give an informed and therefore valid consent to participation in research – but can the same be said of a child? The Declaration of Helsinki specifically mentions the 'legally incompetent' participant in research, stating that the consent of the guardian should be procured; this approach is also adopted in the guidelines on experimentation issued by the British Paediatric Association,[2] the Medical Research Council[3] and the Royal College of Physicians.[4] All these influential bodies accept that non-therapeutic research on children is justified in that it is intended to benefit other children – although it should not be carried out if it could be done equally well using adults. Such research should not be instigated before parental consent has been obtained; in the view of the Royal

---

1 B Dalens et al 'CSF Levels of Lactate and Hydroxybutyrate Dehydrogenase as Indicators of Neurological Sequelae after Neonatal Brain Damage' (1981) 23 Devl Med Child Neurol 228 cited in R H Nicholson (ed) *Medical Research with Children: Ethics, Law and Practice* (1990) p 19.
2 British Paediatric Association *Guidelines for the Ethical Conduct of Medical Research Involving Children* (1992).
3 Medical Research Council *The Ethical Conduct of Research on Children* (1991).
4 Report of the Royal College of Physicians of London *Research Involving Patients* (1990) p 19.

College of Physicians, parental consent is required in respect of children under 16 years old and also in the case of 'some older children'.

The Institute of Medical Ethics studied the question in depth[5] and recommended that parental consent should be ethically acceptable only when the risks involved in the research are minimal – this being defined by the institute as a risk of death lower than 1:1,000,000, a risk of major complications less than 1:100,000 and a risk of minor complications of less than 1:1,000. In addition, the institute thought that the consent of the child should be obtained after the age of seven years. This concern was shared by the Royal College of Physicians, which felt that a child who is capable of giving a consent should also be allowed to refuse to participate in a research procedure – even if parental consent had been obtained. The college does not rule out proceeding with research involving a child who objects but is too young to give consent but it suggests that, in such circumstances, investigators should reconsider whether it is appropriate to go ahead.

Obtaining parental consent is clearly important but the fact that it has been given does not, of itself, justify carrying out research on children. Our first concern here must be with the welfare of the child and it need hardly be said that parental consent to something which is obviously to the detriment of the child is unacceptable. Parents do not have an absolute, unfettered right to regulate their children's lives; it is implicit in the modern concept of parenthood that the aim of such parental powers as there are is to protect and enhance the status of the child.[6] It follows that the researcher cannot simply say: 'The parents have consented and this means that I can go ahead'; parental consent may justify the involvement of children in non-therapeutic research but it will do so only because it points to the acceptability of the research in terms of some interest of the child.

One way of assessing parental consent is to see it as a substitute for the child's own judgment which cannot, as yet, be expressed. Under this theory, parental consent does no more than voice what the child would be expected to state had he the ability to do so. Acceptance of this approach salves any qualms the researcher might have – in effect, the child consents to what is done, the only complication being that this cannot be expressed personally. Critics of theories of proxy consent point out that this involves a blatant fiction. It would be more honest, they argue, to accept that this constitutes non-consensual research and to admit the need to justify it on other grounds. The difficulty cannot be avoided by attempting to justify the child's involvement in terms of his 'future identification' with the decision made on his behalf.[7] It is difficult to see any distinction between 'identification' and 'consent' and, whatever terms one uses to imply future assent, there is no certainty that the child will, in fact, subsequently endorse what his parents have decided.

The matter may, however, be approached from an entirely different perspective – one which focuses not on any imagined consent of the child but on what is in that

---

5   Institute of Medical Ethics 'Medical Research with Children: Ethics, Law and Practice' (1986) Bull no 14, p 8. For discussion of the recommendations, see R J Robinson 'Ethics Committees and Research on Children' (1987) 294 BMJ 1243.

6   See B M Dickens 'The Modern Function and Limits of Parental Rights' (1981) 97 LQR 462; also A McCall Smith 'Is There Anything left of Parental Rights' in E Sutherland and A McCall Smith (eds) *Family Rights* (1991) ch 1.

7   R B Redmon 'How Children Can Be Respected as Ends Yet Still Be Used as Subjects in Non-therapeutic Research' (1986) 12 J Med Ethics 77.

child's best interests. This test would allow the parents to involve the child in that which is in – or, alternatively, that which is not manifestly against – the child's best interests. The first of these would require that the non-therapeutic research secures some benefit for the child – a difficult, though not impossible, case to make. A child is a member of a class within the community – the class of children – and the individual can be said to be a potential beneficiary if research will benefit the class as a whole. It is also possible to extrapolate the reasoning used to justify organ donation (see ch 14) and to argue that participation in research related to a disease from which, say, a sibling is suffering will benefit the normal child – it being in his interests that his sibling should recover.

An allied benefit-based theory focuses on the altruistic nature of participation in non-therapeutic research.[8] Here, the issue is, at base, whether or not parents have the right to involve their children in projects by way of imposed unselfishness. Such co-operation is undoubtedly good for the subject but this would apply only if the child were sufficiently mature to understand the philanthropic nature of what he was doing. An older child may later derive satisfaction from the fact that he helped others when younger but the same objection applies here as to proxy consent – how can we be sure that this is what he would feel?

The alternative interpretation of the best interests test, which allows for measures which are not to the actual detriment of the child, clearly licenses the child's involvement in non-therapeutic research so long as the risks involved are negligible. This assessment gives a wider discretion to the parent, who may choose to interpret his duty to society as including a duty to engage his children in pro-social activities. Such parents act within their rights, and cannot be regarded as abusing their position, until such time as the child suffers actual harm or runs an appreciable risk of harm.[9]

Even if this were not accepted and the child's interest in non-participation were to be seen as being more significant than any parental social duty, the non-interventionists could still hold that this is an area of the family's activities in which the law has no right to interfere. State intervention may be justified if a child's life is threatened through neglect or through a parental decision which is going to lead to great danger – but these are not the stakes involved in comparatively harmless research. The protagonist of individual self-determination is unlikely to approve of a justification based on relative values but the inevitable consequence of the extreme individualistic position would be the suspension of all non-therapeutic medical research on children – which would benefit nobody, least of all the children themselves.

Discussion thus far has proceeded on the assumption that the child in question is not of an age to give any meaningful consent. Even so, many children of relatively tender age will be able to understand the issues involved and the question then arises as to the weight to be given to any agreement they might give. The age at which a child can appreciate the implications of what he is doing will obviously vary, but some generalisations may be made.[10] Children under the age of seven are usually

---

8 See A McCall Smith 'Research and Experimentation Involving Children' in J K Mason (ed) *Paediatric Forensic Medicine and Pathology* (1989) p 469.
9 The test of acceptability then becomes one of the 'reasonable parent'; see J K Mason *Medico-legal Aspects of Reproduction and Parenthood* (1990) p 291.
10 See J Berryman 'Discussing the Ethics of Research on Children' in J van Eys (ed) *Research on Children* (1978) p 85.

considered to be incapable of that degree of morally sophisticated thought required to make consistent altruistic decisions but, above that age, a child may be perfectly able to understand that he is helping doctors to cure others by taking part in the research programme. A child who was not able to grasp the general idea of medical research by the age of 15 would probably be an exception today. This view is supported by a study which was designed to assess the ability of groups of 9- and 14-year-olds to make decisions relating to medical treatment. The 14-year-olds were shown to have the same general level of capacity to make this sort of decision as did adults and a surprising degree of competence was shown in the 9-year-old group.[11]

The ethical issues might be clarified to an extent if the law could give a clear answer to this question. Unfortunately, the law itself is uncertain in this area and this has not eased the difficulties of those involved in paediatric research. In 1962, the Medical Research Council stated that: 'in the strict view of the law, parents and guardians of minors cannot give consent on their behalf to any procedures which are of no particular benefit to them and which may carry some risk of harm.'[12] This was followed by a Department of Health circular which confirmed that interpretation in a negative way:

> Health authorities are advised that they ought not to infer [from a Royal College of Physicians' recommendation that children can be used in certain forms of research provided the consent of the guardian has been obtained] that the fact that consent has been given by the parent or guardian and that the risk involved is considered negligible will be sufficient to bring such clinical research investigation within the law as it stands.[13]

The advice of the Department of Health was roundly attacked by doctors. Lawyers were also critical of this strict view of the law, pointing out the paucity of authority on the point.[14] In these conditions – almost amounting to a legal vacuum – the proper way of approaching the issue is to look at general legal principles governing the parent/child relationship and to infer from these what a court might decide if the matter were to come before it.

We have already seen that the consent of a minor to medical treatment may be adequate even without parental ratification provided that the child has sufficient understanding and intelligence to appreciate what is involved. The judgment of the House of Lords in *Gillick v West Norfolk and Wisbech Area Health Authority*[15] has confirmed this view. 'Parental rights', said Lord Scarman, 'exist only so long as they are needed for the protection of the person and property of the child'. It is not certain whether the *Gillick* principle, which is concerned with consent to treatment, would be applied to cases of non-therapeutic experimentation. Much would, of course, depend on the severity of the procedure – this being one of the factors to be balanced

---

11 L A Weithorn and S B Campbell 'The Competency of Children and Adolescents to Make Informed Treatment Decisions' (1982) 53 Child Develop 285. For discussion, see R H Nicholson (ed) fn 1, at p 146.
12 Report of the Medical Research Council for 1962-63 (Cmnd 2382) pp 21-25.
13 Supervision of the Ethics of Clinical Research Investigations and Fetal Research' HSC (5) 153.
14 See, for example, discussion by G Dworkin 'Law and Medical Experimentation: Of Embryos, Children and Others with Limited Legal Capacity' (1987) 13 Monash Univ LR 189.
15 [1986] AC 112, [1985] 3 All ER 402, HL.

in the assessment of '*Gillick*-competence'. As to statute, it is clear that the Family Law Reform Act 1969, s 8, refers only to diagnosis and treatment[16] – the statutory age of 16 years has, therefore, no relevance as to consent to experimentation. To infer from this that consent to non-therapeutic investigations is impossible below the age of majority would be, again, to accept a total embargo on paediatric research. It is not unreasonable to extrapolate Lord Donaldson's interpretation of the law in *Re R*[17] and to infer that anyone who is capable of doing so may give consent but that demurral by the minor would be a very important consideration in judging whether to carry out the research. Moreover, this would be even more significant than it would be in relation to treatment – to such an extent that it would be improbable in the extreme that a responsible doctor would ignore the minor's negative attitude. The problem then becomes that of deciding whether there is any age below which a person is deemed incapable of consent and, while there is no law on the point, it would be unwise, in our opinion, for a researcher to accept the unendorsed consent of a child under the age of 16; indeed, the circumstances in which such a consent would be acceptable would be exceptional. Hazardous experimentation authorised by the consent of a minor alone might, in fact, be unlawful and actually *restrained* by statute.[18]

To say that a procedure is legal is not to say that it is necessarily morally acceptable; furthermore, there is no reason to assume that the court, if asked, would approve an action which was unethical. The position is, therefore, still delicately balanced. Anticipating a judicial reaction is a matter for ethical committees who may assume that the court would act as a wise parent would act – giving first consideration to the child but being, at the same time, hospitable to good research.[19] Thus, the essential measure is the 'risk-benefit ratio' of the investigation – but, within this, the 'risk' factor must, without doubt, retain primary control. We would also suggest that, notwithstanding what the true legal position may be, it would be, in practice, improper to proceed with an experiment involving a child against the wishes of its parents. The only arguable exception might be when that refusal was clearly unreasonable and was jeopardising an otherwise essential trial to which a child who was capable of understanding – the 'mature minor' of *Gillick* – had already consented. Such conditions must be extremely rare; in the event of their materialising, a decision to go ahead would be taken only after very careful consideration – and, probably, not even then.

It must not be thought that an ethical assessment of a project is always clear cut. A most apposite example was an experiment in preventive medicine which entailed the deliberate infection with the virus of hepatitis of children in a home for the

---

16 It is problematic as to whether this limitation applies in Scotland in so far as the Age of Legal Capacity (Scotland) Act 1991, s 2(4) refers to consent to 'any surgical, medical or dental *procedure* or treatment' (our emphasis).

17 *Re R (a minor)(wardship: medical treatment)* [1991] 4 All ER 177, (1991) 7 BMLR 147.

18 Lord Donaldson distinguished between medical treatment and a severely damaging operation which gave no benefit to the subject: *Re W (a minor)(medical treatment)* [1992] 4 All ER 627 at 635, 639, (1992) 9 BMLR 22 at 31, 35.

19 G Dworkin 'Legality of Consent to Nontherapeutic Medical Research on Infants and Young Children' (1978) 53 Arch Ds Childh 443. The author notes the transition in legal thinking from paramount interests to first consideration of the child – the latter indicating that other interests are admissible.

mentally handicapped. Although the chances of the children being infected naturally were as high as 60% within six months of admission, the project was castigated by some writers.[20] Others disagreed with such an analysis – one of Britain's most respected paediatricians described the experiment as: 'a small, carefully controlled trial for which the director also deserves a great deal of credit for his scrupulous care in securing the truly informed consent of the children's parents.'[1] It is clear that there can be no generalised approach to a subject such as childhood experimentation, the practice of which is governed, in the end, by humane pragmatism.

Fetal research and experimentation

Several of the legal and moral attitudes to fetal life have already been discussed. The possibilities of fetal research and experiment, which are repugnant to many, extend the area of debate and merit further discussion. Research on the fetus is of considerable importance: just as children are, medically, more than little adults so – or rather more so – are fetuses not just immature children. The environment in which they exist is wholly different and, as has already been discussed, it is within that environment that something in the region of half the morbidity and mortality of infancy is fashioned.[2] Major areas of disease will never be properly understood in the absence of fetal research. Nor will the outstanding dilemma of drug therapy during pregnancy be fully resolved.

Sources of fetal material and the problems of consent

Other than those which are born alive prematurely and with which we are not currently concerned, fetuses become available either through spontaneous miscarriage or as a result of therapeutic abortion. It is axiomatic that any necessary consent to research can only be given by the mother and both her attitude and that of her physicians may be different in the two cases.

The position seems clear in the case of miscarriage. The mother is distressed and, normally, wants everything possible done for her offspring. It seems unlikely in the circumstances that a research project will be contemplated but, were it so, the informed consent of the mother would be required. The therapeutic abortion situation is rather different. In the majority of cases, the mother will have requested termination and it could be held that, in so doing, she has effectively abandoned her fetus. The Peel Committee made the following recommendation:

> There is no legal requirement to obtain the patient's consent for research but, equally, there is no statutory right to ignore the parent's wishes – the parent must be offered the opportunity to declare any special directions about the fetus.[3]

20 See, for a good review, L Golman 'The Willowbrook Debate' (1973) 9 World Med (1) (79).
1 A W Franklin 'Research Investigation on Children' (1973) 1 BMJ 402 at 405.
2 The Peel Committee, reporting in 1972, listed 53 ways in which fetal research could be valuable, a catalogue which will have increased in the interim: *Report of the Committee on the Use of Fetuses and Fetal Material for Research* (London, HMSO).
3 At para 42.

This recommendation would now be considered inadequate. The very strict rules as to consent to research on the abandoned embryo should, in theory, be extrapolated to the abandoned fetus.[4] Moreover, the Peel Report has now been overtaken by that of the Polkinghorne Committee,[5] which detected no material distinction between the results of therapeutic or spontaneous miscarriage (para 2.9). It was firmly recommended that positive consent be obtained from the mother before fetal tissue is used for research or treatment in either circumstance (para 3.10) – for it was thought to be too harsh a judgment to infer that she has no special relationship with her fetus that has been aborted under the terms of the Abortion Act 1967 (para 2.8). The mother should, also, have counselling and her consent should include the relinquishing of any property rights – this latter to eliminate any controversy over, for example, cell lines as is discussed at p 367. Interestingly, the committee rejected the notion of any control by the father over the disposal of his child – this being on the grounds that paternal consent was not required for an abortion and that his relationship to the fetus is less intimate than is that of the mother (para 6.7).[6] We have already referred to what we see as an unreasonable denial of paternal interests in the fetus (see p 119) and this seems to be another questionable extension of the principle of the woman's right to self-determination.

The Polkinghorne Committee was established mainly in response to concerns over fetal brain implants (which we discuss as a separate issue at p 310), and, as a consequence, one of its main concerns was that the research worker seeking consent should be wholly independent of the caring gynaecologist. Every moral and public policy principle dictates that it be made absolutely clear that abortions are not being performed in order to provide research or therapeutic material; the timing of a therapeutic abortion should be subject only to considerations of care for the pregnant woman.

The status of the fetus

The Polkinghorne Committee was fully alert to the fact that conditions for fetal research are not uniform and, in particular, that the fetal subject may be alive or dead – or it may be killed during the process of abortion. The living human fetus should be accorded a profound respect – a conclusion which is based upon its potential for development into a fully formed human being (para 2.4). In so saying, the committee clearly differentiated the dead fetus but still thought that this commanded respect. Research on the living fetus should be considered in a way broadly similar to that pertaining to children and adults and it was, therefore, recommended that it should not be undertaken if the risk to the fetus was more than minimal; research or experimentation carrying a greater risk should be limited to that which was of direct benefit to the subject. Respect for the dead fetus was recognised by the belief that research in that area should also be considered by ethics committees (para 7.3).

4   Human Fertilisation and Embryology Act 1990, Sch 3.
5   *Review of the Guidance on the Research Use of Fetuses and Fetal Material* (Cmd 762, 1989).
6   For this and several other criticisms of the recommendations, see J Keown 'The Polkinghorne Report on Fetal Research: Nice Recommendations, Shame about the Reasoning' (1993) 19 J Med Ethics 114. The father's consent may be even more significant in the event of fetal ovum or ovarian tissue donation in which his genes are being used (see p 312).

Somewhat surprisingly, the committee did not seek that the law be used to impose their restrictions. Rather, fetal research was to be overseen by local ethical research committees (para 2.3) and here, as we discuss at p 352, conditions are not uniform. Definitions of minimal or of direct benefit are likely to differ – as, indeed, are doctors' interpretations of research and experimentation and of the need for reference to an ethics committee. The general ethical and legal principles involved still merit some discussion.

Some useful research is non-invasive and may be coupled with patient care but even then there is no simple answer. Thus, the experimental use of X-rays, at least in the first trimester, would be unethical; ultrasonic investigations seem, by contrast, to be wholly safe – but we cannot yet know, for example, whether fetal ultrasonic investigations will affect the subject at retiring age. Our more immediate concern is with invasive investigations and these, once again, focus attention on the uncertainties surrounding the legal status of the unborn child (see chapter 5, above).

It has been argued that no action exists in the United Kingdom in respect of 'wrongful death' of the fetus; the stillbirth has no right of action of itself and the only redress available is to the parents on the grounds of distress, inconvenience, etc[7] – but this is not to deny the trend towards a moral and legal acceptance of fetal rights which are comparable to those of a self-existent child.[8] If the fetus were born deformed, it would clearly have right of action against a research worker whose defence, assuming causation to have been proved, would rest on the standard of reasonable care having been observed. The matter of consent then becomes paramount and must be judged in the same light as has been discussed in relation to children.

Assuming that the mother has a right of proxy consent to research procedures, the risk/benefit test would have to be very stringently applied because, whereas the child has at least minimal understanding, the fetus can certainly have none. A negligence action based on a lack of informed consent would be more likely to succeed in these conditions than in many others; if, by contrast, parental consent is impossible, the damaged infant has a cause of action for trespass which will be virtually indefensible other than on issues of causation. In practice, the nature of any invasive experiment of this type is strictly limited on clinical grounds.

But what if the fetus should die? The fetus not being a legal person, it may well be that there is no offence of feticide as such; but, should the fetus die prior to or during a resultant miscarriage, an offence may lie under the Offences Against the Person Act 1861, s 58 or under the Infant Life (Preservation) Act 1929, s 1 if the subject were capable of being born alive. Both these sections, however, include a requirement of intent, in the former to procure a miscarriage and in the second to destroy life. To prove an offence, it would then be necessary to show that the action amounted to constructive intent – that is, something was done when it was known that fetal death was a very high probability – and this seems a very doubtful

---

7   See, for example, *Bagley v North Herts HA* [1986] NLJ Rep 1014; *Grieve v Salford HA* [1991] 2 Med LR 295. In the United States, however, actions for wrongful death of the fetus have succeeded and a new form of tort – with a largely punitive motivation – appears to be being developed: *Amadio v Levin* 501 A 2d 1085 (Pa, 1985).

8   The constitutional protection of the fetus may be less extensive than that provided by private law – particularly when the issue is that of abortion: M L McConnell 'Sui Generis: The Legal Nature of the Foetus in Canada' (1991) 70 Can BR 548.

proposition. It is, however, quite clear that intentional or reckless intra-uterine injury which results in neonatal death can attract a charge of manslaughter or of culpable homicide;[9] it is at least likely that disregard of the recommendations of the Polkinghorne Committee would give rise to an inference of recklessness. We do, however, see such eventualities as becoming increasingly rare.

The pre-viable fetus

Perhaps it is the pre-viable fetus which attracts most emotion in the general issue of fetal research. Pre-viability implies that the fetus as a whole is incapable of a separate existence but that, nevertheless, there are signs of life in some organs. There can be no doubt that this is the fetal state which offers the greatest research potential; it is also true that the time available for such research is limited and so, therefore, is the opportunity for abuse. But, again, one must ask – is this an ensouled human being with the rights of a human being? And, moreover, do we know that it has no feeling and is incapable of pain and suffering? The Polkinghorne Committee was unable to discern any relevant ethical distinction between the pre-viable and the viable fetus – thereby diverging from the Peel Report. None the less, the status of the pre-viable fetus in relation to the criminal law needs consideration and the door is not quite closed on the moral concerns of the researcher.

We suggest that the criminal law is inadequate in this area. To destroy a fetus outside the terms of the Abortion Act is to destroy life. But in doing so, what offence is being committed? By no stretch of the imagination could a fetus which is incapable of an independent existence be described as a 'reasonable creature in being' – it cannot be murdered. The discussion may seem sterile in present conditions but, in the event of extension of techniques being coupled with a deterioration in professional standards, it might, as has already been suggested in chapter 3, be necessary to invent an offence of feticide. The moral dilemma is clear from the questions posed above and, equally, turns on the definition of 'life'. We suggest that the moral problem may be resolved by considering, first, whether or not a placenta is present and whether there is or is not a competent fetal/maternal connection. If there is, the fetus is clearly alive and destructive research or experimentation would be morally unacceptable; it should be disallowed on these grounds alone. If, however, the pre-viable fetus is separated from its mother, it is no longer capable of an existence; it is, therefore, possible to argue that its state is one of somatic death. Experiments or research conducted on the body are, by this reasoning, conducted during the interval between somatic and ultimate cellular death which has been described in chapter 13. Accordingly, we suggest that the processes involve neither moral nor legal culpability.

The dead fetus and fetal parts

Much useful research can be done on fetuses which are clearly dead or are incomplete and this would seem to raise neither legal or ethical problems. The only differentiating

9   *Kwok Chak Ming v R* [1963] HKLR 349; *McCluskey v HM Advocate* 1989 SLT 175. For further discussion, see J Temkin 'Prenatal Injury, Homicide and the Draft Criminal Code' (1986) 45 CLJ 414.

factor is how the fetus came to be dead – any objection on principle to the use of tissue from dead fetuses is most probably grounded on an overall objection to abortion.[10] The tissues can be regarded as abandoned biological specimens and treated accordingly. This is subject only to the mother's ultimate discretion. An exception must be made in respect of such material being sold for commercial purposes. The concept was condemned out of hand by the Polkinghorne Committee and is foreign not only to the ideals of a national health service but to public opinion in general. There are no rules governing the disposal of fetuses other than those related to offences against public decency; at the present time, the sale of fetal tissues clearly comes into the latter category.

Fetal materials

Fetal materials – which the Polkinghorne Committee preferred to call 'other contents of the uterus' – are those parts of the products of conception which are discarded by both the mother and the fetus and comprise the placenta and its membranes and the umbilical cord. The placental membranes and the cord are both valuable in therapy and their use in that way is not subject to the Human Tissue Act 1961.

As a consequence, their disposal seems to present no difficulty. The Polkinghorne Report was concerned to distinguish, in general, conditions pertaining to the human fetus from those applying to the other contents of the uterus (para 3.12). In our view, the latter, once discharged from the mother, represent a classic example of res nullius and, thus, can become the property of the first person into whose hands they rightly fall. It is proper, and desirable, that such a person should harvest the material for the benefit of the community. The only proviso we would suggest is that, again, there should be no direct sale of biological materials – and the Polkinghorne Committee deprecated even the acceptance of 'administrative costs' in their collection. It is true that an 'intermediary body' might be financially responsible for the collection and distribution of fetal tissues and materials but, pending the establishment of such a body, the suggested policy seems over-conservative – if for no other reason than that it would lead to a shortage of therapeutic material. The committee did, however, draw attention to an important exception to their negative attitude to control of the placenta and membranes. Clearly, the mother's consent would be needed were the materials to be tested for HIV or hepatitis B infection – for the effects of testing would be identical to those of testing her own body tissues.

Embryonic research

Research into human infertility and an understanding of embryonic development and implantation are inseparable. Embryonic research is also essential to the study and conquest of genetic disease. Systematic study in both these fields depends upon a supply of human embryos for there always comes a time when animal models are

10 For discussion of attitudes and practices in relation to fetal tissue research in various countries, see 'Fetal Tissue Research around the World' (1992) 304 BMJ 591.

inadequate for human research purposes. Essentially, there are two adoptable attitudes – either one can be totally opposed to research and experimentation on what are considered to be living human beings who cannot refuse consent to manipulation, or one can hold that the benefits to mankind are likely to be so great that the opportunity for study must be grasped if it is presented. Given that the case for human research is agreed – and we believe that it must be – the problem then arises as to how the necessary material is to be obtained within an acceptable moral framework. There are, again, two possibilities which are by no means mutually exclusive – either one can use the inevitable surplus or embryos that are produced for infertility treatments or one can go one stage further and create embryos in vitro for the explicit purpose of using them for research. It is, first, necessary to look at the general proposition.

Arguments against a policy of prohibiting embryo research rely, ultimately, on the view that, although the embryo may have human properties, it is not a human being invested with the same moral rights to respect that are due to any other living members of the human community.[11] This approach has a familiar ring to it; indeed, it introduces the same concepts of personhood that have been so much a part of the abortion debate. There is, however, a crucial distinction to be made between lethal embryo research and abortion. The life of the aborted fetus is extinguished because its interests are outweighed by a more powerful and tangible set of interests – namely, those of the pregnant woman. The embryo subjected to experimentation, by contrast, dies because of the far less obvious interests of society in the pursuit of medical knowledge. The justification of feticide in abortion does not necessarily license the taking of in vitro embryonic life – and the legislative concern for the latter in the face of a liberal abortion policy may not be as unreasonable as is sometimes argued. [12]

Yet, if we consider, first, the surplus embryo, we have to ask: 'what is the alternative to embryocide?' The techniques in IVF and the welfare of the patient demand that more embryos are created than are strictly necessary; to say that all must be implanted[13] is to fly in the face of the reality that there are insufficient wombs available for the purpose. The alternatives then lie between embryocide and reduction of multiple pregnancy – of which the former is clearly the less objectionable. We have discussed elsewhere (p 311) the ethics of obtaining good from a morally poor or doubtful fait accompli. It is only the innate public fear of the 'scientist'[14] which stands against the acceptance of such a principle – one which we believe to be valid, perhaps particularly so in respect of the undifferentiated embryo.

But this can only hold so long as the basic tenet of the doctrine of double effect – that the good result must not be achieved by means of the ill-effect – is observed and it is this that distinguishes research on the surplus embryo from that undertaken on the embryo that has been created for the purpose; it follows that the latter needs further justification. The proponents of unrestricted research would reply that it is

11 For a statement of this position, see J Harris 'Embryos and Hedgehogs: On the Moral Status of the Embryo' in A Dyson and J Harris (eds) *Experiments on Embryos* (1990) p 65.
12 See, for example, Mason, fn 9, p 371 at p 209.
13 As seems to be the case in the Infertility (Medical Procedures) Act 1984 (Victoria), s 6(5). But the section can be read as being directed only at the creation of embryos for non-therapeutic research purposes which is certainly unlawful in Victoria.
14 M Warnock *A Question of Life* (1985) p xiii.

acceptable not only because the embryo fails to satisfy the requirements of personhood which the fetus, similarly, fails to satisfy but also because, at least in its earlier stages,[15] its cells are pluripotential. In other words, until the development of the primitive streak, the conceptus is not a single, identifiable individual; any of its cells can develop along a number of lines – into a placenta, a hydatidiform mole, into a human being or, indeed, into several human beings. The early embryo, according to this argument, thus lacks the essential qualities which go to make the human individual unique and worthy of moral respect.

The counter-assertion is, of course, that the embryo is the first stage of the human being that is born at the end of pregnancy – and that this holds from the moment of syngamy. It has been pointed out that the embryo stage is an essential part of life and that it makes no sense to argue that a person's life begins only with the appearance of the primitive streak on about the fourteenth day after conception.[16] It follows that the use of an embryo for any purpose that does not bear upon its future good constitutes a wrong; the embryo is, otherwise, being treated as a means to an end rather than as an end in itself – a process which offends a fundamental principle governing the way in which we treat other persons. To create human life in the full knowledge that it can have only the most limited future is seen by many opponents of embryo experimentation as an example of amoral exploitation and a first step on yet another slippery slope.

Between the two 'extreme' positions – that of a total rejection of embryo research on the grounds of its inescapable immorality and that of its acceptance in the case of any embryo, however derived – lies the middle view that, whereas research on surplus embryos is acceptable, the creation of embryos for that purpose is not. This is a view which is held by many and one with which we have very great empathy. Even so, it is not easy to establish a valid moral basis for the claim – for, in so far as the ultimate outcome is their destruction, the harm done to the embryos is the same in each case. A possible philosophical solution depends on distinguishing harm from wrong. No *wrong* is done to the embryo at the time it is formed with a view to implantation; a later failure to achieve that goal is due to circumstances which are, to a large extent, beyond the control of the person who has brought it into being. By contrast, the embryo which is developed with the express intention of harming it is clearly *wronged* at the moment of its formation. Thus, while the harm done to each is the same, the wrong done is of a different quality. But do those who take the middle road adopt such reasoning in reality? It seems more probable that they accept instinctively that a utilitarian argument which holds that the benefit to mankind exceeds the harm done to what are the unfortunate rejects of a legitimate therapeutic activity cannot be substantiated in the case of specially created research subjects. This problem has raised what has been, perhaps, the most difficult hurdle for the world's legislatures.[17] We see below that the United Kingdom Parliament, in contrast to that of Victoria, has opted in favour of the similarity of in vitro embryos however

---

15 The use of the term 'pre-embryo' is suggested for this stage of development. We feel, however, that this smacks of using words to establish a moral bolt-hole.

16 A Holland 'A Fortnight of My Life Is Missing: A Discussion of the Status of the Pre-embryo' (1990) 7 J Appl Philos 25.

17 The UK debate is well summarised in D Morgan and R G Lee *Blackstone's Guide to the Human Fertilisation and Embryology Act 1990* (1991) ch 3.

they originate; could it be that this disparity mirrors the public intuition unearthed by the intense involvement of community, or peoples', organisations in the deliberations of the preparatory Australian committee?

The legal response

The legal regulation of embryo research in the United Kingdom is embodied in the Human Fertilisation and Embryology Act 1990. The debate on the Bill was a free one in both the House of Lords and the House of Commons and there is no doubt that moral, rather than political, loyalties determined the position of the individual legislators.

We have already discussed this Act at length in chapters 3 and 5. For present purposes, it is to be noted that, so great was the dilemma posed by the issue of embryo experimentation, that the unusual step was adopted of introducing three mutually exclusive clauses relating to the point in the Bill. As we have seen, the most important overall effect of the Act is to establish an authority which is responsible for overseeing fertilisation treatment and research services in the United Kingdom. The fundamental principles to be adopted are now clear. It is illegal to conduct any research on human embryos except under licence from the authority. The authority can only issue such a licence if the project is thought to be desirable for the purposes of advancing the treatment of infertility, for increasing knowledge of the causes of congenital disease, for studying the causes of miscarriage, for developing methods of contraception or for developing methods of detecting the presence of genetic or chromosomal abnormalities in embryos before implantation; other reasons may be added by regulation (Sch 2, para 3(2)). In the absence of further regulation, no licence may authorise altering the genetic structure of a cell while it is part of an embryo and, while the hamster test for the normality of human sperm is allowed, all products of such research must be destroyed not later than the two-cell stage. There are strict regulations as to the maintenance of experimental records (s 15). Overall, licences cannot authorise keeping or using an embryo after the appearance of the primitive streak – taken as being not later than 14 days after the gametes were mixed – nor may any embryo be placed in any animal (s 3). Most importantly, in decreeing that research may be carried out, Parliament placed no restrictions on the source of the embryos used; there is no evidence that the authority will impose an overall embargo on the creation of embryos for that specific purpose.

A tight regime of licensing and regulation will satisfy those who feel that research of this nature, while being permissible, needs close monitoring. Even so, the 1990 Act demonstrates a legislative approach which is probably more liberal than that existing elsewhere. Much will depend upon the ability and motivation of the Human Fertilisation and Embryology Authority; it is doubtful if the current legislation will go far to quietening the concern of those who feel that we are now allowing the use of human life in a way that is contrary to the spirit of, for example, the Declaration of Helsinki. One thing is certain – the mere existence of an authority will not end the debate and may, in fact, generate controversy of its own. Even as we go to press, the authority is being asked to decide whether treatment licenses should include restrictions on the age of the patient and whether research should extend to the use of gametes derived from aborted fetuses. It is arguable that it is wrong for an unelected body – or, come to that an elected government – to interfere in what many would see as a private matter between doctor and patient. Others will be grateful for the existence of a ready-made form of control of a form of reproductive engineering. The authority's response to such demands will be awaited with interest.

Psychiatry and the law

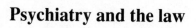

18 Human rights, psychiatry and the law

The practice of psychiatry is more vulnerable to criticism than any other area of medicine. The reasons for this are complex; one factor, however, stands out – while treatment for physical conditions almost always depends upon the consent of the patient, the psychiatrist may be called upon to treat the unwilling. The associated powers may involve the involuntary detention of a fellow being for a considerable time, something which is usually reserved to the judiciary in a state governed by law. In addition, psychiatric treatment is likely to be aimed at ameliorating a disturbance of mood or behaviour. In so doing, it sets out to alter the functioning of the human mind and this can be seen as an interference in human autonomy which will be justified only in the most exceptional circumstances. Thus, in the view of some critics,[1] the powers accorded to psychiatric medicine give rise to unnecessary and unwanted intervention in the lives of persons whose beliefs and views, albeit bizarre, should be left undisturbed. This criticism of psychiatry became fashionable in the 1960s and 1970s, but is now more muted. The civil liberties concerns of the critics have, to an extent, been addressed by reforming legislation of the early 1980s, and it is now difficult to find psychiatrists who are not acutely aware of the dangers of excessive intervention in the lives of mentally ill people.

Society has favoured the institutional or asylum approach to the management of mental illness throughout most of this century. Those diagnosed as suffering from a psychiatric illness have been sent usually to 'mental hospitals' where in-patient treatment would be provided. The growth of a large group of patients whose only home was hospital was an inevitable result of such a policy and there grew up increasing calls for the release into the community of as many long- and short-term psychiatric patients as possible. This movement was motivated principally by the desire to save those with mental disability from the indignities of forced 'removal' from the community but the cause was, in due course, taken up by governments which were anxious to keep health costs as low as possible; as a result, many psychiatric hospitals were closed. Thus, the debate on psychiatry and human rights is entering a new phase. Whereas, in the past, the emphasis has been on protecting the patient from what might be considered over-zealous enthusiasm for therapy, the focus has now turned to how the right to proper treatment can be secured. This is not to say that the civil libertarian aspects of the rights of the unwilling individual are no longer a matter for concern; these issues are still important and occupy much of the time of lawyers involved with mental health. Equally important, however, is the plight of those who, while being mentally ill, find help hard to obtain because of

---

1 For a classic example of the radical view of mental illness, see T S Szasz *The Myth of Mental Illness* (1972) and, more recently, T S Szasz 'Diagnoses are not Diseases' (1991) 338 Lancet 1574. For a general survey of this issue, see P Millar and N Rose *The Power of Psychiatry* (1986).

the inadequacy of community care arrangements.[2] Prisons have always contained more than a chance proportion of those with mental health problems, whether by way of illness or handicap[3] – and this is now exaggerated simply because, with the closure of psychiatric wards, other places become more limited. It is not at all uncommon for those who are discharged from hospital to find themselves quite incapable of living in the community and ending up in prison as a result.[4] Such injustices should be every bit as much a matter for concern for civil libertarians as are the rights of those who do not seek treatment.

Proper community care is undoubtedly an attractive option for many mentally ill people – and indeed the concept meets with wide support amongst psychiatrists and patients. Yet the danger with such a change is that adequate resources will not be available and that some patients – particularly the more difficult ones – will have inadequate arrangements made for them. A solitary bed-sit with none of the facilities or diversions of hospital life, no programme of rehabilitation and nothing but four walls to stare at is not real community care; it is more a washing of the hands on the part of the state.

This issue is essentially a political one but human rights considerations resulted in legal attention being given to community care in *R v Ealing District Health Authority, ex p F*.[5] The patient in this case had been detained in a secure psychiatric hospital after he had been convicted of causing grievous bodily harm. Some three years later a Mental Health Review Tribunal had ordered his discharge, subject to the relevant health authority making arrangements for him to be supervised in the community. The health authority declined to make these arrangements, offering instead to manage him for 18 months in a regional secure unit. The court held that once the patient had been conditionally discharged, then it was the duty of the health authority to make every effort to ensure that he was able to meet the condition of his discharge. The court accepted, however, that this obligation had to be considered within the limits of the authority's resources. Further support for the community care principle came in the unlikely guise of a Lands Tribunal decision holding that a covenant restricting the use of a domestic dwelling could be discharged in favour of allowing the house to be used for psychiatric patients in community care.[6] This decision affirms the public interest in community care.

The grounds for intervention

The mere presence of a psychiatric condition will not, of itself, be sufficient to justify compulsory treatment: a person may suffer from psychiatric illness and yet still be able to reach a reasoned decision as to whether or not to undergo therapy. Compulsory treatment is justified only if a person's remaining untreated poses a threat to his own health or safety or to the safety of others.

2   E Murphy 'Commuity Mental Health Services: A Vision for the Future' (1991) 302 BMJ 1064.
3   R Bluglass 'Mentally Disordered Prisoners: Reports but No Improvements' (1988) 296 BMJ 1757.
4   For discssion, see B G A Weller and M P I Weller 'Prison, the Psychiatric Dumping Ground?' (1989) 139 NLJ 1335 who cite a study of prisoners on remand for violent offences which revealed an incidence of schizophrenia 22.5 times higher than the epidemiological expectation. See also, by the same authors, 'Mental Illness and Social Policy' (1989) 139 NLJ 1382.
5   [1993] 4 Med LR 101.
6   The decision, sub nom *Lloyd*, is discussed by G Thornicroft and A Halpern 'Legal Landmark for Community Care of Former Psychiatric Patients' (1993) 307 BMJ 248.

Danger to others

One problem confronting psychiatrists in this field is the definition of mental illness and, particularly, what practical distinction – in terms of treatment and disposal – is to be made between psychosis and psychopathy (sociopathy). The clinical differentiation may be very difficult; moreover, the two conditions are by no means mutually exclusive. In one study which is, admittedly, rather old, 24 out of 100 psychopathic prisoners had been diagnosed alternatively at some stage in their criminal careers and the author commented on the ease with which the diagnosis could be changed;[7] the diagnostic conflict with schizophrenia lay at the heart of the important decision in *W v Egdell*[8] which is discussed in detail at p 171. Legislation has, however, gone some way to easing the problem. Psychopathy – defined as abnormally aggressive or seriously irresponsible conduct resulting from a persistent disorder or disability of mind – is now included in a definition of mental disorder which may be treatable;[9] moreover, even if there is no specific therapy available, treatment can be limited to nursing, care and rehabilitation for the purposes of the Mental Health Act 1983, s 72.[10] There is, thus, comparatively little to prevent the compulsory admission of psychopaths for assessment and treatment and, whatever one's views as to the use or abuse of such powers in social terms, this facility is clearly desirable – at least some psychopaths are, by definition, likely to expose the public to physical danger.

There is wide social acceptance of the proposition that those who are dangerous should be contained in a way which will prevent their causing harm to others. This principle is observed regularly by the courts when heavy custodial sentences are imposed on violent offenders in the interests of public safety. It is, nevertheless, axiomatic that a person who is dangerous but has not yet committed a crime is entitled to his liberty whatever his potential for future harm may be. We are then left with a paradox – why would so few people argue against the prophylactic detention of a dangerous person who is suffering from a mental illness? The answer must be that, in contrast to the case of the mentally 'healthy' violent person, the illness itself may provide a basis for asserting that certain forms of violent or irrational conduct may be reasonably foreseen.

Even so, the prediction of dangerousness is an imprecise – and, perhaps, fruitless – exercise. Many attempts have been made to determine an objective concept of dangerousness but none has succeeded in allaying all doubts as to the strong element of subjectivity that is inherent in such judgments.[11] Disparities are frequently detected; in one such study, 60% agreement between a group of assessors was

---

7 D Power 'Psychopathic Disorder' (1988) 12 The Criminologist 202.
8 [1990] Ch 359, [1990] 1 All ER 835, CA.
9 Mental Health Act 1983, s 3(2).
10 Mental Health Act 1983, s 145; *R v Mersey Mental Health Review Tribunal, ex p D* (1987) Times, 13 April.
11 P E Mullen 'Mental Disorder and Dangerousness' (1984) 18 Austral NZ J Psychiat 8. Opinions differ amongst psychiatrists as to the ethical implications of making predictions of dangerousness. Not all psychiatrists are reluctant to do so; see, for example, T Grisso and P S Applebaum 'Is it Unethical to Offer Predictions of Future Violence?' (1992) 16 Law and Hum Behav 621. Legislators might prove ready to act on such predictions, providing for the detention of those who *might* offend: M A Bochnewich 'Prediction of Dangerousness and Washington's Sexually Violent Predator Statute' (1992) 29 Cal West Law R 277.

achieved in only four out of 16 case appraisals.[12] Psychiatric assessment of dangerousness must not, therefore, be considered an exact science – although the fact remains that reliable prediction is exactly what courts, parole boards and tribunals may be expecting. It is, indeed, possible that dangerousness is best established retrospectively by way of a history of recidivism; the problem then becomes one for the criminologist rather than the psychiatrist.[13]

The position of the psychiatrist is, thus, difficult and, in all but a few exceptional cases, it will be impossible for him to say with any degree of certainty whether violent conduct is to be expected. Harm to others may result from premature release; yet excessive caution may cause injustice to the patient himself. This issue has provoked litigation in the United States where the courts have imposed civil liability upon psychiatrists when patients have been released and have subsequently harmed others.[14] The American courts have, in fact, been unrelenting in their demands. In *Lipari*,[15] the court was not persuaded that the inherent difficulties in predicting dangerousness justify denying the injured party relief regardless of the circumstances. Not surprisingly, the psychiatric reaction to such developments results in a tendency to err on the side of caution.[16] The issue of dangerousness also raises questions of psychiatric confidentiality which is discussed more fully in chapter 8. *Tarasoff v Regents of the University of California*[17] is, perhaps, the best known of the relevant cases and is one which has given rise to widespread debate in North America and elsewhere. In this case, a patient had confessed to a therapist that he intended to harm a woman who had rejected his advances. The therapist failed to warn her of the danger and she was later killed by the patient; her family then sued the therapist's employers successfully. *Tarasoff* concerned a threat to a specific individual but subsequent cases have extended the principle so as to impose liability on psychiatrists who fail to detect and warn of danger on a general scale. A similar dilemma of confidentiality arose in England in *W v Egdell*.[18] Here, a psychiatrist, who was invited by a patient's solicitors to examine him with a view to an application for transfer from a secure hospital, sent his report to the Home Office in order to prevent what he saw as a danger of the patient's premature release. This action was held to be justified in the public interest – a decision which was upheld in the Court of Appeal. The trial judge, however, made some disturbing observations – in particular:

> I accept that [the conclusion that the weight of public interest prevails over the private right to confidence] places W and persons like him in a position in which the duty of confidence owed by their psychiatrists is less extensive than the duty that would be owed by psychiatrists to other members of the public.[19]

12 G Montadon and T Harding 'The Reliability of Dangerousness Assessments: A Decision-making Exercise' (1984) 144 Brit J Psychiat 149.
13 D J Gee and J K Mason *The Courts and the Doctor* (1990) p 138.
14 T J Rudegeair and P S Applebaum 'On the Duty to Protect: An Evolutionary Perspective' (1992) 20 Bull Amer Acad Psychiat Law 419.
15 *Lipari v Sears, Roebuck & Co* 497 F Supp 185 (Neb, 1980).
16 For a discussion of criteria for release, see D J Power 'When not to Release Potentially Dangerous Patients' (1992) 16 Criminologist 2.
17 529 P 2d 55 (Cal, 1974); on appeal 551 P 2d 334 (Cal, 1976).
18 Fn 8, p 387 above.
19 [1990] Ch 359 at 393, [1989] 1 All ER 1089 at 1135, per Scott J.

Why, it may be asked, was W not an ordinary patient? Was it because he was in a secure hospital or because he had killed several persons? If it was the latter, the opinion raises doubts as to the rights of any prisoner convicted of violent crime. Or was it because he was now labelled as a psychopathic personality? While the outcome of *Egdell* would probably be approved by the majority, the implications the case raises for the psychiatrist/patient relationship are clearly considerable.

Paternalistic intervention

The compulsory treatment of mental illness in those who pose no threat to others is based on the notion of justified paternalism.[20] A paternalistic act is one which is not sought by the patient but which is provided with the intention of protecting him from harm. Ordinarily, paternalistic action will be considered wrong because it offends the principle of autonomy. It may be justified, however, when the person for whose benefit the act is performed is unable to make an informed choice for himself. Thus, paternalism towards a child is accepted on the grounds that a child may not be sufficiently mature to make important decisions about his or her life. The mentally impaired and the mentally ill may be similarly incompetent in that their ability to understand the reality of their situation is compromised by their mental state. The absence of rationality in such cases then warrants action directed towards preventing their being harmed. One approach to the problem is by way of the question: 'Would the patient, were he or she rational, consent to the treatment proposed?' There may be grounds for involuntary treatment if the answer is Yes. This is the American 'substituted judgment' test which is, effectively, autonomy-based in so far as intervention is directed to the higher goal of restoring the patient's already compromised autonomy. The relief of suffering would never be a sufficient justification for paternalistic intervention *by itself* – otherwise, the imposition of medical treatment would be permissible whenever a person refused palliation.

An alternative way of justifying intervention in the face of mental illness is to invoke the doctrine of implied consent. Someone who cannot consent to a procedure while incompetent may later be able to endorse what was done, thereby providing a form of retrospective consent. There are serious objections to this approach. To begin with, there is the difficulty of predicting whether subsequent consent will be given. Many patients who resent involuntary intervention continue to do so after their treatment – and, indeed, may never change their attitude to psychiatric interference. It is also possible that any post hoc consent will be a product of the intervention itself – as, for example, where treatment results in increased docility, compliance or even dependence on the person providing it. For these reasons, it is safer to rely on the autonomy-based arguments identified above.

All such means depend, however, upon the patient having ever had a meaningful degree of autonomy through which to exercise the decision-making function – it is philosophically impossible to appeal to substituted judgment in the absence of such a resource. Moreover, it is an ethically dubious ruse to invoke the doctrine of implied

---

20 There is a major survey of paternalism in general in D VanDeVeer *Paternalistic Intervention* (1976). Other contributions include: B Gert and C M Culver 'Paternalistic Behavior' in M Cohen, T Nagel and T Scanlon (eds) *Medicine and Moral Philosophy* (1981) p 201.

consent in the near certainty that there will be no recovery phase in which implication may become reality. In such circumstances, it is more honest to take the opposite, frankly paternalistic, route and apply a 'best interests' test. This is the way followed in statute whereby, subject to the safeguards discussed in detail below, treatment for the mental disorder that has occasioned compulsory admission to hospital may be given without specific consent. In recent years, the courts have increasingly been using a best interests rule to justify non-consensual treatment of a non-psychiatric nature[1] and there is no doubt that doctors will continue to rely upon it. The patient, however, is unconcerned in such esoteric argument; the fact is that legitimating paternalism in this way carries the danger of licensing excessive interference in the lives of those afflicted by mental illness. There must, therefore, be limits both as to the determination of incompetence and the extent of treatment. Competence is not necessarily entirely compromised by mental illness and the fact that a psychiatric diagnosis has been made does not mean that the patient, thereafter, loses all capacity to decide upon treatment for himself. On the other hand, there will be conditions which deprive the patient of all insight into his plight and where the effect of the illness is so profound as to deny him all chance of an autonomous life. Intervention on a major scale may be justified in the latter case; it may be difficult to accept any paternalistic intervention at all in the former instance.

The happiness of the patient is another limiting factor. One who is psychotically ill, but relatively contented, may dread incarceration in a hospital or may dislike the effects of a drug he has been prescribed. There will be a case for abandoning therapeutic goals if these can only be attained at the expense of extreme and long-lasting unhappiness – therapy should not be allowed to eclipse all other considerations. This is just another way of saying that the mentally ill have their rights which are significantly affected by their status. Rights may have to be considered, and adapted, in the light of limitations imposed by the illness but the wishes of the patient must always be taken into account when determining a therapeutic regime. Sometimes these wishes will put a stop to a promising line of treatment; at others, they may properly be overruled in the interests of the patient's future happiness.

Pure theory will not necessarily provide the right answer in such a dilemma. An unequivocal commitment to the consensual rights of the mentally ill may result in their being denied treatment on civil libertarian grounds. It may also lead to unnecessary suffering by the families of those afflicted; calls for the recognition of the psychiatric patients' right to reject treatment may well sound hollow to those struggling to cope with their demands in a domiciliary situation. Enthusiasm for a rigid and one-sided doctrine of rights may amount to misplaced kindness, as became apparent in the United States. There, a movement to de-institutionalise the mentally ill resulted in limitation of involuntary admission for those who were a danger to themselves or others; as a consequence, there was strong backlash pressure to reintroduce compulsory paternalistic treatment including those who were not dangerous. The American Psychiatric Association bowed to these demands in their 1982 Guidelines for Legislation on the Psychiatric Hospitalization of Adults.[2]

---

1   For example *Re B (a minor)* [1981] 1 WLR 1421; *Re F (mental patient: sterilisation)* [1990] 2 AC 1, sub nom *F v West Berkshire Health Authority* [1989] 2 All ER 545, HL.

2   For discussion of the reaction against involuntary commitment in the United States, see A E Buchanan and D W Brock *Deciding for Others* (1989) p 312.

In Canada, civil liberties considerations have significantly eroded the paternalistic claim of society to treat those who are suffering from mental disorder. In *Fleming v Reid*,[3] the appellants, who had committed crimes of violence, had been diagnosed as suffering from schizophrenia. Their doctor had decided that the appellants were incompetent and proposed to treat them with neuroleptic drugs, a proposal which was vetoed by the patients' substitute decision-maker. The latter pointed out that the patients had had previous experience of this form of treatment and had objected to it at a time when they were competent. Under the relevant mental health legislation, the Ontario Mental Health Act, the substitute decision maker's refusal to consent could be overridden by a review board and it was the decision by a review board to do just this that led to the legal challenge. In due course, the Ontario Court of Appeal held that this decision contravened s 7 of the Charter of Rights and Freedoms, which protects the right to bodily integrity and personal autonomy. It was only in the absence of any indication of the patient's previously expressed, competent rejection of treatment, that a best interest argument might be used to justify imposing involuntary treatment on an incompetent person. This means, in effect, that if one expresses an antipathy to any form of drug treatment, and if one subsequently becomes incompetent, psychiatric medicine may be powerless to attempt a cure. Psychiatric treatment is, thus, put on the same footing as the treatment of physical illness, an approach which fails to distinguish those features which make psychiatric disease a special case – namely, that it distorts or destroys the ability to make a *rational* decision.

Controlling treatment

The framework for the treatment of mental illness in the United Kingdom is to be found in the Mental Health Act 1983 and the Mental Health (Scotland) Act 1984.[4] These two statutes introduced major reforms which related principally to the regulation and review of involuntary treatment and to consent to certain forms of treatment. The English Act also established a Mental Health Commission[5] which was structured along the lines of the long-standing Scottish Mental Welfare Commission[6] – both have the general power to monitor procedures for admission to hospital and to scrutinise the conditions in which patients are detained.

Informal treatment

Treatment for mental illness is provided on either a voluntary or an involuntary basis. Informal – that is, voluntary – treatment may be provided by any registered medical practitioner or, indeed, by any layman provided that the provisions of the Medical

3   (1991) 82 DLR (4th) 298.
4   Discussion here is principally in terms of the Mental Health Act 1983. The 1984 Act is similar in many respects but has some important differences – for example, in the role of the sheriff in compulsory admission (s 21). There is a full treatment of the Scottish provisions in J Blackie and H Patrick *Mental Health: A Guide to the Law in Scotland* (1990).
5   Mental Health Act Commission Regulations 1983 (SI 1983/894).
6   Established by the Mental Health (Scotland) Act 1960, s 2.

Act 1983 as to impersonation are observed. Informal hospital treatment is regulated by s 131 of the 1983 Act, which states that a patient may enter hospital for psychiatric treatment without any order being made for that purpose and with freedom to leave at will. Informal patients can object to any particular treatment; they have unhindered access to the courts and enjoy certain other privileges which are denied to those who are detained compulsorily. The proportion of informal patients has increased markedly over the last three decades, this being an objective which was first expressed legislatively in the Mental Health Act 1959.

Although the informal patient in a psychiatric hospital is in much the same position as a patient in any other hospital, his status may be changed to that of compulsory detention (s 5(1)). This can be effected by the 'doctor in charge' of the patient on the grounds that it appears to him that 'an application ought to be made' for compulsory admission (s 5(2)). Detention under this provision expires after 72 hours. Nurses may also restrain a patient from leaving hospital if this is deemed to be immediately necessary and if it is not practicable to secure the immediate attendance of the doctor in charge or his delegate (s 5(4)). This form of detention may last for only six hours or until a doctor entitled to act under s 5(2) is able to attend.

Compulsory admission

There are three routes to involuntary admission to hospital under the Mental Health Act 1983. These are:

(1) *Admission for assessment under section 2*. Application for such admission must be made either by the patient's nearest relative – or by a person authorised by him or by a court to act on his behalf – or by an approved social worker. It is essential that the applicant has seen the patient within the past 14 days; the application must also be supported by two registered medical practitioners, one of whom must be qualified in psychiatry. Responsibility for getting the patient to hospital rests upon the applicant although this may be delegated to others such as ambulance staff; force may be used to this end provided it is not excessive.

The grounds for admission under s 2 are that a patient is suffering from a mental disorder of a nature or degree which warrants detention in hospital for assessment for at least a limited period and that he should be detained in hospital 'in the interests of his own health or safety or with a view to the protection of other persons'. Patients admitted for assessment may be kept in hospital for up to 28 days and such admissions cannot be renewed.[7]

Patients must be informed of their legal position and rights and may apply to have the case reviewed by a Mental Health Review Tribunal during the first 14 days of detention. The procedures for admission under s 3 (see below) must be invoked if it is proposed to detain the patient for a further period.

(2) *Emergency admission*. A patient may be admitted in an emergency under s 4 (1984, s 24). This form of admission can be effected on the recommendation of one doctor and is valid for only 72 hours. The doctor need not be a specialist in mental

---

7   For Scots law and the common law power of detention, see the House of Lords case *Black v Forsey* 1988 SC 28.

illness but he must, if practicable, have known the patient beforehand (s 4(3)); the applicant must have seen the patient within the previous 24 hours. Emergency admission may be converted to admission for treatment (28 days) by obtaining an additional opinion from a specialist in mental illness; the formalities required for s 2 admission must be complied with at this stage.

(3) *Admission for treatment*. Longer-term compulsory detention for treatment is governed by s 3. Application procedures are similar to those used for admission for assessment although, under s 3, the nearest relative must be consulted when admission is being sought by a social worker. Court authority for admission will be needed if the relative objects. The grounds for admission for treatment are that, in the opinion of the doctors recommending admission, the patient is: (a) Suffering from mental illness, severe mental impairment, psychopathic disorder or mental impairment and his mental disorder is of a nature which makes it appropriate for him to receive medical treatment in a hospital; and (b) in the case of psychopathic disorder or mental impairment, such treatment is likely to alleviate or prevent deterioration in his condition; and (c) it is necessary for the health or safety of the patient or for the protection of other persons that he should receive such treatment and it cannot be provided unless he is detained under this section. Treatment for sexual disorders is excluded.

Admission for treatment allows for detention for up to six months. This period is renewable for a second period of six months and, thereafter, for periods of a year at a time. Detention under s 3 can, therefore, last indefinitely; however, on renewal, the responsible medical officer must believe that further treatment is likely to alleviate or prevent deterioration in the patient's condition or that the patient would be unable to care for himself or would be liable to serious exploitation were detention to be ended (s 20(4)(a) and (b)).

The practice of using s 3 to enforce treatment on out-patients has been expressly rejected.[8] It is, therefore, not now possible to admit to hospital under s 3, to provide necessary intermittent treatment and to release on licence until the next treatment schedule. There is some concern that these court decisions make it more difficult for patients to be treated in the community as powers of compulsion will not be available in those cases not requiring continuous in-patient management. The response of the Royal College of Psychiatrists was initially to press for the introduction of community treatment orders and, more recently, for community supervision orders. The idea behind the community supervision order would be to allow patients to be supervised in the community and to ensure compliance with suggested treatment by allowing recall to hospital in the event of a refusal to co-operate. Although this scheme would have the benefit of allowing essential treatment to be carried out within the community – without resorting to the expense and distress of compulsory admission – it would be important to monitor the civil liberties aspect of such an arrangement. In particular it would be vital to ensure that patients had adequate opportunity to appeal for review of what could be very long term compulsory treatment.[9]

8   *R v Hallstrom, ex p W; R v Gardner, ex p L* [1986] QB 1090, [1986] 2 All ER 306.
9   P Fennell 'Arrest or Injection' (1993) 143 NLJ 395.

Persons without physical illness who are compulsorily detained in hospital – and particularly those who are mentally disturbed – are likely to see themselves as victims of paternalistic injustice. The strong possibility exists that they may institute proceedings against those responsible for their committal to and/or detention in hospital. This was foreseen in s 139 of the 1983 Act which states:

> No person shall be liable . . . to any civil or criminal proceedings . . . in respect of any act purporting to be done in pursuance of this Act . . . unless the act was done in bad faith or without reasonable care.

Bad faith or negligence would, however, be something that the proceedings were designed to establish and sub-s (2) gives further protection in stating that no civil proceedings may be brought against any person without the leave of the High Court. Section 139 thus leaves two questions open: has the patient any legal redress in the absence of bad faith or negligence and by what criteria should the High Court grant leave to proceed? As to the first, it has now been held that Parliament must have intended to retain the court's inherent power to protect the rights of the individual; application for judicial review does not constitute 'civil proceedings' for the purposes of the Act and remains open to an aggrieved patient.[10] The answer to the second 'chicken and egg' problem is of even greater significance to the patient. The Court of Appeal in *Winch*[11] overturned the trial judge's ruling that leave to proceed depended upon there being a prima facie case to bring. The change of wording between the 1959 and 1983 Acts was considered deliberate and the court was no longer required to establish that there were substantial grounds for the patient's contention; the issue was simply whether or not the complaint appeared to be such that it deserved the fuller investigation which would be possible if the applicant was allowed to proceed – in Miss Winch's case, the court went so far as to deny any suggestion that the proceedings were likely to succeed. Section 139 relates only to actions against individuals. No such protection is afforded, say, to the Department of Health; this, however, is generally a matter of the criminal law to which we refer later.

It is, none the less, clear that detention in hospital for long periods is open to abuse without some form of independent review. This is provided for in the establishment of mental health review tribunals to which patients who wish to have their cases considered can apply.[12] The tribunals have been subject to considerable criticism in the past – a low incidence of appeals has been alleged and patients are said to have experienced difficulty in obtaining adequate representation; current procedures for automatic review and the availability of legal aid now answer many of these shortcomings. It has also been held that tribunals must state their reasons for their

---

10 *Ex p Waldron* [1986] QB 824, sub nom *R v Hallstrom, ex p W* [1985] 3 All ER 775, CA. Discussed by Legal Correspondent 'Actions by Psychotic Patients' (1986) 292 BMJ 128.

11 *Winch v Jones; Winch v Hayward* [1986] QB 296, [1985] 3 All ER 97, CA. Discussed by Legal Correspondent 'Legal Proceedings by Mental Patients' (1986) 292 BMJ 820.

12 P F Mawson 'The Function of Mental Health Review Tribunals under the Mental Health Act' (1986) 26 Med Sci Law 291. For an account of the way in which the tribunals interpret their role and of the supervision by the courts of the process of review, see G Richardson *Law, Process and Custody: Prisoners and Patients* (1993) p 278 et seq.

decisions,[13] a proposition that provides considerable protection against decisions based on surmise or suspicion. Hospital authorities are now duty bound to explain to patients their right of appeal to a tribunal; a case is now referred automatically if this right is not exercised within the first six months' detention. Hospital managers are also obliged to refer patients to the tribunal when detention has been renewed and the case has not been considered for three years. In all of this, though, the onus lies on the patient to prove that his continued detention is unjustified, whereas it might be argued that the reverse should be the case.

Conditions justifying compulsory admission

A major civil rights concern in this area is that the boundaries of mental illness should not be drawn so widely as to embrace forms of behaviour that are no more than non-conformist. Compulsory admission should be limited to conditions which amount to an illness that can be said to compromise the mental health of the sufferer. In this respect, the Act distinguishes between admission for assessment and admission for treatment.

In the former case, the patient may be admitted under compulsion if he is thought to be suffering from a 'mental disorder'. This term is widely defined. Not only does it include mental illness, arrested or incomplete development of mind and psychopathic disorder – it embraces, too, 'any other disorder or disability of mind' (s 1(2)). The term 'disorder' could potentially include a number of deviations from the psychiatric norm and its application to conditions such as alcoholism, drug addiction or sexual deviation of themselves is expressly excluded by s 1(3). Admission for treatment is more closely controlled and the Act requires that the patient be suffering from one of four specifically identified disorders: mental illness, severe mental impairment, psychopathic disorder or mental impairment. Those suffering from the first two conditions may be admitted irrespective of the likely effect of treatment; those suffering from psychopathic disorder or mental impairment can be detained only if their condition is 'treatable'. None the less, the definition of 'treatability' – or of the appropriateness of detention – is wide. *R v Canons Park Mental Health Review Tribunal, ex p A*[14] concerned an appeal, under s 72 of the 1983 Act, from a decision of the relevant mental health tribunal that the patient should continue to be detained in an interim secure hospital. The Divisional Court held that detention of a person suffering from psychopathic disorder was lawful only if treatment in hospital was appropriate and was likely to be effective; this was not achieved in the present case – due, at least in part, to the patient's refusal to take part in group therapy. The Court of Appeal, however, concluded that whether or not the condition was treatable was little more than a factor in assisting the tribunal to decide as to the appropriateness of hospitalisation. Treatment which was likely to prevent a deterioration in the condition – rather than to alleviate it – satisfied the wording of the Act; moreover, such treatment included nursing and rehabilitation under medical supervision which might, as in the present case, lead to greater therapeutic co-operation on the part of

---

13 *Bone v Mental Health Review Tribunal* [1985] 3 All ER 330.
14 [1994] 1 All ER 481, QBD; (1994) Times, 2 March, CA.

the patient. In passing, the case adds weight to the difficulties attending psychiatric diagnosis to which we have alluded at p 387 – the patient had been re-admitted in the time between the trial and the appeal following recategorisation from psychopathic disorder to mental illness.

The Act does not define mental illness.[15] There is a wide consensus that it includes psychoses such as schizophrenia but neurotic conditions may well be considered to be in the same category as personality disorders and, therefore, beyond its scope. The problem was neatly put by Roth and Kroll[16] who cited the case of a young man who courted disaster through compulsive risk-taking; this involved having dangerous masochistic sexual encounters with violent men and, ultimately, led to his death. Such conduct is an 'illness' in so far as it affects the subject's health and is beyond his control much as an organic illness would be; it would be classified as illness were it due, say, to hormonal imbalance but not if it were psychological in origin – which, say the authors, is illogical.[17] Personality disorders may be distinguished from mental illness on a variety of grounds. It is very doubtful that organic factors play any part in the former;[18] moreover, if one of the criteria of illness is that it 'overlays' the normal self, this cannot be said of a personality disorder which lies at the core of 'self'. There is, in fact, considerable debate as to the categorisation of psychopathy (or sociopathy). The condition, which was identified by psychiatrists of the nineteenth century,[19] is listed as a mental disorder in the American Psychiatric Association's DSM-III-R. Yet the precise criteria defining psychopathy are unclear[20] and there is some concern that the tendency to label a wide range of anti-social conduct as psychopathic may lead to an undue medicalisation of deviant behaviour. One Scottish judge, having listened to a description of the symptomatology of psychopathy, remarked:

> It is, to my mind, descriptive rather of a typical criminal than of a person . . . regarded as being possessed of diminished responsibility.[1]

15 A judicial attempt to do so is to be found in *W v L* [1974] QB 711 at 719, [1973] 3 All ER 884 at 890, CA where it was said that the words 'mental illness' were ordinary words of the English language with no particular medical significance which should, therefore, be construed in the way in which 'ordinary sensible people would construe them' per Lawton LJ.

16 M Roth and J Kroll *The Reality of Mental Illness* (1986) p 79.

17 In one view, conditions such as self-destructive behaviour are merely matters of choice. One opponent of the disease model is H Fingarete who, in his *Heavy Drinking: The Myth of Alcoholism as a Disease* (1988) argues strongly against the genetic theory of alcoholism. For a view of drug abuse as chosen, rather than compelled, behaviour, see J Davis *The Myth of Addiction* (1992).

18 A genetic factor may, however, be operating: M Roth 'Psychopathic (Sociopathic) Personality' in R Bluglass and P Bowden (eds) *Principles and Practice of Forensic Psychiatry* (1990). Roth also cites research revealing EEG abnormalities in psychopaths.

19 The historical background is discussed in N Walker and S McCabe *Crime and Insanity in England and Wales* (1973) at II, p 205. See also P Pichot 'Psychopathic Behaviour: A Historical Overview' in R D Hare and D Schalling (eds) *Psychopathic Behaviour: Approaches to Research* (1978).

20 The category of personality disorder is now more differentiated - and refined. For a survey of advances in the diagnosis of conditions of this nature, see P Tyrer, P Casey and B Ferguson 'Personality Disorder in Perspective' (1991) 159 Brit J Psychiat 463.

1 *Carraher v HM Advocate* 1946 JC 108 at 117, per Lord Normand.

This is an unscientific view but, in a sense, it points to the difficulty which many people have with the concept of psychopathy – namely, how it is to be distinguished, if at all, from uncomplicated anti-social conduct.

The personality traits which feature most commonly in attempts to characterise psychopathy are a tendency to disruptive or selfish behaviour, inability to form relationships or to learn from experience and an inadequate moral sense. It is doubtful if there is any point in trying to treat the psychopath on an involuntary basis; certainly the Butler Committee[2] took the view that prison is the proper place for the psychopath who has offended and many psychiatrists are unwilling to admit them to their wards.

Mental impairment and severe mental impairment are both defined in the Act (s 1(2)). Mental impairment is not, of itself, a sufficient ground for admission for treatment. To satisfy the requirements, the patient's condition must be associated with 'abnormally aggressive or seriously irresponsible conduct' – the object and effect being to limit compulsory treatment to those who pose a threat to others.

Sexual deviancy is specifically excluded as a sole ground for intervention under the Act (s 1(3)). This means that a person may engage in outrageous sexual practices but will not be liable to compulsory treatment unless he also manifests one of the qualifying mental disorders discussed above. In *Clatworthy*,[3] the appellant had been detained by reason of psychopathic disorder. He argued, successfully, that the only ground for the diagnosis was his sexual behaviour and that this could not, by itself, constitute the basis for his detention by virtue of the explicit exclusion of sexual deviance as a statutory form of mental disorder. Contemporary psychiatry is cautious on this subject following the acrimonious debate on the classification of homosexuality as a psychiatric illness.[4]

Consent to treatment

Previous legislation made no direct reference to the conditions under which a person compulsorily admitted could be given hospital treatment. The 1983 and 1984 statutes remedy this by, in particular, delimiting the degree of invasion which is permitted. It is important to note that the Mental Health Acts refer only to treatment given for the mental condition itself. The rules evolved to regulate the treatment of physical illness in psychiatric patients have been discussed in chapter 10; here we are concerned purely with the treatment of mental disorder in involuntary patients, for which statutory authority is provided in the mental health legislation – circumventing the problem that mental disorder is, itself, likely to inhibit the giving of a true consent.

Non-consensual treatment of mental disorder is permitted by statute (s 63) but this is subject to the limitations imposed by s 57 and s 58. Section 57 refers to what are loosely known as irreversible procedures which include destruction of brain

2 Report of the Committee on Mentally Abnormal Offenders (Cmnd 6244) 1975.
3 *R v Mental Health Review Tribunal, ex p Clatworthy* [1985] 3 All ER 699.
4 M Ruse *Homosexuality* (1988) p 202. The equivalent philosophical debate has focused on whether homosexuality can be considered a perversion: S Ruddick 'Better Sex' in R Baker and F Eliston (eds) *Philosophy and Sex* (1975); R Scruton *Sexual Desire* (1986).

tissue or of its function and the surgical implantation of hormones for the control of the male sex drive;[5] it applies to both voluntary and involuntary patients. Consent is needed before such treatment can be given and this must be verified and certified by an appointed doctor and two non-medical witnesses who have, also, been appointed for the purpose.[6] Furthermore, the appointed doctor must certify that the treatment is likely to benefit the patient; he can do this only after consultation with two persons concerned professionally with the patient, one of whom is a nurse and the other neither a doctor nor a nurse. It is apparent that this section presents some difficulties. First, consent is essential. It follows that a patient who cannot consent cannot have treatment even though it may appear appropriate; the regulations can be waived only when the treatment is regarded as life saving (s 62(1)(a)). Secondly, the two confirmatory opinions must be *professionally* involved and a suitable non-health carer may be hard to find. The whole scenario must, however, now be extremely rare. The fact and results of irreversible treatments must be notified to the Mental Health Act Commission who may withdraw the certificate issued by the appointed doctor (s 61(3)).

Section 58 controls 'hazardous' treatments which, currently, include electroconvulsive therapy and long-term drug treatment – which is defined as continuing for three months or more. These may only be given if the patient has consented and either his responsible medical officer or an appointed doctor has verified that consent or if an appointed medical practitioner has certified that the patient cannot give valid consent but that the treatment would be of benefit to him; again, the doctor must consult two other persons as above who have been professionally concerned with the patient. Hazardous treatment can be given in the absence of certification only if it is needed to save the patient's life or, provided it is not irreversible, to prevent a serious deterioration in his condition (s 62(1)(b)). Treatment covered by ss 57 or 58 may be given in circumstances of urgency if it is neither hazardous or irreversible and is either necessary to alleviate serious suffering on the patient's part or represents the minimum interference necessary to prevent the patient from behaving violently or being a danger to himself or others.[7] The patient may withdraw his consent to s 57 or s 58 treatments at any time – once he does so, the process of certification must start again (s 60).

Behaviour modification

Several methods may be employed by psychologists and psychiatrists in an effort to alter undesirable behaviour. These may be non-intrusive, in the sense that they involve no physical intervention, or they may be very invasive – psychosurgery being the most extreme example. Several ethical problems arise in either case: Are coercive techniques ever acceptable? To what extent has the therapist the right to

---

5   The specific limitations of ss 57 and 58 are laid out in Mental Health (Hospital, Guardianship and Consent to Treatment) Regulations 1983 (SI 1983/893).
6   The procedures to be followed in such cases are laid out in the *Code of Practice* approved by Parliament in 1990, para 16.
7   Section 62 (1)(c) and (d).

impose his model of desirable behaviour on the patient?[8] Can consent ever be given to such treatments if they are offered in the form of an inducement – for example, as an alternative to punishment? These questions are posed most dramatically in relation to psychosurgery which merits separate discussion.

The essential claim of psychosurgery is that it can change behaviour patterns in reasonably predictable ways. Modern techniques avoid the crudities of leucotomy and may involve localised interference with parts of the brain which influence feelings and sexuality. Psychosurgery may be offered for a variety of conditions, most frequently for affective illnesses such as depression. Other indications for such surgery have included aggressive behaviour, intractable pain and unacceptable sexual urges.[9] Any discussion of the effectiveness of the procedure raises, of course, the question of the standpoint from which success is measured. It is important to distinguish the concept of therapeutic success – removal of symptoms without incurring unacceptable side-effects – from that of manageability. It is hardly proper to regard a treatment as successful if its main effect is merely to render the patient passive and compliant. In one sense, this constitutes little more than the 'neutralising' of the patient. Psychosurgery as a method of making uncontrollable patients more quiescent is open to the challenge that it is primarily a means of social control. As one writer has put it, 'Life in "Brave New World" may be more pleasant for all, but only John the Savage is fully human'.[10]

The success of psychosurgery is debated. A number of surgeons have reported good results. Depression seems to be the condition in which there is the best chance of success; positive improvement, however, has also been claimed in the case of patients whose unacceptable anti-social behaviour prior to the operation made it difficult for them to live successfully in society. It is rarely used, however, even if considerable claims are made for it: in the two years between June 1987 and June 1989, 46 applications for second opinions on psychosurgery were made to the Mental Health Act Commission.[11] In the United States, the National Commission for the Protection of Human Subjects of Biomedical Behavioral Research, which considered the subject of psychosurgery in detail, concluded that such surgery should no longer be considered experimental and, although it suggested safeguards in the form of review boards, the commission recommended that psychosurgery should be available to those institutionalised.[12] The commission explicitly rejected the *Kaimowitz* decision[13] in which it was held that an institutionalised person could not give a free consent to psychosurgery by virtue of the fact of being detained there involuntarily.

---

8 S Fairbairn and G Fairbairn (eds) *Psychology, Ethics and Change* (1987); A McCall Smith 'Changing the Offender: Ethical Issues in Behaviour Modification' (1988) Acta Juridica 169; J Holmes and R Linley *The Values of Psychotherapy* (1989).
9 E S Valenstein 'Who Receives Psychosurgery' in E S Valenstein (ed) *The Psychosurgery Debate* (1980) p 89.
10 J Kleinig *Ethical Issues in Psychosurgery* (1985).
11 Mental Health Act Commission *Third Biennial Report 1987-1989* (1989) para 7.10.
12 United States, National Commission for the Protection of Human Subjects of Biomedical and Behavioral Research Report 1976.
13 *Kaimowitz v Michigan Department of Mental Health* 42 USLW 2063 (1973).

Even if one accepts that the patient is capable of giving a consent which is valid, in that it is informed and uncoerced, that fact alone may not be sufficient to justify the treatment. Consent to a grossly maiming operation which achieves no therapeutic purpose may not justify the operation in the eyes of the law; similarly, psychosurgery could well be seen as a procedure which is unacceptable on grounds of public policy. The patient who is incapable of consenting may not now be given irreversible and hazardous treatments. He may therefore suffer, yet Parliament feels that this is an acceptable price to pay for the protection of the majority from what could turn into abuse were it uncontrolled.

Objections to psychosurgery focus on its drastic and irreversible nature. The consequences of drug therapy, while possibly unpleasant, are usually reversible and a mistake, or a change of mind, can be rectified. Any alteration in behaviour following psychosurgery is likely to be permanent and it is this which gives rise to misgivings. To make out a case for the procedure, the central issue of the aim of treatment must be confronted. If it is seen principally as a means of controlling behaviour, then there are sound reasons for objecting to it as representing a Draconian and ethically unacceptable method of control. A different conclusion may result if, on the other hand, the therapeutic intention is predominant. There is no reason why patients should be denied a potentially effective treatment purely because it is open to abuse or is hazardous. Such treatments should, of course, be subjected to control – preferably control which embodies an element of outside, lay opinion – but they should not be excluded from the range of those available by virtue only of their nature.

Controversy of almost equal intensity surrounds the use of chemical methods to control the behaviour of actual or potential sex offenders.[14] Opponents of these procedures have described them in such terms as 'chemical castration' and have been especially concerned as to their inherent coercive nature. Certainly, Parliament has expressed this view in specifically including surgical implantation of hormones to control the male sex drive in those 'irreversible' treatments controlled by s 57 of the 1983 Act. On the other hand, it is perfectly possible to see behaviour modification of this type in a properly therapeutic light. The person troubled by sexual inclinations which he cannot control may look upon drug treatment as his only hope of a normal life in the community.[15] On this analysis, the refusal of treatment to someone who genuinely seeks it can amount to unacceptable paternalism.

Just such an instance arose in *R v Mental Health Commission, ex p W*.[16] W was a compulsive paedophile who sought medical help. Standard antiandrogen treatment was unsuccessful and he was transferred to a new and relatively untried synthetic compound with the proprietary name of Goserelin; this was administered monthly by the subcutaneous insertion of a thin cylindrical implant. A satisfactory response was obtained with three insertions; however, the Mental Health Commission was now concerned as to the validity of his consent and withdrew its approval of the relevant certificates. W applied for judicial review – as a result of which, the commission's decision was quashed. The court's opinion raised several interesting points; some were, to an extent, peripheral to the main question but they merit note. First, it was held that, despite its action, a synthetic chemical compound could not be described as a

14 Mental Health (Hospital, Guardianship and Consent to Treatment) Regulations 1983 (SI 1983/893).
15 S L Halleck 'The Ethics of Antiandrogen Therapy' (1981) 138 Amer J Psychiat 642.
16 (1988) Times, 27 May, sub nom *R v Mental Health Commission, ex p X* (1988) 9 BMLR 77.

'hormone'; second, the subcutaneous injection of a substance through a needle, albeit of wide bore, was not a 'surgical implant'. Most importantly, however, the court noted that sexual deviance is expressly excluded from the definition of mental disorder for the purposes of the 1983 Act (s 1(3)); Goserelin was used for the treatment of such deviance and, although success in this respect would inevitably lead to improvement in any associated mental condition, it was not a treatment for mental disorder and was not subject to the controls of s 57. The Commission's decision was wholly unreasonable.[17] Although some of the observations may be seen as bordering on the casuistic, we feel that the case demonstrates that, if it is possible to do so, the courts will disapprove a bureaucratic attempt to separate a patient from the treatment he genuinely seeks and that they will support the doctors who are supplying it in good faith.

An even more poignant case is that of K, a 59-year-old paedophile who had served considerable periods of imprisonment following a series of sexual offences against children.[18] K had been offered Goserelin treatment while in prison, but had refused this, expressing a strong preference for surgical castration. The efficacy of this method of reducing sexual impulses is controversial – we return to this briefly at p 423 – but K insisted that it would give relief. The opinion of the Mental Health Act Commission was sought, and, to date, no decision has been taken. This case, however, is one over which views could differ markedly. To allow such an operation could be to do no more than acknowledge the right which the individual has to subject his body to such procedures as he sees fit – short of consenting to his own death or serious injury. In this view, there is no difference between this procedure and other forms of surgery which may be attended by a similarly dubious success rate. Alternatively, it might be held that allowing such a procedure is condoning a treatment which will not address the real nature of K's problem – psychosexual maladaptation – and which will do no more than perpetuate the cycle of failure in which he is trapped. The determining factor should be the likely effect on K's condition – it would be wrong to exclude this option if the treatment, even though theoretically of doubtful value, would help him to change his behaviour – even on no more than psychological grounds.

Thus, we have effectively come full circle in this chapter and are left with the unhappy conclusion that prognosis in psychiatry can often be assessed only after the event. Each person is a unique individual whose response is so uncertain that every treatment borders on the experimental and carries with it comparable practical and ethical implications.

17 For discussion of the case see P Fennell 'Sexual Suppressants and the Mental Health Act' [1988] Crim LR 660; C Dyer 'Mental Health Commission Defeated over Paedophile' (1988) 296 BMJ 1660.
18 M Alexander et al 'Should a Sexual Offender be Allowed Castration?' (1993) 307 BMJ 790.

19 Psychiatry and the criminal law

The psychiatrist may become involved with criminal law at a number of points in the process of trial. Most dramatically, he may be called upon to provide evidence to the court of the accused person's mental state and this intimately involves the psychiatrist in the essential function of any criminal trial – the determination of guilt or innocence. In addition to fulfilling this need, psychiatric evidence may be invoked to assist the court in the exercise of its sentencing power. Psychiatric reports on an offender may persuade the court to impose a more lenient custodial sentence or may point to what would be a more appropriate means of dealing with the offender; moreover, the court may ensure, as a result, that an offender gets further psychiatric or other medical treatment. The psychiatrist may be called upon to assist the court in other ways. Even when the sanity of the accused is not in question, evidence may be called as to the mental state of a witness, if that is relevant to the issue of the reliability of his or her evidence.[1] Attempts have been made to introduce psychiatric evidence which is aimed at demonstrating that an accused person's disposition was such that he could not have formed the necessary intention to commit the offence with which he is charged, but the courts have generally been reluctant to allow what they see as the usurpation of their exclusive power to decide such issues of mens rea.

The grounds for strictly limiting the scope of psychiatric evidence were spelled out in *R v Turner* in which the Court of Appeal warned that:

> The fact that an expert witness has impressive scientific qualifications does not, by that fact alone, make his opinion on matters of human nature and behaviour within the limits of normality any more helpful than that of the jurors themselves; but there is a danger that they think it does.[2]

This sceptical view of psychological or psychiatric evidence has resulted in the rejection by courts of attempts to use expert evidence to interpret the conduct of the accused. In *Weightman*,[3] the appellant had confessed to the police that she had murdered her young child. The defence sought to adduce psychiatric evidence to the

---

1 This was accepted in *Toohey v Metropolitan Police Comr* [1965] AC 595, [1965] 1 All ER 506, HL. See also *R v MacKenney* (1980) 72 Cr App Rep 78.
2 [1975] QB 834 at 841, [1975] 1 All ER 70 at 74, per Lawton LJ. For discussion, see D H Sheldon and M D MacLeod 'From Normative to Positive Data: Expert Psychological Evidence Re-assessed' [1991] Crim LR 811; D Sheldon 'The Admissibility of Psychiatric and Psychological Evidence' 1992 SLT 301. For an interesting analysis of the defects in the 'common sense' view of human conduct, see R D Mackay and A M Colman 'Excluding Expert Evidence: A Tale of Ordinary Folk and Common Experience' [1991] Crim LR 800.
3 [1991] Crim LR 204.

effect that the appellant suffered from a histrionic personality disorder which inclined her to make theatrical statements intended to draw attention to her herself – a condition which would obviously call her confession into question. The exclusion of this evidence was upheld by the Court of Appeal on the grounds that evidence which disclosed anything less than mental disorder or mental abnormality was not relevant; the reliability of a confession would be determined by the jury on the basis of its own experience of human nature rather than on the basis of any psychiatric insight. A similar view has been taken in provocation cases, where the effect of the decision in *Turner* has been to exclude psychiatric evidence of the likely effect of stressful circumstances on a particular individual. In *Roberts*,[4] for example, the defence was precluded from relying on psychiatric evidence to establish that an immature person, affected by a particular form of deafness, will react in an abnormal way when subjected to certain forms of stress. It will be different if it can be shown that the accused suffers from a mental disorder or mental handicap which places him in the category of the 'abnormal'. In *R v Masih*,[5] it was held that psychiatric evidence could be admitted in order to throw light on the state of mind of a mentally defective defendant – with an IQ of less than 70 – because mental abnormality would not be within the jurors' experience. The clarity of the rule has, however, been clouded by later judicial willingness to consider evidence as to mental capacity in the case of defendants who were not classified as being mentally handicapped.[6] The dividing line then between the normal and the abnormal is by no means clear and, certainly, a reference to an arbitrary IQ criterion will not resolve the issue. This was made evident in *Raghip*[7] where the Court observed that it would be impossible to regard as normal an accused aged 19 years who functioned at the level of a child of nine, even if such a person had an IQ which was just within the borderline range.

Other jurisdictions – to their credit – have shown themselves readier to invoke the insights of psychiatry and psychology. In *Murphy v R*,[8] the High Court of Australia distanced itself from the restrictive view expressed in *Turner* and allowed psychological evidence to call into question the admissions made by a defendant who was intellectually limited but not mentally retarded. A similarly receptive view was taken by the Supreme Court of Western Australia which allowed psychiatric evidence to establish that the defendant was not an 'ordinary man' and could not be expected to form the same intentions as the ordinary man.[9] In the Canadian case of *R v Lupien*,[10] psychiatric evidence as to the accused's strong antipathy to homosexuality was held to be admissible in a charge involving a homosexual offence. Such evidence could, of course, be categorised as character evidence – which is admissible in the United Kingdom. Character evidence does not, however, question the ability

---

4 [1990] Crim LR 122.

5 [1986] Crim LR 395.

6 See M Beaumont 'Psychiatric Evidence: Over-rationalizing the Abnormal' [1988] Crim LR 290.

7 *R v Raghip, R v Silcott, R v Braithwaite* (1991) Times, 9 December, CA.

8 (1989) 86 ALR 35. This case is discussed in J Hunter and J Bargen 'Diminished Responsibility: "Abnormal" Minds, Abnormal Murderers and What the Doctor Said' in S Yeo *Partial Excuses to Murder* (1991) p 125.

9 *Schultz v R* [1982] WAR 171.

10 (1970) 9 DLR (3d) 1. Of course, overt antipathy to something does not mean that one will not do precisely that thing. Psychological insights here might promote suspicion for the person who makes much of his distate.

of the judge or jury to determine the issue according to their own understanding of human nature; by contrast, psychiatric evidence, being expert evidence, clothes its conclusions in scientific language and, thereby, inevitably acquires a superior status in the eyes of the layman.[11]

The current role of the psychiatrist in the criminal process has its ethical snares. In theory, the psychiatric witness should be required to do no more than pronounce on the presence or absence of a mental abnormality but, in practice, the danger exists that he will be encouraged to address himself to the question of responsibility. There is also the risk that psychiatric questions will be unduly simplified in order to provide the 'key' to the unlocking of certain pleas. This has happened in relation to that of diminished responsibility (see below), in respect of which medical evidence frequently goes unchallenged; the court may be looking for a pretext for the exercise of leniency. It is doubtful if psychiatrists should lend themselves to procedures which might involve moral and professional compromise.[12] The psychiatrist gives evidence to the court as an expert. He does not provide an irrebuttable conclusion as to the state of mind of the accused but, rather, tenders an expression of opinion which will ultimately be decided upon by the judge or jury as the case may be. As a Scottish judge said of expert witnesses:

> Their duty is to furnish the judge or the jury with the necessary scientific criteria for testing the accuracy of their conclusions, so as to enable the judge or jury to form their own independent judgment by the application of these criteria to the facts proved in evidence.[13]

While a jury does not have to accept psychiatric evidence, it is not justified in discounting such evidence when it is not contradicted in any way. This has been clearly laid down in a number of cases[14] but forensic psychiatric evidence is sometimes ignored in spite of this legal acknowledgment.[15] Certainly, psychiatric evidence which is favourable to the accused is more likely to be accepted in a case where the accused attracts sympathy – where, for example, a woman is charged with the killing of a tormenting and violent husband – rather than in those where such sympathy is unlikely – as in a brutal murder committed for purposes of sexual gratification.

---

11 See R Bluglass 'The Psychiatrist as Expert Witness' in R Bluglass and P Bowden (eds) *Principles and Practice of Forensic Psychiatry* (1990) p 161.

12 D Chiswick 'Use and Abuse of Psychiatric Testimony' (1985) 290 BMJ 975. See also J R Rappeport 'Ethics and Forensic Psychiatry' in S Bloch and P Chodoff (eds) *Psychiatric Ethics* (2nd edn, 1991) p 391.

13 *Davie v Edinburgh Magistrates* 1953 SC 34 per Lord Cooper at 40.

14 *R v Matheson* [1958] 2 All ER 87, [1958] 1 WLR 474, CCA; *Taylor v R* (1978) 22 ALR 599.

15 Psychiatric evidence was discounted by the jury in the trial of Peter Sutcliffe, the so-called 'Yorkshire Ripper'. For discussion, see G Silverman 'Psychiatry after *Sutcliffe*' (1981) 125 SJ 518. Also, H A Prins 'Diminished Responsibility and the Sutcliffe Case: Legal, Psychiatric and Social Aspects (A "Layman's" View)' (1983) 23 Med Sci Law 17.

Mental illness and crime

At the heart of this issue is the question of the extent to which mental illness affects responsibility for criminal conduct. At one extreme is the view that a great deal of such conduct is explained by the psychopathological factors present in the offender's background – the 'crime as disease' position. At the other is the notion that the vast majority of mentally ill offenders are, in fact, responsible for their crimes, on the grounds that their mental abnormality does not necessarily impair their ability to understand the difference between right and wrong and to choose accordingly. Most supporters of the latter position would agree, however, that there can be no question of responsibility where illness is so severe as to distort fundamentally the offender's perception of reality. The controversial cases, then, are those which involve the less serious conditions, such as neuroses or personality disorders.

The problem here is essentially that of identifying a causal relationship between mental illness and crime. Such a relationship cannot be conclusively established, although the association of certain psychiatric conditions with criminal conduct appears to be strong. A proportion of those suffering from neurotic depression, for example, may engage in violent conduct directed against persons or property; the most likely explanation of this conduct lies not in any defect of character so much as in the irritability which stems directly from the illness. Similarly, a number of shop-lifting incidents, particularly those which are markedly out of character, are thought to be associated with depression.[16] Certain crimes attract a psychiatric explanation by virtue of their unusual nature. Arson may be motivated by a financial motive or by a desire for revenge but it is apparently motiveless in some cases. This suggests that there is a psychopathological explanation, a hypothesis which is borne out by the frequently abnormal psychiatric profile of arsonists – particularly younger ones.[17] In the case of sex offences, the nature of the crime may be so bizarre as to make sense only in terms of a psychiatric explanation. Once again, the backgrounds of many sex offenders reveal a range of defects and abnormalities, many of which are rooted in highly stressful experiences in early life. It is significant that many child abusers were themselves sexually abused as children.

The presence of psychiatric abnormality does not of itself provide grounds for exculpation unless it can be established that the abnormality caused the commission of the offence. Even then, there remains the question of whether the defendant could have chosen not to do as he did. A person may have a strong urge to commit an anti-social act, but society may expect such urges to be controlled. Is it unreasonable to expect similar self-control on the part of the mentally abnormal person? It is certainly not such a person's fault if a desire to commit an offence is prompted by illness – but neither is it the fault of the mentally normal person if he experiences a similar strong anti-social desire, which may spring from his unconscious. In fact, society may expect both to conform to the provisions of the criminal law, provided that both are aware that these provisions exist. What lies at the heart of responsibility is the *ability* of a person to conform, because we do not (or, at least, should not) hold people responsible for that which they cannot do. If the condition from which the mentally

16 R Bluglass, 'Shoplifting' in R Bluglass and P Bowden (eds) *Principles and Practice of Forensic Medicine* (1990) p 787.
17 H Prins, G Tennant and K Tirck 'Motives for Arson (Fire Raising)' (1985) 25 Med Sci Law 275.

abnormal person suffers is such as to prevent him from conforming to the provisions of the law, then it is wrong to hold him to account. The test, then, should not be whether a particular label can be put on the condition from which a defendant suffers but whether the effect of his illness was to put him in a position where he either did not know what he was doing or could not help doing it. Such a test satisfies the criteria of a humane theory of criminal responsibility but, as will be seen below, the law has not found it easy to apply.

The insanity plea

The plea of not guilty on the grounds of insanity is the most 'extreme' plea available to the mentally disordered offender. Such pleas were quite common in the days of capital punishment for murder, as a verdict of 'not guilty by reason of insanity' provided an escape route from possible execution. In the decade prior to the passing of the Homicide Act in 1957, and the consequent availability of the plea of diminished responsibility, the proportion of those committed to trial for murder in England who were found to be either guilty but insane or insane on arraignment averaged over 40% of the total. Between 1971 and 1973, the proportion of offenders whose mental state affected the verdict still remained at about 40%. However, the plea involved was that of diminished responsibility in 97% of the latter group.[18] The insanity plea has thus become comparatively rare, although it is still the catalyst of fierce controversy.

The belief that the insane should not be punished because they are not responsible for punishable acts lies at the root of the insanity defence in criminal law.[19] In simple language, the insane are not 'to blame' for what they do, and for many laymen that intuitive moral assessment will be sufficient. At a more theoretical level a variety of grounds can be postulated as the justification for acquittal in such cases. By measuring the behaviour of the insane offender against the behaviour of the sane person who commits the same offence, it will become apparent that the state of mind of the insane person is likely to be different in many significant respects and, therefore, mens rea may be absent. The insane offender may be ignorant of the fact that what he is doing is wrong, in either moral or legal terms, or he may be unaware of the consequences of his actions. His intentions or his motives in acting might likewise differ from those of the sane offender. The mental state of the man suffering from the delusion that he is about to be poisoned by his wife colours the nature of his actions; an attack on her then becomes, from the subjective viewpoint, an act of self-defence. The acts of the insane may also be analysed in terms of involuntariness. That an act should be voluntary is a prerequisite for the attribution of responsibility: if it is not willed by the actor, the law takes the view that there is no actus reus and that there can, then, be no criminal liability.[20] The insane offender can therefore be

---

18 Report of the Committee on Mentally Abnormal Offenders (Cmnd 6244, 1975) p 316.
19 For a useful discussion of the theoretical basis of the insanity defence, see J Radden *Madness and Reason* (1985).
20 On voluntary acts, see A R White *Grounds of Liability* (1985) p 48.

exculpated either on the grounds of lack of mens rea – in that he did not act with the requisite criminal intent – or because there was no actus reus.

Involuntariness is, however, a difficult concept in the criminal law and is generally used to describe only those acts over which the actor has no muscular control. A nervous spasm is classically an involuntary act in the criminal law, as is an act performed while asleep. The status of acts falling into the category of irresistible impulses is, however, different. A mental disorder may well have prompted an accused to steal or set fire to property but, although this may be something over which he (or his reflective ego) really has no control, it would not be accepted as an involuntary act in terms of the criminal law if it were shown that the act was performed consciously. It is only in those states where somebody is so disturbed as to be 'out of control' that his actions might fit into the usual criminal law category of involuntary acts.

In many cases, a mentally abnormal offender may act in a way which would not exculpate him prima facie in terms of the mens rea and actus reus requirements. The accused may know exactly what he is doing and intend to achieve a very specific and intelligible objective in acting as he does. And yet, in the background, there may be a grossly disturbed personality or a long-standing mental illness. As the Royal Commission on Capital Punishment pointed out, there are many offenders who know what they are doing and who know that it is wrong but who are none the less clearly insane and should not therefore be held responsible for their actions.[1] In considering such cases, there may be an inclination to treat the accused in a way which is different from the way in which we treat sane offenders. The reason for this difference in treatment might lie not so much in the absence of the constituent elements of mens rea but, rather, in the assumption that there is a causal link between the mental disorder and the criminal act. The crime may be seen as the product of a mental disorder and it is arguable that the accused would not have acted as he did if he had not been suffering from the mental condition.[2] This is the theory of the matter; practice, as will be seen, can be different.

The place of deterrence is also an important consideration. If it be accepted that one of the principal purposes of the criminal law is to impose sanctions aimed at deterring offenders, then there is no point in convicting the insane because the deterrent effect is unlikely to have significant personal impact. As Barry J put it:

> It is useless for the law to seek to deter persons from committing crimes if they cannot be influenced by the possibility or probability of subsequent punishment because of their psychotic condition. The kind of mental awareness which justly exposes the person to punishment for a criminal act is thus sane awareness not the distorted or confused or unreal awareness of a diseased mind.[3]

---

1 (Cmnd 8932, 1953) para 295.
2 For further discussion of the theoretical basis of the defence of insanity, see H Fingarette and A Hasse *Mental Disabilities and Criminal Responsibility* (1979).
3 *R v Weise* [1969] VR 953 at 964.

The McNaghten rules

Merely being insane does not, in itself, qualify as a defence to a criminal charge in English law. In order to benefit from the special verdict, an accused person must satisfy the test laid down in the McNaghten rules, the controversial text which has dominated English law on the subject since the mid-nineteenth century. The rules originate in the pronouncement of the House of Lords in 1843 in the case of *Daniel M'Naghten*[4] who had been charged with the shooting of the Prime Minister's secretary in the belief that the secretary was the Prime Minister himself. The House of Lords laid down the basic test that acquittal on the grounds of insanity was appropriate if, firstly, the accused 'was labouring under such a defect of reason, from disease of the mind, as not to know (1) the nature and quality of the act he was doing, or, if he did know it, (2) that he did not know he was doing what was wrong'. This test, variously formulated and interpreted, has since been applied throughout the Commonwealth as well as in the United States.

Criticism of the McNaghten rules has been forceful and continuous. At the root of the problem is the very antiquity of the rules; nineteenth-century psychiatry differed from modern psychiatric notions in terminology and in substance, and it seems remarkable that Victorian concepts should still dominate the modern test of insanity. At the outset, the rules place too great an emphasis on reason as the controlling element in human behaviour. Second, the concept of disease of the mind, which forms a vital part of the Rules, is one which is no longer in favour amongst psychiatrists. Nor is there an accepted legal definition of what constitutes such a disease – and this raises the question as to the status of a host of conditions including psychopathy and other personality disorders. The judges, however, have not necessarily been deterred by this uncertainty. In *R v Kemp*[5] for instance, the court held that arteriosclerosis was a disease of the mind and could, therefore, provide a defence to a criminal charge. *Bratty v A-G for Northern Ireland*[6] provided another example of a judge determining what is a disease of the mind; Lord Denning considered that this question was one for judicial resolution – but the propriety of bending medical diagnosis to suit judicial policy is doubtful. We discuss this further under the heading of automatism.

More important than the objections on the point of reason are those which refer to the emphasis in the rules on the knowledge of the accused. The controversy here has focused on the interpretation of the word 'know'. Narrowly interpreted – and the majority of the critics of McNaghten have assumed that it is the narrow interpretation which will be favoured by the courts – the word 'know' implies cognitive awareness rather than broader emotional understanding. As a result of this, many insane offenders might be held to fail the McNaghten test on the grounds that, in this sense, they would probably know what they were doing. In fact, courts have tended to take a broader view of the knowledge requirement and have often required something more than an intellectual knowledge of the nature and quality of the act in question. In Canada, s 16 of the Criminal Code essentially embodies the McNaghten test of insanity but states that the defence may be established if it is shown that the accused

---

4   *M'Naghten's Case* (1843) 10 Cl & Fin 200, HL. McNaghten – to use the conventional spelling of his name – experienced delusions of persecution and would probably be diagnosed today as suffering from paranoid schizophrenia.
5   [1957] 1 QB 399, [1956] 3 All ER 249.
6   [1963] AC 386, [1961] 3 All ER 523.

failed either to know or to appreciate the nature and quality of his act.[7] In interpreting this provision, the Canadian courts have ruled that, in order to be said to appreciate the nature and quality of his act, an accused person must not only know what he is doing but also must be able to understand the consequences of his act. As the Supreme Court of Canada held in *Cooper v R*,[8] appreciation involves emotional as well as intellectual awareness and, thus, is not the same as knowledge as conceived in the McNaghten test.

There has been some judicial debate over the significance of the term 'wrong' as it is used in the context of the McNaghten rules. Does the accused have to know that his act is morally wrong or does he have to know that it is legally wrong? English courts have come down in favour of the latter; a successful defence must show that the accused did not know that the act was legally wrong.[9] In theory, at least, this might lead to the absurd result of the denial of the insanity defence to an accused who heard voices commanding him to commit murder and, although he knew murder to be illegal, thought that the voices came from God and acted accordingly.

One avenue of escape from the limitations of McNaghten is to adopt a test which emphasises the actor's control over action. This test concentrates not on the cognitive aspects of the matter but on volitional features – an accused is not to be held responsible if he is shown to be incapable by reason of mental disorder of conforming his conduct to the requirements of law. These theories have long enjoyed support, and indeed a control test is written into a number of statutory statements of the defence, sometimes alongside other criteria. The Criminal Code of Western Australia, for example, allows the defence where the accused can establish either lack of capacity to understand what he is doing, lack of capacity to know that what he is doing is wrong or lack of capacity to control his actions.[10] One form of the control test is the irresistible impulse doctrine, which was rejected in English law in *Sodeman v R*[11] and, again, in *R v Rivett*[12] and which has attracted sparse support elsewhere.[13] Control theories need not, however, always be tied to the irresistible impulse concept; this is demonstrated by some American decisions in which the suddenness of the prompting to act has not been regarded as significant.

A final, and wider ranging, difficulty associated with these tests of responsibility which focus on ability to control behaviour lies in the fact that such theories view the cognitive and volitional functions of the mind as being quite separate and isolated. Modern psychiatry rejects this and regards the human personality as an integrated whole – one cannot distinguish these functions and view them in isolation from other mental processes.

---

7   The application of s 16 of the Canadian Criminal Code is discussed by S V Verdun-Jones, 'Tightening the Reins: Recent Trends in the Application of the Insanity Defence in Canada' (1991) Med Law 285.
8   (1980) 110 DLR (3d) 46.
9   *R v Windle* [1952] 2 QB 826, [1952] 2 All ER 1, CCA.
10 Section 27. For discussion of the Western Australian provisions, see Law Reform Commission of Western Australia, *Report on the Criminal Process and Persons Suffering from Mental Disorder* (1991).
11 [1936] 2 All ER 1138, PC.
12 (1950) 34 Cr App Rep 87, CCA.
13 For the fate of the irresistible concept in Canada, see *R v Wolfson* [1965] 3 CCC 304; *R v Borg* [1969] SCR 551.

Alternative attitudes

The American experience of the insanity defence has been particularly interesting. Criticism of the McNaghten rules in the United States has been especially intense and the courts have responded by experimenting with a variety of alternative approaches. One test which, although not widely applied, occasioned much discussion was developed in *Durham v United States*,[14] in which the Court of Appeals of the District of Columbia abandoned the McNaghten approach in favour of what appeared to be the more scientific test of linking the crime with a diagnosed 'mental disease or mental defect'. The problem with this test is twofold: how has a mental disease to be defined – the test takes us no further in this direction – and how can one ascertain a firm causal link between the criminal act and the disease? The mere fact of mental illness need not exculpate; the criminal act must be attributable in some way to the illness and this may be a difficult, if not impossible, task.[15] A more helpful solution was suggested by the American Law Institute in its Model Penal Code.[16] The test outlined in the code is a conventional one, involving a combination of the cognitive and control criteria: an insanity defence will be available if, in the presence of mental disorder, there is a failure to appreciate the criminality of the act or, even in the event of an appreciation of this sort, there is an inability to conform conduct to the requirements of the law. There has been a successful move to limit and, in some cases, even to abolish the insanity defence in many parts of the United States. There has always been a degree of grass-roots scepticism about the exculpatory role of forensic psychiatry and this was given a considerable boost after the acquittal of John Hinckley, who has now achieved in an American context much the same sort of immortality as did Daniel McNaghten. Hinckley attempted to assassinate President Reagan; he was acquitted on the grounds of insanity after a long trial, in which psychiatric evidence figured prominently. Public outrage at this outcome resulted in the abolition of the distinct defence of insanity in a number of States where the issue of insanity was subsequently restricted to the role of deciding whether or not there was mens rea. Other states left the insanity defence in place but either reverted to strictly McNaghten-style tests[17] or introduced additional verdicts of 'guilty, but mentally ill'. Such verdicts allowed for the psychiatric treatment of disturbed offenders without denying their responsibility.

An apposite example of legislation in this area is the Insanity Defense Reform Act 1984 (a Federal Act) which states:

> It is an affirmative defense to a prosecution under any Federal statute that, at the time of the commission of the acts constituting the offence, the defendant, as a result of severe mental disease or defect, was unable to appreciate the nature and quality or the wrongfulness of his acts. Mental defect does not otherwise constitute a defense.

---

14 214 F 2d 862 (1954).
15 In those jurisdictions where the *Durham* rule was applied, the courts became disenchanted with its effect and the rule was abandoned; see G Fletcher *Rethinking Criminal Law* (1978) p 840.
16 Model Penal Code, 4.01. See also *US v Brawner* 471 F 2d 969 (1972).
17 American developments are summarised by R D Mackay 'Post-Hinckley Insanity in the USA' [1988] Crim LR 88.

It is significant that this provision abandons the volitional part of the American Law Institute's Model Penal Code and it is, therefore, no longer a defence that the defendant was 'unable to conform his conduct to the requirements of the law'. It also refers to 'severe' mental illness or defect, thereby apparently excluding neuroses, behavioural disorders and other conditions falling short of psychotic illness.[18]

The courts in Scotland now seem to have developed a fairly simple test of insanity. The McNaghten Rules have never been part of Scots criminal law and the courts have, therefore, been tied to no specific formula. In *HM Advocate v Kidd*,[19] the judge's instruction to the jury, although couched in terms of reason and of alienation – which are not terms which would necessarily be accepted by psychiatrists today – stated quite simply that the defence would be available if the accused was considered to be of unsound mind at the time of the offence. That is language which anybody can understand and, although a psychiatrist might argue that it begs a lot of questions, at least the psychiatrist himself should find it quite possible to give an opinion to a court in terms of mental soundness or unsoundness.

The reform of English law was considered at length by the Butler Committee, which reported in 1975.[20] The committee accepted the fact that there were major flaws in the McNaghten rules and proposed that a verdict of 'not guilty on evidence of mental disorder' should be introduced; this would be appropriate if there was adequate psychiatric evidence of the existence in the accused of a sufficiently severe degree of mental disorder at the time of the commission of the offence charged. This recommendation is embodied in the Draft Criminal Code, prepared by the Law Commission, which provides for a defence where the accused suffers from severe subnormality or, at the time of the offence, a severe mental illness.[1] It would also be a defence under this draft code if mental disorder is proved to negate the fault element in the offence, the grounds upon which this is to be done being left open. Severe mental illness is defined in clause 38(e) of the draft and embraces those conditions which lead to significant thought disorder – particularly delusions.

The main attraction of this proposal is that, at least where severe conditions are involved, there is no need to tie the condition to any putative mental state of the accused in relation to the act in question; it will suffice that he has been diagnosed as suffering from a sufficiently serious mental disorder. Another attractive feature of the proposed defence is that diagnostic labels are avoided and the criteria laid out are intelligible to the layman. Any attempt at a statement of an insanity defence will have its critics – but the provisions in the draft code seem to be very much better than many.

Unfortunately, the code remains a draft; the McNaghten rules continue to be the governing test of insanity in English criminal law, although the Criminal Procedure (Insanity and Unfitness to Plead) Act 1991 allows a broader range of options to a court once the special verdict has been reached. Under this Act, a court is no longer

---

18 For criticism of the removal of the volitional aspect of the test, see R J Simon and D E Aronson *The Insanity Defense* (1988) p 49.

19 1960 JC 61. For an analysis of the development of the Scottish cases, see G H Gordon *The Criminal Law of Scotland* (2nd edn, 1978) pp 364ff. Also, R A A McCall Smith and D Sheldon *Scots Criminal Law* (1992) p 20.

20 Report of the Committee on Metally Abnormal Offenders (Cmnd 6244).

1 *Codification of the Criminal Law* (Law Com No 143).

obliged to order detention in a secure hospital under a restriction order (which had no limit of time); it may choose from a number of options, including a supervision or treatment order, guardianship or the absolute discharge of the defendant. This removes the inflexibility of the previous system and will also help to avoid the absurdity of, say, detaining a diabetic or somnambulist in a psychiatric hospital under the Draconian shadow of a restriction order – which is what would have happened following upon a successful defence of insane automatism under the previous system.[2]

Unfitness to plead

In addition to the criticism directed against the actual criteria of the insanity defence, there has been frequent criticism of the rules governing fitness to plead. Until the implementation of the Criminal Procedure (Insanity and Unfitness to Plead) Act 1991, a person who was deemed incapable of standing trial by reason of mental disorder would be sent to hospital under a restriction order without any trial as to whether or not he committed the offence with which he was charged. Now there must be a trial of the facts in order that the jury may decide whether the accused actually committed the offence in question. The 1991 Act makes no changes in the grounds upon which there may be a finding of unfitness to plead. The basis of the plea is an inability to understand proceedings and to defend oneself, but the way in which the criteria for the plea are applied varies greatly.[3]

Diminished responsibility

The plea of diminished responsibility was devised as a means of allowing the court to avoid a conviction for murder where the mental condition of the accused made the attribution of full responsibility inappropriate. The doctrine was first used in Scotland in the case of *HM Advocate v Dingwall*[4] in 1867 and was eventually introduced into English law in the Homicide Act 1957, s 2(1). This provides that, in cases of homicide, there should be no conviction for murder if the accused is found to be suffering from —

> such abnormality of mind (whether arising from a condition of arrested or retarded development of mind or any inherent causes or induced by disease or injury) as substantially impaired his mental responsibility for his acts and omissions in doing or being a party to the killing.

The doctrine is justified because of the fixed penalty of life imprisonment for murder; it is not required elsewhere because the degree of culpability can be

---

2   See I Mackay 'The Sleepwalker is not Insane' (1992) 55 MLR 714.
3   D Grubin ' Unfit to Plead in England and Wales 1976-1988: A Survey' (1991) 158 Brit J Psychiat 540; 'What Constitutes Fitness to Plead?' [1993] Crim LR 748.
4   (1867) 5 Irv 466.

considered in sentencing. The reduction of the offence to one of manslaughter allows this discretion to be exercised in a homicide charge and the court can then choose a sentence ranging from the leniency of a probation order on the one hand to life imprisonment on the other.[5] Sentencing discretion already exists in respect of most other offences and, as a result, the case for extending the application of the plea is hardly strong. Some have criticised the whole concept of a diminished responsibility plea, arguing that we are either responsible or not responsible for our actions and that there should be no half-way house. It has been pointed out that the killing is both premeditated and intended in many cases where homicide occurs in conditions accepted as qualifying for diminished responsibility. Self-control in such circumstances is still a possibility; it is quite unlike the situation, say, where there is a disorder of thinking as a result of psychotic illness. Such iconoclasm discounts the fact that we do regularly make allowances which influence the extent to which we hold people to account for their acts. More usually, such allowances are described as mitigating circumstances rather than as factors influencing responsibility, but the ultimate effect will be the same. The usefulness of the concept of diminished responsibility lies in its flexibility; through its operation, those who are accused and for whom sympathy is felt can be treated in a lenient fashion on conviction without there being any condoning of their offence. A plea of diminished responsibility will, for example, enable the courts to look with equal mercy on cases of 'mercy-killing'. Inferring diminished responsibility in such circumstances does not involve any diminution of the seriousness with which the taking of life is viewed; what it does say is that something other than a long prison sentence may be appropriate by virtue of the accused's mental condition.

The conditions which may give rise to a successful plea of diminished responsibility vary considerably.[6] Disabilities such as reactive depression or hysterical disassociation, which are unlikely to qualify as mental disorders requiring prolonged psychiatric treatment, have been so accepted on occasion and, at the other end of the scale, psychopathy has also succeeded as the basis of a plea.[7] General guidance as to what constitutes abnormality of mind for the purposes of the Homicide Act 1957, s 2(1) was given by Lord Parker CJ in *R v Byrne*[8] where he stated that such abnormality existed when there was a state of mind: 'so different from that of ordinary human beings that the reasonable man would term it abnormal'. This concept, it was stressed, was wide enough to cover 'the mind's activities in all its aspects', including both the ability to form a rational judgment as to right and wrong and the ability to control behaviour in accordance with that judgment.

The wording of s 2(1) excludes abnormality of mind that derives from the working of the emotions. A person who kills another in a state of rage, or who

---

5 S Dell *Murder into Manslaughter* (1984); S Dell, 'The Mandatory Sentence and Section 2' (1986) 12 J Med Ethics 28.
6 For an Australian survey which reveals the wide range of conditions on which pleas of diminished responsibility have been based, see K L Milte, A A Bartholomew and F Galbally, 'Abolition of the Crime of Murder and of Mental Condition Defences' (1975) 49 A LJ 160 – in the cases studied, the conditions included epilepsy, paranoia, reactive depression and alcoholism.
7 G H Gordon *The Criminal Law of Scotland* (2nd edn, 1978) p 395.
8 [1960] 2 QB 396, [1960] 3 All ER 1, CCA. See also *Rose v R* [1961] AC 496, [1961] 1 All ER 859 and *R v Seers* (1984) 79 Cr App Rep 261, CA where it was stressed that there need not be a condition 'on the borderline of insanity' in every case.

commits homicide out of passionate hatred or jealousy, will not succeed with a plea of diminished responsibility. Alcoholic intoxication may justify the plea but only if the intoxication (a) has caused an abnormality of the mind by way of organic damage or (b) it results from an uncontrollable compulsion to drink caused by the fact that the person is dependent on alcohol.[9] The evidence of mental abnormality may need only to be slight in 'meritorious' cases in which the courts may be prepared to clutch at whatever psychiatric straws are available to avoid the consequences of a conviction for murder. Yet, such a process has its dangers and there have been occasional judicial reactions to what is seen as the over-extension of the concept. In Scotland, where the plea of diminished responsibility lies at common law, the High Court has emphasised that, to be successful, there must be clear psychiatric evidence of mental illness; psychiatric expressions of opinion on the issue are worthless in the absence of such evidence. This severe approach is based on a relatively old case, the meat of which is:

> ... it has been put in this way: there must be aberration or weakness of mind; that there must be some form of mental unsoundness; that there must be a state of mind which is bordering on, though not amounting to, insanity; that there must be a mind so affected that responsibility is diminished from full responsibility to partial responsibility – in other words, the prisoner in question must be only partially accountable for his actions. And I think one can see running through the cases that there is implied . . . that there must be some form of mental disease.[10]

All of which may sound a touch archaic; yet, not only has it been restated recently as the law of Scotland, but it has been emphasised that the passage must be read as a whole and that the four criteria cannot be regarded as alternatives.[11]

There have been many suggestions made for reform of the doctrine of diminished responsibility, ranging from arguments in favour of its extension to cover offences other than murder to calls for its abandonment – along with the abolition of the fixed penalty for murder. The Criminal Law Revision Committee favoured a less radical change and its suggestions have now been embodied in the Law Commission's Draft Criminal Code.[12] Clause 58 of this draft avoids the term 'diminished responsibility' and provides instead for the reduction of a charge of murder to one of manslaughter when the accused is suffering from a form of mental abnormality substantial enough to warrant such reduction. Mental abnormality is defined as: 'mental illness, arrested or incomplete development of mind, psychopathic disorder and any other disorder or disability of mind, except intoxication'.

Difficult cases: infanticide and the abused woman
'Infanticide' has both a general and a technical legal meaning. In its general sense – as used, for example, in the United States – it means no more than the killing of an

9　*R v Tandy* [1989] 1 All ER 267, [1989] 1 WLR 350, CA.
10 *HM Advocate v Savage* 1923 JC 49 per Lord Alness LJ-C at 51.
11 *Connelly v HM Advocate* 1990 SCCR 504.
12 Fn 1, p 411 above.

infant; in its English legal sense it is restricted to the killing of a child by its mother within the terms of the Infanticide Act 1938. This Act, which was based on earlier statutory provisions and which does not run to Scotland, takes such killing out of the ambit of murder into which it would otherwise fall in the absence of any special factors – such as diminished responsibility. This special treatment is based on the sympathy traditionally shown by the courts to women in this position and on the resulting disinclination to apply the full rigour of the law in such cases.[13] This attitude is dressed up in medical language of very doubtful scientific validity. According to the Act, the crime will be charged as infanticide when the death occurs within 12 months of the birth of the child and the mother is suffering from an imbalance of the mind caused by her not having recovered from the effects of childbirth or by reason of the effects of lactation. Such maternal homicidal behaviour can result from various reasons and psychiatric abnormality cannot be presumed in them all. d'Orban, in his major study of British maternal filicide, categorises six causes of infanticide including battering in angry response to behaviour on the child's part; mental illness, in the form of depressive psychosis or personality disorder, was a factor in only 24 of the 89 cases studied.[14]

Infanticide is an uncommon crime and there is real doubt as to the need to preserve it as a separate offence. The doctrine of diminished responsibility appears to cope adequately with the problem in Scotland, where the matter will be dealt with in the same way as other cases of culpable homicide when there is evidence of a psychiatric abnormality. The specific question is whether it should be dealt with even more leniently than is the 'average' case of culpable homicide. There is a case for retaining the separate crime if this is the true objective of legal policy – and infanticide, as it stands, attracts very lenient sentences. An objection to this approach, however, is that there will be cases in which the mother deserves to be convicted of murder and it is difficult to justify special treatment for women on grounds of gender. Maternal filicide results probably often from the special stresses experienced by women and this conclusion must attract a deal of sympathy. Yet, to allow such factors to mitigate homicide in some cases but not in others would be to establish a fundamental inconsistency in the law.

Claims that women should be treated differently from men in matters of criminal responsibility tend to be based on the idea that the existing criminal law is significantly biased in favour of a male of the world. This issue has been most actively debated in the context of provocation, where it has been suggested that the plea of provocation, with its insistence on an immediate response to provocative conduct, fails to take account of the way in which women respond to ill-treatment. The matter has been medicalised by the concept of the battered woman syndrome, a feature of which is the development of helplessness on the part of the victim of prolonged physical and psychological torment. The concept of the syndrome is

13 For general discussion of the background to the offence, see J K Mason *Medicolegal Aspects of Reproduction and Parenthood* (1990) p 331 et seq.
14 P T d'Orban 'Women who Kill Their Children' (1979) 134 Brit J Psychiat 560. See also P J Resnick 'Murder of the Newborn: A Psychiatric Review of Neonaticide' (1970) 126 Amer J Psychiat 1414; D Maier-Katkin and R Ogle 'A Rationale for Infanticide Laws' [1993] Crim LR 903.

controversial,[15] but it has now been recognised in Canada and Australia.[16] The Court of Appeal in England has also accepted that the features of the syndrome may be taken into account as characteristics of the victim when assessing the response to provocation.[17]

The emergence of a realistic defence for abused women will satisfy the undoubted need for a more sympathetic legal response to the plight of those who are subjected to intolerable conduct on the part of their partners or spouses. If psychiatry can achieve this by the creation of a new syndrome, then the courts can at least avoid having to impose mandatory life sentences on those who kill in these extraordinary circumstances. It might, however, be preferable to approach the matter from the point of view of self-defence; this would avoid the creation of a further psychiatry-based ground of non-responsibility which could, logically, be applied to many others who take life when exposed to intolerable conditions. This could lead to the abandonment of basic notions of responsibility which form the essential foundation of criminal justice and without which systems of criminal law simply could not operate.

The problem of psychopathy

Psychopathy, which is variously known as sociopathy or anti-social personality disorder, is a condition over which there has been considerable disagreement among psychiatrists. Some deny the value of the concept altogether, arguing that it does no more than describe those who behave consistently in an anti-social fashion. The term appears, however, in diagnostic manuals and in mental health legislation and it has been accepted by the courts as grounds for a plea of diminished responsibility.[18] What, then, is psychopathy and is the psychopath to be held legally responsible for his acts? According to the International Classification of Diseases, Injuries and Causes of Death of the World Health Organisation, psychopathy involves: 'deeply ingrained maladaptive patterns of behaviour, generally recognisable by the time of adolescence or earlier, and continuing throughout most of adult life, although becoming less obvious in middle or old age.'[19] The Mental Health Act 1983 defines psychopathic disorder as a 'persistent disorder or disability of mind (whether or not including impairment of intelligence) which results in abnormally aggressive or seriously irresponsible conduct on the part of the person concerned'.[20]

Psychopathy has caused some difficulty for the criminal courts.[1] One response has been to deny its relevance to the question of criminal guilt – a sceptical approach

---

15 There are those who feel that it perpetuates stereotypes of women: D Nicolson and R Sanghvi 'Battered Women and Provocation: the Implications of *R v Ahluwalia*' [1993] Crim LR 728. See also K O'Donovan, 'Defences for Battered Women Who Kill' (1991) 18 J Law & Soc 219.
16 S Yeo 'Battered Women Syndrome in Australia' (1993) 140 NLJ 1380.
17 *R v Ahluwalia* [1992] 4 All ER 889.
18 See G Williams *Texbook of Criminal Law* (2nd edn, 1983) p 691. Professor Williams sums up the doubts at p 654: 'The term [psychopathy] can be regarded as a declaration of interest in the subject of habitual criminality by the medical profession.'
19 World Health Organisation ICD 9 (1978).
20 Section 1(2).
 1 For discussion, see M Roth, 'Psychopathic (Sociopathic) Personality' in R Bluglass and P Bowden, fn 16, p 405 above, at p 437.

based on the notion that all that a diagnosis of psychopathy does is to confirm that the patient behaves in a deviant fashion. Legal scepticism can be understood in the absence of more specific clinical features; while a judge or jury may be prepared to accept the presence of insanity when the condition of the accused is described in terms of delusions, hallucinations or blunting of affect, they may be less swayed by a general term such as personality disorder.

The fate of the psychopath in the British criminal process has varied. Psychopathy would have to be accepted as a mental disease in order to justify an insanity plea in McNaghten terms in England or to satisfy the test of insanity in Scots law; the issue has not, however, been decided in a United Kingdom case.[2] In *R v Cooper*,[3] the Supreme Court of Canada decided that a personality disorder could fit within the concept of a 'disease of the mind' for legal purposes but, even were this to be generally accepted, it is most unlikely that psychopathy would have such an effect on cognitive capacity as to relieve the accused of responsibility. Indeed, personality disorders are specifically excluded from the scope of the insanity defence in a number of jurisdictions.[4] This being so, the only practical implications of psychopathy for the criminal courts relate to the plea of diminished responsibility and, here, there has been occasional willingness to allow evidence of the condition to reduce murder to manslaughter. More usually, however, the courts have declined to accept it as grounds for the plea and the psychopath will most probably be sentenced in the same way as any other offender.[5] This is not to say that such persons will always elude psychiatric attention during their incarceration; in 1990, it was estimated that 143 out of the 577 mentally disordered persons in prison establishments in England and Wales were classified as psychopaths.[6] The Butler Committee concluded that 'the psychopath is, in general, untreatable, at least in medical terms'. That being so, he could expect to find little haven in the psychiatric hospital but whether this view is generally held is unclear since the Mental Health Act 1983, s 3(2)(b) now includes the psychopath amongst those who may be compulsorily admitted – subject to a treatability test (see p 395).

Although the Butler Committee condoned the sending of psychopaths to prison, another view holds this to be unacceptable. Such persons, it is argued, are suffering from a personality disorder and are therefore not fully responsible for their actions. Conviction and imprisonment are quite different qualitatively from acquittal and admission to a psychiatric institution and it is inadmissible to impose the former on

2   The diagnosis was not clearly established in *A-G for Northern Ireland v Gallagher* [1963] AC 349, [1961] 3 All ER 299, HL.
3   (1979) 13 CR (3d) 97.
4   As in the American Law Institute's Model Penal Code, which provides that the term 'mental disease or defect' excludes an abnormality 'manifested only by repeated criminal or anti-social conduct' (s.4.01). For further discussion, see P A Fairall and P W Johnston 'Anti-social Personality Disorder (APD) and the Insanity Defence' (1987) Crim L J 78.
5   See, for example, *R v Jennion* [1962] 1 All ER 689, [1962] 1 WLR 317, CCA. In *R v Aarons* [1964] Crim LR 484 a reduction to manslaughter was allowed by way of a diagnosis of psychopathy; nonetheless the accused was sentenced to life imprisonment. For the Scottish position, see D Chiswick 'Criminal Responsibility in Scotland' in R Bluglass and P Bowden, fn 16, p 405 above, at p 313. Chiswick suggests that the rejection of the term psychopathic disorder in favour of a synonymous description may increase the chances of this form of personality disorder being accepted as grounds for a plea of diminished responsibility.
6   A Ashworth and J Shapland 'Psychopaths in the Criminal Process' [1980] Crim LR 628.

those who offend for that reason. The refutation of this argument takes one to the heart of the issue of responsibility. There is no obvious reason why a personality disorder of this nature should be treated as being any different from what one might loosely term a 'criminal or anti-social disposition' (which is a matter of character). The aetiology of psychopathy is certainly controversial but the psychopath will probably always have been what he is at the time of the offence – that is his 'nature'. By contrast, the person who is mentally ill is not anti-social 'by nature' – his anti-social behaviour is likely to be connected with his illness. And this leads one to the question as to whether it is wrong to punish somebody for what their character dictates. If one argues that it is wrong, then the entire basis of the system of criminal justice must be seen as being immoral. People are regularly punished because their conduct is bad. The reasons why they are bad may be of some criminological interest but do not affect the basic issue of accountability in the courts; only the determinist will be inclined to argue otherwise. This view may seem unsympathetic but its critics will have to contend with the realities of the penal and hospital systems. If psychiatrists can do little or nothing for the psychopath and, at the same time, the psychopath will be a highly disruptive element within the hospital, then the viable alternatives are those of prison or freedom – in excluding the latter on grounds of public safety, one is left only with prison and with such attempts at psychotherapy as might be possible within that framework.

Automatism

The difficulty of reconciling legal requirements with medical insights into the nature of human action is also illustrated by the development of the automatism defence in criminal law. Like the insanity plea, this is a controversial defence which raises some awkward problems of balancing justice for the individual against the protection of society.

The basic principle of the criminal law that only voluntary acts will result in criminal liability clearly indicates acquittal if the accused has acted automatically. Automatic behaviour consists of acts of which an actor is not conscious or over which he has no control. Actions of somnambulistic type provide a classic illustration of this sort of behaviour.[7] Sleep-related violence may take place within the context of night terrors, which occur during slow-wave sleep, or it may occur in the course of somnambulistic activity itself. In a night terror, the subject may awake to find his hands round the throat of his sleeping partner and he may have no recollection of events preceding this. The same type of amnesia will occur when he has been sleep-walking. He may have performed complicated actions – operated machinery, opened doors or even fired a gun – and yet none of these will have been executed consciously. It is obvious that there should be no responsibility for such behaviour although it has been observed that somnambulistic behaviour does, in fact, involve a higher level of consciousness than has been supposed previously. Automatic behaviour can result from a number of other causes. These may arise

---

7   The possibility of violence during sleep is discussed by P Fenwick 'Murdering while Asleep' (1986) 293 BMJ 574. See also R A A McCall Smith, C M Shapiro and A Moscovitch 'Legal Aspects of Sleep and Alertness' in C M Shapiro (ed) *ABC of Sleep Disorders* (1993) p 84.

from well-established patho-physiological conditions such as hypoglycaemia, the encephalopathies and post-traumatic states. Cerebral function may also be affected by the state of the blood vessels (arteriosclerosis)[8] and by the ingestion of alcohol and drugs, but offences committed while intoxicated are usually considered in a different context. More legally – and, indeed, morally – controversial are states of dissociation resulting from acute emotional stress; these are sometimes categorised as non-organic automatism.

The main problem with the defence of automatism lies in the difficulty of establishing with certainty that a given physical condition actually produced automatic behaviour. Idiopathic epilepsy may be taken as an example. It is beyond question that complicated actions, of which the subject may later have no recollection, may be performed either during a seizure or in the post-ictal period. These actions are clearly unconscious and are therefore involuntary from the point of view of the law. That, unfortunately, is as far as certainty can go. There is very little concrete evidence of the occurrence of violence in such states[9] but automatism at least provides an explanation of otherwise inexplicable behaviour; its rejection in such circumstances would be substantially unfair to the accused. Whether an acquittal is appropriate in such cases or whether some other form of disposal is to be preferred involves complicated policy issues.

In principle, a finding that the criminal offence was committed automatically should result in an acquittal. This will, in fact, be the result in some cases but, in others, the reluctance of the courts to release potentially dangerous offenders has led to the development of two conceptual categories of automatism – insane and non-insane. If the automatic behaviour is classified as insane, the court will then be able to deal with the offender in the same way as it deals with other insane offenders and so ensure that society is protected from potential danger. The question which the courts have, thus, set for themselves is: in what circumstances will automatism count as insanity?

A useful starting point for discussion is Lord Denning's judgment in *Bratty v A-G for Northern Ireland*.[10] The accused in this case was charged with the murder of a girl whom he strangled when what he described as 'a feeling of blackness' came over him. The basis for deciding whether automatic behaviour should be classified as insane, according to Lord Denning, depended upon the question of whether or not it resulted from a disease of the mind. Clearly, if a criminal action derives from a disease of the mind it is appropriate to raise the question of insanity, with all that this entails. In *Bratty*, Lord Denning chose to define disease of the mind in terms of a mental disorder which had manifested itself in violence and which was prone to recur. These criteria indicate the main policy objective behind the distinction – the protection of the public. But the decision is open to criticism in that its logical corollary is that a non-recurrent disorder would not be a disease of the mind; the reasoning is also somewhat circular in that the definition of mental disease depends

---

8 *R v Charlson* [1955] 1 All ER 859, [1955] 1 WLR 317; *R v Kemp* [1957] 1 QB 399, [1956] 3 All ER 249.

9 The form of association between epilepsy and violent or aggressive behaviour is controversial. See P Fenwick 'Automatism' in R Bluglass and P Bowden, fn 16, p 405 above, at p 271; also P Fenwick 'Aggression and Epilepsy' in M Trimble and T Bolwiq (eds) *Aspects of Epilepsy and Psychiatry* (1986) p 31.

10 [1963] AC 386, [1961] 3 All ER 523, HL.

upon the inference of mental disorder which is, itself, not defined. The case of *R v Quick*[11] highlights the difficulties faced by the courts when trying to evaluate complex medical problems within the framework of a public protection policy. The appellant in *Quick* was a diabetic who, having injected himself with insulin and then failed to eat, went into a hypoglaecemic state during which he committed an assault. The court declined to hold that hypoglycaemia resulting from incorrect therapy was a disease of the mind and ruled that the defence of non-insane automatism was available. The injection of insulin, it was held, was an external factor in the same sense as a blow to the head is an external factor in those cases in which concussion leads to automatic behaviour. Recklessness in failing to eat could, of course, mean that the defence of non-insane automatism would not be available, a point which was stressed in the later case of *R v Bailey*.[12] In this case, the court, by implication, took the view that the defence of insane automatism would be appropriate in those cases where a state of *hyper*glycaemia resulted from failure of the medical regime; in such cases the abnormal state is produced by disease and not by an external cause such as the injection of insulin. Once again, the court stressed the role of recklessness and emphasised that knowledge of the risks of non-compliance with medical advice in such a case would exclude the defence of non-insane automatism. An attempt to circumvent the strictures of this rule was made in *R v Hennessy*,[13] a decision which, also, denied the defence of non-insane automatism to a diabetic who failed to inject himself with insulin. The appellant in this case argued that his condition of automatism was caused not only by this failure but also by stress, anxiety and depression. It was held that these were not external causes for the purposes of the automatism defence but were states of mind that were prone to recur; they were, therefore, relevant to insane rather than to non-insane automatism.

The position of the epileptic is somewhat clearer.[14] In *R v Sullivan*,[15] the House of Lords dealt with the case of an epileptic who had been convicted of assault during an alleged seizure. The judgment of Lord Diplock in this case is unambiguous: any disease-induced state of mind which satisfies the requirements of the McNaghten Rules – in that it impairs the faculties of reason, memory and understanding – amounts to insanity for legal purposes. The permanence or transience of the impairment is irrelevant, as is the question of its having been caused functionally or organically. Acts performed as a result of an epileptic seizure amount, therefore, to insane automatism. This will be the case even if the offence in question is not one involving violence; in this respect the decision in *Sullivan* broadens the concept of insane automatism beyond Lord Denning's definition in *Bratty*, where the condition was required to manifest itself in violence.

The problem of somnambulistic automatism came before the Court of Appeal in *R v Burgess*.[16] The appellant had alleged that an attack he made on a friend was committed while he was asleep. The jury accepted that he was not conscious at the time of the attack but returned a verdict of insane automatism rather than non-insane

11 [1973] QB 910, [1973] 3 All ER 347, CA.
12 [1983] 2 All ER 503, [1983] 1 WLR 760, CA.
13 [1989] 2 All ER 9, [1989] 1 WLR 287, CA.
14 K J M Smith 'Epileptic Action and Criminal Responsibility' (1983) 99 LQR 506.
15 [1984] AC 156, [1983] 2 All ER 673, HL.
16 [1991] 2 QB 92, [1991] 2 All ER 769.

as was claimed. The Court of Appeal upheld this verdict on the grounds that the somnambulistic behaviour was a product of a disease of the mind rather than of any external cause. This decision maintains the principle that automatism will be treated as insanity if it results from a mental disorder that is prone to recur – with or without manifestations of violence. The concern of the courts over the acquittal of persons who might pose a future danger are understandable but the difficulty will always be that of predicting dangerousness in such cases. One episode of somnambulistic violence may provide weak grounds for prolonged detention, particularly when the causative factors in relation to such behaviour are so difficult to identify – and the evidence given in *R v Parks*[17] was that there is no recorded instance of repeated violence during sleepwalking. A conclusion opposite to that in *Burgess* was reached in *Parks*, a Canadian case involving homicide; it was confirmed on appeal that the loss of mental faculties in somnambulistic automatism is caused by the normal condition of sleep rather than by disease of the mind – it was pointed out that, otherwise, all children and some 2.5% of adults could be said to be affected.[18] The words of Watt J, the trial judge in this case, have a persuasive ring:

> There may be any number of appropriate responses . . . in the control and treatment of those who have caused serious social harm while in a somnambulistic state, but a mischaracterization of the disorder as a disease of the mind and the use of the blunt instrument of indefinite confinement by warrant under a special verdict of not guilty by reason of insanity is not one of them.[19]

The Supreme Court of Canada upheld the findings in the lower courts.

Non-organic automatism, or psychogenic automatism, has been viewed very much more sceptically by some courts. Such automatism may occur when there is subjection either to prolonged stress or to a sudden shock. In each case, a state of dissociation may result in which actions are performed without the exercise by the subject of conscious control. In a series of decisions, the Canadian courts recognised what became known as 'psychological blow automatism' as being grounds for acquittal as non-insane automatism; more prolonged states of dissociation were treated as insanity.[20] In *R v K*,[1] for example, the accused, who had been undergoing treatment for a severe neurotic condition, killed his wife after the shock of hearing that she planned to leave him. Psychiatric evidence to the effect that the killing took place while he was in a state of automatism was accepted by the jury and the accused was acquitted. Similarly, in *R v Gottschalk*[2] the accused was acquitted of assault after psychiatric evidence was led of his state of depersonalisation which was productive of automatism. A reverse in the trend of the Canadian decisions occurred, however, with the decision of the Supreme Court of Canada in *Rabey v R*,[3] in which it was held that dissociation resulting from a psychological shock should be treated as insanity

17 (1990) 73 OR (2d) 129, Ont CA; (1993) 95 DLR (4th) 27, SCC.
18 Per Brooke JA at OR 147.
19 Quoted by Brooke JA at OR 147.
20 Se M E Schiffer *Mental Disorder and the Criminal Process* (1978) p 101.
  1 (1971) 3 CCC (2d) 84.
  2 (1974) 22 CCC (2d) 415.
  3 (1980) 114 DLR (3d) 193.

rather than as non-insane automatism. It is significant in this case that the accused, who assaulted a woman after she had rejected him, did not have the sort of psychiatric record which was produced by the defendants in *K* and *Gottschalk*. It may be suspected, too, that the court wished to restrict defences of psychogenic automatism for policy reasons, as the whole concept is an obvious candidate for abuse and non-meritorious defences.[4]

The High Court of Australia considered the issue of psychogenic automatism in *R v Falconer*,[5] a case involving the killing by a woman of her violent and abusive husband. The High Court ruled that psychiatric evidence of the dissociative state in which the accused had acted should have been admitted – and it was also observed that there was no reason in principle why the law should allow automatism following upon physical trauma and yet disallow it if it proceeds from a psychological cause. In England, the possibility of a non-insane automatism defence based on dissociation was rejected in the Court of Appeal decision in *R v Isitt*.[6] The accused in this case failed to stop after an accident and had attempted to evade the police. In considering his claim to have been in a state of shock, the court took the view that, although the accused's mind might have been 'shut to the moral inhibitions which control the lives of most of us', there was no suggestion that his mind was not working at all and the defence of automatism was, therefore, not available. This concept of 'diminished awareness' has, only recently, been again rejected by the Court of Appeal in a driving case.[7] A driver caused the death of two pedestrians while driving in a state in which his awareness of his surroundings was impaired due to fatigue. The court held that this failed to qualify as automatism as some conscious control of his actions was still retained.

Psychiatry and the sex offender

Sex offenders present particularly difficult problems in the field of behaviour modification. They are most commonly dealt with by way of imprisonment on the grounds that the prime consideration in sentencing policy must be the protection of potential victims.[8] Such disposal works as a temporary measure but release may well bring a fairly rapid return to anti-social behaviour. Imprisonment of sex offenders also involves more than the usual measure of cruelty because isolation from other prisoners is often needed in order to protect the offender from violence. Successful treatment of the abnormal sexual urge may well be regarded as preferable to simple segregation of the subject.

Psychiatric assistance aimed at overcoming anti-social sexual behaviour may be offered either before the patient has come into conflict with the criminal law or, following conviction of an offence, within the context of punishment and rehabilitation.

4   For a criticism of *Rabey*, see R D Mackay 'Non-organic Automatism – Some Recent Developments' [1980] Crim LR 350.
5   (1990) 65 ALJR 20.
6   (1977) 67 Cr App R 44, CA.
7   *A-G's Reference (No 2 of 1992)* [1993] 4 All ER 683.
8   Howard League Working Party *Unlawful Sex* (1985) p 87.

It may also be available, of course, in the case of a person whose sexual impulses are not necessarily anti-social but which, nevertheless, cause him or her – almost always him – distress or embarrassment. Most homosexuals are satisfactorily integrated into society and are content with their sexual orientation; others, however, regret their preference, and a few even seek to develop heterosexual impulses. Sex therapy may provide the only route to personal adjustment in the latter cases. The fundamental ethical implication underlying any attempt to alter the sexual behaviour of another person is whether intervention of any form is justified.[9] Conventional punishment of offenders presupposes the ability to make free choices and leaves the personality untouched other than by the environment. Inducements to moral change may be offered but the subject's capacity to reject the opportunity is not compromised. Behaviour therapy goes considerably further than this. The essence of such treatment is an attempt to change responses to and relationships with the world at large – that is, to effect something which is different in kind from a reformed moral outlook. The aim is to create a different personality and the point from which the patient deals with others shifts significantly if the therapy succeeds.

It would need a rather rigid adherence to the principle of the sanctity of personality to deny the legitimacy of any attempt of this sort. The more acceptable viewpoint would, perhaps, involve accepting the ideal while rejecting any behaviour modification programmes which are not undertaken in the knowledge of – and quite voluntarily – by the patients. As discussed in chapter 10, this requirement might rule out all such programmes being applied to prisoners or to others threatened with penal sanctions on the grounds that consent must contain an element of coercion. But a denial of opportunity might, at the same time, deny the possibility of a genuine change of heart following conviction and of a real desire to undertake treatment which would obviate future offending. There may be doubts as to voluntariness even in the case of the person who is not an offender but who seeks release from sexual inclinations which do no more than trouble him. The search for such treatment by a homosexual may be inspired by pressures from his family or others who have an interest in his conforming to perceived social norms. The same may be true of one whose unfulfilled sexual fantasies are those which might be expected to attract strong societal disapproval – a pederast, for example – but who does not translate his sexuality into practice. He is then likely to seek treatment through externally induced shame or self-disgust and it might be argued that, in such circumstances, it is more appropriate that treatment should be aimed at self-acceptance and understanding than be of a type which is intended to suppress the emotions. But, given the supposition that we accept the propriety of therapeutic intervention in sexuality, the question then arises as to what can be achieved in practice. The most radical form of attempted therapy is that which involves surgery by way of castration or psychosurgery – and both are of dubious value. There are some reported successes in reducing the rate of recidivism in sex offenders subjected to castration[10] but it is

9 For discussion, see J Bancroft 'Ethical Aspects of Sexuality and Sex Therapy' in S Bloch and P Chadoff *Psychiatric Ethics* (2nd edn, 1991) p 215. Intervention, in any event, may be pointless, given the difficulties inherent in changing sexual proclivities: A Kaul 'Sex Offenders – Cure or Management' (1993) 33 Med Sci Law 207.
10 For a European review, see N Heim and C Hirsch 'Castration for Sex Offenders: Treatment or Punishment' (1979) 8 Arch Sex Behav 281.

naive to assume, as the lay public often does, that a person whose sexual impulses have led him into trouble can be 'neutralised' merely by removing his gonads. There may be a reduction in libido after such an operation but it is seldom completely destroyed and some sexual urge commonly remains. The fallacy is to regard sexuality as being purely a product of the body rather than being, in part at least, a product of the mind. As Meyers put it so graphically: 'The cause of, and answer to, the sexual psychopath's abnormal urges lie in his cranium, not in his scrotum.'[11]

Even so, by extrapolation from the discussion in chapter 18, we see no place, in our current state of knowledge, for psychosurgery in the prophylaxis of abnormal sexuality. Chemical methods which are so targeted are, however, more acceptable and are fairly widely used today. These methods involve the use of anti-androgen drugs which are given either by mouth or through subcutaneous implants; their action is to counter the effects of the male hormones and, as a result, it is hoped they will diminish the male sex drive. The drugs have several, sometimes distressing, side-effects – notably impotence, enlargement of the breasts and loss of body hair – and it is these which constitute the major drawback to what would, otherwise, be an attractive option in the management of potential recidivists who have not responded to less severe forms of therapy.[12]

Aversion therapy involves less serious physical intervention but may, none the less, make a major inroad into the integrity of the personality. The standard techniques consist, essentially, of an attempt to induce the patient to associate the desired sexual object or situation with pain or discomfort and, thus, to make them less attractive. Some successes have been reported but aversion is nowadays less widely used than is the opposite approach – that is, of positively rewarding appropriate reactions. Psychotherapy involving individual or group counselling is widely used in an attempt to modify anti-social sexual behaviour and treatment in special units designed for this purpose has, in fact, been offered in the United Kingdom. The success of the methods depends upon the patients' self-awareness and willingness to participate. Some sexual offenders are simply too recalcitrant to respond to psychotherapy but others may be successfully dealt with or, at least, 'defused' by such treatment.

A delicate balance?

All forms of 'mental defence' give rise to the same general dilemma. While the non-punishment of the mentally disordered is seen as an attractive goal, the need both for a certain degree of scepticism and a measure of social defence have constantly to be borne in mind. A broad, sympathetic view of excusing conditions of this sort may prevent the unjust punishment of those who are truly not responsible for their actions,

11 D W Meyers *The Human Body and the Law* (1970) p 46.
12 D Torpy and A Tomison 'Sex Offenders and Cyprotene Acetate – A Review of Clinical Care' (1986) 26 Med Sci Law 279; S S Yang 'Treatability of the Sex Offender: Considerations of Etiology, Pathology, and Treatment in Repealing Sexually Dangerous Offender Status' (1989) 8 Med Law 319. The legality of the use of clinical methods of libido suppression arose in the case of *R v Mental Health Commission, ex p W* discussed at p 400 above. The issue is dealt with by P Fennell 'Sexual Suppressants and the Mental Health Act' [1988] Crim LR 6.

but it may also have the effect of blunting our conceptions of responsibility and of imposing upon psychiatric institutions a group of people who should not be there. At the same time, too fine a net will deny a defence to meritorious cases and that, too, is socially damaging. The inescapable task of the criminal law then becomes one of charting a course between Scylla and Charybdis. To achieve this, the criminal law should adhere to a broad definition of insanity (such as in the Scottish formula) which allows maximum leeway for a court to take into account expert evidence while at the same time avoiding necessarily being bound to an acceptance of psychiatric notions of responsibility. The matter is thus ultimately left in lay hands which, although fettered to an extent by theoretical guidelines, may none the less exercise such discretion as the situation demands. In the final analysis, the question : 'Is the accused responsible for his acts?' is answered not in terms of a McNaghten-style dissection of mental states but in terms of our reaction to the question: 'Should the accused be punished?' Finding the answer to that question, of course, will, in many cases, be as perversely difficult and unsettling as ever.

Appendices

Appendix A
The Hippocratic Oath

'I swear by Apollo the physician, by Aesculapius, Hygiea and Panacea, and I take to witness all the gods, all the goddesses, to keep according to my ability and my judgement the following Oath:

'To consider dear to me as my parents him who taught me this art; to live in common with him and if necessary to share my goods with him; to look upon his children as my own brothers, to teach them this art if they so desire without fee or written promise; to impart to my sons and the sons of the master who taught me and the disciples who have enrolled themselves and have agreed to the rules of the profession, but to these alone, the precepts and the instruction. I will prescribe regimen for the good of my patients according to my ability and my judgement and never do harm to anyone. To please no one will I prescribe a deadly drug, nor give advice which may cause his death. Nor will I give a woman a pessary to procure abortion. But I will preserve the purity of my life and my art. I will not cut for stone, even for patients in whom the disease is manifest; I will leave this operation to be performed by practitioners (specialist in this art). In every house where I come I will enter only for the good of my patients, keeping myself far from all intentional ill-doing and all seduction, and especially from the pleasures of love with women or with men, be they free or slaves. All that may come to my knowledge in the exercise of my profession or outside of my profession or in daily commerce with men, which ought not to be spread abroad, I will keep secret and will never reveal. If I keep this oath faithfully, may I enjoy my life and practice my art, respected by all men and in all times; but if I swerve from it or violate it, may the reverse be my lot.'

Appendix B
Declaration of Geneva
(As amended at Sydney, 1968)

At the time of being admitted as a member of the medical profession:

I will solemnly pledge myself to consecrate my life to the service of humanity;

I will give to my teachers the respect and gratitude which is their due;

I will practise my profession with conscience and dignity;

The health of my patient will be my first consideration;

I will respect the secrets which are confided in me, even after the patient has died;

I will maintain by all the means in my power the honour and the noble traditions of the medical profession;

My colleagues will be my brothers;

I will not permit considerations of religion, nationality, race, party politics or social standing to intervene between my duty and my patient;

I will maintain the utmost respect for human life from the time of conception; even under threat, I will not use my medical knowledge contrary to the laws of humanity.

I make these promises solemnly, freely and upon my honour.

Appendix C

International Code of Medical Ethics

English text

Duties of Doctors in General
A DOCTOR MUST always maintain the highest standards of professional conduct.
A DOCTOR MUST practise his profession uninfluenced by motives of profit.
THE FOLLOWING PRACTICES are deemed unethical:

(a) Any self advertisement except such as is expressly authorised by the national code of medical ethics.
(b) Collaboration in any form of medical service in which the doctor does not have professional independence.
(c) Receiving any money in connection with services rendered to a patient other than a proper professional fee, even with the knowledge of the patient.

ANY ACT OR ADVICE which could weaken physical or mental resistance of a human being may be used only in his interest.
A DOCTOR IS ADVISED to use great caution in divulging discoveries or new techniques of treatment.
A DOCTOR SHOULD certify or testify only to that which he has personally verified.

Duties of Doctors to the Sick
A DOCTOR MUST always bear in mind the obligation of preserving human life.
A DOCTOR OWES to his patient complete loyalty and all the resources of his science. Whenever an examination or treatment is beyond his capacity he should summon another doctor who has the necessary ability.
A DOCTOR SHALL preserve absolute secrecy on all he knows about his patients because of the confidence entrusted in him.
A DOCTOR MUST give emergency care as a humanitarian duty unless he is assured that others are willing and able to give such care.

Duties of Doctors to Each Other
A DOCTOR OUGHT to behave to his colleagues as he would have them behave to him.

431

A DOCTOR MUST NOT entice patients from his colleagues.

A DOCTOR MUST OBSERVE the principles of 'The Declaration of Geneva' approved by the World Medical Association.

Appendix D
Declaration of Tokyo, 1975

Statement on torture and other cruel, inhuman or degrading
treatment or punishment

Preamble
It is the privilege of the medical doctor to practise medicine in the service of
humanity, to preserve and restore bodily and mental health without distinction as to
persons, to comfort and to ease the suffering of his or her patients. The utmost respect
for human life is to be maintained even under threat, and no use made of any medical
knowledge contrary to the laws of humanity.

For the purpose of this Declaration, torture is defined as the deliberate, systematic
or wanton infliction of physical or mental suffering by one or more persons acting
alone or on the orders of any authority, to force another person to yield information,
to make a confession, or for any other reason.

Declaration
1. The doctor shall not countenance, condone or participate in the practice of
torture or other forms of cruel, inhuman or degrading procedures, whatever the
offence of which the victim of such procedures is suspected, accused or guilty, and
whatever the victim's beliefs or motives, and in all situations, including armed
conflict and civil strife.

2. The doctor shall not provide any premises, instruments, substances or
knowledge to facilitate the practice of torture or other forms of cruel, inhuman
or degrading treatment or to diminish the ability of the victim to resist such
treatment.

3. The doctor shall not be present during any procedure during which torture or
other forms of cruel, inhuman or degrading treatment is used or threatened.

4. A doctor must have complete clinical independence in deciding upon the care
of a person for whom he or she is medically responsible. The doctor's fundamental
role is to alleviate the distress of his or her fellow men, and no motive whether
personal, collective or political shall prevail against this higher purpose.

5. Where a prisoner refuses nourishment and is considered by the doctor as capable of forming an unimpaired and rational judgement concerning the consequences of such a voluntary refusal of nourishment, he or she shall not be fed artificially. The decision as to the capacity of the prisoner to form such a judgement should be confirmed by at least one other independent doctor. The consequences of the refusal of nourishment shall be explained by the doctor to the prisoner.

6. The World Medical Association will support, and should encourage the international community, the national medical associations and fellow doctors to support, the doctor and his or her family in the face of threats or reprisals resulting from a refusal to condone the use of torture or other forms of cruel, inhuman or degrading treatment.

Appendix E
Declaration of Oslo, 1970

Statement on therapeutic abortion

1. The first moral principle imposed upon the doctor is respect for human life as expressed in a clause of the Declaration of Geneva: I will maintain the utmost respect for human life from the time of conception.

2. Circumstances which bring the vital interests of a mother into conflict with the vital interests of her unborn child create a dilemma and raise the question whether or not the pregnancy should be deliberately terminated.

3. Diversity of response to this situation results from the diversity of attitudes towards the life of the unborn child. This is a matter of individual conviction and conscience which must be respected.

4. It is not the role of the medical profession to determine the attitudes and role of any particular state or community in this matter, but it is our duty to attempt both to ensure the protection of our patients and to safeguard the rights of the doctor within society.

5. Therefore, where the law allows therapeutic abortion to be performed, or legislation to that effect is contemplated, and this is not against the policy of the national medical association, and where the legislature desires or will accept the guidance of the medical profession, the following principles are approved:

(a) Abortion should be performed only as a therapeutic measure.

(b) A decision to terminate pregnancy should normally be approved in writing by at least two doctors chosen for their professional competence.

(c) The procedure should be performed by a doctor competent to do so in premises approved by the appropriate authority.

6. If the doctor considers that his convictions do not allow him to advise or perform an abortion, he may withdraw while ensuring the continuity of (medical) care by a qualified colleague.

7. This statement, while it is endorsed by the General Assembly of the World Medical Association, is not to be regarded as binding on any individual member association unless it is adopted by that member association.

Appendix F
Declaration of Helsinki

(Revised 1975)

Recommendations guiding medical doctors in biomedical research involving human subjects

Introduction

It is the mission of the medical doctor to safeguard the health of the people. His or her knowledge and conscience are dedicated to the fulfilment of this mission.

The Declaration of Geneva of the World Medical Association binds the doctor with the words: 'The health of my patient will be my first consideration,' and the International Code of Medical Ethics declares that, 'Any act or advice which could weaken physical or mental resistance of a human being may be used only in his interest.'

The purpose of biomedical research involving human subjects must be to improve diagnostic, therapeutic and prophylactic procedures and the understanding of the aetiology and pathogenesis of disease.

In current medical practice most diagnostic, therapeutic or prophylactic procedures involve hazards. This applies *a fortiori* to biomedical research.

Medical progress is based on research which ultimately must rest in part on experimentation involving human subjects. In the field of biomedical research a fundamental distinction must be recognised between medical research in which the aim is essentially diagnostic or therapeutic for a patient, and medical research the essential object of which is purely scientific and without direct diagnostic or therapeutic value to the person subjected to the research.

Special caution must be exercised in the conduct of research which may affect the environment, and the welfare of animals used for research must be respected.

Because it is essential that the results of laboratory experiments be applied to human beings to further scientific knowledge and to help suffering humanity, the World Medical Association has prepared the following recommendations as a guide to every doctor in biomedical research involving human subjects. They should be kept under review in the future. It must be stressed that the standards as drafted are only a guide to physicians all over the world. Doctors are not relieved from criminal, civil and ethical responsibilities under the laws of their own countries.

I. Basic Principles

1. Biomedical research involving human subjects must conform to generally accepted scientific principles and should be based on adequately performed laboratory and animal experimentation and on a thorough knowledge of the scientific tradition.

2. The design and performance of each experimental procedure involving human subjects should be clearly formulated in an experimental protocol which should be transmitted to a specially appointed independent committee for consideration, comment and guidance.

3. Biomedical research involving human subjects should be conducted only by scientifically qualified persons and under the supervision of a clinically competent medical person. The responsibility for the human subject must always rest with a medically qualified person and never rest on the subject of the research, even though the subject has given her consent.

4. Biomedical research involving human subjects cannot legitimately be carried out unless the importance of the objective is in proportion to the inherent risk to the subject.

5. Every biomedical research project involving human subjects should be preceded by careful assessment of predictable risks in comparison with foreseeable benefits to the subject or to others. Concern for the interests of the subject must always prevail over the interest of science and society.

6. The right of the research subject to safeguard his or her integrity must always be respected. Every precaution should be taken to respect the privacy of the subject and to minimize the impact of the study on the subject's physical and mental integrity and on the personality of the subject.

7. Doctors should abstain from engaging in research projects involving human subjects unless they are satisfied that the hazards involved are believed to be predictable. Doctors should cease any investigation if the hazards are found to outweigh the potential benefits.

8. In publication of the results of his or her research, the doctor is obliged to preserve the accuracy of the results. Reports of experimentation not in accordance with the principles laid down in this Declaration should not be accepted for publication.

9. In any research on human beings, each potential subject must be adequately informed of the aims, methods, anticipated benefits and potential hazards of the study and the discomfort it may entail. He or she should be informed that he or she is at liberty to abstain from participation in the study and that he or she is free to withdraw his or her consent to participation at any time. The doctor should then obtain the subject's freely-given informed consent, preferably in writing.

10. When obtaining informed consent for the research project the doctor should be particularly cautious if the subject is in a dependent relationship to him or her or may consent under duress. In that case the informed consent should be obtained by a doctor who is not engaged in the investigation and who is completely independent of this official relationship.

11. In case of legal incompetence, informed consent should be obtained from the legal guardian in accordance with national legislation. Where physical or mental incapacity makes it impossible to obtain informed consent, or when the subject is a minor, permission from the responsible relative replaces that of the subject in accordance with national legislation.

12. The research protocol should always contain a statement of the ethical considerations involved and should indicate that the principles enunciated in the present Declaration are complied with.

II. Medical Research Combined with Professional Care (Clinical research)

1. In the treatment of the sick person, the doctor must be free to use a new diagnostic and therapeutic measure, if in his or her judgment it offers hope of saving life, re-establishing health or alleviating suffering.

2. The potential benefits, hazards and discomfort of a new method should be weighed against the advantages of the best current diagnostic and therapeutic methods.

3. In any medical study, every patient - including those of a control group, if any – should be assured of the best proven diagnostic and therapeutic method.

4. The refusal of the patient to participate in a study must never interfere with the doctor-patient relationship.

5. If the doctor considers it essential not to obtain informed consent, the specific reasons for this proposal should be stated in the experimental protocol for transmission to the independent committee.

6. The doctor can combine medical research with professional care, the objective being the acquisition of new medical knowledge, only to the extent that medical research is justified by its potential diagnostic or therapeutic value for the patient.

III. Non-therapeutic Biomedical Research Involving Human Subjects (Non-clinical biomedical research)

1. In the purely scientific application of medical research carried out on a human being, it is the duty of the doctor to remain the protector of the life and health of that person on whom biomedical research is carried out.

2. The subjects should be volunteers – either healthy persons or patients for whom the experimental design is not related to the patient's illness.

3. The investigator or the investigating team should discontinue the research if in his/her or their judgment it may, if continued, be harmful to the individual.

4. In research on man, the interest of science and society should never take precedence over considerations related to the wellbeing of the subject.

Appendix G

Specimen living will

To my family, my physician and my solicitor

This declaration is made by me . . . .
(Full name and address)

. . . .
at a time when I am of sound mind and after careful consideration

I, the said . . . .
in the event of my being unable to take part in decisions concerning my medical care
due to my physical or mental incapacity, and in the event that I develop one or more
of the medical conditions listed in clause (3) below and in the event that two
independent physicians conclude that there is no reasonable prospect of my making
a substantial recovery, do hereby **DECLARE** that my wishes are as follows. VIZ:—

(1) I request that my life should not be sustained by artificial means such as: life
support systems, intravenous fluids and/or drugs, tube feeding.

(2) I request that distressing symptoms caused either by illness or by lack of food
or fluid should be controlled by appropriate sedative treatment, even though
such treatment may have the incidental and secondary effect of shortening my
life.

(3) The said medical conditions are:—
1. Severe and lasting brain damage sustained as a result of an accident or
injury.
2. Advanced disseminated malignant disease.
3. Advanced degenerative disease of the nervous and/or muscular systems
with severe limitations of independent mobility, and no satisfactory response
to treatment.
4. Stroke with extensive persisting paralysis.
5. Pre-senile, senile or Alzheimer type dementia.
6. Other conditions of comparable gravity.

(4) I request that, in the event of my becoming incapable of giving or withholding
consent to any medical treatment or procedures proposed to me, the Court of
Session be petitioned to appoint as my tutor the following person:—

. . . .
whom failing:—

439

. . . .

whom failing: such other person as may be deemed by the Court to be a fit person. It is my specific request that in exercising his or her powers to consent or withhold consent on my behalf to any medical treatment or procedures, my tutor shall take into account, in any determination of what is in my best interests, the requests which I solemnly make in clauses (1) and (2) of this document.

And I declare that I hereby absolve my medical attendants of all legal liability arising from action taken in response to and in terms of this declaration,

I reserve the right to revoke this declaration at any time, before witnesses, in writing or orally.

. . . .
(Signature)   (Town/Place)   (Day/Month/Year)

The above specimen of a 'living will' was drafted by one of the authors of this volume. It is distributed, on request, by the Voluntary Euthanasia Society of Scotland. Clause (4) refers to the appointment of a tutor – who has the power under Scots law to make decisions relating to the person of an *incapax*.

Index